PSYCHOPATHOLOGY A Source Book

PSYCHOPATHOLOGY

A Source Book

EDITED BY

CHARLES F. REED, Ph.D.
Upstate Medical Center
State University of New York

IRVING E. ALEXANDER, Ph.D.
Duke University

SILVAN S. TOMKINS, Ph.D.
Princeton University

With an Introduction by
ROBERT W. WHITE, Ph.D.
Harvard University

SCIENCE EDITIONS®
John Wiley & Sons, Inc., New York

Publication as a Science Editions paperback authorized by
Harvard University Press

First Science Editions printing 1964

Science Editions Trademark Reg. U. S. Pat. Off.

Library of Congress Catalog Card Number 58–10405
Printed in the United States of America

PREFACE

This book arose from a mutual wish on the part of its three editors, who in successive years taught the undergraduate course in abnormal psychology at Princeton University. Each of us felt a need for a single source of current periodical literature to supplement the text we used. Hence this joint effort.

We intended this source book as a secondary text for courses in abnormal psychology and psychiatry. It consists of papers selected from the psychological and psychiatric literature, primarily of the period 1952–1957. In a few instances outstanding contributions of an earlier vintage were also included.

The criteria of selection employed were diverse. Foremost we stressed the excellence of the work. Our only compromise here was the rejection of some papers which demanded a degree of technical knowledge beyond that of our intended audience.

Representativeness as such was not a criterion to which we attached much significance. The primary text ordinarily meets this demand. As a corollary, some excellent papers devoted to areas of research which have been thoroughly explored and evaluated were excluded. Thus we did not include papers on shock therapy and lobotomy. We favored the more recent developments, stressing novelty, promise and suggestiveness.

Our primary obligation and thanks are due to the authors and publishers whose material we have reprinted. In each case permission was granted by both the author and the publisher. We wish to thank Dr. John N. Rosen and Dr. Peter Witt for preparing new and additional material specifically for this volume.

C. F. REED
Princeton, New Jersey   I. E. ALEXANDER
August 1957   S. S. TOMKINS

CONTENTS

INTRODUCTION · Robert W. White

III. SCHIZOPHRENIC PSYCHOSES

IV. SOMATIC FACTORS IN PSYCHOPATHOLOGY

Contents

V. PSYCHOPATHOLOGY AND THE SOCIAL CONTEXT

INTRODUCTION

When one undertakes to teach abnormal psychology at the college level there are several ways in which the project can go astray. One danger is that students will learn the subject-matter as a set of abstract principles without opening their minds to the events in people's lives upon which the whole thing is based. This trouble can best be met by the regular use of case material, supplemented when possible by visits to institutions. Another danger is that students will fail to realize the importance of scientific method in the study of psychopathology. Once the case history has become real to them they may succumb to its charms and hopefully conclude that everything can be discovered by looking at single cases. Today the hunches of the consulting and examining rooms are being put under the sharp scrutiny provided by experimental methods. Case studies are only starting points on the rough and twisting road toward systematic knowledge. The news of recent research, however, lies awkwardly scattered through professional journals which can rarely be made available to college classes. This is the situation which the editors of this book have resolved to correct, thus making it possible for students to read at the very frontiers of scientific advance.

Having set this as their goal, the editors have wisely refrained from taking their readers to every frontier. To do so would have created the kind of blur which results from a quick trip around the world. Leaving coverage to conventional textbooks, they have chosen five areas, in each of which there is time to talk with a number of experts and to observe a variety of experimental programs. It is appropriate that the first stop should be made at that part of the frontier where workers are attacking the important problem of the effects of early experience upon pathological development. Ten papers devoted to various aspects of this problem are followed by eleven in the general area of psychosomatic disorders and neurosis. Then come nine papers on the schizophrenic psychoses, seven on somatic factors in psychopathology, and a final nine which deal with the social context and its effects on the incidence and treatment of disordered behavior. If it be objected that this by no means exhausts the field of psychopathology, one can properly reply that an undergraduate, not to mention a graduate student, who has studied these forty-six papers will have had an unforgettable experience of what is involved in scientific exploration — in any field.

What the student gains from an experience of this kind can be illustrated by considering the first group of papers. The effects of early experience upon psychopathological development were first discerned through intensive studies of individual patients, especially those patients who happened into the consulting room of Sigmund Freud in Vienna. The head of the couch subsequently proved itself to be a peculiarly choice observation post for detecting the traces of the past in present behavior and fantasy. Can we generate the whole genetic story of psychopathology out of reports issued from this one location? The ten papers chosen by the editors will certainly force the student out of any such comfortable optimism. He will find that inquiry has been pushed from the free associations of adult patients to the direct study of children and even infants, that the family circle is included in the study, that child patients are being followed up in later years, and that animals are being requisitioned as subjects in order to test hypotheses under conditions of experimental control. If this exposure leaves him with a feeling that many problems remain unsolved and even seem to elude definition, then we can say that he has been properly introduced to the science of psychopathology as it is today.

So persistently have the editors looked for the latest work that we can use these selections as indicators of contemporary trends in psychopathology as a whole. Only two papers were written before 1951; more than half carry a date of 1955 or later. Had the selections been made a little earlier they would probably not have included a major section on the social context, and it is doubtful that research on somatic factors in psychopathology would have seemed challenging enough to occupy a main category. But even under the more standard headings the atmosphere has changed in the course of a decade. There is no longer an air that the problem of schizophrenia, or of neurosis, or of psychosomatic disorder is going to be solved by a stroke of insight and a simple theory. Where once it was hoped to unlock the secret of a disorder, we now know that we must creep up slowly upon its many secrets and that we must use to the utmost the help provided by scientific method. In this new climate the present book is an indispensable teaching aid.

Robert W. White

Harvard University
Cambridge, Massachusetts
January 1, 1958

Part I

PSYCHOPATHOLOGY AND EARLY EXPERIENCE

1

EARLY INFANTILE AUTISM, 1943–1955

LEON EISENBERG, M.D., AND LEO KANNER, M.D.

Children's Psychiatric Service, Harriet Lane Home, Johns Hopkins Hospital, Baltimore, Maryland

In 1943, under the title "Autistic Disturbances of Affective Contact" (1), eleven children were reported, whose clinical features appeared to constitute a unique syndrome, later termed "early infantile autism" (2). Since this publication of the original paper, more than 120 children so diagnosed with reasonable certainty have been observed at the Children's Psychiatric Service of the Johns Hopkins Hospital. The syndrome is now recognized as having clinical specificity, as is attested by numerous case reports and discussions of its theoretical and dynamic aspects. Preliminary data from follow-up studies at this clinic have further verified the uniqueness of the syndrome. It seems appropriate at this point to review briefly the nature of the original conception, to consider the modifications necessitated by greater knowledge, and to evaluate the present status of infantile autism.

In the original paper, the pathognomonic disorder was seen as "the children's inability to relate themselves in the ordinary way to people and to situations from the beginning of life" (1). The extreme nature of their detachment from human relationships separated the appearance and behavior of these children in a fundamental fashion from other known behavioral disturbances. It was noted that the process was not one "of withdrawal from formerly existing participation" with others, as is true of the older schizophrenic child, but rather "from the start an extreme autistic aloneness" (1). This could be discerned from the almost universal report by parents that these children, as infants, had failed to assume an anticipatory posture before being picked up and never displayed the plastic molding which the normal child shows when cradled in his parent's arms. Initially pleased by the child's "goodness" — that is, his ability to occupy himself for long periods without requiring attention — parents later became distressed by the persistence of this self-isolation and by their observation that their coming or going seemed a matter of complete indifference to the child.

A second distinctive feature was noted as the failure to use language for the purpose of communication. In 3 of the 11 cases, speech failed to develop altogether. The remaining 8 rapidly developed a precocity of articulation which, coupled with unusual facility in rote memory, resulted in the ability to repeat endless numbers of rhymes, catechisms, lists of names, and other semantically useless exercises. The parroting of words intellectually incomprehensible to the child brought into sharp relief the gross failure to use speech to convey meaning or feeling to others. The repetition of stored phrases, while failing to recombine words into original and personalized sentences, gave rise to the phenomena of delayed echolalia, pronominal reversal, literalness, and affirmation by repetition.

A third characteristic was described as "an anxiously obsessive desire for the maintenance of sameness" (1), resulting in a marked limitation in the variety of spontaneous activity. Regularly displaying fear of new patterns of activity, these children, once having accepted a new pattern, would incorporate it into the restricted set of rituals which then had to be endlessly iterated. Thus, a walk had always to follow the same prescribed course; bedtime to consist of a particular ritual of words and actions; and repetitive activities like spinning, turning on and off lights and spigots, or flushing toilets could preoccupy the child for long periods. Any attempt to interfere with the pattern would produce bursts of rage or episodes of acute panic.

Fourthly, as distinct from the poor or absent relation to persons, there could be discerned a fascination for objects which were handled with skill in fine motor movements. So intense was this relationship that minor alterations in objects or their arrangement, not ordinarily perceived by the average observer, were at once apparent to these children who might then fly into a rage until the change had been undone, whereupon tranquility was restored.

Finally, it was argued that these children had "good cognitive potentialities" (1). In the speaking group this could be discerned in the extraordinary, if perverted, use of language, manifesting feats of unusual memory. In the mute children, this was concluded, though with less confidence, from their facility with performance tests, particularly the Seguin formboard, at or above their age level.

Thus a syndrome had been delineated which was differentiated from childhood schizophrenia by virtue of detachment present no later than the first year of life, and from oligophrenia by the evidence of good intellectual potentialities. Physical examination failed to reveal any consistent organic abnormality that could be related to the clinical picture. Family background was striking in the universal presence of high intelligence, marked obsessiveness, and coldness. But the extreme aloneness *present from the beginning of life* led to the tentative conclusion that this group of children comprised "pure-cultural examples of inborn autistic disturbances of affective contact."

In the light of experience with a tenfold increase in clinical material, we would now isolate these two pathognomonic features, both of which must be present: extreme self-isolation and the obsessive insistence on the preservation of sameness, features that may be regarded as primary, employing the term as Bleuler did in grouping the symptoms of schizophrenia (3). The vicissitudes of language development, often the most striking and challenging of the presenting phenomena, may be seen as derivatives of the basic disturbance in human relatedness. Preoccupation with simple repetitive activities may be seen at times in severely retarded children and may offer a diagnostic problem, but the presence of elaborately conceived rituals together with the characteristic aloneness serves to differentiate the autistic patients. The case material has expanded to include a number of children who reportedly developed normally through the first 18 to 20 months of life, only to undergo at this point a severe withdrawal of affect, manifested by the loss of language function, failure to progress socially, and the gradual giving up of interest in normal activities. These latter cases have invariably been severe and unresponsive. When seen, they could not be differentiated from the children with the more classical account of detachment apparently present in the neonatal period. But even these cases are much earlier in onset and phenomenologically distinct from cases of childhood schizophrenia.

When this conception was set forth 12 years ago, it met with a reception very similar to that which greeted the reports of childhood schizophrenia advanced in the previous decade. Workers in the field, limiting their thinking to the conventional lines prescribed by the then current notions of adult schizophrenia, had had difficulty in accepting as schizophrenic a clinical picture in children which necessarily had distinctive differences dictated by the much younger age of these patients. Within the past six years confirmatory reports have appeared with increasing frequency so that now the term infantile autism is rather widely — and often not too accurately — employed. Despert was perhaps the first in a personal communication to note the similarities between this group of children and others she had studied (4, 5). Mahler suggested the useful division between autistic and symbiotic infantile psychoses (6, 7). Rank (8), Weil (9), Sherwin (10), Murphy (11), in this country, Cappon (12) in Canada, Creak (13) in England, Stern (14) and Stern and Schachter (15) in France, and van Krevelen (16, 17) in Holland added significant case reports. Recently, the Dutch Society for Child Psychiatry organized a symposium on infantile autism (Grewel 44). A number of other workers have discussed the theoretical implications for language and perceptual function of the phenomena shown by the autistic child (18, 19, 20). It therefore seems justified to state that the specificity of early infantile autism is now rather commonly accepted, with, of course, inevitable differences in diagnostic allocation: van Krevelen placing it with oligophrenia, most workers in this country with schizophrenia, Stern and Schachter and Grewel regarding it as a syndrome *sui generis*, and so on.

The preliminary results of our follow-up studies are of interest in that they, too, emphasize the phenomenologic uniqueness of the syndrome. Of the some 50 children followed for a mean period of 8 years, none is reliably known to have exhibited hallucinations. The major pathology remains in the area of inability to relate in the ordinary fashion to other human beings. Even the relatively "successful" children exhibited a lack of social perceptiveness, perhaps best characterized as a lack of *savoir faire*. This can be illustrated by the following incident involving one of our patients who has made considerable progress. Attending a football rally of his junior college and called upon to speak, he shocked the assembly by stating that he thought the team was likely to lose — a prediction that was correct but unthinkable in the setting. The ensuing round of booing dismayed this young man who was totally unable to comprehend why the truth should be unwelcome.

This amazing lack of awareness of the feelings of others, who seem not to be conceived of as persons like the self, runs like a red thread through our case histories. We might cite a four-year-old boy whose mother came to us with the account that on a crowded beach he would walk straight toward his goal irrespective of whether this involved walking over newspapers, hands, feet, or torsos, much to the discomfiture of their owners. The mother was careful to point out that he did not intentionally deviate from his course in order to walk on others — but neither did he make the slightest attempt to avoid them. It was as if he did not distinguish people from things or at least did not concern himself about the distinction. This failure to recognize others as entities separate from oneself was exhibited by the 28-year-old patient retrospectively diagnosed as autistic and reported by Darr and Worden (21). To mention one example of her behavior: "On one occasion she spilled ink on the floor of a dormitory room, dashed out to ask the first person she met to wipe it up, and became angry on being refused." The existence of feelings or wishes in other people that might not accord with the patient's own autistic thoughts and desires seemed beyond recognition.

On clinical grounds, it is now useful to differentiate between the children who have learned to speak by the age of five and those who have no useful language function by that age (3). Of the former group, about half have made some sort of scholastic adjustment and participate in a limited way in the social life of the community, though we are none too sanguine about their future. Of the latter group — the nonspeakers — only one out of twenty subsequently developed language and is making at least a mediocre adjustment in a protected school setting. The remainder are either in institutions or remain at home, functionally severely retarded. Interestingly, a number of these emotionally isolated children, though confined to institutions for the feebleminded, are still distinguishable from their fellow patients, as is attested by reports of psychological testing that bewilder the observer in the conjunction of social imbecility with the preservation of isolated areas of unusual intellectual performance.

The information obtained from long-term study of these children is beginning to supply us with a natural history of the syndrome, against which therapeutic efforts will have to be evaluated. Thus, it would appear on the basis of current information that, if we consider the cases in aggregate, about one third appear able to achieve at least a minimal social adjustment to school and community. This percentage of improvement without extensive psychiatric treatment is comparable with the data reported on a much larger group of schizophrenic children treated with electric shock by Bender (21), allowing for differences in diagnostic categories and in indices of improvement. It should be stressed that, insofar as our data permit evaluation, psychotherapy seems in general to be of little avail, with few apparent exceptions. If one factor is significantly useful, it is a sympathetic and tolerant reception by the school. Those of our children who have improved have been extended extraordinary consideration by their teachers. They constitute a most trying group of pupils. School acceptance of behavior that elsewhere provokes rejection is undoubtedly a therapeutic experience. Obviously, it is feasible only in the case of the less severely disturbed children.

Etiologic investigations have centered about organic, genetic, and psychodynamic factors. Thorough pediatric examinations of all the children who have passed through our clinic have failed to reveal any more than occasional and apparently unrelated physical abnormalities, unless one considers relevant the consistent preponderance of boys over girls in a ratio of 4 to 1. Careful medical histories of pregnancy, delivery, and development are negative insofar as any consistent pattern of pathological complications is concerned. Electroencephalographic studies have been carried out only sporadically; of the 28 cases on which reports are available, 21 were stated to be negative, 3 definitely abnormal, and 4 equivocal. It must be recognized, however, that neurologic investigations of the integrity of central function remain as yet in their clinical infancy and a negative result with current methods cannot be regarded as a conclusive demonstration of the lack of central nervous system pathology.

If we turn to a study of the families, we learn that, of 200 parents, there are only 6 with clinical psychiatric disorders, only one of whom had a psychotic episode. Among 400 grandparents and among 373 known uncles and aunts, 12 were afflicted with mental illness. This low incidence of psychotic and neurotic relatives, even if we double the figures to allow for the relative youth of these families, contrasts sharply with the high incidence in the families of older childhood schizophrenics reported by Bender (22) and in adult schizophrenics reported by Kallmann (24). Similarly, of 131 known siblings of 100 autistic children, 3 can be regarded as probably autistic on the basis of the information supplied and 7 others as emotionally disturbed. Thus, if one limits his search for genetic factors to overt psychotic and neurotic episodes in family members, the results would appear to be negative. If one considers the personalities of the parents who have been described as "successfully autistic," the possibility suggests itself that they may represent milder manifestations and that the children show the full emergence of the latent structure. One of the fathers in this group, a physician engaged in research, stressed the mildly schizoid trends in his own grandparents, more strongly evident in his father, fairly marked in himself and to some degree in all of his progeny, and full-blown in his autistic child.

One of the striking features of the clinical histories remains the unusually high percentage of these children who stem from highly intelligent, obsessive, and emotionally frigid backgrounds. Eighty-seven of the fathers and seventy of the mothers had been to college. A large number are professional people who have attained distinction in their fields. A control study of the parents of private patients selected solely by virtue of being next in call number to each of the first 50 autistic cases revealed levels of educational attainment and professional status that were considerably lower. In the control group one does not find the dramatically evident detachment, obsessiveness, and coldness that is almost a universal feature of parents of autistic children. Yet one must admit that some 10 per cent of the parents do not fit the stereotype and that those who do have raised other normal, or in any event, nonpsychotic children. Moreover, similarly frigid parents are seen who do not give rise to autistic progeny.

The emotional frigidity in the typical autistic family suggests a dynamic experiential factor in the genesis of the disorder in the child.

The mechanization of care and the almost total absence of emotional warmth in child rearing may be exemplified by the case of Brian, who was one of twins born despite contraceptive efforts, much to the distress of his parents whose plans centered about graduate study and had no room for children. Pregnancy was quite upsetting to the mother and caused the father, who was already immersed in study, to withdraw still further from the family. The mother, a psychology graduate student, decided that the children were to be raised "scientifically" — that is, not to be picked up for crying, except on schedule. Furthermore, an effort was made to "keep them from infections" by minimizing human contact. What little care was dispensed was centered upon Brian's twin who was physically weaker and, according to the mother, more responsive. At five months of age, the twin was found dead after an evening in which both infants had been crying loudly but had not been visited, in accordance with rigid principle. Following this tragedy, the mother withdrew from the remaining child even more completely, spent her days locked in the study reading, and limited her concern almost exclusively to maintaining bacteriological sterility, so that Brian was isolated from children and almost all adults until he was well over two. During this period he was content to be alone and to occupy himself, just how the parents rarely bothered to inquire. It was only when he reached the age of four without the development of speech and began to display temper tantrums when his routines were interrupted that they began to recognize the fact that he was ill. So distant were the members of this family each from the others that the parents failed to be concerned about, if they did not actually prefer, Brian's indifference to them. One might accurately state that this was an environment that rewarded preoccupation with autistic interests and that provided the barest minimum of human contact compatible with the maintenance of physical health. Stimuli that might have fostered attention to or interest in the human environment were almost entirely absent. This case, an extreme instance chosen for emphasis, can serve as a paradigm of the "emotional refrigeration" that has been the common lot of autistic children.

Psychiatrists are rather widely agreed that emotional deprivation has profound consequences for psychobiological development (25). Infants subjected to impersonal care in institutions for prolonged periods in the first years of life display both psychomotor retardation and physiological dysfunction, a syndrome that has been termed hospitalism (26, 27). Longer periods of exposure are correlated with depression of intellectual function, as measured by scores on developmental and intelligence tests (28, 29). Analogous data are available from controlled animal experiments, in which poverty of environmental stimulation in the neonatal period produces apparently irreversible loss in adaptive ability (30, 31, 32). Moreover, children exposed to prolonged affective deprivation are likely to display antisocial and psychopathic behavior traits (33, 34, 34). It has been contended that the personality pattern of such children as adolescents is typically "affectionless" (36). The most recent study by Dr. Lewis casts doubt on the concept of a specific personality pattern in the child who has suffered from lack of mothering, but does confirm the significant correlation between disturbed, usually antisocial behavior and early separation from the mother without adequate substitution (37).

Experience in Israel with communally reared children casts cross-cultural light on the nature of the emotional needs of infants and children (38). From six weeks of age, Kibbutz infants live full time in communal nurseries, and though identification with their parents is maintained by frequent visits, the great preponderance of their care is given by permanent nursery workers. They are raised as a group under a common roof until late adolescence. These children grow into mature and capable adults as far as clinical evaluation can determine. Stress should be placed on the fact that the Kibbutz culture is child-oriented, and while the mother is not the main dispenser of care, the children are reared by warm and demonstrative trained people — as it were, in an atmosphere of affectionate interest.

Thus it is evident that affectionate care and a consistent relationship to one or more adults in the mothering role is a prerequisite for normal growth in infancy and childhood.

The case histories of autistic children reveal that in almost all instances they were raised by their own parents. Obvious mistreatment, overt rejection, or abandonment, usual in the life experience of the children who are classified as emotionally deprived, is the exception. But the formal provision of food and shelter and the absence of neglect as defined by statutory law are insufficient criteria for the adequacy of family care. The role of "parent" is not defined merely by the biological task of giving rise to progeny. In the typical autistic family it is as if the Israeli experiment had been repeated in reverse: in having parents, but not a warm, flexible, growth-promoting emotional atmosphere. These children were, in general, conceived less out of a positive desire than out of an acceptance of childbearing as part of the marital contract. Physical needs were attended to mechanically and on schedule according to the rigid precepts of naïve behaviorism applied with a vengeance. One can discern relatively few instances of warmth and affection. The usual parental attitude is cold and formal; less commonly, it is laden with great anxiety. The child's worth seemed to lie in the extent to which he conformed to predetermined parental expectations: "perfect" behavior, cleverness, "self-sufficiency," and so on. Their parents, who were themselves preoccupied with careers and intellectual pursuits to the exclusion of interest in other people, had little more feeling for their own children. It may be a measure of the intellectual aptitude of some of these children that they were able to parrot long and resonant lists of meaningless words, but it even more clearly bespeaks the emphasis placed at home on such useless activities which were a source of pride to the parents.

It is difficult to escape the conclusion that this emotional configuration in the home plays a dynamic role in the genesis of autism. But it seems to us equally clear that this factor, while important in the development of the syndrome, is not sufficient in itself to result in its appearance. There apears to be some way in which the children are different from the beginning of their extrauterine existence. Indeed, it has been postulated that the aberrant behavior of the children is chiefly responsible for the personality difficulties of their parents who are pictured as reacting to the undoubtedly trying situation of having an unresponsive child (39). While we would agree that this is an important consideration, it cannot explain the social and psychological characteristics of the parents which have a history long anteceding the child.

There is little likelihood that a single etiologic agent is solely responsible for the pathology in behavior. Arguments that counterpose "hereditary" versus "environmental" as antithetical terms are fundamentally in error. Operationally defined, they are interpenetrating concepts. The effects of chromosomal aberrations can be mimicked in the phenotype by environmental pathogens, and genetic factors require for their complete manifestation suitable environmental conditions. It is not possible to distinguish between biochemically mutant microorganisms until we expose them to nutrient media deficient in appropriate metabolites. Conversely, the full effect of environmental agencies cannot be seen unless the genotype is adequate. A culturally rich environment will be little different from a culturally poor one in its influence on the intellectual development of phenylketonuric children.

The dualistic view implicit in a rigid distinction between "organic" and "functional" is no longer tenable. The pharmacologic production of psychosislike states simulating certain features of schizophrenia (40, 41) — and the recent hint that analogue blockade will interfere with chemically induced "model psychoses" (42) — serves to reassert the obvious fact that biochemical change is accompanied by alterations in thought processes. Nevertheless, the disordered thoughts obey the laws governing psychic processes and lend themselves to psychological analysis. It is equally important to recognize that originally psycho-genic forces must by their enduring action transform the physiological substrate, as the conditioned reflex so clearly demonstrates (43). The finding of biochemical or psychological abnormalities is only the start-ing point in a search for etiology.

Early infantile autism is a total psychobiological disorder. What is needed is a comprehensive study of the dysfunction at each level of integration: biological, psychological, and social. The supposition of an innate difference in the autistic child will mean relatively little until we can specify the nature and meaning of that difference. Cur-rently, research sponsored by the League of Emotionally Disturbed Children is attempting to uncover metabolic and electrophysiologic abnormalities, research that complements the psychodynamic investi-gations at this and other clinics.

In summary, early infantile autism has been fully established as a clinical syndrome. It is characterized by extreme aloneness and pre-occupation with the preservation of sameness, and is manifest within the first two years of life. The history, early onset, and clinical course distinguish it from older childhood schizophrenia, to which it is prob-ably related generically. The degree of aloneness constitutes the im-portant prognostic variable since those children sufficiently related to the human environment to learn to talk have a significantly better outlook for future adjustment. Present knowledge leads to the infer-ence that innate as well as experimental factors conjoin to produce the clinical picture. It remains for future investigation to uncover the precise mode of operation of the pathogenic factors as a basis for rational treatment.

References

1. Kanner, L. Autistic Disturbances of Affective Contact. *Nerv. Child*, 2: 217–250, 1943.

2. ———. Early Infantile Autism. *J. Pediat.*, 25: 211–217, 1944.

3. Kanner, L., and L. Eisenberg. Notes on the Follow-Up Studies of Autistic Children, in *Psychopathology of Childhood* (P. H. Hoch and J. Zubin, Eds.), pp. 227–239. Grune & Stratton, New York, 1955.

4. Despert, J. L., quoted by L. Kanner. Problems of Nosology and Psycho-dynamics of Early Infantile Autism. *Am. J. Orthopsychiatry* 19: 416–452, 1949.

5. ———. Some Considerations Relating to the Genesis of Autistic Behavior in Children. *Ibid.*, 21: 335–350, 1951.

6. Mahler, M. S. On Child Psychosis and Schizophrenia: Autistic and Symbiotic Infantile Psychoses, in *The Psychoanalytic Study of the Child*, Vol. VII, 286–305. Internat. Univ. Press, New York, 1952.

7. Mahler, M. S., J. R. Ross, Jr., and Z. De Fries. Clinical Studies in Benign and Malignant Cases of Childhood Psychosis. *Am. J. Orthopsychiatry*, 19: 295–305, 1949.

8. Rank, B. Adaptation of the Psychoanalytic Technique for the Treatment of Young Children with Atypical Development. *Am. J. Orthopsychiatry*, 19: 130–139, 1949.

9. Weil, A. P. Clinical Data and Dynamic Considerations in Certain Cases of Childhood Schizophrenia. *Am. J. Orthopsychiatry*, 23: 518–529, 1953.

10. Sherwin, A. C. Reactions to Music of Autistic (Schizophrenic) Children. *Am. J. Psychiatry*, 109: 823–831, 1953.

11. Murphy, R. C., and C. E. Preston. Three Autistic Brothers. Presented at the 1954 Annual Meeting of the American Orthopsychiatric Association.

12. Cappon, D. Clinical Manifestations of Autism and Schizophrenia in Childhood. *Canad. Med. Assoc. J.*, 69: 44–49, 1953.

13. Creak, M. (a) Psychoses in Childhood. *Proc. Royal Soc. Medicine*, 45: 797–800, 1953. (b) Psychoses in Childhood. *J. Ment. Sci.*, 97: 545–554, 1951.

14. Stern, E. A propos d'un cas d'autisme chez un jeune enfant. *Arch. Franç. de Pediatrie*, 9: 1952.

15. Stern, E., and M. Schachter. Zum Problem des frühkindlichen Autismus. *Prax. Kinderpsychol. Kinderpsychiat.*, 2: 113–119, 1953.

16. van Krevelen, D. A. Een Geval van "Early Infantile Autism." *Ned. Tijdschr. voor Geneeskunde*, 96: 202–205, 1952.

17. ———. Early Infantile Autism. *Z. für Kinderpsychiatrie*, 19: 91–97, 1952.

18. Arieti, S. Some Aspects of the Psychopathology of Schizophrenia. *Am. J. Psychotherapy*, 8: 396–414, 1954.

19. Norman, E. Reality Relationships of Schizophrenic Children. *Brit. J. Med. Psychol.*, 27: 126–141, 1954.

20. Ritvo, S., and S. Provence. Form Perception and Limitation in Some Autistic Children, in *The Psychoanalytic Study of the Child*, Vol. VIII, 155–161. Internat. Univ. Press, New York, 1953.

21. Darr, G. C., and F. G. Worden. Case Report Twenty-Eight Years After an Autistic Disorder. *Am. J. Orthopsychiatry*, 21: 559–570, 1951.

22. Bender, L. Childhood Schizophrenia. *Psychiatric Quart.*, 27: 1–19, 1953.

23. Kanner, L. To What Extent Is Early Infantile Autism Determined by Constitutional Inadequacies? *Res. Publ. Ass. Nerv. Ment. Dis.*, 33: 378–385, 1954.

24. Kallman, F. J. *Heredity in Health and Mental Disorder*. Norton, New York, 1953.

25. Bowlby, J. Maternal Care and Mental Health. *W.H.O. Monogr.*, Geneva, 1951.

26. Bakwin, H. Emotional Deprivation in Infants. *J. Pediat.*, 35: 512, 1949.

27. Spitz, R. A., and K. M. Wolf. Anaclitic Depression: An Inquiry into the Genesis of Psychiatric Conditions in Early Childhood, in *The Psychoanalytic Study of the Child*, Vol. II, 313–342. Internat. Univ. Press, New York, 1946.

28. Steels, H. M., and H. B. Dye. A Study of the Effect of Differential Stimulation on Mentally Retarded Children. *Proc. Amer. Assn. Stud. Ment. Def.*, 44: 114–136, 1939.

29. Gesell, A., and C. Amatruda. *Developmental Diagnosis*. 2nd ed., Hoeber, New York, 1947.

30. Thompson, W. R., and W. Heron. Effects of Restriction Early in Life on Problem Solving in Dogs. *Canad. J. Psychol.*, 8: 17–31, 1954.

31. ———. Exploratory Behavior in Normal and Restricted Dogs. *J. Comp. Physiol. Psychol.*, 47: 77–82, 1954.

32. Beach, F. A., and J. Jaynes. Effects of Early Experience on the Behavior of Animals. *Psychol. Bull.*, 51: 239–263, 1954.

33. Goldfarb, W. Effects of Psychological Deprivation in Infancy and Subsequent Stimulation. *Am. J. Psychiatry*, 102: 18–33, 1945.

34. ———. Variations in Adolescent Adjustment of Institutionally Reared Children. *Am. J. Orthopsychiatry*, 17: 449–457, 1947.

35. Bender, L. Psychopathic Conduct Disorder in Children, in *A Handbook of Correctional Psychiatry* (R. M. Lindner, Ed.). Philosophical Library, New York, 1947.

36. Bowlby, J. Forty-Four Juvenile Thieves: Their Characters and Home Life. *Int. J. Psychoanal.*, 25: 19–53, 1944.

37. Lewis, H. *Deprived Children: A Social and Clinical Study*. Oxford Univ. Press, New York, 1954.

38. Caplan, G. Clinical Observations on the Emotional Life of Children in the Communal Settlements in Israel, in *Problems of Infancy and Childhood: Seventh Conference* (M. S. E. Senn, Ed.). Josiah Macy, Jr. Foundation, New York, 1954.

39. Peck, H. B., R. D. Rabinovitch, and J. B. Cramer. A Treatment Program for Parents of Schizophrenic Children. *Am. J. Orthopsychiatry*, 19: 592, 1949.

40. Hoch, P. H., J. P. Cattell, and H. H. Pennes. Effects of Mescaline and Lysergic Acid (d. LSD 25). *Am. J. Psychiatry*, 108: 579–584, 1952.

41. Hoch, P. H., H. H. Pennes, and J. P. Cattell. Psychoses Produced by the Administration of Drugs. *Res. Publ. Ass. Nerv. Ment. Dis.*, 32: 287–296, 1953.

42. Fabing, H. D. New Blocking Agent against the Development of LSD-25 Psychosis. *Science*, 121: 208–210, 1955.

43. Gantt, W. H. Principles of Nervous Breakdown — Schizokinesis and Autokinesis. *Ann. N. Y. Acad. Sci.*, 56: 143–163, 1953.

44. Grewel, F. (Ed.). *Infantiel Autism*. J. Muusses te Purmerend, Amsterdam, 1954.

2

THE AUTISTIC CHILD IN ADOLESCENCE

LEON EISENBERG, M.D.

Children's Psychiatric Service, Johns Hopkins Hospital, Baltimore

Early infantile autism was first described by Kanner in 1943 on the basis of 11 cases whose features were sufficiently unique to constitute a new and previously unreported clinical syndrome (1). Subsequent publications by the same author have reported extensive experience with a much larger series of cases (2), analyzed the clinical phenomenology (3, 4), discussed its nosological allocation (5), and inquired into its genesis (6). Since the original papers, there have been numerous publications, both in this country (7–15) and abroad (16–22), which attest to the widespread recognition of infantile autism as a clinical syndrome (23). It remains a challenging problem, both because of its position as the earliest psychosis known to occur in childhood and because of its similarities to, and differences from, childhood schizophrenia. It becomes a matter of especial interest, therefore, to study the subsequent careers of children so diagnosed at an early age in order to determine the "natural history" of the syndrome. This may serve to shed light on the question of its specificity and contribute to an understanding of its psychopathology (24).

METHOD

The problems besetting follow-up studies have recently been critically reviewed by Robins (25). In order to facilitate an evaluation of this study, its definitions and its methods will be described in some detail. The cases were selected from the files of the Children's Psychiatric Service of the Harriet Lane Home of The Johns Hopkins Hospital. The original diagnosis was based upon the conjunction of the two cardinal symptoms which are to be regarded as pathognomonic for early infantile autism: extreme *self-isolation*, present in the first years of life, and *obsessive insistence on the preservation of sameness* (23). All of the children exhibited distortions of language functions, ranging from mutism and delayed onset of speech, through echolalia, affirmation by repetition, and pronominal reversal, to highly metaphorical language, employed with little intent to communicate mean-

From *The American Journal of Psychiatry*, February 1956.

ing to others (3, 4). Very few of the cases had organic abnormalities of the central nervous system, discernible either to physical examination or laboratory studies; where they did exist, they were inadequate to explain the clinical phenomenology (23).

An attempt was made to follow all of the children, 80 in number, who were known to the clinic for at least 4 years and who had attained an age of 9 or over. Sixty-three of the 80, or 79%, were traced. The 17 cases whose precise outcome is unknown to us were largely patients seen during the war years and for whom only temporary addresses were available. The cases lost comprise only 21% of the total and do not appear to have been selected on any systematic basis; indeed, incomplete (2–3 years) follow-up information on 10 of the 17 exhibits the same pattern as do our over-all results. We feel, therefore, that our data permit the construction of a reliable measure of the course of autism.

Of the 63 cases, 34 are in full-time residential settings and 29 at home with parents or foster parents. We have accurate institutional reports on the first 34, 10 of whom have also been reexamined. Of the remaining 29, 20 were reevaluated at the clinic. In 9 cases living at some distance, our information is limited to letters from the parents, supplemented by school and physician's reports. Follow-up letters from parents, it must be admitted, can be accepted only cautiously, but the usual doubts seem to be less applicable in our cases. We have been repeatedly impressed with the almost uncanny objectiveness and obsessive accuracy of parents of autistic children. In summary, the following analysis is based upon reexamination plus supplementary reports in 30 cases, institutional abstracts in 24 cases, and parents', physicians', and school reports in 9 cases.

Both the median and the average age of the children is 15 years, the range from 9 to 25.[1] Both the median and the average length of the follow-up period is 9 years, the range from 4 to 20. The range is admittedly wide, but the cases are clustered about the medians. Our figures may underestimate the number of children who will get into subsequent difficulties and do not, of course, permit extrapolation into the future. The ratio of girls to boys is 13 to 50, or about 1 to 4, which corresponds to the ratio in our total clinical experience, and there was no significant difference in clinical course between boys and girls.

The follow-up evaluation was classified into 3 categories: "poor," "fair," or "good" outcome. By "poor," we mean a patient who has

---

[1] There are 13 children between 9 and 12 years of age in our group of 61; all into the "poor" outcome category. Since our case histories reveal that signs of improvement are evident early, if improvement is to occur at all, we feel justified in including these not yet adolescent cases in our totals.

not emerged from autism to any extent and whose present function is markedly maladaptive, characterized by apparent feeblemindedness and/or grossly disturbed behavior, whether maintained at home or in an institution. By "fair," we mean a patient who is able to attend regular classes in public or private school at a level commensurate with age and who has some meaningful contacts with other people, but who exhibits schizoid peculiarities of personality, sufficient to single him out as a deviant and to cause interference with function. By "good," we mean a patient who is functioning well at an academic, social, and community level and who is accepted by his peers, though he may remain a somewhat odd person. In only 2 cases, both finally classified as poor, was there any question as to which category applied.

RESULTS

Of the total group of 63, 3 can be said to have achieved a good adjustment, 14 a fair one, and 46 a poor one. Thus, a little less than a third are functioning at a fair to good social level, a figure which corresponds to Bender's findings on a larger group of schizophrenic children (26). It is of some historic interest to note that all but Case 4 of the original series of 11 have been followed (1). Of these, all but Case I are doing poorly.

It soon became apparent, however, that those children who were so isolated from human contact that they failed to develop, or, once having developed, lost the ability to communicate by speech, did much more poorly than the others. If we choose as the line of demarcation the presence of *useful* speech at the age of 5, the total series can be divided into 32 "speaking" and 31 "nonspeaking" children.[2] The outcome of the first group of 32 can be classified as good in 3, fair in 13, and poor in 16 instances. Contrariwise, the outcome of the 31 nonspeaking children was fair in one and poor in 30 cases. Thus 16 of 32 children with useful speech at 5 years of age have been able to achieve a fair to good social adjustment, whereas only one of 31 nonspeaking children can be so classified. Chi square for this difference equals 15.19, with 10.83 equivalent to a probability value of 0.001, so that the difference between the 2 groups is highly significant (Table 1).

Our follow-up study fails to reveal any correlation between formal psychiatric treatment and the clinical outcome. Of the 16 cases with fair or good outcome, 2 had brief periods of psychiatric hospitalization and only 2 others were followed intermittently on an outpatient basis.

[2] The category "nonspeaking" includes mute children, those who exhibit only echolalia, and those who may possess in addition a few words, usually employed in a private sense. Its meaning in this context is "unable to communicate verbally with others."

TABLE I

Category	Poor outcome	Fair or good outcome	Total
"Speaking"	16	16	32
"Nonspeaking"	30	1	31
Total	46	17	63

$$X^2 = \frac{N([AD - BC] - N/2)^2}{(A+B)\ (C+D)\ (A+C)\ (B+D)}$$

$$= \frac{63\ ([16 - 480] - 31.5)^2}{32 \times 31 \times 46 \times 17}$$

$$= 15.19$$

$$p < 0.001$$

In the cases with poor outcome, a full range of psychiatric treatment — hospitalization, intensive psychotherapy, electroshock, CO_2, and even, in one case, an orgone box — had been applied with only at most temporary change which failed to interrupt the down-hill course. We have, however, been impressed by the prodigious efforts expended by both schools and parents for those children who have improved. We cannot escape the feeling that the extraordinary consideration extended to these patients was an important factor in the amelioration of their condition.

ILLUSTRATIVE CASE HISTORIES

CASE A. — Classification: "speaking," favorable outcome. Donald T., reported as Case 1 in the original series (1), has been followed by this clinic since 1938. Able at 2 to repeat by rote the 25 questions and answers of the Presbyterian catechism, at 5 he was described by his parents as "oblivious to everything about him . . . to get his attention almost requires one to break down a mental barrier between his inner consciousness and the outside world." On examination, he exhibited the pathognomonic features of autism. Distance from the clinic resulted in infrequent revisits through 1941. Some increase in awareness of others was noted as well as gradual use of the first person pronoun, but his modes of thought and expression remained highly idiosyncratic. His inability to participate in family life, his precarious school adjustment, and his anomalous position in a small town where his family was socially prominent led to the recommendation that he be placed with a warm and unsophisticated farm couple without intellectual pretensions. Donald remained in this rural setting for 3 years; moderate improvement was noted, though while on vacation with his parents during this period, his mother reported that his chief interest on the trip was to record carefully the mileage between towns. The boarding arrangement had to be terminated when Donald, at 14, developed an undiagnosed illness manifested by fever, chills, and joint pains.

He became bedridden and developed joint contractures. On the basis of a tentative diagnosis of Still's disease, he was placed empirically on gold therapy with marked improvement. After 18 months he was once again ambulatory. He emerged with little residual deficit from a second episode of arthritis 2 years later. The clinical improvement in his behavior, first observed during his rural placement, was accelerated during and after his illness and convalescence at home. He was able to enter and graduate from high school. At present he is doing well in his studies at a Junior College, where he was elected a class officer. He plans to attend a small local liberal arts college. He remains, however, "matter of fact and tactless," little aware of the response of others. His parents, though delighted with his progress, complain that he exhibits "little initiative" and "requires to be prodded" into activities.

CASE B. — Classification: "speaking," poor outcome. Charles, Case 9 of the original series (1), was 4½ when his mother brought him to the clinic with the distressed complaint, "I can't reach my baby." The history of precocious intellectual accomplishments, pronominal reversals, obsessive behavior, and marked detachment presented the classical features of autism. Charles "related" to the examiners only in so far as he made demands or became enraged at interference from without. His excellent vocabulary was manifested by the ejaculation of words and phrases that had no function as communication to others. He was referred to the Devereux Schools. During his year of residence there, definite though limited improvement could be noted in his social responsiveness. His parents, however, dissatisfied with the slowness of his progress, removed him against advice in order to hospitalize him at another institution where he was given a course of electroconvulsive therapy. Almost at once, marked regressive trends were noted and it became necessary to place him in a state hospital because of outbursts of aggressive behavior, soiling and smearing, and further withdrawal. At 8 he was transferred to an intensive therapy center in a children's unit. There he displayed "disorganized and regressive behavior . . . incoherent and irrelevant speech . . ." His failure to respond to therapeutic efforts led to his removal to a state hospital at 13. Now 15, he exhibits "schizophrenic deterioration . . . emotional blunting interrupted by periods of excitement . . . [he is] withdrawn, disoriented, unclean, destructive, and frequently depressed . . ."

CASE C. — Classification: "nonspeaking," fair outcome. George O. was so withdrawn and inaccessible that, at 3, institutionalization for severe retardation had been recommended. When seen at 4, he stood on his toes rocking and humming, oblivious to his surroundings. Only his detachment and the history of obsessiveness served to distinguish him from a feebleminded child. His father, a very successful physician, had little to do with his children. Interaction between mother and child was graphically illustrated when she was requested to place him on her lap. The two sat much like an Assyrian statue, rectangular, distant, rigid. The mother herself hardly looked the role of a prominent person in the community; she was bedraggled, vague, and defeated. She showed the first sign of awakening interest when foster placement for her child was suggested. This stirred obvious resentment and resulted in a decision to take over George (and herself) as her own responsibility. Over the ensuing years, with infrequent counselling at the clinic, a remarkable change in both mother and child could be observed as a symbiotic relationship developed. Mother took interest in her appearance, became more animated, and much more alert to her child's needs. George began to speak, was able to attend a small private school and learned to simulate social relations with other children. He became sufficiently accessible to be tested and one year ago achieved a Binet I.Q. of 91. Now 13, he has just entered 7th grade in a public junior high. Some initial difficulties in the classroom situation were resolved when "other children were taught to treat him right." He illustrated his artistic proficiency, much to his mother's pride, by sketching a lovely landscape while sitting in the waiting room; characteristically, his drawings never include people. He is a wooden, uncomfortable child who exhibits facial grimaces and avoids looking directly at people. He cannot bring himself to shake hands, initiates little conversation, but responds appropriately and intelligently. He can still be recognized as a disturbed child, but the change from the 3-year-old child who was diagnosed as severely retarded is impressive and gratifying.

CASE D. — Classification: "nonspeaking," poor outcome. Virginia, case 6 of the original series (1), at 11 exhibited almost total indifference to her surroundings, uttering not a sound and responding to no verbal requests. So detached had she been as a child that deafness had been suspected by a number of physicians but careful audiometric examination revealed normal threshold to sound. At 5 she had been placed in a state training school for the feeble-minded. There she stood out from the group because of her self-imposed isolation and her single-minded pursuit of her own interests (such as puzzle solving) for hours. Yet at 7 she achieved an I.Q. of 94 on Merrill-Palmer performance tests, which, in the opinion of the examiner, "underestimated her capacities." He stated: "Her performance reflected discrimination, care and precision . . ." At 8 on the Pintner-Patterson "her performance was never inferior to her own chronological age . . . with some scores in the superior range." Repeated efforts by staff members to reach this child over the years have been unavailing. She exhibits no concern about her personal appearance and makes no effort to communicate or socialize with her cottage mates or institutional personnel. She remains on the periphery, hardly bothering to watch when group activities occur. Testing her has become increasingly difficult. Nevertheless, at 21, she scored in the upper 10% of the population on the Kohs Blocks, completing 17 designs correctly, receiving time bonuses on the first 12. On the other hand, she treated the manikin with disregard for content, reversing arms and legs, and could not be induced to attend to it further.

DISCUSSION

Clinically, the degree of disturbance in language function emerges clearly as an important guide to prognosis. In effect, we have an index of the extent of autistic isolation, for the development of language obviously bespeaks a meaningful interchange with other people. The intrinsic severity of the autistic process thus appears to be the significant determinant of the outcome. In the absence of speech, the probability of emergence is vanishingly small, apparently without regard to which of the currently available treatment methods is employed. There is, however, no justification for the converse assumption that psychiatric supervision is superfluous and that recovery will necessarily occur when verbal communication is present. The child's subsequent experience will have no less profound an influence on the course of his development in this syndrome than in any other. All of the customary indications for psychiatric guidance will still apply here: therapy for the child, help for the parents, proper choice of school, and so on.

The separation of early infantile autism from other cases of childhood schizophrenia continues to be justified clinically. The early age of onset and the classical early history has already been reported in the literature (3, 4); the low incidence of psychotic progenitors (6) contrasts sharply with the rate reported for childhood schizophrenics (26). To these factors, we can now add the observation that clinically detectable hallucinations or delusions are extremely rare or nonexistent in these patients. The striking disability in interpersonal relations and the severe obsessive-compulsive mechanisms remain the pathognomonic features of autism. The peculiarities of language and thought, while somewhat different, share the general features of schizophrenia, so that the syndrome can be logically classified as one of the schizophrenias (but cf. 15, 22, 27). Its relative specificity, however, does not necessarily imply a common etiology. What we are dealing with is a behavior pattern that is shared by a number of patients but which may represent a response to any one of several underlying inciting factors. In view of the heterogeneity of the schizophrenias, it would seem wise to isolate clinically distinct groups for purposes of study.

Most of the adolescent autistic children who have not emerged from their illness are now functioning at what to all intents and purposes is a severely retarded level, though they remain distinguishable from cases of "simple" retardation by their affective isolation, a point that has already been developed by Mahler (8). It can, of course, be argued that their cognitive potentialities were, from the first, limited. But it would seem inevitable that a child whose contact with the human environment is so severely restricted must undergo irreversible intellectual deterioration when opportunities for growth are barred by the exclusion of normal experience, a concept that is supported by animal studies (28–33). Intellectual development can occur only in the most limited sense in the absence of language. The evolution of thought runs *pari passu* with the incorporation of the viewpoints of others, as the child assimilates his cultural heritage and substitutes consensual

logic for the egocentric logic of his private world (34). The tenuous
nature of the relationship of the autistic child to those about him
constricts and distorts this process.

Severely autistic children exhibit a preoccupation with the sensory
impressions stemming from the world about them, but seem unable
to organize perceptions into functional patterns. A small change in
the positioning of what to another observer would appear to be a randomly arranged group of toys may be at once apparent to them, but
the use of a doll or a toy car and its homology to people or automobiles
may escape them entirely. At one level this is reminiscent of the behavior of brain-damaged children (35) but certain important qualitative differences exist. The disability of the brain-damaged child
resides at a perceptual level, but once the "gestalt is closed," classification is made on the basis of function. Indeed, one of the difficulties
apparent in sorting tests is the very tendency of such a child to see
things as similar if they are functionally associated (36). The autistic
child, on the other hand, may solve relatively difficult abstract tasks
but the use of objects is not grasped (37). The jig-saw puzzle is assembled by the shape of its parts, but without respect to its content.
At a higher level of function, a similar disability may be observed.
The child may acquire a large vocabulary, but with little or no intent
to communicate meaning (38, 39). He may memorize astronomical
charts or maps of street car systems, but with no interest in principles
or practice of astronomy or transportation. The guiding principle of
purpose is lacking, recalling Bleuler's concept of the disorders of association in schizophrenia: "Only the goal-directed concept can wield
the links of the associative chain into logical thought" (40).

In those patients with a relatively favorable outcome, behavior is
still characterized by a failure to subordinate individual concerns to
social necessity. There appears to be little ability to empathize with
the feelings of others. The successful patients seem to have acquired,
painfully, the ability to simulate the behavior spontaneously exhibited
by their peers. One recalls Donald T., who, called upon to speak as
a student leader at a football rally, stated that the team was going to
lose. The ensuing round of boos led him finally to modify his initially
correct prediction, but the experience bewildered him. In a similar vein,
Jay S. commented, "I've never been able to get along with people. I
don't like 'diplomacy.' I come out and say what I think." The painful
nature of their contact with others leads them to prefer a solitary
existence. David G's first wish was "to be a forest ranger and live
in a cabin alone, far off in the woods"; David W.'s was that "they stop
building new houses in our neighborhood for people to move into."

In a sense, the primary psychopathologic mechanism in infantile autism might be described as a disturbance in social perception, analogous to, but more complex than, perceptual difficulties at a sensorimotor level. Affective contract assures in other children the precedence of things human over things inanimate. Thought and behavior are integrated by the driving force of human purpose, both individually and socially determined. It is this force that assigns the affective value to incoming sensory impressions and organizes the perceptual field into a socially meaningful whole. Its dysfunction in autism results in perceptions that are diffuse and stimulus-bound, thinking that is tangential to human goals, and behavior that is maladaptive. There can be no anatomical "locus" for such a disability; it can only be a reflection of the failure of cortical integration of the affective and cognitive components of behavior. One wonders if there may not be, parallel to intellectual inadequacy, a syndrome of affective inadequacy. Just as intellectual inadequacy may be the outcome of structural limitations or of cultural deprivation, so may affective inadequacy reflect organic dysfunction, affective deprivation, or a combination thereof.

Summary

Sixty-three autistic children have been re-evaluated at a mean age of 15 years after a mean follow-up period of 9 years. Almost one third have achieved at least a moderate social adjustment. The prognosis has been shown to vary significantly with the presence of useful speech at the age of 5, taken as an index of the severity of autistic isolation. Half of those who possessed meaningful language by the age of 5 improved, whereas only 1 of 31 without the ability to communicate verbally by that age has shown significant improvement. The clinical course of these children justifies the segregation of early infantile autism as a clinical entity, probably to be included within the group of schizophrenias. The psychopathology of autism has been reviewed and the suggestion offered that the fundamental feature is a disturbance in social perception.

References

1. Kanner, L. Nerv. Child, 2: 217, 1943.
2. ——— J. Ped., 25: 211, 1944.
3. ——— Am. J. Psychiat., 103: 242, 1946.
4. ——— Ibid., 108: 23, 1951.
5. ——— Am. J. Orthopsychiat., 19: 416, 1949.
6. ——— Res. Publ. Ass. Nerv. Ment. Dis., 33: 378, 1954.
7. Despert, J. L. Am. J. Orthopsychiat., 21: 335, 1951.
8. Mahler, M. S. The Psychoanalytic Study of the Child, 7: 286, 1952.

9. Mahler, M. S., Ross, J. R., Jr., and DeFries, Z. *Am. J. Orthopsychiat.*, 19: 295, 1949.

10. Murphy, R. C., and Preston, C. E. *Am. J. Orthopsychiat.* In Press.

11. Rank, B. *Am. J. Orthopsychiat.*, 19: 130, 1949.

12. Sherwin, A. C. *Am. J. Psychiat.*, 109: 823, 1953.

13. Weil, A. P. *Am. J. Orthopsychiat.*, 23: 518, 1953.

14. Darr, G. C., and Worden, F. G. *Ibid.*, 21: 559, 1951.

15. Ritvo, S., and Provence, S. *The Psychoanalytic Study of the Child*, 8: 155, 1953.

16. Cappon, D. *Canad. Med. Assoc. J.*, 69: 44, 1953.

17. Creak, M. *Proc. Royal Soc. Med.*, 45: 797, 1953.

18. —— *J. Ment. Sc.*, 97: 545, 1951.

19. Stern, E. A Propos d'un cas d'autisme chez un jeune enfant. *Archives Francais de Pediatrie*, 1952, 9.

20. Stern, E., and Schachter, M. Zum Problem des frühkindlichen Autismus. *Praxis der Kinderpsychologie und Kinderpsychiatrie*, 2: 113, 1953.

21. van Krevelen, D. A. Een Geval van "Early Infantile Autism." *Nederlandsch Tijdschrift voor Geneeskunde*, 96: 202, 1952.

22. —— Early Infantile Autism. *Z. für Kinderpsychiatrie*, 19: 91, 1952.

23. Eisenberg, L., and Kanner, L. Early Infantile Autism 1943–1955. *Am. J. Orthopsychiat.* In Press.

24. Kanner, L., and Eisenberg, L. Notes on the Follow-up Studies of Autistic Children. *In* Hoch and Zubin, eds. *Psychopathology of Childhood.* New York: Grune & Stratton, 1955.

25. Robins, A. J. *Am. J. Psychiat.*, 111: 434, 1954.

26. Bender, L. *Psychiatric Quart.*, 27: 1, 1953.

27. Grewl, F. (ed.) *Infantiel Autism.* (Symposium of the Dutch Society for Child Psychiatry). Amsterdam: J. Muusses te Purmerend, 1954.

28. Riesen, A. H. *Science*, 106: 107, 1947.

29. Nissen, H. W., Chow, K. L., and Semmes, J. *Am. J. Psychol.*, 64: 485, 1951.

30. Hebb, D. O. *Organization of Behavior*, New York: Wiley, 1949.

31. Thompson, W. R., and Heron, W. *Canad. J. Psychol.*, 8: 17, 1954.

32. —— *J. Comp. Physiol. Psychol.*, 47: 77, 1954.

33. Beach, F. A., and Jaynes, J. *Psychol. Bull.*, 51: 239, 1954.

34. Piaget, J. Principal Factors Determining Intellectual Evolution from Childhood to Adult Life. *In* Rapaport, D., Ed. *Organization and Pathology of Thought.* New York: Columbia University Press, 1951.

35. Eisenberg, L. Psychiatric implications of brain damage in children. *Psychiat. Quart.* In Press.

36. Strauss, A. A., and Werner, H. *J. Nerv. Ment. Dis.*, 96: 153, 1942.

37. Norman, E. *Brit. J. Med. Psychol.*, 27: 126, 1954.

38. Despert, J. L. *Psychiat. Quart.*, 12: 366, 1938.

39. —— *Nerv. Child*, 1: 199, 1942.

40. Bleuler, E. *Dementia Praecox or the Group of Schizophrenias.* Zinkin, J. (trans.). New York: International Universities Press, 1950.

3

THE INFLUENCE OF DEGREE OF FLEXIBILITY IN MATERNAL CHILD CARE PRACTICES ON EARLY CHILD BEHAVIOR

ETHELYN H. KLATSKIN, PH.D., EDITH B. JACKSON, M.D., AND LOUISE C. WILKIN, M.S.S.

Department of Pediatrics, Yale University School of Medicine, New Haven, Connecticut

The present paper is a report on the analysis of a selected group of cases from the files of the Yale Rooming-in Research Project, a longitudinal study of parent-child relationship focused on observing the effect of certain specific parental child care practices on child behavior. The research program has utilized a team approach to collect data on the developing family unit during the prenatal period, in the hospital during the puerperium, and during the first three years of the child's life. The details of the development of the Project and the methodology of data collection and organization have been reported elsewhere (3).

The study had its inception during a period which marked a cultural shift from rigid to permissive practices in child training. For the previous twenty years, medical trends and Watsonian behaviorism had influenced pediatricians and educators to advocate inflexible techniques in child training (2). Beginning around 1935, increasing familiarity with Freudian analytic tenets and the necessity to deal with an apparently increasing number of behavior problems led a number of child psychiatrists to propose the use of more flexible practices in early child care. This orientation was in large part due to the conviction that many of the then observed problems in early child development were the result of rigid parental child care practices. The ensuing twenty years have witnessed an almost complete shift in popularity from inflexible to flexible practices, both as advocated by specialists in the field (4, 6) and as accepted by the general public (5).

In neither the preceding period of rigidity nor the current period of permissiveness, however, has any body of statistical evidence been presented to substantiate the claims of the proponents of either type of child training. The present research was organized to amass just such a body of data. In general, the Project has been predicated on

From *The American Journal of Orthopsychiatry*, January 1956.

the hypothesis that a demonstrable relationship can be shown to exist between parental child care practices on the one hand and the child's behavior on the other. Specifically, the hypothesis investigated was that either extreme of rigidity or permissiveness in parental practices would be associated with problem behavior in the child, within the area of the parental deviation.

SUBJECTS AND PROCEDURE

The subjects of the present study were 50 mothers and infants chosen from the families followed for three years through the research project. Two factors determined selection of this group: the mother's parity and the completeness of the case history. In order not to obscure the initial parent-child interaction, the records of primiparae were chosen for analysis. The first 50 records were then selected which met the requirements of including all of the major research procedures: office visit and psychological examination, social worker's home visit, and parental report by questionnaire, at one, two and three years.

The socioeconomic composition of this subgroup is given in Tables 1 and 2. In defining the occupational groupings, the categories of the United States Census were used. In both tables, students in training were classified according to educational and occupational expectation. In Table 2, the mother was classified according to either previous or present type of employment; actually, only 11 of the 50 mothers studied were working during any period of the three year follow-up.

The tables show that approximately half of the group was composed of families in which both parents had college or advanced degrees, and that in one-third of the group both parents were at some time in professional or managerial positions. There was no representation from the highest or lowest socioeconomic groups. The relationships within the sample can best be described in terms of Hollingshead's socioeconomic grouping for the New Haven area (1): Class II (professional and managerial), 19; Class III (white collar and skilled workers), 19; and Class IV (semiskilled and unskilled workers), 12.

A rating scale technique of analysis was used to reduce the data contained in the fifty case histories to statistically manipulable form.[1] Independent scales were constructed for rating both parental and child behavior in the areas of feeding, sleeping, toileting, and socialization. Additional scales were constructed for the data on mother's adjustment to the maternal role, and for evidences of emotional disturbance in the child, other than those which might be included in the four behavior areas. Since the data broke logically at the child's first,

---

[1] For details of method of construction of these scales, see (3).

second, and third birthdays because of the timing of the research procedures, each year was scaled separately.

In scaling the areas of feeding, sleeping, toileting, and socialization,

TABLE 1. PARENTS' EDUCATION *

		Mother's Education			
		Grammar School	High School	College	Advanced Degree
Father's Education	Grammar School	3	1		
	High School		16	6	
	College			6	
	Advanced Degree			13	5

* Classified according to attendance at or completion of the given level.

the major variable for the mother's behavior was defined as degree of rigidity in handling the child, and for the child's behavior, degree of problem. The scales of maternal behavior ranged from extreme rigidity (point 1) at one end of the scale to extreme permissiveness at the other (point 5), with flexible handling as the mid-point (point 3). The scales of child behavior ranged from severe problem at one end of the scale (point 1) to absence of problem at the other (point 5), with "problem within normal limits" as the mid-point (point 3). Either extreme of the scale of maternal behavior was assumed to represent deviant handling leading to the development of problems in the child, while the mid-point of the maternal behavior scale was assumed to represent optimal handling associated with normal development. The one exception to this assumption occurred in the evaluation of maternal behavior in toileting during the first year. In this instance, any rating below the mid-point of the scale was regarded as rigid and any rating above the mid-point as optimal.

TABLE 2. PARENTS' OCCUPATION

		Mother's Occupation *				
		Professional-Managerial	White Collar	Skilled	Semi-skilled	None
Father's Occupation †	Professional-Managerial	10	9			
	White Collar	2	9	1	1	2
	Skilled	1	2			1
	Semiskilled	1	2		1	2
	Unskilled		2		2	2

* Classified according to present or previous occupation.
† Classified according to present occupation or occupational expectation.

The scale for rating the mother's adjustment to the maternal role ranged from complete rejection at one end, to complete absorption at the other, with "balanced adjustment" as the mid-point. The scale for other evidences of emotional maladjustment in the child ranged from severe and/or numerous problems at one end to absence of problems at the other, with mild and/or infrequent problems as the mid-point.

Two considerations determined the application of the scales to the evaluation of the case records: the necessity to have an independent rating for mother and child; and to have a rating which would be both reliable and valid. To meet these requirements, six raters were used,[2] who were assigned in groups of three to either mother or child. Both assignment to a group and to a subject was successively randomized among the six raters. In this way, three independent judgments for each segment of behavior were available for both mother and child, except in those instances where insufficient information was available in the record. A reliable judgment was assumed to be one on which two or more raters agreed, and only those were recorded for subsequent correlation. The assignment of raters to successive groupings provided a measure of the extent to which any given rater consistently deviated from the other two, it being assumed that the ratings were more valid if no significant variability occurred within the group. That is, if no rater was found to deviate consistently from the others, the probability would be increased that all were using the same bases for their judgments. The alternation between rating mother and child was planned to focus the raters on the scales themselves as a reference point, rather than on the consecutive records. No significant differences were found between the raters in either number of times they deviated from the group, or number of times they reported insufficient data.

RESULTS

The initial step in analysis of the data was to plot the distribution of the consensus judgments for both mother and child for each segment of the four behavior areas. With two exceptions, both in the area of toileting, the ratings tended to assume a normal distribution around the mid-point (3) of the scale. In the area of toileting, when the mothers' ratings were plotted, it was found that at the first year, only 15 mothers fell below the mid-point of the scale, and at the third year, no information was returned by 21 of the group. In these 21 cases, the mothers replied that the child was trained, although accord-

[2] Nilda Shea, M.N.; Betty Casher, B.A.; Marjorie W. DeGooyer, M.S.; and the authors.

ing to the scale for the child's behavior, only 11 were rated as being trained. The handling of these data therefore constituted an exception to the type of analysis described below.

Since the various points on the mother's and child's scales did not correspond directly to each other (as the mother's scale represented a progression from undesirable rigidity through optimal handling to undesirable overpermissiveness, while the child's scale represented a progression from undesirable to desirable behavior), this fact had to be taken into account in analyzing the relationship between the two. A chi-square rather than correlational analysis was therefore planned. The mothers' scales represented a fairly absolute judgment of deviant behavior, since the extremes of overpermissiveness and rigidity for the various areas were defined so as to take into account marked departures from the normal attitude. In each area, approximately half of the group (between 43% and 60%) fell into the optimal category, while the position of the remaining half varied somewhat according to the behavior area rated. The mothers were therefore initially divided into those obtaining ratings of 1 or 2 (rigid), ratings of 3 (optimal), and ratings of 4 or 5 (overpermissive). The child's scale, however, was found to indicate a more relative degree of disturbance. When the ratings for the various areas were plotted, all tended to assume a normal distribution, but the mode varied slightly for the different years and variables. Thus, the modal score for socialization, first year, was 4.0; for socialization, second year, it fell to 3.5; and for socialization, third year, it was 3.0. In order to maintain a consistent reference point, ratings for the child in each area were therefore dichotomized at the median of the group, dividing the children into those with more or less problem behavior in a given area. Dividing the children's group in this way arbitrarily resulted in a range of incidence of "problem" behavior for the various areas of 33 to 53 per cent. It should be kept in mind throughout the subsequent presentation of results that when "presence of problem behavior" or "absence of problem behavior" is discussed, the child is being assessed relative to his position in the present group of subjects, and not in terms of more absolute standards which might be applied to "problem children" in a child guidance clinic.

The data for maternal attitude toward toileting in the first and third years were treated as follows: at the first year, the mothers were dichotomized into those falling below the mid-point of the scale and those at or above the mid-point. For the third year, in view of the lack of data, the mothers' ratings at two years were correlated with the child's behavior at three years.

Chi-square was then computed for all the relationships, with the exception of first year toileting, on the basis of a six-cell table, tri-chotomizing the mothers' group into rigid, optimal, and overpermissive, and dichotomizing the group of children into those above and below the median incidence of problem behavior. Of the 12 possible relationships, 7 were found to be significant at or below the .01 level. However, it was apparent that because of the small number of cases, some relationships between deviant maternal behavior and the development of problem behavior in the child were obscured. The chi-squares were therefore recalculated on the basis of a four-cell table, dichotomizing the mother's handling into optimal and deviant, without regard

TABLE 3. SIGNIFICANT VALUES OF CHI-SQUARE BETWEEN DEVIANT OR OPTIMAL
MATERNAL HANDLING AND PRESENCE OR ABSENCE OF PROBLEM
BEHAVIOR IN THE CHILD

Year	Area			
	Feeding	Sleeping	Toileting	Socialization
1	—	$\chi^2 - 11.77^*$ $p < .001$	$\chi^2 - 9.91$ $p < .01$	—
2	$\chi^2 - 13.00$ $p < .001$	$\chi^2 - 8.42$ $p < .01$	$\chi^2 - 12.74^*$ $p < .001$	$\chi^2 - 7.18^*$ $p < .01$
3	$\chi^2 - 5.75$ $p < .02$	$\chi^2 - 15.25^*$ $p < .001$	$\chi^2 - 13.97^*$ $p < .001$	$\chi^2 - 12.58^*$ $p < .001$

* $p < .01$ for six-cell table.

to direction. The results of these latter calculations are given in Table 3; those values of chi-square significant when computed on the basis of the six-cell tables are also indicated. Because of the number of significance tests calculated in analyzing the data, the criterion for a "significant" relationship was set as probability of occurrence by chance less than twice in a hundred. Consequently, only those relationships significant at or below the .02 level of confidence will be reported here.

The direction of the maternal deviation associated with "problem" behavior in the child is indicated in Table 4. It is apparent from this

TABLE 4. DIRECTION OF MATERNAL DEVIATION SIGNIFICANTLY ASSOCIATED
WITH PROBLEM BEHAVIOR IN THE CHILD

Year	Area			
	Feeding	Sleeping	Toileting	Socialization
1		Overpermissive		
2	Rigid	Overpermissive	Both	Rigid
3	Rigid	Overpermissive	Both	Rigid

table that a consistent relationship exists between type of maternal deviation and the behavior area in which this is shown.

Tables 3 and 4 indicate that the relationship between maternal behavior and child behavior tends to be a discrete one, in that the child develops "problems" in response to specific deviations from optimal handling. As a further check on this conclusion, interarea relationships were tested to determine whether maternal deviation in one area was associated with problem behavior in the child in a different area. For example, maternal behavior in feeding was related to the child's behavior in sleeping. No significant relationships of this type were found.

The question might still be raised as to whether some over-all factor of adjustment or maladjustment in the child resulted in the presence or absence of problem behavior. The child's ratings on the scale of "Other Evidences of Emotional Maladjustment," which had been designed to assess the child's general emotional stability, were therefore analyzed in relation to his ratings in each of the four areas for the three years. The only relationships found (p < .02) were in the area of socialization, where during the first and third years, children with "problems" in socialization tended to fall below the median of the group in evidencing "emotional maladjustment." Because of the possibility that this relationship might have arisen from use of the same data in rating both areas, the ratings at the third year were checked for such duplication. Of the 307 individual items of behavior listed by the judges as the basis for their ratings of the child's social adjustment in the 50 cases, only 39, or 13 per cent, were repeated as evidence for additional emotional maladjustment.

Finally, major environmental events in the child's life were related to his behavior in the four areas as well as to his rating with respect to the "emotional maladjustment" scale. The factors studied were: intelligence, dividing the children into below average (5 cases), average (30 cases), and above average (15 cases); duration of breast feeding, dividing the group at the median duration (3 months); birth of a sibling (20 cases); nursery school attendance in the third year (16 cases); and severe and/or recurrent illness (10 cases). The only positive relationship found was that between birth of a sibling during the second year and the presence of greater emotional maladjustment $(\chi^2 - 8.75, p < .01)$.

Since it appeared from the foregoing data that the mother's handling of the child was the major variable in influencing his behavior, the next step in data analysis was to investigate what factors might be influencing the maternal attitude. These fell into three general categories — the mother's general emotional stability, as measured by her adjustment to the maternal role; environmental factors current in the home situation; and the mother's social class membership. When the mother's adjustment to the maternal role was related to her behavior toward the child, significant relationships were found in the areas of handling of sleep and socialization. The chi-square values for these, based on dichotomizing the mother's adjustment as deviant or balanced, and her handling of the child as deviant or optimal, are given in Table 5. In the case of sleep, rejection of the maternal role tended to be associated with rigid practices in this area, and absorption tended to be associated with overpermissive practices. The most striking relationships, however, were found in the area of socialization. During the first year, of the 16 mothers judged as rejecting of the maternal role, 13 used rigid methods of socialization; in the second year, of 20 judged as rejecting, 17 used rigid practices; and in the third year, of 17 judged as rejecting, 15 used rigid practices.

An attempt was next made to evaluate the importance of environmental factors in influencing both actual handling of the child and the mother's adjustment to the maternal role. The following "deviant home situations" were selected for analysis: marked discrepancy in

TABLE 5. RELATIONSHIP BETWEEN ATTITUDE TOWARD MATERNAL ROLE AND MATERNAL BEHAVIOR

Year	Area			
	Feeding	Sleeping	Toileting	Socialization
1	—	$\chi^2 - 8.16$ $p < .01$	—	$\chi^2 - 24.42$ $p < .001$
2	—	$\chi^2 - 11.94$ $p < .01$	—	$\chi^2 - 12.09$ $p < .001$
3	—	$\chi^2 - 5.92$ $p < .02$	—	$\chi^2 - 14.28$ $p < .001$

parental background, inadequate housing, prolonged illness of either parent, atypical employment hours for father, and mother working or out of the home. It was found, however, that these variables occurred too infrequently to permit statistical analysis, and though the presence of any one or constellation of them was of obvious importance for the dynamics of the individual case, such analysis is not within the scope of the present paper.

Because much emphasis has been placed on the mother's social class membership as a determinant of maternal child care practices, the mothers' behavior in the four areas was analyzed for the three classes represented in the present group of subjects. Here, definite trends were observed which, because of the small number of subjects, were not statistically significant. A summary of these data is presented in Figure 1, which was arrived at in the following manner. Since 12 attitude ratings were available for each mother (one for each of the four areas for each of the three years), a total score could be assigned to her based on the category into which the majority of the ratings fell. For purposes of the present summary, a mother was assigned that score into which two-thirds (8 out of the 12) of her ratings fell. On this basis, she could be classed as rigid, optimal, overpermissive, or inconsistent (no two-thirds majority). It will be seen from Figure 1 that the majority of the Class II mothers fell into the optimal category, the majority of the Class III mothers fell into the rigid category, and the majority of the Class IV mothers showed no consistent pattern, but varied in optimal, rigid, or overpermissive behavior from area to area.

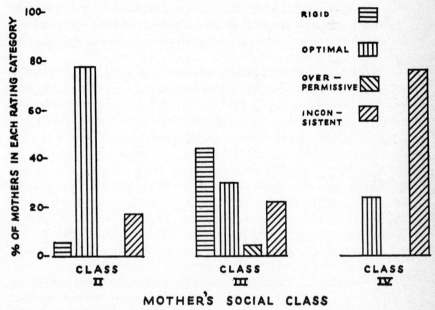

Fig. 1. Relationship between mother's social class membership and her predominant type of child care practice.

Two questions which have been raised about the present data are 1) the relationship between the consistency of the mother's behavior and the development of problems in the child, and 2) the effect on the child of deviant maternal attitudes in those mothers who were judged as well adjusted to the maternal role as opposed to those mothers who were judged as rejecting or overabsorbed.

In order to assess the cumulative effect of maternal consistency or inconsistency, the data were analyzed for each of the four major behavior areas. The child's status at three years (above or below the median of his group with reference to degree of problem behavior) was related to the mother's behavior throughout the three years. The mothers were classed as consistently optimal, rigid, or overpermissive (those who received the same rating at all three years) and inconsistent (those who received a different rating for any or all of the three years). When the consistent mothers were contrasted with the inconsistent mothers, no difference was found in incidence of problem behavior in the children. However, when contrasts were drawn within the group of consistent mothers, significant differences were found in incidence of problem behavior between the children of consistently optimal mothers on the one hand and the children of consistently rigid or overpermissive mothers on the other. In each instance, the children of the consistently optimal mothers had a significantly lower incidence of problem behavior. The chi-square values for the four areas are as follows: feeding — 4.24, p < .05; sleeping — 8.69, p < .01; toileting — 12.62, p < .01; and socialization — 4.24, p < .05.

The hypothesis has been advanced that fewer problems would develop among children handled deviantly by mothers who were well adjusted to the maternal role than among those whose mothers were rejecting or overabsorbed. Because of the small number of cases in the present sample, and the high correlation obtained between maternal adjustment and optimal handling, it was not possible to contrast the effect on the child of deviant handling by the different types of mothers. It was hoped that this type of breakdown would yield information as to the effect on child development of overpermissiveness or rigidity in mothers who felt at ease in such practices (that is, those mothers adjusted to the maternal role), as opposed to deviation which was the outgrowth of superficial adherence to "popular" advice or represented rejection of the child (that is, those mothers overabsorbed or rejecting of the maternal role). Of the 50 cases, 14 mothers were judged as adjusted to the maternal role at all three years; 20 were judged as maladjusted at all three years; and in 16 cases the mother's type of adjustment varied from year to year. As might be anticipated from the data given in Table 5, the majority of the well-adjusted mothers showed optimal handling, and the majority of the maladjusted mothers showed deviant handling. Consequently, no contrasts were possible.

DISCUSSION

The present results show that child behavior during the first three years is more consistently influenced by maternal handling than by other environmental factors. However, in view of the stress which has been placed on the role played by early infancy experience in subsequent development, it is notable that fewer significant relationships were found within the first year than for the two subsequent years. Not only was no significant relationship found in the first year between maternal practice and child behavior in the areas of feeding and socialization, but when the mother's first year practices were related to the child's behavior in the second year to determine whether a delayed effect could be shown, no significant relationships appeared.

There is no ready explanation to account for the fact that in these areas the type of maternal handling during the first year does not here have the same obvious effect on the child's behavior as it does during the second and third. However, three possibilities suggest themselves. The first is that the present techniques were not sufficiently sensitive to detect greater individual variation among the children in these areas than was found during the first year. This is suggested by the fact that although in the first year about the same number of mothers fell into the categories of rigid, optimal, and overpermissive as during the second and third years, a higher proportion of the children fell above the mid-point of the scale (point 3) in the first year than during the second and third years. Using the present techniques of dividing the children's group at the median and thus making a relative judgment as to presence or absence of problem, in the area of feeding, 19 fell below the median and 27 above; in the area of socialization, 22 fell below the median and 26 above. However, dividing the group at the mid-point and thus making a more absolute judgment as to presence or absence of problem, in feeding only 5 fell below the mid-joint, with 40 above it; in socialization, only 7 fell below the mid-point, with 42 above it. Thus, while it appears that this group of children were relatively problem free in these two areas during the first year, it is possible that if finer discriminations could have been made between them, a stronger relationship to type of maternal care might have been found. According to this hypothesis, incipient problem behavior actually existed among the children, but the research techniques were not sensitive enough to detect it.

An alternative explanation is that while this group of mothers showed variation in type of maternal handling, none showed the gross distortions in child care that have previously been correlated with the development of feeding and socialization problems during the first year. It is plausible to assume that, as in the area of toileting, overpermissiveness during the first year in feeding and socialization may not represent the gross mishandling that it does during the second and third years. On the other hand, it is possible that the judgment of rigidity made for the present mothers did not represent the same extreme of control that characterized child care practices 20 years ago. Both interpretations would decrease the probability of finding a significant relationship between maternal care and child behavior. According to this hypothesis, the group of children would be regarded as relatively problem free in these two areas because minor variations in handling among an essentially homogeneous group of mothers would be less likely to produce problem behavior during the first than during subsequent years.

A third possibility is that, because of the nature of the group and the amount of pediatric supervision received, less variation existed among the mothers' attitudes toward the child in the first year than in the second and third. It will be recalled that the present group of subjects were drawn from an "average" population of women routinely attending an obstetrical clinic. In all but 14 of the 50 cases, the baby was planned, and was presumably desired and responded to with affection and acceptance at his birth. During the first year, the mothers — either through attendance at a Child Health Conference of the Visiting Nurse Association or through a private pediatrician — received more intensive supervision than during the second and third years of the child's life. A situation therefore arose in which the mothers received more help in understanding the child when the needs to be met were the basic ones of feeding, sleeping, and protection from injury, than subsequently when he became more independent and active in exploring his environment and the cultural pressures for his "socialization" were increased. Although the mothers could be categorized as rigid, optimal, or overpermissive during the first year, it seems plausible to assume that less variation in underlying attitudes would be found during the child's infancy than later in his life, when his demands became more individual. As a result of the necessity for increased discipline, and for meeting the demands of society that he be toilet trained, learn appropriate techniques in eating, and acquire recognition of the distinction between his property and that of others, the degree of interaction between mother and child is heightened, and presumably a wider range of maternal attitudes are elicited. According to this hypothesis, the attitudes underlying the child care practices during the first year within this group would be more homogeneous than during the second and third years, when the mother's own anxieties and conflicts would be aroused by the child's increasing independence and by the increasing demands of society, and when, because of less intensive pediatric supervision, she would have to deal with him more in terms of her own individual personality and previous experiences.

Another striking aspect of the data which requires explanation is the discreteness of the relationships found between maternal handling and the child's reaction. It is apparent that poor handling in any given area is likely to be associated with "problem" behavior in the child in that area, but that this does not generalize in the child to other areas. It is also apparent that the type of maternal deviation varies in effect in the different areas of child behavior. Thus, in the area of sleep, overpermissiveness produces problems, while in the areas of feeding and socialization, rigidity produces problems. Here again, there are several possible explanations. One is that such specificity is due in part to the structure of the group. Thus, on the one hand, very few of the mothers were rated as falling at the extremes of the scale (points 1 and 5), so that the rigid and overpermissive groups were composed largely of mothers who received intermediate ratings between the mid-point and the extremes. If the mothers had shown more gross deviation from what would be regarded as acceptable child care practices, greater spread of effect might have been found among the children. This interpretation derives some support from the fact that few of the present group of children evidence any severe emotional disturbance of the kind that would lead to a pervasive disruption of behavior. The hypothesis that greater generalization of problem behavior would occur if the child were more generally disturbed is borne out by further analysis of the present data. If, at each year, the children are divided at the median of the scale of emotional maladjustment into those more or less emotionally maladjusted, the median number of problems is always greater in the group judged as more maladjusted. Thus, at the first and second years, the median number of problems for the more maladjusted group fell between 2 and 3, for the less maladjusted, between 1 and 2; at the third year, the median for the more maladjusted group again fell between 2 and 3, but for the less maladjusted group, between 0 and 1.

It can also be hypothesized that the relationships between child behavior and parental child care practice may be more discrete at the time of origin of problems than later in the child's life. The observation that certain neurotic components of personality represent anxiety displaced from early childhood experience is undoubtedly a valid one, but it has been deduced for the most part from the treatment of older children and adults. The present direct observations of early childhood suggest that initially the effect of deviant parental handling is more discrete than has been supposed.

Although some of the results of this study lead to conclusions which seem obvious at the present date to psychiatrists, psychologists, pediatricians and other educators in the field of child development, their apparent clarity is probably more the result of hindsight based on ten years' experience than foresight in predicting the effects of a pendulum swing from rigidity to permissiveness in child care. At the formulation of the research in 1946, no actual documentation existed as to the effects of various types of maternal practices on child development. In the ensuing years, two main difficulties arose which probably could not have been anticipated. The first of these was the focus of teaching on the early infancy period, because of professional interest in changing maternity routines, the encouragement of breast feeding, and the emphasis on "ad lib." care during the neonatal period. As a result, although the limits of permissiveness were tacitly implied, they were not explicitly stated. A situation was thereby created in which the mothers were encouraged to handle the child permissively during his infancy, but received less professional assistance in setting limits on such practices as the child grew older. The second difficulty was the rapidity with which the concept of permissiveness was popularized in lay publications. However, here a misinterpretation arose in equating permissiveness with license and in exaggerating the applicability of the new concept. Because of this trend toward overpermissive practices by many mothers, it was possible to document the effects of extremes in maternal care as well as of optimal handling.

Other of the results — particularly the finding of fewer significant relationships in the first year and the discreteness of relationships in the second and third years — may come as a suprise. Whatever explanations may be advanced to account for these results, the fact remains that they are the product of an objectively collected body of data, amassed at the time of origin of the behavior in question. This may in itself account for the disparity between the conclusions of the present study and current theoretical formulations. That is, most of the data which stress the importance of early mother-child interaction and the pervasiveness of problem behavior have been collected from older patients in psychiatric treatment or from a few intensive longitudinal case histories. While not discounting the value and contribution of information obtained from such sources, it is plausible to assume that differences in methods of data collection would lead to emphasizing different aspects of personality development. Where data are collected from patients through retrospective recall, the emphasis is on pathological processes and may include unconscious distortion and falsification of time relationships. Where minute observations of the effect of many individual variables are available, the influence of factors common to all may be obscured. The present study represents one of the first attempts of which the authors are aware to observe and correlate maternal and child interaction in a "normal" population of subjects, with emphasis on the central tendency of the group.

SUMMARY

Fifty records of primiparous mothers were selected from the files of the Yale Rooming-In Project. The data (prenatal interviews; hospital record data; pediatric posthospital follow-up; psychological examination and interview, social worker's home visits, and mother's report by questionnaire at one, two and three years) were analyzed statistically. A rating scale method of analysis was used, with three raters independently rating the mother's child care practices and three the child's behavior. The areas scaled for the mother were: practices in feeding, sleeping, toileting, and socialization, and her adjustment to the maternal role. For the child, the areas scaled were: behavior in feeding, sleeping, toileting, socialization, and evidences of his emotional maladjustment. The scales for maternal child care practice were continua ranging from extreme rigidity at one end to extreme permissiveness at the other, with optimal handling as the mid-point; adjustment to the maternal role was scaled on a continuum ranging from extreme rejection to extreme absorption. All of the scales for the child's behavior were continua ranging from severe problem to absence of problem, with "problem within normal limits" as the mid-point.

The relationships between the consensus judgments of the two groups of raters for mother's practices and child's behavior were analyzed for every area during each of the three years. Tripartite chi-square was first used, dividing the mother's behavior into rigid, optimal, and over-permissive practices, and the child's behavior into degree of problem above or below the median of the group. It was found that the direction of the difference in the mother's scales was of no significance in relation to the degree of problem manifested by the child, and in the final analysis, bipartite chi-square was used, dividing the mother's scales into optimal and deviant practices.

The following statistically significant relationships were found: within the first year, deviant maternal practices in sleep were associated with problem behavior in the child, though no relationships were found between practices and behavior in the areas of feeding, toileting, and socialization. In the second and third years, significant relationships were found between deviant maternal practices and problem behavior in the child in all four areas. Deviant adjustment to the maternal role was found to be related to deviant practices in sleep and socialization during all three years. Similarly, children showing other evidences of emotional maladjustment were found to have a significantly higher proportion of sleep and socialization problems.

Other aspects of the case history (social class, housing conditions, illness in either parent or child, birth of siblings, nursery school attendance, etc.) were analyzed with respect to both maternal practices and child behavior. The only significant relationship found was that between birth of a sibling in the second year and the presence of greater emotional maladjustment in the child. Trends were observed between the mother's social class membership and her type of child care practices.

The significance of this type of cross-sectional statistical study is discussed.

REFERENCES

1. Hollingshead, August B., and Fredrick C. Redlich. Social Stratification and Psychiatric Disorders. *Am. Sociol. Rev.*, 18: 163–170, 1953.

2. *Infant Care*. U. S. Department of Labor, Children's Bureau. U. S. Government Printing Office, Washington, 1914, 1929, 1938, 1942.

3. Klatskin, Ethelyn H., and Edith B. Jackson. Methodology of the Yale Rooming-in Project on Parent-Child Relationship. *Am. J. Orthopsychiatry*, 25: 81–108, 373–397, 1955.

4. Senn, Milton J. E. (Ed.). *Problems of Early Infancy: Transactions of the First and Second Conferences*. Josiah Macy, Jr. Foundation, New York, 1947 and 1948.

5. Stendler, Celia B. Sixty Years of Child Training Practices. *J. Pediat.*, 36: 122–134, 1950.

6. Witmer, Helen L. (Ed.). *Pediatrics and the Emotional Needs of the Child*. Commonwealth Fund, New York, 1948.

4

A STUDY OF THE EMOTIONAL REACTIONS OF CHILDREN AND FAMILIES TO HOSPITALIZATION AND ILLNESS

DANE G. PRUGH, M.D., ELIZABETH M. STAUB, M.A., HARRIET H. SANDS, EdM., RUTH M. KIRSCHBAUM, M.S., AND ELLENORA A. LENIHAN, B.S., R.N.

Children's Medical Center, Boston, Massachusetts

To most children comes a time of illness; in Western society today, a child's experience with disease carries with it the probability of at least one period of hospitalization. Such a contact with contemporary hospital practices may be brief or prolonged, isolated or repeated, pleasant or disturbing. With current improvements in medical management has come an increasing awareness among pediatricians of the importance of the psychological aspects of hospital care. As Moncrieff (45) has said, "The emotional needs of the sick child need as much consideration as his food or drug therapy."

In recent years, a number of studies of the emotional significance of illness to children of varying ages and levels of development have appeared in the literature. Some of these contributions have derived from the work of thoughtful pediatricians, others from more specialized approaches by child psychiatrists and pediatricians with special training in psychiatry. The exploratory work was done by Beverly (9), Jackson (32), Senn (51), Langford (37), Bakwin (5), and others (6, 40), who described the psychological impact and physiologic reverberations (16) of hospitalization for acute illness and the consequent separation from parents. Important contributions to the understanding of emotional reactions to specific operative procedures have been made by Levy (38) and Jessner and Kaplan (35), in regard to tonsillectomy, as well as Pearson (47) and Deutsch (21), in regard to other surgical procedures.

The effect of long-term hospitalization on children with chronic illness has been discussed by Bibring (10), Beverly (9), Bakwin (5), and others (37, 42, 51). Distortion of personality development as the result of institutionalization in infancy and early childhood has been

From the Children's Medical Center and the Departments of Pediatrics, Psychiatry, and Public Health, Harvard Medical School, Boston, and published in *The American Journal of Orthopsychiatry*, January 1953.

the subject of such important investigations as those of Anna Freud
(23), Freud and Burlingham (24), Spitz (56), Goldfarb (28), Lowrey
(41), Clothier (17), Bakwin (4), and Chapin (15). A recent study
by Roudinesco and co-workers (50) has pointed up the immediate responses in young infants to the separation from their mothers which is
involved in placement procedures.

On the basis of the body of data already at hand, programs of ward
management have been organized in various hospitals in the United
States and abroad, with the total goal, as Senn (51) defines it, "of
restoring physical function and mental well-being and of preventing
as much as possible all psychological and somatic residua." In addition
to Senn, Jensen (34), Langford (37), Jackson (32), Jessner and
Kaplan (35), Bakwin (3), Beverly (9), Parry (46), Powers (48),
Crothers (19), Spence (55), and MacLennan (43) have either
established or collaborated in the use of experimental techniques providing flexibility of management as well as vital emotional support for
the hospitalized child.

Among other methods, frequent visiting and participation in ward
care by parents have been regarded as keystones of such preventive
programs. In an extensive survey of institutional practices, Bowlby
(12) has pointed out that in some instances, more frequently in
European hospitals, mothers have been encouraged, where facilities
allowed, to stay with small children and to take over the major part
of their care throughout the period of hospitalization. Techniques of
psychological preparation for admission to the hospital as well as for
diagnostic or therapeutic procedures with potentially traumatic emotional effects, such as anesthesia (54) or surgical operations, have been
employed also on hospital wards; in certain instances, these measures
have included the use of a preparatory booklet for parents or children
(27). Relatively similar techniques of preparation and support in a
pediatric outpatient clinic have been described by Huschka and Ogden
(30). The use of occupational therapy (49) and the provision of educational facilities (2, 33, 42) and special play opportunities (7, 8, 20,
36, 51) have found important places in the roster of preventive and
therapeutic psychological practices. Also under scrutiny have been the
psychotherapeutic aspects of the grouping of children in regard to age
level and other factors (14, 34, 43, 49) and the over-all group therapeutic effect of planned activities (7, 8, 39).

Much creative thought has been devoted to a consideration of the
need for special planning of the physical characteristics of pediatric
services (14, 44, 53, 55). Topics under study in this area have ranged
from possible provision for the overnight presence of parents through
the psychological aspects of color programming (11, 53).

Of obviously greater importance than the preventive techniques themselves are the attitudes and qualifications of the ward personnel who apply them. Significant clarification of the nature of potentially psychotherapeutic relationships between physician and patient has come from many of the studies cited. More recently, the vital position of the ward nurse in relation to patient and parents has been brought into focus in the writings of Wallace and Feinauer (59), Stevens (57), Wessel (61), and others (1, 51, 55, 58). The contributions of specially trained and variously designated "play supervisors," often nursery-school teachers or persons with training in child development, have received recent attention (59). In their role as "mother substitutes" who administer no medical treatments, thus causing no pain and evoking little resentment, they have been able to utilize play experiences as an attractive avenue toward a therapeutic and even educational relationship with child and parents. The function of the social group worker (18) and the psychological aspects of the role of the dietitian (22) have also received important consideration.

For a variety of reasons, the investigations cited have dealt largely with the emotional reactions of the children experiencing hospitalization or illness, rather than with the reactions of their parents or families. Due recognition has been given, however, to the fact that disturbances in the behavior of the child arising from illness and hospitalization may reflect the attitudes and anxieties of the parents before and after the child's discharge, and may also set off reverberations in the emotional climate of the family group to which the child returns. For other realistic reasons, carefully controlled or longitudinal studies have been difficult to erect. To some extent, these limitations have stemmed from the retrospective character of some of the earlier work in this area. In most instances, the correlation of observations on the hospital ward and in the home has not been feasible. Other difficulties, including the rapidly changing conditions of a busy medical ward and the manifold ramifications of human behavior, are inherent in research of this kind. Even under relatively well-controlled circumstances, the thorny problems of methodology and the multiple character of possible interpretations of observed data have superimposed formidable limitations upon the quality and veracity of final conclusions.

The impetus for a study of the kind undertaken came originally from the nursing service of the hospital, which, in collaboration with an affiliating unit [1] and with the original support of the Children's Bureau, had adopted a year earlier an experimental type of ward nursing practice on the children's medical ward. In cooperation with the Medical

[1] Boston University School of Nursing. The program was under the immediate supervision of Miss Elizabeth Hall, Associate Professor of Nursing.

Service, traditional visiting frequencies had been altered from once weekly to daily, with other changes in the direction of a more individualized and supportive program of management. (Such measures were generally similar to those employed previously by Crothers and Dawes [19] on the Neurological Service of the same hospital.) In the face of inexact impressions about the efficacy of particular techniques, it was felt that a research study would more clearly elucidate the actual results of such an approach, providing at the same time information of a more far-reaching and fundamental character.

OBJECT OF THE STUDY

The present investigation was designed to evaluate: 1) the nature of the immediate reactions and modes of adaptation of children and parents to the impact of hospitalization on a medical ward in a children's hospital; 2) the incidence and character of long-range emotional reactions of children and families to the experience of hospitalization; 3) the degree of modifiability of such reactions with the use of an experimental program of ward management.

As the objectives imply, the purpose of this study was to clarify the nature of the effects of the experience of brief rather than prolonged hospitalization upon children and parents, differentiating these effects insofar as possible from the more basic and currently better understood reactions of children to the specific influences of illness itself. It was recognized that these two functions of the total experience could not be completely separated, and that in most instances these two variables interact in such a way as to accentuate the effects of one or the other.

The main objectives are listed above. Other facets of the approach presented themselves before and during the investigation, such as the differences between reactions to brief and long-term hospitalization, the variation in nature of experience for children and parents among ward settings on different services of a general hospital for children, and numerous other possibilities. A study broad enough initially to encompass all such obviously related aspects, however, would of necessity have been so diffuse as to defy organization and to destroy the meaningfulness of results. The present researches were therefore limited to a relatively uniform type of experience on a single medical ward.

METHODS OF STUDY

A. CRITERIA FOR SELECTION OF PATIENTS

Two groups of 100 children each were selected for study, one designated as the *control* and the other, the *experimental* group. These were patients admitted for varying reasons to a ward given over to the care of children from two to twelve years of age, requiring medical methods of diagnosis and treatment. The bulk of these patients had been hospitalized for relatively acute illnesses and remained in the hospital for a comparatively short period of time. A few children in each group suffered from chronic illnesses, and had been admitted for diagnostic study rather than long-term care.

An attempt was made to match these two groups as closely as possible, in relation to age, sex, diagnosis, and other factors. Because of the need for a base-line period of observation for each patient, no child was included in either group who did not remain in the hospital for longer than 48 hours. Since it was not possible, with groups of this size, to select only patients who had never previously undergone hospitalization, the investigation was restricted to children who had encountered hospitalization briefly and occasionally, with a minimum of experience with hospitalization during the year preceding the current hospitalization and no rehospitalization within at least six months.

Tables 1 and 2 summarize the essential characteristics of both groups.

TABLE 1. RELEVANT STATISTICS FOR BOTH GROUPS

Age	Control Group			Experimental Group		
	Male	Female	Total	Male	Female	Total
2–4 years	8	10	18	7	9	16
4–6 years	5	5	10	7	7	14
6–10 years	9	10	19	8	9	17
10–12 years	3	0	3	1	2	3
Total	25	25	50	23	27	50

	Control Group	Experimental Group
Average length of stay	8.08 days	6.01 days
Number of children with previous hospitalizations	21	20
Nature of adjustment prior to hospitalization		
Maximal	56%	34%
Limited	42%	54%
Inadequate	2%	12%
	100%	100%

Because of the difficulty in fulfilling the above criteria, as well as in carrying out follow-up studies, a total of only 50 children in each group was available for final study. The matching of illnesses between the two groups was necessarily somewhat inexact, and was restricted, because of the circumstances of the study, to a number of larger categories, embracing illnesses involving similar organ systems and relatively identical pathogenic agents.

As may be seen from the tables, the only significant differences between the two groups lay in the somewhat greater number of previously well-adjusted children in the control group and the slightly shorter average hospital stay of those in the experimental group.

B. CIRCUMSTANCES OF STUDY

1. *Control period.* A base-line study of the control group was carried out initially, covering a period of approximately four months. The circumstances under which hospitalization was encountered by children during this period were those involving traditional practices of ward management, existing prior to the experimental nursing program described earlier. Under these "rolled-back" conditions, weekly visiting periods of two hours each had been permitted for parents. Little encouragement had been given to parents to participate in the ward care

TABLE 2. DIAGNOSIS ON DISCHARGE FROM HOSPITAL

Chief Diagnosis	Number of Children	
	Control Group	Experimental Group
Infection (respiratory, systemic, gastrointestinal, etc.)	21	19
Renal disease (nephritis, congenital abnormalities, etc.	8	4
Cardiac disease (congenital anomalies, etc.)	4	8
Central nervous system disease (meningitis, convulsive disorders, cerebral palsy, etc.)	4	6
Emotional disturbance (including psychosomatic disorders)	2	2
Miscellaneous (including diabetes, arthritis, dental disorders, allergy, trauma, blood dyscrasias, physical trauma, etc.)	11	11
Total	50	50

of the child. Clearly, no organized program involving a preventive approach to problems in adjustment had existed, even though valuable emotional support had been provided to children and parents by individual physicians, nurses, occupational therapists, and other ward personnel.

2. *Experimental period.* Following an interval sufficient to allow complete turnover of patients who had been in the control study, an experimental program of ward management was put into effect. This

involved many of the practices employed in other hospitals and included daily visiting periods for parents, early ambulation of patients where medically feasible, a special play program employing a nursery-school teacher, psychological preparation for and support during potentially emotionally traumatic diagnostic or therapeutic procedures, an attempt at clearer definition and integration of the parent's role in the care of the child, and other techniques. Attention was paid to the handling of admission procedures, with parents accompanying the child to the ward to meet the staff and to assist in the child's initial adjustment. As a part of admission routine, parents were given a pamphlet prepared especially to enhance their understanding of their child's needs and their own role in his care.

In order to coordinate the activities of the professional staff in the management of patients, a weekly Ward Management Conference was held, directed by a pediatrician with psychiatric training. In attendance were the ward physician, head nurse, play supervisor, occupational therapist, dietitian, social worker, psychologist, and frequently a public health nurse. An attempt was made to discuss the adjustment of each child on the ward, although children presenting particular difficulties in adaptation received the most attention. Among other measures discussed and implemented in this interdisciplinary conference were: the assignment of one nurse to the principal care of a particularly anxious child; the scheduling of injections or other medical procedures at times other than feeding, nap, or play times; the use of appropriate psychological preparation for forthcoming procedures by physician, nurse, or play supervisor; the selection of particular play activities designed to meet the emotional needs of particular children, the special handling of feeding or other activities; the flexible arrangement of visiting periods or the encouragement of parental participation in ward care; and the provision of special psychological support for particular parents. Psychiatric consultation and psychological appraisal were provided where indicated, but the essential approach was in the direction of the coordination and potentiation of the efforts of all professional personnel involved in the care of the ill child.

C. INVESTIGATIVE METHODS

During both control and experimental periods, similar techniques of study and recording of data were employed in order to facilitate comparison of results.

(I.) An extensive anamnesis was obtained as soon as possible following admission, through one or more interviews with the parent or parents by the ward social worker. This material, often expanded or supplemented during follow-up contacts, dealt with the child's reaction to the illness prior to hospitalization, the context of circumstances immediately preceding admission, the nature of parental anxieties or attitudes, the child's personality structure and previous modes of adaptation, the character of family relationships, and other important factors. Additional data were garnered from the reports of ward personnel.

2. Detailed observations of the child's behavior on the ward, his relationships with personnel and patients, his reactions to various procedures, and the behavior of child and parents on admission and during visiting were recorded independently by psychologist, play supervisor, head nurse, and other professional ward personnel. The material from play and verbal interviews with individual children by psychiatrist, psychologist, and play supervisor was recorded carefully, as were the results of interviews with parents. In the interviews, an attempt was made to gain, through play or fantasy, an understanding of the child's interpretation of his illness and hospitalization, his personality structure and currently employed defense mechanisms, and other factors.

3. Correlation of the effects of changes in physical condition upon the child's emotional state, level of intellectual function, and other aspects of his adjustment on the ward was made, with the use of informal psychological appraisals where possible. Material of this kind was supplemented by observations of ward personnel, and included data on the level of growth and development, the response to ambulation, the possible evidence of cross-infection between children and visiting parents, etc.

Follow-up studies were carried out at three weeks, at three months, and at later intervals following the child's discharge from the hospital. Some unevenness in following this schedule of contacts was inevitably encountered for geographical and other reasons. In early contacts, an interview with the parents by the social worker was employed, together with psychiatric interviews with the child when possible. Because of the size and dispersed character of both groups, later contacts at times had to be made by telephone or mail. Data were obtained on all children covering a period of at least six months following discharge; for nearly one half of the patients, this period covered one year. Particular attention was paid to the child's state of health and the nature of his adjustment following discharge, the continuation or alteration of fantasies or defensive maneuvers exhibited by the child in the hospital, the parental attitudes toward and handling of the child, and possible psychological reverberations in the family constellation as the result of changes in the child's behavior.

D. DEFINITION OF CRITERIA EMPLOYED

A number of criteria were utilized in an attempt to elucidate the influence of different variables upon the handling of the hospitalization experience by child and family. Examples of the clinical application of these criteria are given in the discussion of the results of the study.

1. *Degree of reaction.* In assessing the influence of hospitalization on both groups, the reactions of the children were divided into severe, moderate, and minimal categories. Reactions were arbitrarily classified as severe if crippling manifestations of anxiety occurred, with interference with the child's adjustment persisting longer than three months following discharge. Minimal reactions were characterized by mild and transient disturbances in adaptation, observable largely in the hospital. Reactions intermediate between minimal and severe, persisting less than three months, were classified as moderate in degree. Comparison with the previous level of adjustment, the nature of personality structure, and in particular, the reaction to the illness on the part of the child prior to admission formed the basis on which all classifications were made.

2. *Degree of stress encountered.* Although the children's interpretations of stressful experiences were obviously individualized, it was felt necessary to estimate the degree and nature of objectively verifiable stress encountered by each child during hospitalization. In arriving at a classification of stress as severe, moderate, or minimal in character, such factors as the type of medical or surgical procedures employed, the degree of discomfort involved in diagnostic tests, the severity and character of the child's illness, the illness of parents completely precluding visiting, etc., were considered. For example, operations or diagnostic procedures requiring anesthesia were assumed to represent severe stresses. Admission for observation for such disorders as chronic cervical adenitis, involving X rays, blood tests and oral medication, was considered minimally stressful.

Obvious limitations apply to this type of classification, which does not take into consideration the child's age level, length of hospital stay, interpretation of illness and of separation from parents, encounters with traumatizing handling by ward personnel, etc. Such factors were considered in the interpretation of the child's reaction, however, and are discussed in a later section. With this arbitrary classification, the stresses encountered by the children in both groups were approximately the same, with over 50 per cent in each group facing severe stress, and less than 10 per cent, minimal stress.

3. *Previous adjustment of the child.* Categorization of the child's capacity for adaptation was based on historical knowledge of his emo-

tional development, level of intelligence, relationships with siblings and contemporaries, degree of independence, handling of sexual and aggressive drives, need for symptom formation or crippling defense mechanisms and capacities for sublimation. (Level of intelligence was difficult to estimate, in the face of the definite regression of many children upon admission to the hospital; it appeared, however, that the groups were approximately equal in this respect, with a very small proportion of moderately retarded children in each group.)

The effectiveness of previous adjustment was classified as maximal, limited or inadequate. Children considered as exhibiting inadequate adjustment (with markedly limited integrative capacity or ego strength) were those who had manifested outstanding difficulties in adaptation from early childhood, with severe neurotic symptomatology, behavior disorders, or somatization reactions.

4. *Nature of mother-child relationship.* According to the degree to which the mother (or, in a few instances, the father or mother-substitute) appeared to have been able to accept the child emotionally and to allow him an appropriate degree of independence prior to hospitalization, the mother-child relationship was classified as satisfying, moderately satisfying, or unsatisfying to the child. As might be expected, a strongly positive correlation was present, in most instances, between the degree of satisfaction provided by this relationship and the estimated previous level of adjustment of the child, even though these two factors had been assessed independently.

5. *Child's adjustment to hospital situation.* Assessments were made of the capacity of each child to adapt to the hospital experience. Rather than symptomatic responses, the over-all capacity of the child to relate successfully to peer and adult members of the ward group was considered, together with his capacity for reality testing and his ability to master anxiety successfully, in accordance with his age level, through verbalization or play. Degree of adjustment was categorized as adequate, difficult or inadequate.

6. *Parents' adjustment to hospital situation.* The capacity of the parent or parents to control their anxiety or guilt over the child's illness, to give emotional support to the child, to accept the realities of the child's illness, and to handle visiting opportunities formed the basis for the classification of their adjustment as adequate, difficult or inadequate.

RESULTS

A. GROUP STATISTICS

1. *Immediate reactions.* All of the children in both groups showed at least minimal reactions to the experiences of hospitalization. Arbitrarily

excluding the minimal category, 92 per cent of the children in the control or unsupported group exhibited reactions of a degree indicating significant difficulties in adaptation (moderate and severe categories). In the experimental group, this figure totaled 68 per cent. In a further breakdown of these categories, the experimental group showed a significantly lower percentage of severe immediate reactions to hospitalization (14% as opposed to 36% in the control group), with a much higher percentage of minimal reactions (32% as opposed to 8% in the control group). Moderate reactions were approximately equal in both groups. (See Fig. 1.)

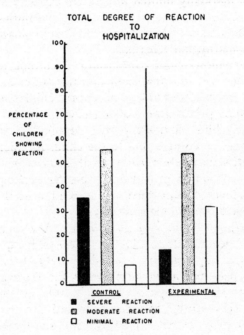

Fig. 1

In analyzing the statistical data within the above framework, some interesting trends were seen, corroborative of the work of other investigators. Immediate reactions to hospitalization were noted to be most marked in children from two through five years of age in both groups (see Fig. 2). Children of three years of age and under showed the highest incidence of reactions of severe degree (50% in the control and 37% in the experimental group; see Fig. 3). From four to six years of age, severe reactions were less common (30% in control and 7% in experimental); the lowest incidence occurred in children from six to twelve (27% in control and none in experimental). Conversely, minimal reactions were approximately five times as frequent in the experimental group as in the control for the total group of preschool children from two through five, as well as for children from six through twelve.

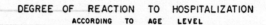

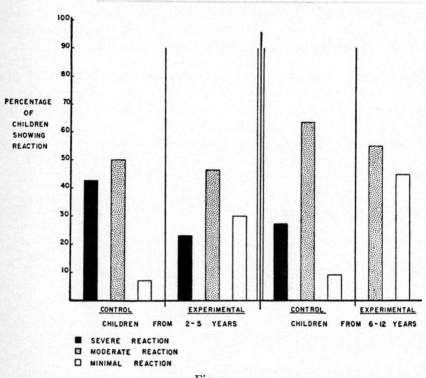

Fig. 2.

From the above statistics, it would appear that a definite prophylactic effect derived from the experimental program, most marked in character for the older children. No striking differences in degree of reaction in relation to the sex of children at any age in either group could be determined, as far as the more diffuse quality of the hospitalization experience was concerned.

The statistics cited so far were checked by the chi-square method with the aid of a consultant statistician; [2] those dealing with the total degree of reaction were found to be highly significant (for Fig. 1, p is

[2] Dr. Jane Worcester, Associate Professor of Biostatistics, School of Public Health, Harvard University.

less than .o1). The other statistics are slightly less significant, although confirmatory trends are present. The necessary assumption that both groups were exactly similar is of course difficult to make when dealing with human personalities, in spite of the relatively comparable character of the groups. The statistical trends cited hereinafter are not regarded as being significant, but represent nonmetrical or semiquantitative approximations of the closest character possible in dealing with components of human behavior.

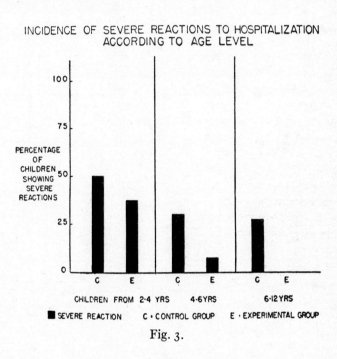

INCIDENCE OF SEVERE REACTIONS TO HOSPITALIZATION ACCORDING TO AGE LEVEL

Fig. 3.

Of the many variables in addition to age which were considered as operative in the confluence of forces impinging upon the child as the result of hospitalization, the highest correlation appeared to exist between the apparent adaptive capacity of the individual child and his adjustment to the immediate ward situation. In general, children with previously limited capacities for adaptation showed the greatest difficulty in adjusting comfortably to the ward milieu and showed as well the most severe reactions to the total experience of hospitalization. There was not always a clear-cut correlation between the child's adjustment on the ward and the total reaction; some children who appeared to adjust relatively successfully while in the hospital exhibited disturbances in behavior of a more crippling character following discharge than did others who had been completely incapable, while on the ward, of handling the anxiety aroused by the current experience.

In the main, the children in both groups who showed the most successful adjustment on the ward were those who seemed to have the most satisfying relationship with their parents, especially the mother, and whose parents accomplished the most balanced adaptation themselves to the experience of illness and hospitalization on the part of their child. Such parents tended to show the most positively expressed response to the more flexible conditions of the experimental program, and appeared to handle the enhanced visiting opportunities with greatest equanimity and benefit to their child (as well as to other children whose parents visited less frequently). As a group, the children in the experimental phase of the study appeared to adjust more adequately on the ward (see Fig. 4).

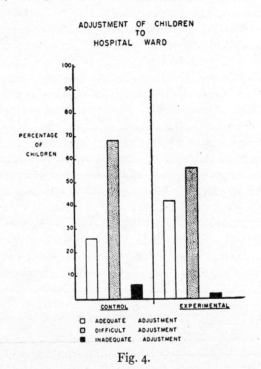

Fig. 4.

As might be expected, the objectively verifiable aspects of the stress encountered during hospitalization bore little specific relationship to the degree of reaction on the part of the children in both groups. The diffuse quality of much of the stress involved, the wide variation in types of medical or surgical procedures employed, and other factors made conclusions difficult in regard to the effect of particular types of stressful experience. In the children under six, however, there was an apparently positive correlation between stress categorized as severe and the number of severe reactions. A relative absence of correlation in regard to severity of response was seen in relation to the specific type of illness faced by the individual child. Even the small number of children, slightly more frequent in the experimental group, who suffered from disturbances in integrity of the central nervous system appeared to fall into no pattern as regards severity of reaction. Here, the number of children fitting into each of the broad diagnostic categories of illness was of a low order of magnitude, rendering generalizations particularly difficult.

From the material at hand, no conclusions can be drawn in regard to the efficacy of psychological methods of preparation of children for admission to the hospital. Approximately 70 per cent of the admissions in both groups were not planned in advance. Nevertheless, nearly one half of the children in both groups received some form of preparation by their parents. Information regarding the extent and character of such preparation in individual instances, however, was fragmentary and incomplete. Unfortunately, the circumstances surrounding admission, at the time of the study, were such that no systematic discussion of the need for preparation was possible in advance, even with parents of children whose admissions were planned. The impression is held by investigators that pediatricians or family physicians took little initiative in encouraging parents to prepare their children. Individual children showed significantly positive responses to preparatory efforts.

No correlation between length of stay in the hospital and degree of reaction or effectiveness of adjustment on the ward could be visualized from the present data, even when considered in relation to age, diagnostic category, integrative capacity, and other factors. Differences in the nature of adaptive response to illnesses of acute as opposed to chronic nature, unrelated to the current hospitalization, were noted, but do not fall within the field of study chosen here.

Although experience with previous hospitalization was fairly common in both groups, particularly in the older children, no general patterns of response could be discerned. Even young children with several hospitalizations prior to the current one showed no constant characteristics in terms of heightened current disturbances in behavior or enhanced ability to handle the experience of hospitalization. It must be noted that accurate information regarding reactions to previous hospitalizations was difficult to obtain.

2. *Long-range reactions.* Assessment of disturbances in adaptation continuing beyond discharge from the hospital was more difficult

than that during hospitalization, principally because of the more limited opportunities for repeated observations and interviews. The material obtained, however, does indicate certain interesting trends, as well as some suggestive differences in the posthospital adjustment of the two groups of children under study.

Surveying the statistics broadly, one sees that, immediately following discharge, 92 per cent of the children in the control group and 68 per cent of the children in the experimental group showed significant disturbances in behavior not present prior to hospitalization (see Fig. 5).

REACTIONS TO HOSPITALIZATION

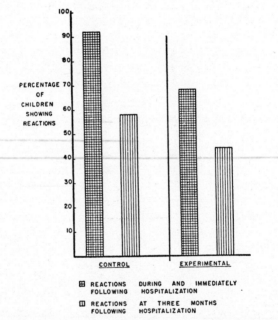

Fig. 5.

After three months had passed, 58 per cent of the children in the control or unsupported group exhibited what were regarded as disturbing reactions of at least moderate degree; in the experimental group this figure totaled 44 per cent (see Fig. 6). Forty-two per cent of the children in the control group and 56 per cent in the experimental group had thus apparently resumed their previous level of adjustment by the time this period had elapsed. Ten per cent or five children in the experimental group were considered to have improved in their adjustment following discharge.

An interesting finding was the fact that, <u>at three months following discharge, nearly one half of the children still disturbed in both groups were under four years of age</u> (41% and 45% in the control and experimental groups, respectively). <u>Including the children from four to six, 54 per cent of the control group and 69 per cent of the experimental group still showing disturbances were under six years of age.</u>

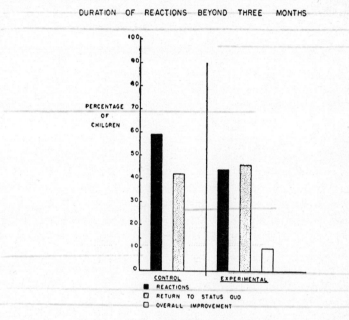

DURATION OF REACTIONS BEYOND THREE MONTHS

Fig. 6.

Additional differences could be seen between the two groups. For example, <u>the severity of the disturbances exhibited by children in the control group at three months following hospitalization was definitely greater than that seen in the experimental or supported group.</u>

Finally, there appeared to be a relatively <u>high correlation between the appearance of crippling disturbances in behavior on the ward and their persistence following the child's discharge from the hospital.</u> Of the 13 children in the control group showing adequate adjustment to the ward situation, only four showed signs of emotional disturbance as long as three months following discharge. A relatively similar proportion of children adjusting adequately on the ward were found to show continued disturbances in the experimental group. In children showing difficult adjustment on the ward, a much higher proportion of persistent disturbances was seen (16 of 34 in the control group and

15 of 28 in the experimental group). Two of three children with estimated inadequate ward adjustment in the control group showed continued disturbances, as did the one such child in the experimental
group.

To summarize, children under four years of age and children who
had relatively unsatisfying relationships with their parents, who had
undergone very severe stress in the hospital, and who had shown the
greatest difficulty in adapting to the ward milieu were those who
tended to show persistent signs of emotional disturbances at three
months following hospitalization.

Follow-up material for periods extending beyond three months
after discharge has been difficult to assemble and to analyze statistically. The scattered geographic background of the patients admitted
to a hospital serving the New England region has presented the major
obstacle. Although contacts were made with all patients at approximately six months following discharge, the fact that a significant
proportion of these could not be by interviews has rendered conclusions open to question. Studies are continuing; at present, the impression is held that a sharp drop in incidence of disturbing reactions in
both groups occurred after six months had passed, with not more than
15 per cent of the children in the control group showing continued
disturbances. Although comparisons between the two groups at this
point are difficult, the impression exists that disturbances in the control
group remained more severe. Furthermore, it is apparent that principally younger children showed disturbances in the experimental
group, as opposed to both younger and older children in the control
group. Thus, although the data are not of statistical value, a continuation of earlier trends is evident. The possibility of delayed reactions is being considered, in relation to subsequent hospitalization
or other experiences.

B. TYPES OF INDIVIDUAL REACTIONS OF CHILDREN IN THE HOSPITAL

The most common manifestation of disturbance in adaptation at
any age level or in either group was that of overt anxiety. Such anxiety
appeared to represent a spilling over the ego's defenses, into behavior
and consciousness, of anxiety arising from the endangerment of the
integrative or "homeostatic" equilibrium of the ego, as the result of
the heightened conflict stemming from increased libidinal drives from
within or overwhelming reality pressures from without. A variety of
defensive maneuvers were employed by individual children in order
to prevent this spilling over of anxiety and possible disorganization of
ego functions. Some of these bore definite relation to age and level of

psychosexual development. Others, as Jessner and Kaplan (35) observed, were used in shifting or exclusive fashion by children at different age levels. As might be expected, nearly all of the restitutive mechanisms at the service of the ego were observed; in individual children, particularly older ones, the mechanisms employed appeared in most instances to have been characteristic of the personality structure prior to hospitalization.

The relative incidence of certain disturbances in adaptation, at different age levels and under control and experimental conditions, is roughly summarized in Figure 7. More detailed discussion of these manifestations and of the various defensive maneuvers follows, taken up according to age and in approximate relation to level of psychosexual development.

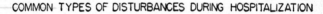

COMMON TYPES OF DISTURBANCES DURING HOSPITALIZATION

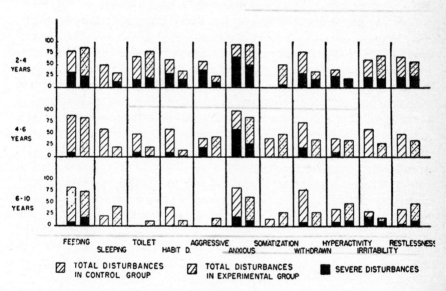

Fig. 7.

1. *Children from two to four years of age. Control group.* At this age level, anxiety over separation from parents was the most common manifestation and the most intense of any age level, occurring equally in both sexes and to some degree in all children. Anxiety was often associated with fear or anger at the time of departure of the parents. Constant crying, apprehensive behavior, outbursts of screaming, and acute panic when approached by an adult were frequent, together with occasional somatic concomitants of anxiety such as urinary frequency,

diarrhea, vomiting, etc. Depression, at times resembling the anaclitic type described by Spitz (56), homesickness and withdrawal were observed in this group more than in older children, particularly at the outset of hospitalization. The need for tangible evidence of home and family, such as dolls, items of clothing, etc., was particularly manifest in this group, as demonstrated by the anxiety of many children over giving them up. At times, shoes and socks, for example, seemed to be incorporated into the body image, with marked anxiety shown whenever they were removed.

Reactions to the experiencing of overwhelming fear or anxiety showed some specificity for the children in this age group, as Figure 7 indicates. Disturbances in feeding behavior, including anorexia, overeating, and refusal to chew food, often combined with regressive smearing of food or the demand for a return to bottle feeding, were more frequent and severe than in any other group. Changes in toilet behavior were next in incidence, involving regressive loss of control of bladder or bowel functions, most marked in the early phases of hospitalization. Fears of the toilet or of the loss of the stool, fear of loss of control of bowel or bladder functions, as well as guilt and fear of punishment over wishes to soil or wet, were handled by mechanisms of denial, projection, and other modes of adaptation available to the child of this age. Fears of the dark or of physical attack were common and were associated with sleep disturbances — insomnia, nightmares and restlessness. Increase of bedtime rituals and other compulsive acts during hospitalization was often seen. In one instance, a boy of three, with limited adaptive capacity and an acute hemolytic anemia, showed persistent depression, and demanded that two chairs be placed by his bed for his absent parents, showing great anxiety if anyone sat upon or moved the chairs.

Open acting-out of infantile wishes and aggressive impulses appeared most frequently in this age group, with wild outbursts of frantic aggression and attendant guilty and anxiety. Marked inhibition of aggressive drives was observed in some children, together with turning inward of hostility. Restlessness, hyperactivity and irritability, with associated rocking, thumb-sucking or aggressive behavior, appeared in many children, particularly if they were confined to bed with the use of a "restrainer," as had been the practice for small or acutely disoriented children in order to prevent their falling from bed. With ambulation, this behavior often disappeared or diminished markedly.

A variety of primitive gratifications of pregenital character (labeled "habit disturbances" on Fig. 7) were employed to greater degree than prior to hospitalization. Thumb-sucking and rocking were common, associated with withdrawal and with masturbation in one third of the children. Head-banging was relatively infrequent. In many instances, as children established parent-surrogate relationships, often with the play supervisor or with one particular nurse, gratifications of this type diminished, no longer interfering with adjustment to the group.

Among the defense mechanisms available to this younger group, regression was the most widespread. Libidinal regression was often uneven, associated with feeding, bowel and bladder symptomatology. Oral components were manifest through enhanced sucking, overeating, and demanding behavior, with occasional biting and other manifestations. Cruelty, sadistic enjoyment of the pain of others, pleasure in handling or smearing feces, and other regressive anal components of behavior were transparently or openly evident, particularly in children isolated for medical reasons.

In some instances, a nearly total regression of the ego to a relatively narcissistic level of psychosexual development, associated with disturbances in reality testing, was manifest, resembling those described by Anna Freud (23). An example of this phenomenon was Anne, aged three years and ten months, a child hospitalized for five days during the control period. Her reaction was classified as a moderate one (because of its disappearance soon after discharge), and included loss of previously attained control over bowel and bladder, a return to infantile feeding habits (requiring feeding by a nurse), withdrawn, passive, and at times apprehensive behavior, intense interest in her own body, particularly her toes, and the reappearance of infantile speech. Her behavior prior to hospitalization had been that of a well-adjusted child of her age, with only a mild feeding disturbance during her illness, even though the cellulitis of her gums, for which she was treated by penicillin injections and tooth extraction promptly on admission, had been fully as painful at home as in the hospital.

Denial of illness or of the loss of the loved object, the mother, was observed in a number of children of this age. For example, one child, a boy of three and a half, insisted for three days that his mother was "downstairs" and that he was "all well now," in spite of the persistence of his dyspnea from a bronchopneumonia.

Experimental group. Among these children, the same types of disturbances in adaptation were noted as among the control or unsupported group. In general, however, manifestations were less severe and lighter in incidence. Depression and withdrawal were less common and less marked, while disturbances in feeding and sleeping and the use of pregenital gratifications were all less common and less severe. Thumb-sucking and rocking were only half as frequent as in the control group. Panic states and marked ego regressions were muted in character, while wildly aggressive behavior was diminished by 50 per cent.

With the greater opportunities for verbalization and acting out in play provided during this period, more frequent expressions of guilt or other feelings were noted. One girl, aged three years and five months, repeatedly begged her parents at visiting periods, "Take me home; I be a good girl now." This was a child who had been somewhat anxious and fearful prior to hospitalization for pyelonephritis, about which her overprotective and anxious mother was both concerned and resentful. The use made by various children of mothers' old purses, items of their fathers' clothing, favorite old toys, or blankets from home, which were made universally available under the experimental program, indicated the extent of their needs for ego support.

2. *Children from four to six years of age. Control group*. In this age group, overt manifestations of anxiety were widespread, but were in general less severe and less frequent than in the younger children. Depression, homesickness and withdrawal were somewhat less common and less disturbing, as were the pregenital gratifications mentioned earlier. Masturbation in both sexes was noted, though less frequently.

Symptom formation at this level showed many similarities to as well as certain differences from the younger group. Restlessness, hyperactivity and irritability were less marked, as were disturbances in feeding, sleeping and toilet behavior. Phobic manifestations were more often observed, particularly in children showing these in mild form prior to hospitalization; one girl, for instance, was constantly afraid of leaving her bed because of the possibility of seeing a cat. Somatization reactions had their highest incidence among the control children in this group, with urinary frequency or urgency, vomiting, diarrhea, dizziness, and other manifestations seen in relation to anxiety-provoking experiences. Obsessive fears were more pronounced. One boy of four, anxious and inhibited, with an unsatisfying relationship with his restrictive parents, talked repetitively of his fear of the possibility of his healthy mother's death while he was in the hospital. His anxiety over this first separation from his mother and his underlying hostility toward her were equally manifest.

Following is an example of a severe reaction to hospitalization in a girl of five years and two months. Janice was admitted to the hospital for the first time without preparation, with acute glomerulonephritis. At home she had shown fever and mild vomiting but no other disturbances in her ordinarily well-adjusted behavior. Her relationship to her parents was a satisfying one, and her only problem had been mild rivalry with a younger sister, three years of age, who had developed acute bronchitis just prior to Janice's admission. She remained in the hospital for nine days, on bed rest and salt-free diet, undergoing lumbar puncture, enemas, and various blood studies, and showing no evidence of severe hypertension or of cerebral edema. In the hospital, Janice was very apprehensive and withdrawn, talking to herself and playing with dolls alone. She fought off diagnostic procedures in stark panic, never submitting and at times vomiting (as she did when her parents left after visiting hours on the two occasions the parents were allowed to visit). She showed consistent refusal of food, repetitive nail-biting and nose-picking, and occasionally wet the bed. To one of the observers, she verbalized her fear of "ponio" and death of crippling. (It was learned later that her mother had told her, early in her illness, that she would have to go to the hospital if she did not eat.) Janice verbalized a fear that a three-year-old child might get this disease, and then cautiously expressed some resentment toward her sister for taking her toys. Repeatedly she spoke of going home "today," and never succeeded in establishing relationships toward personnel or other children. She was markedly resentful over being placed in a crib. Her symptoms continued for four months after discharge, gradually abating.

As in Janice's case, regressive phenomena were still present in many children at this age level, although not so severely or frequently as in younger children. One boy of four years was aggressive and anxious on the ward, with severe feeding difficulties, showing in general an intensification of symptoms seen prior to his admission (for cardiac catheterization as an aid in evaluating his congenital cardiac anomaly of moderate degree). After undergoing the procedure, he appeared passive, subdued and withdrawn, constantly lay on his back, sucking his thumb and hugging a teddy bear in a way that he had not done for more than a year. Other children of four or five years showed temporary disturbances in reality testing similar to those of three-year-olds, one boy of five fearing that he would have "tomato juice put in and blood taken out" in a transfusion.

Acceptance of dependent needs was more difficult for these children between four and six years of age, particularly the boys, who denied such needs more frequently than girls and produced more vivid fantasies of helplessness and of imminent attack. One boy of five-and-a-half years, with a previously well-adjusted personality and a current respiratory infection, did not cry and openly denied feeling unhappy when his parents left after visiting hours, but refused supper and wet his bed that night for the only time during his stay. He projected unacceptable impulses onto other children, telling a nurse that he wanted to "tell the doctor that girl swore," immediately after feeling angry at the doctor for paying little attention to him. This boy, like numerous others, showed an identification with Hopalong Cassidy, clinging even at night to his hat and gun; certain more anxious children showed this type of behavior still more intensely.

Possibly because of regressive tendencies, little striking difference in fantasy formation could be determined between boys and girls in this age group. Children of both sexes who were able to verbalize successfully or felt free to play out their feelings seemed preoccupied at times with fantasies of mutilation and punishment, involving genitals, eyes, head and extremities. Deeply unconscious fantasies or affects were of course beyond the scope of this study. Much evidence of displacement was seen, as in the case of the five-year-old boy mentioned earlier, who drew a number of pictures of men and boys without arms and showed great concern over pencils, inquiring anxiously whose they were, and if they needed new erasers.

In this age group, aggressive behavior, appearing diffusely or in response to treatment procedures, was less widespread and less uncontrolled than among the younger children. As with the children under four, little difference could be detected overtly between boys and girls in this regard. Identification with the aggressor, combined with acting out, projection and displacement, was seen frequently. One boy pretended to stick needles in other children, later stating that this was because "I had one and I hate it." Turning inward of hostility, inhibition, and other mechanisms were also seen.

Experimental group. In this group, overt anxiety was definitely less widely manifest, and was present in severe degree in only half as many instances as in the control group. Pregenital gratifications and symptom formation were generally less pronounced, even in the face of regression. Inhibition and turning inward of hostility seemed less marked. Total aggressive behavior was actually increased over both the control group at this age level and the experimental group of younger children. Most of this aggression was not destructive or crippling in character, however, but appeared frequently during the working through of anxieties in play activity, combined with verbalization of hostility, permitted more freely in the relationship to the play supervisor and other personnel. One girl, aged 4½, with somewhat limited capacities for adaptation, tore a doll to pieces after receiving a transfusion, and punished it by spanking it repeatedly. This same girl, with two other children, spent one afternoon playing "doctor and nurse," using several dolls provided by the play supervisor. The children gave "needles" to the dolls, and the girl in question mentioned repeatedly, "Take that, you bad doll, you bad doctor, you."

3. *Children from six to ten years of age. Control group.* In the children in early latency, anxiety still remained a common manifestation,

although there were fewer panic reactions than in the younger groups. Some anxiety over separation from the parents was apparent, but in general anxiety seemed more free-floating or definitely attached to potentially painful or new and frightening experiences. In this group, marked anxiety was noted more directly in conformity with such factors as the previous personality structure and integrative capacity, the degree of adjustment on the ward, and the nature of the parent-child relationship, rather than in relation to the degree of stress or the specific type of experience encountered in the hospital. Withdrawn behavior remained surprisingly common, but depression and homesickness were milder, except in previously poorly adjusted children.

Symptom formation showed definite differences from younger age groups. Feeding disturbances still were common, but were generally milder in character. The need for pregenital gratifications dropped off sharply, as did significant disturbances in bowel or bladder function and in sleep, although nightmares were frequent. Somatization reactions were less frequent and more clearly related to previous modes of adaptation, as with one anxious, inhibited boy of eight who vomited before every treatment procedure. Another boy frequently developed nasal congestion if anxious or excited, as he had done occasionally for the year preceding admission. Conversion symptoms were more frequent; for example, one girl of seven developed abdominal pain whenever approached by a physician.

Openly aggressive behavior was less evident in daily behavior in these children, even in response to painful or threatening treatment procedures. Hyperactivity and restlessness were frequent and more intense than in children from four to six. Compulsive behavior appeared more frequently, as did obsessive fears of death from illness during sleep. Denial and rationalization were strenuously employed, particularly by boys who appeared afraid of losing control of aggressive or libidinal impulses. Libidinal regression was seen surprisingly frequently, but appeared in milder form, being most striking in previously disturbed children. A few showed occasional masturbation, with much guilt and secrecy.

Fantasies of these children involved possible mutilation or death. One boy of nine, with limited adaptive capacity, had been told by his rigid and ambivalent mother that if he did not cooperate in the treatment of a cellulitis of the left leg, he would have to go to the hospital and have it cut off. On the ward, he seemed somewhat depressed and withdrawn, fought off injections or medications, and said he didn't want to get well when told why he was being subjected to such procedures. As he left the hospital, he said, with great relief, "Well, I never expected to get out of there with both legs." Another boy of eight resisted

desperately preoperative preparation for a debridement of an osteo-
myelitic lesion of his leg, finally verbalizing, with the help of a nurse
to whom he had developed a mother-surrogate relationship, his fear
that his leg would be cut off and thrown away.

Many children in this age group tended to interpret their illnesses
as a type of magical retribution for unacceptable impulses or acts.
One boy of seven, a diabetic patient, said, in regard to the causation of
his illness, "I think it was something I did." A girl of six said, "God
makes you sick because you're bad; I'm not bad." Projection, denial
and rationalization were utilized frequently to handle the accompanying anxiety and guilt.

Experimental group. In general, this group showed a lighter incidence of anxiety than the children in the control group and less need
to utilize in as strenuous a fashion the defense mechanisms described.
More children appeared able to master their anxieties by acting out
in play or by verbalizing their fantasies or feelings of hostility and
fear. The greater utilization of the enhanced opportunities for sublimation and development of temporary superego identifications under the
experimental program was evident in the more frequent and ambulatory acting out of the roles of "doctor," "nurse," "sheriff and bad
men," etc. Fantasies, expressed more freely than under the control
conditions, embraced, in addition to those mentioned, fears of "broken
fingers" or of "losing teeth" in boys; more frequent in girls were fears
of dying, being "poisoned," or of "never getting well."

C. REACTIONS TO SPECIFIC TYPES OF TREATMENT OR DIAGNOSTIC
PROCEDURES

Because of the small number of children at any particular age level
undergoing such diversified procedures as cardiac catheterization,
pneumoencephalogram, proctoscopy, abdominal paracentesis, spinal
puncture, prolonged intravenous drip or transfusion, and other major
diagnostic or therapeutic procedures, it is impossible to say whether
there was any characteristic form of response. The impression was
gained that any or all of these procedures seemed to be interpreted by
a child at a particular level of libidinal development in terms of the
specific anxieties and fears characteristic of that level, and to be
dealt with by means of his own previously developed defenses, rather
than in terms of the exact nature of the procedure itself. The type of
illness, the particular organ or organ system involved, the nature
of the immediate handling by and relationship with the physician
performing the procedure, the degree of support gained from parent-
surrogate relationships with ward personnel, the child's previous expe-

rience with illness or pain (on his own part or that of other children observed on the ward), and a host of other variables appeared also to play a role. With cardiac catheterization, at least, the impression was gained that, in individual instances, sound preparation by the parents for the procedure was of significant supportive value. Both groups showed approximately the same total number of children (two thirds) with disturbing immediate reactions to treatment procedures of all kinds. Qualitative differences did exist, and will be described in relation to age level.

In the main, the younger children tended to react to such threatening procedures as to hostile attacks, often interpreted as punishment. Primitive reactions such as wild, aggressive behavior, stark panic, and virtual temporary paralysis of ego functions resulted, with sharp regression often following the procedure. At times, children under four showed much guilt over loss of control of feelings and exhibited subsequent temporary inhibition of unacceptable impulses, pointing out to physicians or nurses how "good" they were. Diagnostic procedures necessitating a departure from the ward and from familiar personnel and objects were particularly disturbing to children in this group, apparently representing a repetition of the separation from the parents. Lesser procedures such as venipunctures, blood counts, injections, etc., produced disturbing reactions but usually of lesser degree. The fear verbalized most frequently was that of needles. In this regard, an undoubted response to a reality factor involving pain was present. The impression was gained, however, that a great deal of the small child's fear of unknown procedures, of separation from the parents, of punishment, and of overwhelming attack was displaced much of the time onto such objectively less threatening but directly visible things as needles, tourniquets, etc. Fears of rectal temperature procedures or of throat sticks, for example, appeared to have such a displaced meaning as well as the more specific meaning in terms of the erotogenic zone involved. In the experimental group, aggressive responses in particular to various procedures were only half as frequent and were less intense than those in the control group; this difference was presumably related to the attempts at preparation for and emotional support during such procedures, even away from the ward whenever possible.

The reactions of children from four to six to diagnostic and treatment procedures were superficially similar to those of the younger children. Aggressive feelings were less uncontrolled, however, as one would expect, and realistic fears of specific procedures were more common. Fantasies about such procedures and the mechanisms of handling anxiety were similar to those described in relation to more diffuse stresses. In the experimental group again, aggressive responses were less pronounced for both sexes and slightly less common in girls than in boys.

In older children, the differences between the reactions of boys and girls appeared more marked, with girls showing less aggression and somewhat greater tendencies toward withdrawal and passive submission during and following procedures. Individual fantasies centered more specifically around certain procedures; in several children, for instance, catheterization appeared to arouse both fears of damage to the genitals and, at times, stimulation of sexual fantasies. In the experimental group, rational explanations of projected procedures were of greater value in limiting distorted interpretations than with younger children.

D. POSTHOSPITALIZATION REACTIONS

Following discharge, most of the regressive manifestations in the younger age group appeared to subside rather promptly. Behavior of an infantile or demanding nature, together with greater dependence on parents, persisted for several months in a number of children under five years of age. Wetting, soiling, and intensified pregenital gratifications, however, were ordinarily given up within three months' time.

The most common manifestations among children showing continuing disturbances were related to anxiety over separation from parents, appearing most intensely in younger children but arising also in latency children. Such anxiety was often combined with "distrust" of the parents, expressed as fear of their "leaving" again. Specific fears of strangers, the dark, cribs, animals, doctors, needles, etc., were more frequent in children from four to six years of age. Disturbances in feeding, of similar nature to those described on the ward, sleep disturbances (including the giving up of afternoon naps), hyperactivity, tantrums, fighting with siblings, and generally aggressive behavior were all seen to a limited degree, principally in younger children. All of these manifestations appeared to be milder in children in the experimental group (e.g., sleep disturbances were five times as common in the control as the experimental group).

In addition to anxiety and specific fears, children from four to six showed hyperactivity and disturbances in feeding and sleeping behavior (nightmares were frequent, at times involving "needles," or "doctors being sick in bed"). Regressive phenomena disappeared more quickly in these and older children than in the younger group. Manifestations seen in older children included withdrawals and fantasy formation, denial of illness or even temporary handicaps, and at times heightened dependence, together with some anxiety, and occasional feeding and sleeping disturbances. Fantasies were similar to those seen in the hospital. In play interviews, anxiety over broken guns and fears that "something was done to me that I don't know about" were encountered.

In general, symptoms which persisted were fewer in number and milder for each child at home than in the hospital. Such symptoms appeared to be related more directly to the personality structure and characteristic patterns of adaptation of the child prior to hospitalization. The impression was gained that the older children in the experimental group tended to verbalize more readily, to their parents and during follow-up contacts, their feelings and memories related to the hospital, acting out such feelings more easily in play as "doctors" or "nurses" than did the children in the control group.

In follow-up visits of a medical nature after discharge, approximately two-thirds of the children in both groups were seen either at the hospital or by a private physician. Most of the children in the control group who were seen in such visits (predominantly children of six years and under) showed increased anxiety, aggressive behavior, or other manifestations at the time of the first return visit. Of the experimental group, approximately half as many children showed such reactions, suggesting that anxiety in this area may have been handled more effectively by those children who had received greater preparation for and support during therapeutic or diagnostic procedures in the hospital.

As mentioned earlier, five children in the experimental group were described by their parents as being improved in their over-all behavior following discharge. A large number (four in the control group and seven in the experimental) were said to have shown improvement in one or more aspects of their behavior. No common characteristics in regard to age, sex, personality structure, previous adjustment, adjustment on the ward, parent-child relationship, stress encountered in the hospital, or other variables could be discerned for any of the five mentioned above. None of the five received psychotherapy while in the hospital, which Jackson (32) has described as bringing about post-hospital improvement. From careful scrutiny of the criteria of improvement held by the parents involved and of the behavior described as "improved," the impression was gained that these five children, as well as the majority of others showing partial improvement, actually had inhibited behavior previously unacceptable to their parents. This is in accord with the impressions of Jessner and Kaplan (35), in regard to the appearance of such improvement in children undergoing tonsillectomy, and casts no light on the possibility, mentioned by Langford

(37), of constructive growth experiences arising as the result of well-handled hospitalizations. It may be significant, however, that no phobic or other manifestations appeared as substitute symptoms in these children.

E. REACTIONS OF PARENTS AND FAMILIES

Certain nuclear affects were manifest among parents, whatever their adjustment on the ward. Realistic fear in proportion to the severity of the child's illness, overt anxiety, guilt over possible involvement in the causation of illness or over previously hostile feelings toward the child, and other feelings were handled in various ways, dependent upon the character structure of the parent, the nature of the relationship with the child, experiences immediately preceding hospitalization, and other factors. Where opportunities were available, the well-adjusted parents were able to participate effectively in ward care, feeding their children, playing with them, and putting them to bed. In some less adequately adjusted parents, anxiety arising from repressed hostility toward the child or from overvaluation of the child as an object reached such proportions that any such participation was blocked, and supportive psychotherapeutic measures were necessary. With some parents, isolation and denial, combined with projection of guilt or a need to use the illness of the child as a punishment, were observed. Defensiveness and projection onto staff members, often combined with rivalry on the part of the mother toward the nurses in particular, occasionally reached such intensity that acceptance of medical recommendations was impossible without psychotherapeutic intervention, not infrequently unacceptable to such parents.

Realistic acceptance of the implications of the child's illness was possible ultimately for the well-adjusted parents. In less well integrated personalities, accounting for the bulk of inadequate parental adjustments, sweeping anxiety, depression, acting out of sadistic impulses toward the child, and the use of a variety of defense mechanisms were observed in the face of serious or possibly crippling illness. Open and complete rejection of the child at any point was rarely seen, even on follow-up study. Marked ambivalence, even on the part of well-adjusted parents, was frequent in the face of behavioral regression on the part of the child, either during or following hospitalization. In the previously well-adjusted children showing reactions beyond three months, such parental ambivalence and overcompensatory indulgence or punitiveness appeared to be involved in the perpetuation of symptoms. In a number of instances, following a period of confusion, resentment, guilt and anxiety, parents intuitively handled posthospitalization reactions in an effective way, the best-adjusted ones giving initially greater emotional support to the children, gradually "weaning" them from increased dependent satisfactions.

Emotional reverberations among other members of family constellations were not infrequently observed. Intensified rivalry on the part of other siblings in the face of parental overindulgence of a regressed, recently discharged child was apparent in some instances. Information in this area was limited to some extent by the frequent defensiveness of parents in follow-up contacts.

Table 3 summarizes the frequency with which parents in the two groups took advantage of the differing visiting opportunities. A variety of factors, including geographic obstacles, home responsibilities, adverse working hours, and parental attitudes toward the child, influenced these figures. Some parents in both groups used control of visiting frequency as a potential threat held over their children. A small number in each group could not bring themselves to visit at all because of anxiety or guilt. In most of the 26 per cent of parents visiting infrequently or not at all in the experimental group, there appeared to be a relationship with the child of only partially satisfying or unsatisfying character. No direct statistical correlation was seen, however,

TABLE 3. PARENTAL VISITING

	Control Group	Experimental Group
Visited regularly (weekly for control, daily for experimental)	80%	74%
Visited infrequently		18%
No visiting observed	20%	8%
Total	100%	100%

between frequency of visiting and the severity of the child's reaction to hospitalization.

In general, the well-adjusted parents whose children were hospitalized under the experimental program seemed more satisfied with visiting regulations than those in the control group, where visiting was strongly curtailed. Culturally derived attitudes, however, stemming from previous contacts with doctors, nurses or friends, operated in a number of instances to produce uncertainty and rationalization about possibly disturbing effects upon the child, such as increased crying, etc. Difficulty in telling children truthfully about times of departure and return was encountered in many parents. Greater opportunities for working through conflicting feelings underlying such behavior were provided under the experimental program; a few parents, however, never succeeded in handling such situations comfortably. In a small number, often parents with limited integrative capacities, strong unconscious or at times conscious ambivalence in regard to more frequent visiting opportunities was apparent. In these instances, guilt often drove such parents to overcompensate by visiting compulsively and clinging to the child, actually producing interference with his adjustment on the ward. In the latter case, supportive work was necessary in order to help such parents limit their visiting and accept their realistic home responsibilities, after superficial guilt and anxiety had been allayed. Such experiences point up the need for flexible application of freer visiting regulations, geared to the needs of parent as well as child.

F. PROBLEMS IN WARD MANAGEMENT

The common conception that crying occurs more frequently among children whose parents visit frequently was found to be erroneous in the experimental phase of the study. It was evident that even very young children, if initial adjustment had been effected, tended gradually to cry less frantically and frequently in the face of their growing certainty that their parents would return in accordance with their statements at the times of departure. This was in the face of the fact that crying and other expressions of feeling were accepted more readily during the experimental program, being regarded as forms of emotional release of generally constructive character.

An apprehension frequently expressed by physicians in regard to flexible visiting has been that cross-infection would be increased. Only one child in each group while on the ward acquired a mild respiratory infection of probable cross-infectious origin. This finding, not completely valid without detailed bacteriological studies on all possible sources of infection, including ward personnel, would tend to support the impression of Bakwin (3) and Watkins and Lewis-Faning (60) that the hazard of cross-infection is not appreciably increased under circumstances involving more frequent contact with parents.

Limitation of space precludes extensive discussion of the manifold problems encountered in the erection of a preventive program of ward management. In the current study, major challenges were posed by limitations in availability and adequate planning of spatial facilities for effective grouping of children or for parental visiting and participation in ward care, as well as by insufficient personnel for close and supportive relationships with a large number of children on a busy ward. The attitudes of the professional staff toward the program varied greatly, from the vital support of the senior medical staff and the positive participation of the nursing personnel to a relatively passive sense of responsibility on the part of many of the younger ward physicians, a few of whom were either openly enthusiastic or definitely resistant and anxious in the face of permissive practices. The need for consideration of the many pressures impinging upon the busy, at times even harassed, ward physician was clearly apparent, as were the indications for a sensitive meshing of the visiting arrangements with other aspects of the hospital program in order to achieve flexible teamwork.

By encouraging participation of ward staff through the weekly Ward Management Conference, it was possible for the personnel to make considerable use of parent-surrogate relationships, to coordinate constructively treatment, feeding, and other schedules, and to put into practice, superficially, methods of psychological preparation and assistance for children in working through disturbing experiences, as for instance the death of a patient. Significant educational potential derived from the role of the play supervisor in particular, in the direction of the avoidance of "good" and "bad" dichotomies of thought in relation to patients, the diminution of traumatic consequences from ward procedures, and of imparting an understanding of the importance of a consideration of the emotional needs of the child and parent. Striking examples of failures to achieve effective teamwork of educational effect, however, were present in a number of areas. The impact upon small children of a large number of adults and the effect of changing shifts of personnel as well as patient assignments could not be completely overcome. For various reasons, including crowded facilities, participation in ward care by parents was not as widely available as had been planned. Limitations on permissive practices had to be set at times because of the anxieties of certain ward personnel (as well as of certain children, who became guilty and more aggressive without firm though broad limits on expression of aggression).

Group interrelationships, with their family-surrogate quality, provided interesting material, not possible to discuss in detail. Group panic over the sudden death of a child, as well as various types of interactive play, increased by early ambulation, provided fertile opportunities for observation and important challenges to preventive work under group living conditions. The more subtle "epidemiological" effects of anxiety among children and the supportive influence of one parent upon the child of another parent represent additional examples. Siblinglike relationships of anaclitic, supportive, rivalrous, and other nature were apparent among subgroups of children. Rivalry with or projection of feelings onto parents on the part of the younger medical staff at times complicated countertransference relationships. Children's reactions to ward rounds or to the overhearing of inadvertent remarks, promoted

by crowded spatial conditions, were striking and at times traumatic. .
For example, one boy of eight, who overheard a physician discussing
the fact that 10 per cent of children died from the illness from which
he suffered, became depressed and frantically tried to leave the ward.

Discussion

In an exploratory study of this nature, only tentative conclusions
may be drawn from the mass of data at hand. Anna Freud (23) has
discussed the limited degree of validity which one can ascribe to observations of behavior in children, even within the framework of a psychoanalytically oriented approach. It is her feeling, however, that research
of this kind, when based upon the body of knowledge already accumulated from thoroughgoing analytic study of individual children,
may be fruitful insofar as it corroborates currently held concepts or
opens up new avenues for more intensive scrutiny. The present investigation does indeed provide corroborative support for working concepts already developed by previous workers. It contributes nothing
new psychodynamically, but may be said to highlight certain areas for
future study and to underline the necessity for and, in some degree,
the effectiveness of current preventive methods.

The impact of hospitalization upon the child and family appears to
carry with it many and varied implications. The results of this study
tend to support the impressions of other investigators, particularly
Levy (38) and Jessner and Kaplan (35), to the effect that the child
of three years and under is the most susceptible to the circumstances
surrounding hospital care. At this level of psychosexual development,
separation from the mother, the loved object, often misinterpreted as
punishment or desertion, appears to pose the chief threat to a still
immature and dependent ego. Such "separation anxiety," however,
appears to occur to some degree in children up through the latency
period at least, being strongest and most devastating, at this older age
level, in neurotic children.

For the average child in the oedipal stage of development, the psychological meaning of the illness and its treatment appears to have greater
potential traumatic effect than the actual separation from the parents.
Reality factors, inviting misinterpretation and fears of mutilation or
death, appear to combine with unconscious anxieties and fantasies to
invest various treatment or diagnostic procedures with punitive significance, reviving or intensifying castration fears in the boy and helping to fixate in the girl fantasies that her genital configuration arose
through mutilation.

To summarize, for the small child in the hospital, "objective anxiety," as defined by Anna Freud (23), is strongest in the absence of the parent as a type of substitute ego. Such "objective anxiety" is enhanced by fears of overwhelming attack, arising from the limited capacities of the young child for reality testing and from his greater tendency toward regression. For the older child, preoccupied with the struggle to internalize controls over instinctual impulses, "superego anxieties" appear to be most intense. The latency child, with his greater repressive capacity, stronger ego defenses, more effective superego controls and identifications and more varied sublimatory outlets, appears to suffer less from the experiences involved in hospitalization and treatment for illness. Certain children in early latency, however, seem to show anxieties similar to those seen in children during the oedipal stage.

In addition to age, sex and level of psychosexual development, a number of variables appear to operate to determine the degree and nature of traumata deriving from the hospitalization experience. Most important of these would seem to be the quality of the child's relationship with his parents, the principal determinant of the capacity of his ego to integrate conflicting forces from within and from without. From the material at hand, however, criteria of limited accuracy only are available for purposes of prompt assessment of such integrative capacity and for prediction of the severity of response. In addition to the character of his previous adjustment, the capacity of the individual child to relate to new adult figures, to test reality, and to master anxiety successfully through verbalization or acting out in play while on the hospital ward would appear to be immediately helpful in this regard. Clearer understanding must first be obtained of the long-range effects of such an experience, however, since anxieties which appear to be handled successfully at the time of hospitalization may be reactivated later within the framework of specifically meaningful situations.

It is impossible to distinguish the most effective components of the preventive program from the data at hand. The fact that there appeared to be little correlation between the frequency of visits of an individual parent and the adaptation of the child during the experimental phase would seem to support the hypothesis that the more diffusely supportive aspects of the program were most prophylactic in effect. This is a puzzling statistical result, however, and may only serve to emphasize the multidetermined character of reactions to hospitalization. Further research is necessary in order to elucidate this point, as well as the effect of psychological preparation for hospitalization. A definite need is apparent for supportive work following the child's discharge, in order to aid parents in dealing with confusing regressive or other behavioral manifestations in their children and thus to prevent the development of more lasting problems.

Lack of space inhibits discussion of future investigative goals or areas of emphasis. The limited validity which can be assigned to the statistical trends cited herein points up the need for repetition of similar studies involving more intensive psychiatric investigations, as well as for further experimentation with specific techniques of ward management, spatial and grouping arrangements and other variables. Finally, the ways in which nonpsychiatrically trained ward personnel can operate most effectively in a preventive or therapeutic fashion remain to be clarified. Certainly, the impression is gained from the current study that, in spite of definite obstacles, a coordinated program of the type described can succeed in bringing to focus already existing or hitherto unsuspected capacities in individuals with varying professional backgrounds, who can thus render important contributions to the psychological welfare of the ill child.

SUMMARY

The study of emotional reactions to hospitalization appears to answer certain questions and to pose others for further investigation. All children in this series showed some observable reaction to the experience of hospitalization and treatment for illness, as distinct from the effect of the illness itself. The majority of children exposed to the traditional program of hospital management exhibited reactions calling for special and at times strenuous modes of adaptation, relatively self-limited in character but often persisting for a number of weeks or months following discharge. Such reactions were apparently more severe and persistent in children of preschool age, where separation from the parents seemed to play a major role, and in children with previously limited capacities for adaptation.

Although a persistently traumatic effect of an emotional nature arising from hospitalization does not seem to be inevitable, the possibility of such an effect appears great enough to warrant the application of special prophylactic measures. An experimental program designed to inculcate such measures and carried out through teamwork on the part of ward personnel appears to have produced a significant lowering of the incidence and severity of reactions at all age levels, most marked among children over four years of age. The use of more frequent visiting on a hospital ward as one of these preventive measures has not appreciably increased the risks of cross-infection.

Parental reactions to the illness and hospitalization of the child are important and may call for special supportive efforts. If opportunity is available, certain parents can make vital contributions to the hospital program through their participation in the ward care of their own children.

The lack of adequate psychological preparation of children for hospitalization shown in this study would support the need for more widespread educational measures designed to bring about this end. The preventive possibilities of the work of pediatricians, public health nurses, and other professional groups in regard to the handling of posthospitalization reactions seem clearly evident.

The foregoing study is regarded as only an exploratory one, leading to future investigations in order to evaluate more delicately the exact prophylactic techniques to be employed, with undoubted variations in different settings and with different age groups. Although many questions remain unanswered, it is hoped that an impetus has been given to the already progressing development of psychologically sound and administratively feasible programs of ward management by all members of the medical "team" concerned with the total care of the ill child. The goal of such programs is the prevention of serious emotional problems of patients through the efforts of professional personnel, harmonized as closely as possible with those of parents and the community.

REFERENCES

1. *A Study of Pediatric Nursing.* National League of Nursing, New York, 1947.
2. *Advancing the Education of the Hospitalized Child.* Conference in Atlantic City, New Jersey, February 26–27, 1948. National Foundation of Infantile Paralysis.
3. Bakwin, H. The Hospital Care of Infants and Children. *Pediat.*, 39: 383, 1951.
4. ——— Loneliness in Infants. *Am. J. Dis. Child.*, 63: 30, 1942.
5. Bakwin, R. M., and H. Bakwin. *Psychologic Care During Infancy and Childhood.* D. Appleton-Century, New York, 1942.
6. Barraclough, W. W. Mental Reactions of Normal Children to Physical Illness. *Am. J. Psychiatry*, 93: 1151, 1937.
7. Bender, L. Group Activities on a Children's Ward as Methods of Psychotherapy. *Am. J. Psychiatry*, 93: 865, 1937.
8. Bettelheim, B., and E. Sylvester. A Therapeutic Milieu. *Am. J. Orthopsychiatry*, 18: 191, 1948.
9. Beverly, B. I. Effect of Illness on Emotional Development. *J. Pediat.*, 8: 533, 1936.
10. Bibring, G. L. The Child First, in *Long-Term Care of Children.* Report of Bi-Regional Conference. Published by Arizona State Department of Health and Public Welfare in cooperation with the Children's Bureau, 1949.
11. Birren, F. Color and Psychotherapy. *Modern Hospital*, 67: 54 (Sept.), 1946.
12. Bowlby, J. Maternal Care and Child Health. *World Health Organization Monog.* Series, No. 2, Geneva, 1951.
13. Burlingham, D. Precursors of Some Psychoanalytic Ideas About Children in the Sixteenth and Seventeenth Centuries, in *The Psychoanalytic Study of the Child*, Vol. VI. Internat. Univ. Press, New York, 1951.

14. Butler, C., and A. Erdman. *Hospital Planning*. Dodge, New York, 1946.

15. Chapin, H. D. A Plan for Dealing with Atrophic Infants and Children. *Arch. Pediat.*, 25: 491, 1908.

16. Clayton, G. W., and J. G. Hughes. Variations in Blood Pressure in Hospitalized Children. *J. Pediat.*, 40: 462, 1952.

17. Clothier, F. Institutional Needs in the Field of Child Welfare. *Nervous Child*, 7: 154, 1948.

18. Coyle, G. L., and R. Fisher. Helping Hospitalized Children Through Social Group Work. *The Child*, 16: 114, 1952.

19. Crothers, B. Personal communication.

20. Davidson, E. R. Play for the Hospitalized Child. *Am. J. Nursing*, 49: No. 3 (March), 1949.

21. Deutsch, H. Some Psychoanalytic Observations in Surgery. *Psychosom. Med.*, 4: 105, 1942.

22. English, O. S. Psychosomatic Medicine and Dietetics. *Am. J. Dietet.*, 9: 721, 1951.

23. Freud, A. Observations on Child Development, in *The Psychoanalytic Study of the Child*, Vol. VI. Internat. Univ. Press, New York, 1951.

24. Freud, A., and D. T. Burlingham. *Infants Without Families*. Internat. Univ. Press, New York, 1944.

25. Freud, A., and S. Dann. An Experiment in Group Upbringing, in *The Psychoanalytic Study of the Child*, Vol. VI. Internat. Univ. Press, New York, 1951.

26. Freud, S. On Narcissism: An Introduction, in *Collected Papers*. Hogarth Press, London, 1950.

27. *Going to the Hospital*. Prepared by Child Development Center, Children's Hospital of the East Bay, Oakland, Calif., 1951.

28. Goldfarb, W. Infant Rearing and Problem Behavior. *Am. J. Orthopsychiatry*, 13: 249, 1943.

29. Hendrick, I. Early Development of the Ego: Identification in Infancy. *Psa. Quart.*, 20: 44, 1951.

30. Huschka, M., and O. Ogden. The Conduct of a Pediatric Prophylaxis Clinic. *J. Pediat.*, 12: 794, 1938.

31. Isaacs, S. *The Nursery Years*. Internat. Univ. Press, New York, 1936.

32. Jackson, E. B. Treatment of the Young Child in the Hospital. *Am. J. Orthopsychiatry*, 12: 56, 1942.

33. Jean, S. L. Mental Windows for Hospitalized Children. *The Child*, 13: 182, 1949.

34. Jensen, R. A., and H. H. Comly, Child-Parent Problems and the Hospital. *Nervous Child*, 7: 200, 1948.

35. Jessner, L., and S. Kaplan. Observations on the Emotional Reactions of Children to Tonsillectomy and Adenoidectomy, in *Problems of Infancy and Childhood* (M. J. E. Senn, Ed.). Macy Fd., New York, 1948.

36. Langdon, G. A Study of the Uses of Toys in a Hospital. *Child Develop.*, 19: No. 4, 197, 1948.

37. Langford, W. S. Physical Illness and Convalescence: Their Meaning to the Child. *J. Pediat.*, 33: 242,1948.

38. Levy, D. Psychic Trauma of Operations in Children, and a Note on Combat Neurosis. *Am. J. Dis. Child.*, 69: 7, 1945.

39. Linde, P. A. Some Factors Aiding the Development of Security in the Institutionalized Child. *Nervous Child*, 5: 85, 1946.

40. Liss, E. Convalescence. *Ment. Hyg.*, 21: 619, 1937.

41. Lowrey, L. G. Personality Distortion and Early Institutional Care. *Am. J. Orthopsychiatry*, 10: 576, 1940.

42. Lucas, W. P. Education for Hospitalized Children. *Med. Women's J.*, 56: 22, 1949.

43. MacLennan, B. B. Non-Medical Care of Clinically Ill Children in a Hospital. *Lancet*, 2: 209, 1949.

44. Moloney, J. C., J. Montgomery, and G. Trainham. The Newborn, His Family, and the Modern Hospital. *Modern Hospital*, 67: 43, 1946.

45. Moncrieff, A. Social Pediatrics. *Courrier du Centre Internat. de L'Enfance*, 1: 3 (No. 3), 1951.

46. Parry, L. A. The Urgent Need for Reforms in Hospitals. *Lancet*, 2: 881, 1947.

47. Pearson, G. H. J. Effect of Operative Procedures on the Emotional Life of the Child. *Am. J. Dis. Child.*, 62: 716, 1941.

48. Powers, G. F. Humanizing Hospital Experiences. *Am. J. Dis. Child.*, 76: 365, 1948.

49. Richards, S. S., and E. Wolff. The Organization and Function of Play Activities in the Set-up of a Pediatric Department: A Report of a Three-Year Experiment. *Ment. Hyg.*, 24: 229, 1940.

50. Roudinesco, J. M. David, and J. Nicholas. Responses of Young Children to Separation from Their Mothers. *Courrier du Centre Internat. de L'Enfance*, 2: 66, 1952.

51. Senn, M. J. E. Emotional Aspects of Convalescence. *The Child*, 10: 24, 1945.

52. Simmel, E. The Doctor Game and the Profession of Medicine, *Psychoanalytic Reader*, 1: 291, 1948.

53. Sloan, R. P. *Hospital Color and Decoration*. Physicians Record Co., Chicago, 1944.

54. Smith, R. Methods of Induction in Pediatric Anesthesia. *New Eng. J. Med.*, 240: 761, 1949.

55. Spence, J. C. *The Care of Children in Hospitals*. The Charles West Lecture, Royal College of Physicians, November 1946.

56. Spitz, R. Hospitalism, in *The Psychoanalytic Study of the Child*, Vol. I. Internat. Univ. Press, New York, 1945.

57. Stevens, M. Visitors Are Welcome on the Pediatric Ward. *Am. J. Nursing*, 49: 233, 1949.

58. Sutton, H. A. Some Nursing Aspects of a Children's Psychiatric Ward. *Am. J. Orthopsychiatry*, 17: 675, 1947.

59. Wallace, M., and V. Feinauer. Understanding a Sick Child's Behavior. *Am. J. Nursing*, 48: 517, 1948.

60. Watkins, A. G., and E. Lewis-Faning. Incidence of Cross-Infection in Children's Wards. *Brit. Med. J.*, 2: 616, 1949.

61. Wessel, M. A. The Pediatric Nurse and Human Relations. *Am. J. Nursing*, 47: 213, 1947.

5

THE CONCEPT OF EGO DISTURBANCES AND EGO SUPPORT

FRITZ REDL, Ph.D.

National Institute of Mental Health

It would be hopeless to try to find a short definition of the term "ego" with which a whole room full of people would easily agree, and which would, at the same time, be precise enough for theoretical speculation. Nor would it be feasible to try to follow the development which this concept has experienced since its earliest formulations by Sigmund Freud. For the sake of creating some kind of starting point for our discussion, however, I shall at least try to suggest what I mean by "ego." By "ego," I refer to that part of our personality which has primarily two duties to fulfill: 1) to establish a relationship with the world in which we live; and 2) to see to it that we behave reasonably in line with it without too serious inner conflict.

This rather crude "job analysis" of our ego obviously suggests that it has a variety of functions available by which to do these jobs. The first basic function seems to be of a cognitive nature. As the "research arm" of the personality, it seems to be the ego's task to perceive, assess, predict, etc., what social and physical reality would do to us if. . . . However, it is not only the "outside world" which must be brought into the realm of ego awareness. In order to do its other job, the research department of the ego must also supply it with adequate data about the dictates of our conscience, the nature and intensity of our strivings, in short, of our "inner reality." At least it seems always tacitly assumed that impulses or superego particles which would not be accessible to the self-perceptive department of the ego would also be outside the reach of its power.

This "research arm" of our ego seems to be coordinated to some sort of "executive branch," which has the task of exerting force, so as to keep our impulses and our behavior in line. Just where it derives the energies to do this still perplexes us.

The importance of the ego, and with it the focal role of ego psychology, has increased tremendously since its early "part-time employment" as a guardian on the border line between inside and outside

From *The American Journal of Orthopsychiatry*, 21:273, 1951.

reality, and the details of this development, as well as the most recent speculations about it, would be a most fascinating story indeed.

This short paper, however, sets itself a limited task: 1) to lure the practitioner into becoming much more impressed with the need to be very specific in the use of the term "ego disturbance"; and 2) to stimulate the clinician to seek a much wider repertoire of techniques, whenever he is confronted with the task of "ego support."

A. DEFICIENCIES OF THE CURRENT CONCEPT OF EGO DISTURBANCE

No matter how elaborate the speculations of the theoretician about ego functions may be, when used in connection with actual clinical material, it seems to me that the concept of "ego disturbances" shrivels up into a rather oversimplified little gadget, hardly able to do the job we expect of it. My main criticisms of the current usage of the term in connection with case material are these:

1. The term "ego disturbance" frequently confuses *qualitative* and *quantitative* aspects and lumps them together as though they were all the same, so much so that the terms "ego weakness" and "ego disturbance" are often used synonymously. It is obvious that this must lead to a great deal of diagnostic and prognostic confusion. If Johnny, for instance, attacks me in a prepsychotic temper tantrum, his attack can be blamed on disturbance of his ego functions. For the clinician, however, it would be of paramount importance to know more specifically just where this disturbance lies. Johnny might, for instance, perceive me correctly as the person I am, with the role I play in his life, but his ego may not have "strength" enough to hold his terrific impulse upsurgence or frustration onrush in check. The same behavior may result with a youngster whose ego might be perfectly able to cope with an onrush of impulsivity, but who would be too "confused" about the difference between present and past, so that the mere role similarity between me, Johnny's camp director, and his foster father of earlier childhood years would stir up old images instead of a correct reality appraisal. In both cases the behavioral results will be highly similar. Clinically, however, the two are very different.

2. The most frequent breakdown of the concept of "ego disturbances" parallels our concept of "ego functions," of course. However, most of these "functions of the ego" have been derived from the psychoanalysis of the neuroses of children from the middle or upper classes. In order to be even amenable to the very basic requirements of analytic therapy, most egos have to be well intact, and their functioning can be described in terms of the usual list of "ego defense mechanisms," which become a disturbance primarily if they get out of hand. The

kind of children I refer to seem to have a variety of functions seriously
disturbed which obviously belong to the realm of the "ego," which
we would never arrive at, however, from the study of the ego of the
neurotic, which is still more or less intact. I think there are many
more "ego functions" than we have assumed in the past, which we
simply take for granted and which may be separately disturbed. I shall
try to describe a few of them.

3. In blaming symptomology on "ego disturbances" we usually automatically assume that things go wrong only if an ego or part of it does
not function, or is too weak to assert its role. We seem to forget a
wide variety of behavioral disturbances which seem to me due to an
overfunctioning of ego activities, at least in certain areas. For example,
I would call it a job of the normal ego to be aware of large parts of
the id. The unusual acuity of self-perception which we find in certain
types of schizophrenic stages has puzzled us for a long time. For,
while obviously part of a pathological state, it seems a hypertrophic
development rather than a "disturbance." Similarly, we find that certain egos which are totally in the service of a delinquent superego have
a terrific overdevelopment of the skill of appraisal of the world as far
as delinquent enterprises are concerned. Some of my toughest customers, for instance, have a skill in "casing the joint," an acuity of observation of job-relevant facts, which is certainly an overdevelopment
rather than a disturbance or underdevelopment of ego functions. The
fact that the subsequent behavior can be called disturbed has misled
us into assuming that they suffer from "ego disturbances," whereas
partial "ego hypertrophy" would be a more correct statement. Not all
disturbances which happen to be connected with a "poor adjustment to
reality" are by that very fact also real "ego disturbances," and before
the term ego disturbance assumes any practical sense, a much more
specific description of symptomology as well as causality is indicated.

B.   EGO DISTURBANCE — JUST WHERE?

It would not do simply to mention obvious and understandable
weaknesses of our present conceptualizations. The job to be done is
really the work on a much more specific psychology of ego disturbances
than we have as yet attained. To arrive at it, we would have to extend
our studies much beyond the usual classical psychoanalytic interview
or play situation, and would have to create settings in which we can
see in operation ego functions and their disturbances even at a time
when conscious or unconscious expression of them within regular
treatment channels is practically not to be had.

We have tried to do just this for the last eight years in our various projects in Detroit. The observations referred to in this paper were all gained in the framework of the following three projects: the *Detroit Group Project*, an agency for group therapy with children on a small-club basis; the *Detroit Group Project Summer Camp*, in operation between 1943 and 1947; and *Pioneer House*, a residential treatment home for ego-disturbed children, in operation between 1946 and 1948. I must forfeit the fascination of dwelling either on the treatment design or on the intake and other details of these projects, and can, of course, not even try to list some of the findings which we hope to submit soon in a larger publication. In a nutshell, I think we can describe around thirty very distinct forms of "disturbance" of ego functions, all of which may be independently observed in varying degrees. For illustration, I shall select only a few.

1. *Inability to Cope with Frustration Aggression.* We frequently, and rightly, consider the inability of a child to "hold his own" under the impact of impulse onrushes as a phenomenon of "ego disturbance." The healthy ego is supposed to have considerable energy and to be able to use it at times of emergency.

What I want to imply here is this: some of our children are able to maintain reasonable ego intactness in the face of certain rather heavy impulse doses, but still lose all control in the face of typical "frustration aggression." For instance, Johnny may successfully cope with the temptation to yield to an urge for the possession of somebody else's toy; he may be able to hold his own under the impact of quite sizable doses of temptation in this realm. However, whenever confronted with the slightest "frustration," by simple interruption of a game when called for a meal, for instance, his ego reacts with a total loss of control. This seems to suggest that the ability to cope with frustration-produced aggression may be a separate function of the ego, and may be disturbed by itself, even though in other areas some other more complex ego functions are well intact.

2. *Loss of Ego Control through Group Psychological Intoxication.* We usually assume that the amount of "ego control" which a child has achieved in a certain area remains reasonably constant for the time being. This is an illusion indeed. We have all the evidence to support a theory to the contrary. It is clearly visible that *under certain group atmospheric conditions* some of our children suffer a total loss of ego control even in areas where their ego otherwise seems to be well intact. For example, a youngster with a considerable desire to "behave reasonably in line with dining-table expectations," especially in the presence of certain staff members, may be thrown totally out of control the moment the "group mood" has reached a certain level of hilarity, and especially if, for a variety of other reasons, the "contagion index"

for the whole group has gone up for the time being. In short, Johnny, who ordinarily wouldn't think of taking a chance by breaking a rule of table behavior which has just been reinforced, is suddenly going haywire under the impact of that element of "group psychological intoxication" which is so familiar to the practitioner and yet so hard to describe.

This item has an importance far beyond the situational implication in each case. In fact, we have arrived at a desire to define something like the "group intoxicational breaking point" of every child's usual ego control, and thus could arrive at the following rather puzzling fact: A child with a relatively *low level of ego control* sometimes has a rather high melting point of whatever level he has achieved; that is, while lower in ego control than his neighbor, whatever ego control he has is group psychologically more indestructible than the other fellow's. Another child with a *very high level of ego control, but a very low melting point* under group atmospheric conditions, will be more of a risk to the practitioner than the first child. Thus, instead of talking about ego strength and ego weakness even in specific areas, we should introduce as a further variable the concept of "group psychological melting point" of whatever ego-function levels are otherwise in action. In short, the highness or lowness of the group psychological melting point of existing ego functions is in itself as important an item clinically as the functioning or disturbance itself.

3. *Apperception of the Inherent Structure of Situations and Things.* Most anybody, if overwhelmed by a sudden onrush of aggressive impulsivity, may suffer a temporary loss of control. In such a state of mind he would most likely use anything at hand as a weapon against his opponent. Such a situation seems so simple, because whatever contribution the ego may have tried to make is flooded by the obvious impulse intensity with which we deal, so it looks as though all that happened was an overpowering of the ego through impulsivity onrush. It becomes easy, however, to see how much more complex the situation really is, if we vary the intensity of the impulsive side of the picture so that the cognitive signal functions of the ego can more clearly emerge. The following illustration may clarify what I have in mind: In the early months at Pioneer House, the children, entering their toy room even in a mild state of restlessness or hilarity, far removed from their usual more dangerous aggressive moods, would have reacted to practically any toy in the same way. A piece of wood, as well as a typewriter, would have suffered the same fate as a piece of clay: it would have been joyously thrown around, banged up, and finally trampled under. In a later development with increased specification of ego function, the same medium degree of restless hilarity would not have led to

the same scene. One of them would have apperceived immediately the potential of the typewriter for typing a "dirty" insult against an opponent or an adult; the piece of wood as a source of fun by cutting a gun out of it first, and then throwing only what was left at the people around. In short, in the second case the youngsters were able to show a more "civilized" reaction to the inherent structure of the toys they were confronted with, not because their impulsivity was reduced, but because the ego function of perceiving the inherent structure of situations and things was improved. It can well be seen of what tremendous importance for the whole problem of sublimation and socialization this very special ability of our ego may become, and it can easily be seen how an attack upon this type of ego disturbance would require entirely different strategy and techniques from any one of the others described here or elsewhere.

4. *Remaining "Reasonable" under the Impact of Unexpected Chance.* Very often the concept of "ego control" is narrowly identified with the task of the ego to visualize the limitations which the "reality principle" sets, and to enforce the limitations of reality against a recalcitrant id. This seems to me a much too narrow definition of its task. What if the ego is suddenly in the embarrassing position of having to set limitations where reality does not set any? Many an ego I know, which does a reasonably good job of "reality limitation enforcement," would miserably flunk this other task. In the children I am thinking of, this other disturbance usually did not become visible until we exposed them to the treatment process itself. Briefly, this is what we saw: Some of our children were reasonably able to take some reality limitations in some areas of their lives. The deficiency of their ego suddenly became overt when limitations were taken away. In that case, their egos proved entirely unable to cope with the task presented to them. The result was that the offering of freedom, presents or love would, in many of them, produce a terrific amount of anxiety. The old, well-known "fear of one's own impulses" would emerge, and reckless, aggressive demands would result.

Example 1. A child who manages well to keep his hostile impulses against other children subdued in the face of a sharp disciplinary regime may become entirely reckless the moment organizational pressures are removed. It would not do to call this youngster simply "ego-disturbed." His ego was good enough to signal clearly and demand submission sharply in the face of direct reality limitations. What it lacked was the resourcefulness to substitute for the sudden dropping out of outside reality limitations a limitational system of its own.

Example 2. Some children have been deeply deprived in terms of love from adults, and of possessions and toys. When given what they have long needed, they may go through a period of partial regression and some exaggerated dependency, but on the whole that is all. Under the impact of the diet they need, their ego soon gains strength and is able to unfold in many ways.

Not so the "toughies" I am thinking of at the moment. They have been equally deprived in terms of adult love, possessions and toys. Of course, because of their disturbance, they also have developed strong defenses against an open acceptance of what they originally needed. So we know it will take quite some time until we can get them to accept our offerings. But that is not the problem I want to concentrate on here. The trouble I want to talk about begins after we succeed in breaking down their defense. At the very point where they are openly and greedily accepting the fact that old reality frustrations have ceased, and where they begin to "take" to our affectionate and giving attitude toward them, we suddenly see their ego in another fit of despair. It had learned somewhat how to deal with some reality limitations, though not too well. It seems entirely at a loss, however, in dealing with a sudden dropping out of limitations. The demands of these children for love and total possession of adults, for gifts and permissiveness, assume such terrific and absolute proportions that nobody could or should try to live up to them. In short, these children, when getting what they obviously need, may suddenly be found lacking in ego functions which are needed by the new, therapeutically created situation. We could not have seen before that these ego functions were disturbed. The ability of the ego to set self-demand limitations where reality is unexpectedly granting seems to be as essential a function of the ego as the old stand-by of signaling barriers from the outside.

I can hardly exaggerate the impact which the functioning or non-functioning of this phase of ego effectiveness must have on the clinician's strategy, and especially on the problem of permissiveness versus interference as well as total treatment design. If this item is not calculated accurately, the basically best treatment design may easily leave the child's ego in a panic which is more than it can handle.

C. WHAT DO WE MEAN BY EGO SUPPORT?

If we are in dire need of a richer and more specific symptomology and etiology of ego disturbances, we certainly could do with more knowledge about possible techniques of "ego support." An attempt to demand more precision in the use of the term itself might be a good beginning.

The importance of giving at least partial ego support even in the most orthodox form of treatment of the most classical anxiety neuroses in children is, fortunately, a demand that can be taken for granted today. Only popularized distortions of psychoanalysis and, unfortunately, some of the earlier theories in group therapy are regressing still to the old model of pre-egoconscious therapy. We know now that we do not treat just by cathartic opportunity lure, interpretation-happy id analysis, or a do-nothing, see-nothing, say-nothing style of group leadership. In any serious treatment of a child's problem, whatever it may be, we have to take into account the state his ego is in at the time of the treatment, the added strain upon the ego during, and in spite of our special treatment goal, and the special problem his ego may be confronted with by the very impact of treatment itself.

Ever since Anna Freud drew the first clear delineation marks along that line, some respect for the shenanigans of the ego has been insisted upon even in cases where the ego itself was not the primary object of treatment. However, I wonder how far we have moved from there. The following seem to me to be the present limitations in our current concept of "ego support":

1. When we talk about ego support, we usually think of something the therapist says by way of interpretation to a child in interview or play situations, or by way of argument in favor of reality issues which the child might tend to ignore or deny. In short, the verbal medium is often considered the domain of ego-supportive help.

2. When we talk about "ego support," we usually assume by implication that the person who gives it has been able to establish a certain type of "positive rapport," whatever we may consider its nature to be, with the child. Thus, ego support assumes a high level of child-adult relatedness in order to become possible at all.

3. When we talk about giving "ego support," we sometimes think of indirect measures, as, for instance, our influence on parental behavior, the manipulation of school situations, the exposure to "supportive" recreational and other experiences. It is easy to see that such manipulation as a marginal addition to the "real treatment" that is supposed to go on in the psychiatric interview with the child is of a much more complex nature, and that in this instance "ego support" means primarily a partial and chance use of the relation of other people with the child, rather than having the meaning indicated by the term "ego support" in the two instances cited above.

The insufficiency of this concept of ego support for our child population at large is easy to see. Let me just raise a few questions to the point: What about children who do not talk, cannot relate to people, are so restless they will not stay put long enough to be given ego support on a rapport interpretive basis? What about children with whom the problem not only is how to give ego support while we treat something else, but who need ego repair before they can even be treated by the usual channels at all? Is it sufficient to consider such children as "not amenable to psychotherapy" and to keep complaining that we cannot do anything with them and that they clog up the channels of detention home, foster home referral and institutional intake?

None of the children we started with at Pioneer House could have been amenable to the usual forms of "ego support," because something else had to be done to their ego first to make them amenable to the usual channels of therapy. And I could point at hundreds like them. What about them? Are there other forms of relationships or activities that could be used with these cases?

At this point I am afraid we may fall into a grave error, that has led us to drift from a fair and realistic apraisal of our ignorance into a sudden and hardly pardonable naïveté. Because we, as therapists, feel at a loss about nonverbal, action-close, toughness-proof, transference-exempt techniques of ego support, we readily think that maybe others know and can do what we are so desperately groping for. It is along this line of naïve illusion that I see many of us impressed by the most unwarranted, foggy and unsubstantiated claims. If therapy hasn't produced much around ego treatment techniques, how about education, institutional work, recreation, group work? And here we are invariably engulfed by the most reckless confusion as to what really constitutes "character training," "reality support," "ego support through authority," and so on, and are in danger of two extremes. One is to fall into the trap of the old educational confusion between enforcement of reality-geared behavior and real treatment. The other is to adopt one or another of the most unsubstantiated claims of those who recommend them as marginal "ego-supportive" measures. I am ashamed to admit that the statements which were made recently even by psychiatrists about issues like physical punishment and child rearing or the confused claims of many trends in group therapy itself bear ample witness to the danger I am trying to describe.

The real way out lies, of course, only in a frank admission of our ignorance, a proudly maintained awareness of the complexity of the issues at hand, and a patient attempt to get research results in specially designed frameworks over the years to come. The difficulty of having to create special — and I might add extremely costly — designs in which to gain data about ego treatment techniques may hold us up for a few decades, but this is still the only way out.

D.   SOME ILLUSTRATIONS OF EGO-SUPPORTIVE TECHNIQUES

In organizing our materials gained in the projects mentioned previously, and especially in the Pioneer House experiment, we can at this time differentiate between about forty techniques, each one of which bears upon the attempt to give ego support or more directly to contribute to ego repair. Needless to say, the number is somewhat arbitrary and may vary in the final writing, depending on later and more adequate chances for subcategorization. These various techniques are obviously on very different levels and are meaningless alone, that is, unless they are presented in a total treatment design. I shall mention only a few for the purpose of illustration.

1. *Manipulation of "Hang-Over" Effects.* When children are engaged in intense activity, it is not just that much "liveliness drained off so they don't get into trouble elsewhere." It invariably makes certain very specific demands on their control systems, as it also offers very specific chances for certain impulse gratifications. In short, it creates a quite unique pattern of internal distribution of impulse-control constellations, and this specific distribution usually does not stop with the discontinuation of the structure itself. It seems to "swing over" into the next phase and, depending on its nature, may create problems and confusion. An illustration may help make this situation clearer. Cabin 7 has just had a lively game of "Capture the Flag," which, however, left a number of emotionally charged issues dangling in mid-air, such as whether or not the umpire had rightly declared Johnny tagged. Assuming that this activity had to be interrupted prematurely, and had to be followed by exposure to a story, within a larger group setting, which required passive listening, we can anticipate some trouble. Some of the youngsters seem to have special difficulties coping with "hang-overs" from previous patterns while the new situation demands an entirely different set of mind. Some youngsters have good ego control over mild impulse quantities as such, but their ego is overwhelmed whenever it is confronted with a transitional job. The result is that if the daily life program contains too many such tasks of special difficult transitional situations, a breakdown of ego function can be observed. If the daily diet of schedule and program is wisely planned, with "transition hygiene" in mind, the sum total of intolerable ego problems will be reduced, which indirectly seems empirically to lead to a total increase in ego resilience. For instance, it was very important in the treatment of the Pioneer House children to plan good supplementation-balanced diets for every hour of the children's day. Confronting them in the early afternoon, after a tense school period, with another competition-loaded situation would have led to ego breakdown where wiser program planning did not exhaust the sum total of available emergency resilience of their ego strength.

2. *Preventive Signal Interference.* The trouble with some children's ego is not so much its inability to cope with ordinary situations. The

trouble is that they get themselves, under the impact of momentary excitement or group contagion, into behavior far beyond the level which their own superego will allow to go fear- and guilt-free. As a result they are suddenly flooded with an upsurgence of guilt feelings. However, this is where their ego disturbance hits them heavily. While they are able to cope with many of the usual ego tasks, the manipulation of guilt feelings is one of the disturbed areas. Therefore, laden with their feelings of guilt, they produce aggression, hostility, anxiety, or whatever the case may be, and from there go into an increased stage of disorganization. In those cases it is important to avoid too many serious guilt-charged situations for a while. In short, interference when Johnny starts getting himself into a stage he will later not be able to control prevents the production of so much excess guilt that new hatred against the adult who left him helpless through his hyperpermissive ways is produced. Therefore, we planfully save them for a while from the production of too heavy guilt situations so that their ego is exposed to having to handle them until is it strengthened all around and we can concentrate on that specific repair task.

3. *Interpretation through Reshuffled Reality.* Some things can be talked down. Others can be listened down. There are a few which have to be lived down or they will not budge. We have the impression that this is true for some of the more serious forms of pathological responses, at a time when rapport or verbal interpretation is still out of the question. For example, Johnny forces us into separating him from the group through skillfully produced behavior which makes his temporary removal from the dinner table morale-essential for the rest of the group. His real design is, of course, production of a situation where the adult is pushed into the role of hostile bouncer, depriver of food, loveless frustrater of little children. Needless to say, we can easily avoid falling into the well-devised trap Johnny hoped to lure us into, but the basic issue of having to go to the other room with him for a while, away from the other children and their contagion-loaded build-up, cannot be avoided. Johnny now sits there, exploiting the rest of his delusions. He daydreams that we hate him, want to starve him, would like to poison him anyway, and so on. At this time, interview rapport and organized verbal interpretation are months away. Falling into Johnny's various delusional traps, on the other hand, would make treatment impossible. The answer is what we might loosely call "interpretation through reshuffled reality." It prescribes as follows:

(a) Avoidance during this time, by careful program diet, impulse drainage, etc., of as many run-ins or potential frustration situations in other areas as possible.

(b) Keeping the crisis situation in which Johnny has embroiled you entirely free of counteraggressions, side issues, etc.

(c) Offering him visibly, with calm reassurance, the very food he claims you want to withhold from him; avoiding being drawn into an argument by his delusional accusations.

(d) Creating ample affection-evidence opportunities with the same person during the same day around other life issues.

If carefully planned, this type of policy has an amazing cumulative effect. Even though Johnny's delusional desires far outbalance his reality insight at the time, the concrete offer of a three-decker sandwich has a chance to sink in where verbal acrobatics would have made no impression. Johnny's ego is being strengthened in its attempt to establish some kind of control over delusional patterns by being offered tangible counterevidence at the right time and in the right amount. It is strong enough to use it when it gets it, but not developed enough to produce it out of its own data regarding human beings. Needless to say, such a technique is meant only as one among a variety of others, and is tied to elaborate conditions without which it would remain an empty and ill-applied "trick."

4. *Exploitation of Group Psychological Securities.* One of the greatest strategic advantages of the group situation, especially the residential one, is the possibility of inserting a variety of direct ego supports into the child's life which are relatively independent of our individual rapport and of verbal communications at the time. We had ample chance, for instance, to be impressed by the great ego-supportive power of *traditionalized routine* — once we got that far. In the beginning, each evening seemed like a new confrontation of their egos with a new accumulation of crises, and became an endless sequence of breakdowns at their attempt to control frustration, aggression, time confusion, transitional anxieties, adult role hostilities all at once. With the establishment of some sort of regime around bedtime — which has to be tailored to fit the situation in all its details — it became quite clear that through the emergence of a "group habitual pattern" their egos had a load taken off their task. The ego seems, then, to have to function only as a signaler of what is proper time and proper avenue of behavior, instead of having to try and produce the whole creative chain of ideas of just how to behave, while being confronted with frustration aggression at the same time. In the same way, it was easy to see that a skillful *exploitation of their native group code* could temporarily, at least, relieve the ego's task. At a time, for instance, when reality insight would not have stood a chance of dealing with the excitement of a fight starting in the middle of a boat ride, the group-code propaganda for an attitude that "we Pioneers wouldn't want to act

that way in a boat" could carry the burden of impulse management for the time being. In short, group-code value tie-ups make it possible to put issues for which actual ego insight cannot yet be expected temporarily under the control of another department. This technique, too, makes sense only as a partial step and in close connection with a total policy of strategic handling.

SUMMARY

1. I think that the concept of "ego disturbances" needs much more specified study; that some of its ramifications become observable especially under group situational conditions; that organized research into all forms of ego functions, over and beyond those customarily summarized under the title of "mechanisms" and the like, is sorely needed.

2. I am convinced that the whole problem of "ego support and ego repair" needs study far beyond the scope available to us in verbal or play interview situations; that some new techniques especially needed for nonverbal, severely ego-disturbed and hyperaggressive children could be obtained by the planful use of group therapy and especially the planful design of residential settings, with their chance for the exploitation of group psychological securities, as well as the strategic advantage of action proximity and total milieu manipulation.

6

A STUDY OF AN INFANT WITH A GASTRIC FISTULA

I. Behavior and the Rate of Total Hydrochloric Acid Secretion

GEORGE L. ENGEL, M.D., FRANZ REICHSMAN, M.D., AND
HARRY L. SEGAL, M.D.

University of Rochester School of Medicine and Dentistry

Since the classic investigations of Beaumont on Alexis St. Martin, a number of individuals with gastric fistula have been studied, mainly from a physiological point of view. Wolf and Wolff's (1) classic study of Tom was the first systematic effort to relate manifest behavior, emotions, and gastric functions in such a patient. Margolin (2) subsequently psychoanalyzed such a patient and attempted to relate gastric activity and unconscious mental processes. Although a few observations of children (3) have been made, to our knowledge no detailed psychophysiologic investigation of an infant with a gastric fistula has been reported. This is a study of an infant girl with a congenital atresia of the esophagus on whom a gastric fistula was established in the fourth day of life. We began our research when the child was 15 months old and made detailed observations of behavior and gastric secretion until she reached the age of 22 months, when substernal colonic anastomosis between esophagus and stomach was formed. During these six months we observed the child in 59 experiments and collected more than 600 specimens of gastric juice. This paper is a report on those data that have been analyzed to date. The literature will be discussed when all the material has been analyzed and prepared for publication.

HISTORY OF THE INFANT

The infant girl, Monica, was born during July, 1952, in a small hospital about 90 miles from Rochester, New York. When it was discovered two days after her birth that she regurgitated all fluids, she

From the Departments of Psychiatry and Medicine of the University of Rochester School of Medicine and Dentistry and the Strong Memorial and Rochester Municipal Hospitals, Rochester, New York, and published in *Psychosomatic Medicine*, September-October 1956. © 1956 by American Psychosomatic Society, Inc.

was referred to the Pediatric Service of the Strong Memorial Hospital, where a diagnosis of congenital atresia of the esophagus was made. The next day a cervical esophageal fistula was established, and the day thereafter a gastric fistula. After a smooth postoperative course Monica was discharged, having been hospitalized for ten days. The mother was instructed to feed the baby through the gastrostomy on a four-hourly schedule. The parents were also told that when she was four to five months old, the child should receive an operation that would allow her to swallow normally.

At the time of Monica's birth her parents and her 20-month-old brother lived in the maternal grandmother's home. Our knowledge of this setting, particularly of the emotions and attitudes of the figures around Monica, is somewhat limited because of the guardedness of the parents in their communication with us and with others interested in the child. The mother was 19 years old when Monica was born. She appeared a child-like, timid woman, obviously dominated by her husband. She usually allowed him to do the talking and when faced directly with a question, often answered in a questioning tone through her husband. The father, 13 years older than the mother, was employed as a long distance truck driver. He spoke volubly and glibly and presented himself as a forthright, solid citizen. We know from other sources that he is considered unreliable and irresponsible. Both parents were brought up on farms, with restricted social backgrounds and limited education, but they seemed to have average intelligence.

Both parents were "frightened" when the malformation was discovered, and particularly by the baby being taken to Rochester. At first they communicated with the doctors at the Strong Memorial Hospital by telephone only and had difficulty comprehending Monica's condition and what was being done for her. When Monica came home from the hospital the mother was squeamish and anxious about the gastrostomy and the gastric tube. She could not reinsert the tube without "feeling faint" and at times could not bring herself to do it at all. Furthermore, she was afraid to fondle and hug the child for fear of disturbing the gastric tube, which she regarded, with some justification, as the baby's lifeline.

For the first five months of her life, while she lived at the grandparents' house, Monica gained weight and to all observers seemed to be developing adequately. During this time the grandmother helped materially with the care of the malformed infant, picking her up when she cried and holding her on her lap for long periods. Toward the end of 1952 the relationship between the father and his in-laws, which apparently had been strained for some time, worsened. An open conflict erupted, particularly over the grandparents' handling of the children, and the parents decided to move. At about the same time, in December, two other events took place. The operation that Monica was to undergo about that time did not take place because, for some administrative reasons, the state aid to cover hospitalization costs did not materialize. Furthermore, the mother discovered that she was pregnant again. Throughout this unplanned and unwanted pregnancy she was afraid that this infant also might be defective.

In December, 1952, the family moved to an isolated farmhouse. During this winter they were snowed-in repeatedly for days at a time, on some occasions when the father was away on one of his trips. It was at this time that Monica started to go downhill. The mother said, "She acted tired out, like a person who is discouraged." Because the parents were quite reticent, we can only conjecture about the relationship between mother and child. We know the mother was a very dependent, immature woman who, in this situation, thrown on her own resources, was afraid to get too close to the child.

Monica's downhill course continued through the spring of 1953, while the parents made several moves in rapid succession (allegedly to avoid payment of rent). Her condition was further aggravated when she contracted chicken pox in May. She was described by the parents as "cranky and irritable" and as "crying all the time." She began to refuse the sugar nipple that the mother had given her to suck before and during gastric feedings, in accordance with the doctor's instructions. The parents began, instead, to give her lollipops. Monica also would become quite excited during meal time and if sitting on a parent's lap would attempt to grab and devour any food she could reach. Swallowed food, of course, ran out through the esophageal fistula. She had failed to gain weight for some time and now began to lose weight. After a brief admission to a local hospital she was again referred to the Strong Memorial Hospital in June, 1953, where she arrived looking marasmic. The nurse described her as "very neglected" and "lethargic." She was not studied by us on this admission.

During a hospitalization of one month Monica improved considerably, both physically and emotionally. She maintained this improvement at home for about one month, until the mother gave birth to a baby girl at the end of August. Following this event Monica's condition again declined sharply. She became very irritable and fretful and seemed particularly disturbed when the baby sister was held or fed. When the baby was held near her, Monica would push her away or claw at her. During this period she was particularly avid for food by mouth. When she heard her mother setting the table she cried to be fed by mouth, and when given juices by spoon, "she couldn't get enough." Within a few weeks she lost the weight she had gained during her hospitalization, and because of her increasing marasmus she was re-admitted to the Pediatric Service on October 12, 1953; she was 15 months old and weighed 4500 grams. She was cachectic and the pediatric house officer described her as "very depressed." She was unable to sit up or even to turn over in bed.

During the first 2½ months in the hospital she gained only 1 kilogram. By the end of 5½ months she showed considerable improvement in strength and her weight had reached 7500 grams. During this time she became quite attached to one of the nurses and to one of the investigators, both of whom became quite attached to her.

During her nine months in the hospital, Monica's parents visited only seven or eight times, three of these visits around the time of the operation. At times the social worker and public health nurse had to make extensive efforts to contact the parents. Because their visits were infrequent and unpredictable, we unfortunately have no direct observations of Monica's response to her parents. The nurses, however, reported that Monica always recognized them and responded with signs of pleasure. We do not know whether this response was immediate or delayed. The father was more active with her and she was reported to be more responsive in general to him than to the mother. The parents' visits were brief and they occasionally left her a small gift.

The nurses and doctors openly expressed their feeling that the parents were not sufficiently interested in Monica and that particularly the father seemed insincere in his display of affection and expression of interest. Some of them looked upon Monica as a deserted waif and were especially attentive to her for this reason. Throughout the prolonged period of hospitalization Monica became something of a celebrity and there was great interest in the outcome of her case. For some ward personnel she became "the darling of the ward"; a few resented the special attention she received. At the outset some of the hospital personnel identified the investigators with Monica's persecutors, but later most considered the interest of the investigators to exert a beneficial effect. At the end of 5½ months she was deemed physically fit for colonic substernal anastomosis between esophagus and stomach. After a somewhat stormy postoperative course, Monica regained her preoperative developmental level, and during the next 6 months she learned to feed herself, to stand, and to walk with help. She also developed some speech. Her subsequent development will be the subejct of another paper.

A summary of the historical data follows:

July 1952   Birth. 2nd day admitted to Strong Memorial Hospital, weight 2700 grams. 3rd day cervical esophostomy. 4th day gastrostomy. 10th day discharged home, weight 2970 grams.

Aug. 1952   At maternal grandparents' home. Cared for by grand-
to   mother and mother. Gained weight.

Dec. 1952   Friction between parents and grandparents. Monica and family move to isolated farm home. Mother pregnant —
to   unplanned. Monica's operation postponed through administrative tangle.

Jan. 1953   Monica begins to go downhill. Tired, irritable, loss of
to   weight. Mother frequently alone with children.

May 1953   Family moves several times. Chicken pox — rapid decline. Admission to Hornell Hospital.

June 1953   Admission to Strong Memorial Hospital, weight 4830 grams. Condition stabilized. Discharged in one month.

July 1953   Return to home weighing 5180 grams.

Aug. 1953   Baby sister born. To grandmother's house for 5 days.
to   Further decline until admission to

Oct. 1953   Strong Memorial Hospital on October 12, 1953.

THE DESIGN OF THE STUDY

Basic to the design of this study is the concept that the experimenter is part of the experiment. An infant with a gastric fistula through which gastric juice is being aspirated manifests behavior in relation to the person withdrawing the gastric juice. The baby is behaving always in some way in relationship to the experimenter, the experimenter in some way to the baby, and the behavior of each is modified thereby. To this extent we are dealing with a transactional system which must itself be observed. We, therefore, regard the more or less naturally developing relationship between the baby and the experimenters as a behavioral variable, not to be controlled, but to be observed carefully and recorded by one or more observers behind a one-way vision screen. A second major premise of this study is that human behavior and associated physiological processes cannot be expected to follow the imposed time schedule of the experimenter. Since a variety of significant events, known and unknown, precede any period of observation, and since to a large degree baby and experimenter influence each other in unpredictable ways from the moment the two come in contact, we discard the concept that regards the initial period of observation of any experiment as a base line or control for what follows. Instead, we assume that we deal with analogical, that is, continuous, functions that are being observed simultaneously in different conceptual frameworks — physiologic, interpersonal, behavioral — and that from these can be derived categories or classes, any two or more of which can be compared. The methodologic problem is to set up categories that are clearly identifiable or measurable by any observer. In this study we measured by chemical techniques a variety of components of gastric juice and by observational techniques a variety of categories of behavior. For each specimen of gastric secretion there were corresponding observations of the behavior during the time that the gastric juice was being secreted and aspirated. The more than 600 specimens of gastric juice obtained provide ample material for statistical analysis.

Actual operation of the study was carried out as follows: During the 5 months there were 59 observation periods during which gastric juice was examined, 44 fasting and 15 after eating. Only the 44 fasting observations are reported in this paper. In nearly all experiments one of us (F. R.) was the experimenter, but on 13 occasions the experimenter was a relative stranger to the baby. The observation periods occurred 2–4 times per week and each lasted from 1–5 hours, making a total of 161 hours. Most of the studies took place in the laboratory, with the observers behind a one-way vision screen; some were in a cubicle on the infant ward with the observer behind a glass partition, visible to the baby. In the latter setting the usual activities of a busy infant ward were visible and audible to the baby, experimenter, and observer (Figs. 1 and 2). Additional sources of psychological data were:

Sources of Psychological Data:

1. Interview with Parents
2. Interview with Public Health Nurse
3. Daily Diary of Miss D., Pediatric Nurse
4. Spot Observations of Pediatric Resident Staff
5. 1–3 Hour Observation Periods on Ward by Mr. Chinchinian and Mr. Wright
6. Multiple Daily Visits by Dr. Reichsman
7. Psychological Testing by Dr. Parsons
8. 1–5 Hour Observation Periods in Ward or Laboratory with Simultaneous Gastric Analyses

Both the experimenter and the observer(s) behind the screen made detailed minute-by-minute notes on the behavior of the baby (and of

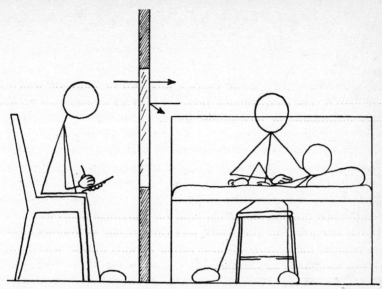

Fig. 1. The experimental set-up in the laboratory. The experimenter withdraws gastric juice and makes behavioral observations. The observer records behavior of baby and experimenter from behind a one-way vision screen.

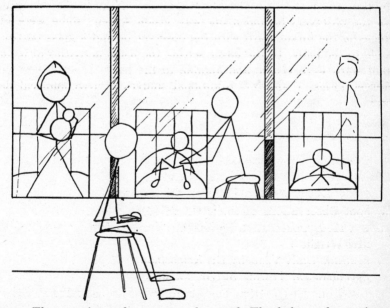

Fig. 2. The experimental set-up on the ward. The baby and experimenter were in a cubicle, while the observer was behind a glass partition. The observer was visible to the baby, as were nurses, doctors, attendants, and other babies concerned in ordinary infant ward routine.

the experimenter) that was apparent to them. The experimenter either made brief notes or dictated his observations to a secretary who was out of the baby's view. Thus for each experiment there were two or more detailed behavioral protocols, which were subsequently analyzed into discrete categories. Clock time was meticulously recorded so that for the period of collection of each gastric juice specimen the corresponding behavioral data were available. (The criteria for the behavioral categories are presented later.)

Particular attention was paid to the development of object relationships between Monica and the various experimenters. F. R. quickly became the favored experimenter, and the relationship became highly invested on both sides. Within the framework of this relationship, Monica manifested her more advanced ego development. When new experimenters were introduced they were first experienced as strangers, from whom Monica withdrew, lapsing into a state that we have called the "depression-withdrawal reaction." This is discussed in more detail elsewhere (4). With repeated contacts, this reaction became attenuated and Monica made efforts to establish contact with the new experimenter. The experimenter was not instructed specifically how he should respond to these overtures. The depression-withdrawal response was always alleviated promptly when the stranger left and F. R. returned. F. R.'s return invariably evoked unmistakable signs of pleasure. These characteristic responses to different experimenters offered a convenient method of studying the behavioral and gastric secretory responses to variations in object relationships. When pediatric care necessitated procedures such as catheterizations we obtained behavioral and secretory data characteristic of such periods of external stress.

Physiological Methods

Our physiological observations were purposely limited to studies of secretion. The small diameter of the gastric stoma would have necessitated interruption of aspiration for the study of mucosal color or of gastric motility; we thought it of greater importance to aspirate gastric secretion as completely as possible.

Gastric aspiration was performed by gentle manual suction on a 20 cc. syringe attached by a metal adapter to a #18 rectal tube which fitted somewhat loosely into the small gastrostomy opening. By alternating the tube between the fundus and plyorus of the stomach secretions were aspirated as completely as possible. Both volume of secretion and the length of time it took to collect the specimen were accurately recorded. During the earlier experiments there were often pauses of 5–10 minutes between the individual gastric specimens, but later aspiration was carried on almost continuously. The volume of the individual specimen was determined by the necessity of obtaining at least 3–4 cc. of secretion for the determination of *p*H, hydrochloric acid, and pepsin. Our physiologic measurements are as follows:

Gastric Analyses

1. Gross Appearance
2. Volume of Secretion in cc./min.
3. *p*H
4. Concentration of Free and Total HCl in m.eq./cc.
5. Rate of Secretion of Free and Total HCl in m.eq./min.
6. Concentration of Pepsin in units per cc.
7. Rate of Secretion of Pepsin in units per min.

Of these we will deal in this paper only with the rate of total hydrochloric acid expressed in milliequivalents per minute. The concentration of total hydrochloric acid was determined by titration with 0.1N NaOH, using phenolphthalein as the indicator. The rates of secretion were calculated only when the stomach had been emptied of gastric juice immediately before the sample was collected and the exact time of collection and the exact volume of the sample were available. In most instances the interval between specimens did not exceed 3–4 minutes, and usually was one minute. We arbitrarily excluded any specimen in which the preceding interval exceeded the duration of the specimen; in most instances the interval was much shorter.

In this paper we are reporting on 389 specimens of gastric juice in which the rates of total hydrochloric acid secretion in the fasting state were calculated.

PSYCHOLOGICAL METHODS

In considering the psychological-behavioral observations, one should keep in mind that we were dealing with an infant with a chronological age of 15–21 months but who was much retarded physically and mentally. Monica was unable to sit up and she did not speak at all. Gesell rating at the age of 16 months was approximately 4–8 months; at 22 months it was 9–15 months.[1] Behavioral observations were therefore limited to recumbent bodily positions and movements, facial expressions, and a variety of inarticulate, but quite expressive, sounds. Although at first glance this may appear a serious limitation of the study, we believe that it was more than offset by the opportunity to observe

[1] We are indebted to Dr. Frances Parsons for these data.

a human being at a level of development at which emotions are expressed without any or with only slight disguise.

Our observations were recorded without preconceived ideas of what behavioral categories should be studied; only at the completion of the study were the various categories established. After criteria had been established, the protocols of the observer and the experimenter were independently analyzed by two of us (G. E. and F. R.), without knowledge of or reference to the results of the gastric analyses. The independent judgments were then compared. With the rare exceptions noted below, there was agreement. The behavioral categories reported in this paper are as follows:

A. Affects
B. Object Relations (OR)
C. Non-Nutritional Oral Behavior (NNOB)
D. Sleep-Walking Status
E. Non-Nutritional Feeding Experiences (NNF)

We shall now discuss our criteria for identifying and classifying the different behavioral categories.

AFFECTS

In this study we consider affects to be revealed by primary behavioral patterns that express the dynamic steady state of the organism and the deviations therefrom. We believe the basic behavioral pattern expressing the affect to be innate and essentially unlearned; it involves innervations of both the autonomic and voluntary nervous systems. Monica being in a preverbal stage no psychic representations of effect or manifestations of secondary process were observable. On the other hand, some affect, evoked by external or internal sources, was manifest during all observation periods except during sleep.

Our criteria for identifying affects were based on observations of posture, movements, facial expression, and vocalization that accompany the affects. The detailed descriptions by Charles Darwin of the external manifestations of affects have been of great help to us (5). Empathic responses of the observer were not unimportant in affect identification. Consistency of audience response to motion picture strips of the various affects has greatly enhanced our belief in the reliability of this method of classification.

In Monica we could identify six affects, which we classify under two major headings: *Pleasure and Unpleasure.* We distinguish two degrees of pleasure: *Contentment* and *Joy;* and four kinds of unpleasure: *Depression, Depression-Unpleasure, Irritation,* and *Rage,* the last two being different degrees of anger. These are illustrated in the accompanying photographs (Fig. 3).

Contentment (Fig. 3a)

This was a state of rather quiet relaxation. The posture was comfortable and uninhibited. It was appropriate for quiet play activity, self-stimulation, or repose. When she was flat on her back, her most usual position, her knees were usually flexed. Movements were generally slight and rather gentle, but occasionally more vigorous waving or reaching occurred. Movements included nodding and shaking the head; self-stimulatory scratching, rubbing, tickling, or oral manipulation; movements for manipulation of inanimate objects; movements toward a person, such as waving, touching with arms or legs, stroking, pinching, and reaching. The facial expression during Contentment was placid, with not infrequent smiles, narrowing of palpebral fissures, and mimicking. Vocalization consisted of occasional cooing or gurgling.

Joy (Fig. 3b)

This was a very active pleasure response. Movement overshadowed posture and usually was vigorous and almost continuous. It included waving, reaching, kicking with stretched legs, arching and turning of trunk. Facial expression was very active and mobile with much smiling and laughing. Vocalization consisted of almost continuous cooing, gurgling, or baby talk. Joy was marked by striking responsivity of the infant to the experimenter.

There was no sharp dividing line between these two degrees of pleasure. In general a period of observation was classified as Joy either when the dominant behavior was as described above or when such behavior repeatedly broke through a background of contented behavior.

Irritation (Fig. 3c)

During this state Monica either had a relatively low tolerance to stimulation or was responding to disagreeable stimuli, as, for example, when intubation through the gastric stoma evoked pain or memory of pain. Under these conditions, stimuli that were ordinarily pleasurable often produced an unpleasurable effect. In this state her posture was relatively hypotonic; the legs often lay flat on the bed with the knees slightly bent. At the same time there was readiness for evasive movements, which were usually quick, slight, and jerky, with a tendency to turn away from the experimenter. Periods of muscular inac-

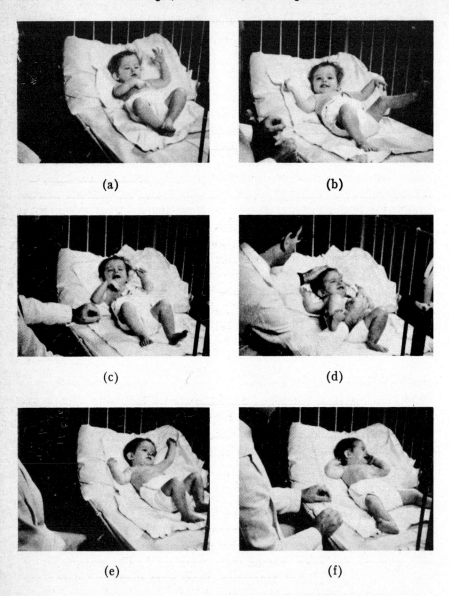

Fig. 3. Affects: (a) Contentment, (b) Joy, (c) Irritation, (d) Rage, (e) Depression, (f) Depression-Unpleasure. It is not possible to illustrate Object Relationship or Non-Nutritional Oral Behavior by photographs since evaluation of these categories depends on the sequence of behavior over a period of time. Motion pictures are the only effective means to do this. It is planned to make available soon a motion picture of the major behavioral data of this study.

tivity were interrupted by occasional self-stimulation. The facial expression was impassive, even to the usual pleasurable stimuli, or she responded with scowling or frowning. Vocalization consisted of whimpers, whines, or complaining grunts from time to time.

Rage (Fig. 3d)

This was a vigorous and sometimes violent response to an excessive stimulus, be it pain or a threat, real or anticipated. Posture was stiff and vigilant at the same time. Movements were those of vigorous resistance and evasion: she arched her back, bounced her hips, and turned from side to side. She pushed, kicked, and hit with her extremities. At times the legs extended and interlocked scissor-like while she used her whole body as a lever. The facial expression was contorted, eyes were wide open or squeezed tightly shut. At times she covered her face with her arms. Her mouth was wide open, she cried, and her face was often reddened and moistened by tears. Loud crying, high-pitched wailing, screaming, and sobbing comprised her vocalizing.

As with Joy and Contentment, at times there was no sharp line dividing Irritation and Rage, and the observation period was classified under the predominant affect.

Depression[2] (Fig. 3e)

The most striking feature of this state was the lack of movement and of any kind of activity. At the point of transition into depression, which always occurred in the presence of a stranger, movement ceased and the limbs tended to fall gravitationally. Posture remained hypotonic and flaccid; the arms were flexed along the head or body, and the legs also were in slight flexion. The extremities usually lay flat on the bed, although at times the knees were slightly elevated.

The trunk was either flat on the bed or slightly turned away from the experimenter. The head was either turned away or straight ahead. Rarely she would look toward the experimenter, sometimes without even turning her head. Either there were no bodily movements or, with less severe degree of depression, there were slight and slow movements, such as fingering inanimate objects, occasional scratching or tickling, or, rarely, turning the body and perhaps glancing at the experimenter. With severe degree of depression she closed her eyes and eventually fell asleep. When she was awake, her facial expression during this state was characteristic: the face sagged flabbily; the

---

[2] This term is used to denote the behavioral pattern of an affect which will be discussed later as the depression-withdrawal reaction. (4)

corners of the mouth were down; the inner parts of the eyebrows were elevated and the brow furrowed; all producing "the omega of melancholy." Although she was usually silent, there were occasional brief whimpers or wails.

Depression-Unpleasure (Fig. 3f)

This reaction occurred during Depression when the child could not entirely avoid external stimulation by withdrawing. Elements of the fight-flight pattern of the anxiety reaction were then superimposed upon the underlying depression. In contrast to Depression, there was more tendency to flex the thighs on the abdomen and to turn away more actively from the experimenter, positions which were regarded as self-protective. Bodily movements were evasive and resistive and included turning, pushing, and arching the back. Such movements, however, were less vigorous and less well-integrated than similar ones during the Rage response. Facial expression and vocalization included crying, wailing, whimpering, and sobbing, added to the underlying expression of depression; the brow became deeply furrowed, the face puckered, and the mouth opened in a square fashion. Occasionally there was flow of tears.

The question may be asked whether what we describe as Depression might be an anxiety state in which the child became frozen with fear instead of showing the more usual hyperkinetic response of anxiety. We investigated this possibility by recording electrocardiographically on four occasions Monica's heart rate while she exhibited the withdrawal response in the presence of a stranger. Although marked tachycardia occurred during Rage and Depression-Unpleasure, during Depression, the heart rate either did not change or slowed slightly. Figure 4 illustrates one of these experiments. We consider this additional evidence that we are not dealing here with the anxiety reaction, in the sense of a preparation for flight or fight, but with some other reaction, which we chose to call Depression-Withdrawal, a matter discussed in more detail elsewhere. (4). We do recognize that free anxiety (anxiety reaction) is indeed present in the affects of Irritation, Rage, and Depression-Unpleasure.

Mixed Affect

When an affect changed during a specimen, this was designated as *Mixed Affect*. The usual change was from Contentment to Irritation or vice versa. The 25 Mixed Affect specimens have not been included in this report; they will be considered at a later time.

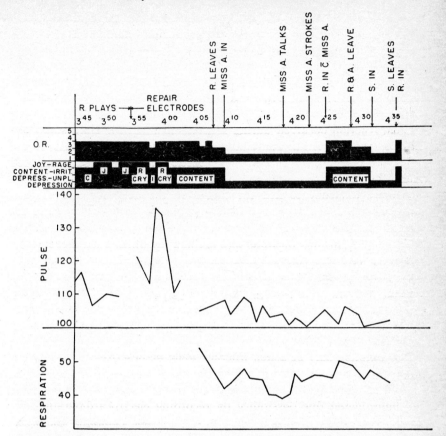

Fig. 4. Respiration and heart rate during the depression-withdrawal reaction. While there was a marked acceleration of heart rate during Rage and Irritation, both of which undoubtedly also included an element of fear, during depression there was no change or even a slight slowing. In this experiment "Miss A" and "S" were strangers, both of whom provoked the typical depression-withdrawal reaction.

Comments

The identifications from the protocols of the major affect categories — Contentment and Joy, Irritation and Rage, Depression-Unpleasure and Depression — presented no difficulties. The investigators (G. E. and F. R.), who independently categorized affects, always agreed on these major categories. There were occasional disagreements between Contentment and Joy and between Irritation and Rage. These disagreements were resolved by mutual discussion of the detailed recorded data. Audiences viewing motion pictures illustrating the various affects also found the affects readily distinguishable.

OBJECT RELATIONS (OR)

Monica's interest in things or persons in the environment, as expressed behaviorally, was classified in different degrees of object relations (ORs). We first established five such degrees but later reduced these to three when it became clear that the finer subdivisions, although easily distinguishable, did not differ materially in correspondence to the secretory data. Thus OR2 and 3 were grouped together to become OR2, and OR4 and 5 became OR3.

Object Relation 1

For the most part the child was motionless and relatively unresponsive. She did not look at the experimenter. Her eyes were often closed, and at most she glanced occasionally toward the observer. No activity could be interpreted as effort to contact the experimenter by either motor behavior or vocalization. Those activities that occurred were usually limited to small movements.

Object Relation 2

For the most part she was actively concerned with looking, examining, manipulating, dissecting, touching, or stroking such objects as a piece of gauze, a clamp, a piece of tubing, or parts of her body such as fingers, the stomal region, face, neck, feet. The motor patterns were appropriate for such activities, and her attention was largely occupied by them. Occasionally she might look toward, smile at, or even touch the experimenter, while continuing the previous activity. More often she appeared oblivious of the experimenter.

Object Relation 3

In this category the child's visual, vocal, and motor behavior all were directed predominantly towards attracting, contacting, or maintaining contact with the experimenter. These included looking, calling, smiling, reaching, touching, grasping, stroking, hitting, pushing, and kicking the experimenter. Although they were infrequent, we regarded placing her fingers in the experimenter's mouth or bringing the experimenter's fingers to her mouth as patterns indicative of high OR.

Comment

Whenever mixtures of patterns occurred during the period corresponding to a specimen of gastric juice, the evaluation was based on the pattern that predominated. The commonest mixture was OR2 and

3. Much less common were occasions when OR1 included short periods of OR2, usually in the form of manipulation of some inanimate object; or mixtures of OR1 and OR3, when the activity of the experimenter evoked evasive movements or struggling. There were few disagreements between the two investigators in their judgments of degrees of Object Relation.

NON-NUTRITIONAL ORAL BEHAVIOR (NNOB)

Mouth activities not related to actual ingestion of food were classified in three categories:

NNOB1 — There was no (or only fleeting) oral behavior during the period of observation.

NNOB2 — The behavior during the observation period fell between NNOB1 and NNOB3.

NNOB3 — At least half the period was occupied with vigorous oral activity, or there was some kind of oral activity during the entire period.

Those classified as oral were activities in which the mouth and adjacent structures alone were involved, such as smacking, sucking, licking, protruding tongue, swallowing, and biting; activities involving fingers or hands and mouth, or objects and mouth, such as touching of lips, teeth, tongue or buccal mucosa, sucking, chewing, biting, and licking. In rare instances there was biting of the favored experimenter's finger, which was always classified as NNOB3.

Comment

There were no disagreements between the identification of NNOB1 as compared to NNOB2 and NNOB3. Disagreements in the judgment of NNOB2 and NNOB3 were few because the duration of oral activity was generally quite accurately recorded.

SLEEP

We classified sleeping periods by (a) depth and (b) the setting. In the latter category we differentiated between *Fatigue Sleep* and *Withdrawal Sleep* on the basis of the following criteria. *Fatigue Sleep* was preceded by yawning, stretching, scratching, seeking a comfortable position, and resisting any disturbance of this comfortable position. After the eyes had begun to close, they reopened only infrequently for an occasional glance. There was a gradual, fluctuating reduction of spontaneous activity preceding sleep, and the affects preceding it were those other than Depression or Depression-Unpleasure.

A relative lack of yawning, stretching, and sleep positioning preceded
Withdrawal Sleep. After the eyes had closed, they would reopen frequently to glance. During this period there was often a sustained, if
quite low, level of activity. The preceding affect was Depression or
Depression-Unpleasure.

In classifying depth of sleep, we regarded arbitrarily as Deep Sleep
all periods during which either no motor activity occurred or not more
than one movement in five minutes. If there was any more activity
the period was classified as Light Sleep.

The first specimen obtained after falling asleep was not included
under *Sleep* unless Monica had been asleep for 10 minutes or longer.

Comment

There was no disagreement between the two investigators in their
independent judgment of depth and kind of sleep.

NON-NUTRITIONAL FEEDING EXPERIENCES (NNF)

Two procedures were followed in observing the responses to feeding
situations in which food did not reach the stomach.

Sham Feeding — Lollipops and crackers were given by mouth, and
the swallowed material was extruded through the esophageal fistula.

Bottle — The baby was shown or permitted to handle a bottle of
her formula that was tightly stoppered so that no contents entered the

TABLE 1. Sample Protocol

Experiment #30   January 14, 1954

Spec.	Time	Observed Behavior	Affect	OR	NNOB	Sleep
	10:16	On E4. M lying on back, knees drawn up. Right hand holding toy, left hand fingering neck. Watches us thru glass partition. Puts both hands to toy. Lies relatively motionless.				
	10:19	Doctors on rounds. M watches.				
	10:21	R arrives. m. stretches legs out to him and smiles. She smiles at him. Exchange. Waves legs at R. R busy getting ready. Lowers bars. M reaches with arms and legs and smiles. R undressing M.				
	12:23	R takes off dressing. She whimpers a little. Watches him prepare tube. Finger at corner of mouth. Then beside head. R tries out glass electrode. M gives a little cry. R pleased and says it will work. M watches.				

TABLE 1. (*Continued*)

Spec.	Time	Observed Behavior	Affect	OR	NNOB	Sleep
#1	10:26	R inserts tube. Gives M paper. She picks up scissors and drops paper.				
	10:26	Specimen. Playing with scissors. Miss D comes in view. M raises arms and legs to her. Miss D walks away. She looks after her. Tongue out. Moves restlessly. Pushes R's hands with foot. Crosses right leg on knee.				
	10:29	Holding scissors. Watching group behind glass. R takes her foot down and she kicks him. Holds scissors up. She smiles and coos. R cos. Smiles broadly. Bites on lower lip, M heads voices and looks behind her. Tongue out. Babies crying.	Content	3	2	—
	10:31	End specimen. Reaching. Tongue out. Finger in mouth. Both hands on mouth. Watching R who had taken scissors. R gives scissors back and after a few seconds takes them out.				
#2	10:33	Specimen. M playing with scissors. Talking — smiles. Hears nurses and looks behind her. Holds scissors in right hand and touches syringe and tube with left. Holds scissors up with both hands. Holds right foot up. Tongue out. Miss D next cubicle. M smiles and reaches toward her. D turns back and M smiles and attends to scissors. D looks at her — they exchange smiles. Smiles at R. Tongue out. Smiles at D. Holds foot up.				
	10:37	Waves hand. Half smile. Wawawa. R answers. Smiles and laughs. R laughs. Miss D talks and she smiles. Handling scissors. Miss D looks and she grins and reaches. She puts scissors in mouth. Chews on them. Miss D reappears. M looks at her — back to her. Continues to chew on scissors. Raises foot toward D. D leaves without looking. She waves foot. Turns scissors around and puts handle in mouth. Smiles at R. He responds. Kicks at syringe. Holds it with left hand. Bites intermittently on scissors.	Joy	3	2	—
	10:41	Puts it to side. Drops it. Tongue out. R gives her paper which she holds up. Leg up in air. Pulls at paper. Looks at R. Eh. R answers and she smiles. Awawawa. Pulls up kimono. Pulling at paper. Babies crying.				
	10:43	End specimen.				
	11:15	In R-146. HS takes over. She looks wide-eyed.				

TABLE 1. (*Continued*)

Spec.	Time	Observed Behavior	Affect	OR	NNOB	Sleep
	11:16	In R-151. M looks wide-eyed. Eyebrows raised. Stares. S comes over. M begins to cry. Frowns. Omega. Hands up. Continues cry. S talks.				
	11:18	She cries vigorously. Tube in.				
#5	11:19	Specimen. M quiet. Staring. Eyebrows raised. Hands beside head. Corners of mouth down. Looks to window. M looks up at S. Frowns. Eh. S answers. Whimper. Holding gauze. S makes noise and she startles. Tube out. Whimpers with tube in. Looks at S. Picks up metal, fingering it. Drops it. Picks up gauze. She whimpers. Red in face.	Depression-Unpleasure	2	1	—
	11:26	End specimen. Watches S. Playing with gauze. 3¾ cc. cloudy bile. S talking to us.				
#7	11:47	Specimen. Looks to window. Looks back to S, stares at him. Looks to window. Staring with slight frown. Looks back. She sighs. Lying quietly. Looks toward S. Hands beside head, legs down. Arched brow. Stares at S. No movement, closing eyes. Eyes closed.	Depression	1	1	—
	11:53	Now is asleep. S says OK. End specimen. M awakens and looks at S. 4½ cc. bile stained. "Eh." Folds arms.				
#8	11:54	Tube in. M whimpers and turns away from S. Cries as S manipulates. Lying on right with left arm over face. Staring toward window. Feet crossed. Lies motionless. Staring — eyes closed — open.				
	11:57	Turns back toward S. Arms out. Closing eyes. Intermittent open and closed, but more closed.	Depression	1	1	—
	11:59	Asleep.				
	12:05	Asleep — turns to right.				
	12:06	End specimen. S talks to us. She doesn't move, opens and closes eyes. Turns to left as S moves about. Puts crib side up and leaves. She looks toward door.				

mouth. Monica was accustomed to seeing her formula before receiving it through the fistula.

The specimens following non-nutritional feeding experiences were not included in the analysis of the behavioral categories in the fasting state.

Table 1 is a sample protocol of primary behavioral data and the corresponding analysis. We realize the inadequacy of providing such a small sample of our raw behavioral data. It is our intention to include all behavioral protocols when the completed study is published as a monograph.

RESULTS

SOME TYPICAL OBSERVATIONS

From the total of 59 observation periods we present four as representative.

Observation #43 (Fig. 5) illustrates spontaneous behavior in the laboratory with the favored experimenter. During the first 1½ hours the predominant affects were Contentment and Joy, Object Relation was mostly high, and there was intermittent Non-Nutritional Oral Behavior. During this period the rate of total hydrochloric acid secretion rose, and free acid appeared. Toward the end of this first period the baby became sleepy and then feel into a light sleep. With this the secretion of acid decreased markedly. During the 28-minute sleep the observer and experimenter disagreed as to how long to continue. The experimenter, who had a 1:00 P.M. appointment, wished to stop for lunch; the observer wished to secure data on the awakening period. The observer prevailed and the experimenter, somewhat disgruntled, resumed

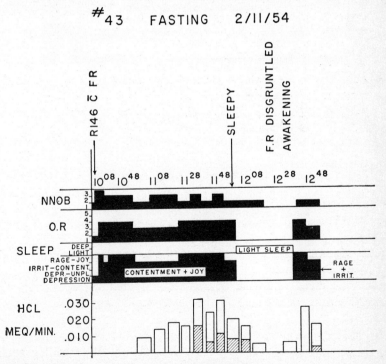

Fig. 5. Experiment #43: See text for description.

aspirating gastric juice. When the baby awakened, t̶h̶e̶ ̶e̶x̶p̶e̶r̶i̶m̶e̶n̶t̶e̶r̶ ̶w̶a̶s̶ ̶r̶e̶l̶a̶t̶i̶v̶e̶l̶y̶ ̶u̶n̶c̶o̶m̶m̶u̶n̶i̶c̶a̶t̶i̶v̶e̶,̶ ̶t̶e̶n̶d̶e̶d̶ ̶t̶o̶ ̶b̶e̶ ̶b̶u̶s̶i̶n̶e̶s̶s̶-̶l̶i̶k̶e̶ ̶a̶n̶d̶ ̶i̶m̶p̶e̶r̶-̶ ̶s̶o̶n̶a̶l̶ ̶i̶n̶ ̶c̶o̶l̶l̶e̶c̶t̶i̶n̶g̶ ̶t̶h̶e̶ ̶s̶p̶e̶c̶i̶m̶e̶n̶,̶ ̶a̶n̶d̶ ̶w̶a̶s̶ ̶r̶e̶l̶a̶t̶i̶v̶e̶l̶y̶ ̶s̶e̶r̶i̶o̶u̶s̶ ̶a̶n̶d̶ ̶u̶n̶s̶m̶i̶l̶-̶ ̶i̶n̶g̶.̶ ̶A̶s̶ ̶t̶h̶e̶ ̶b̶a̶b̶y̶ ̶r̶e̶s̶p̶o̶n̶d̶e̶d̶ ̶w̶i̶t̶h̶ ̶R̶a̶g̶e̶ ̶a̶n̶d̶ ̶I̶r̶r̶i̶t̶a̶t̶i̶o̶n̶,̶ ̶s̶e̶c̶r̶e̶t̶i̶o̶n̶ ̶o̶f̶ ̶a̶c̶i̶d̶ ̶i̶n̶c̶r̶e̶a̶s̶e̶d̶ ̶s̶h̶a̶r̶p̶l̶y̶.̶

Observation #47 (Fig. 6) illustrates the typical behavior with a stranger. C̶o̶n̶t̶e̶n̶t̶ ̶a̶n̶d̶ ̶o̶u̶t̶g̶o̶i̶n̶g̶ ̶f̶o̶r̶ ̶t̶h̶e̶ ̶f̶i̶r̶s̶t̶ ̶1̶0̶ ̶m̶i̶n̶u̶t̶e̶s̶ ̶w̶i̶t̶h̶ ̶t̶h̶e̶ ̶f̶a̶v̶o̶r̶e̶d̶ ̶e̶x̶p̶e̶r̶i̶m̶e̶n̶t̶e̶r̶,̶ ̶s̶h̶e̶ ̶l̶a̶p̶s̶e̶d̶ ̶i̶n̶t̶o̶ ̶t̶h̶e̶ ̶D̶e̶p̶r̶e̶s̶s̶i̶o̶n̶-̶W̶i̶t̶h̶d̶r̶a̶w̶a̶l̶ ̶s̶t̶a̶t̶e̶ ̶w̶h̶e̶n̶ ̶t̶h̶e̶ ̶s̶t̶r̶a̶n̶g̶e̶ ̶e̶x̶p̶e̶r̶i̶m̶e̶n̶t̶e̶r̶ ̶a̶r̶r̶i̶v̶e̶d̶ ̶t̶o̶ ̶t̶a̶k̶e̶ ̶h̶e̶r̶ ̶t̶o̶ ̶t̶h̶e̶ ̶l̶a̶b̶o̶r̶a̶t̶o̶r̶y̶.̶ During

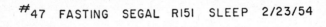

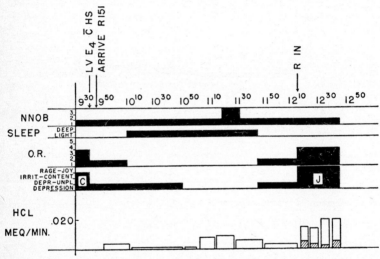

Fig. 6. Experiment #47: See text for description.

the entire period with this experimenter she remained relatively motionless, turned away from the experimenter; her facial expression was sad. The affect was Depression and the Object Relation was 1. There was no Non-Nutritional Oral Behavior. She closed her eyes; in about 30 minutes she was asleep and remained asleep for 96 minutes. The secretion of acid was extremely low until the last 30 minutes of sleep, during which there was a slight rise; during this last 30 minutes of sleep there was active sucking. Upon awakening and finding the stranger still present, she remained in the Depressed-Withdrawn state and gastric secretion again fell to very low levels. With the return of the favored experimenter there was a joyful response and a prompt and sustained rise in the rate of acid secretion.

Observation #45 (Fig. 7) also illustrates response to a stranger. It is of interest that the same response of Depression-Withdrawal was elicited and the rate of acid secretion was strikingly reduced; however, very active sucking behavior developed during the sleep period and acid secretion rose notably. Before her awakening the secretion of acid again diminished. After awakening the baby remained in the depressed state, but now made cautious overtures to the stranger. These consisted of slight rubbing and touching movements of her foot and hand. Although the experimenter did not respond, the secretion of acid increased.

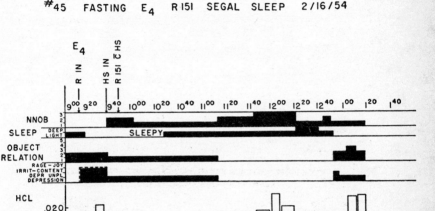

Fig. 7. Experiment #45: See text for description.

Observation #46 (Fig. 8) illustrates the high secretion of acid during a period of sustained Irritation and Rage. For reasons that were not clear, Monica had been fretful and irritable for two days. The skin around the stoma appeared somewhat reddened and may have been sensitive. The experimenter was firm in overcoming Monica's resistance to intubation. She responded with a vigorous rage reaction alternating with periods of irritation. When no aspiration was attempted, she was relatively content. The rate of hydrochloric acid secretion was high.

AFFECTS

Figure 9 illustrates the range of rates of total hydrochloric acid secretion in m.eg./min. during the six affects. Each circle represents the rate of total hydrochloric acid secretion in one specimen of gastric juice collected during the period of the affect noted on the left. N refers to the total number of samples in each category. Mw is the mean secretory rate corrected for the mean collection time in each category.

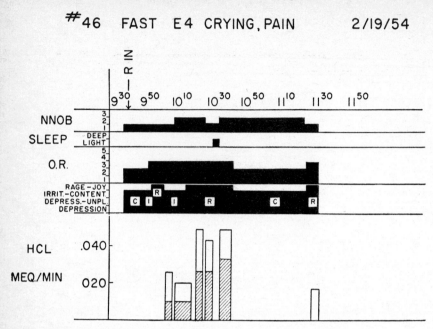

Fig. 8. Experiment #46: See text for description.

While there is considerable spread within each affect, the data reveal that the secretion was lowest during Depression (Mw=.007±.001 m. eq./min.; N=31) and highest during Rage (Mw=.027 ±.003; N=28). Statistical analysis by t-test[3] shows that the mean rate during Depression was significantly less than during all other affects. These differences are significant at .01—.001 levels, except for that with Depression-Unpleasure, which is significant only at the .02 level. The mean rate during Rage was significantly higher than the mean rates during all other affects. The significance again is at the .01—.001 levels except for the differences between Irritation and Rage which are significant only at the .02 level.

There were no statistically significant differences between rates of hydrochloric acid secretion during Irritation, Depression-Unpleasure, Contentment and Joy.

OBJECT RELATIONS

These data are presented in Fig. 10. This reveals that the mean rate of total hydrochloric acid secretion during OR1 (Mw=.006±.001;

[3] We are grateful for advice on statistical methods to Dr. S. Lee Crump, Associate Professor of Radiation Biology and Chief of Section (Statistics), Atomic Energy Project, University of Rochester.

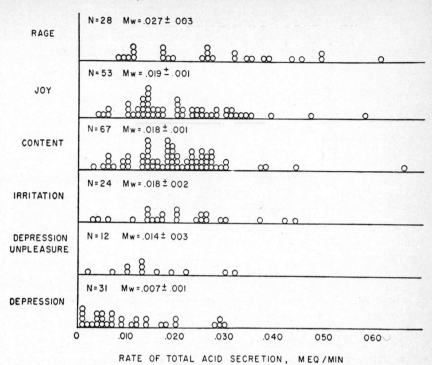

Fig. 9. Rates of total hydrochloric acid secretion in m.eq./min. during the various affects. Each circle represents one specimen of gastric juice. N = the number of specimens. Mw = the mean weighted for the duration of the specimen. See text for significance of results.

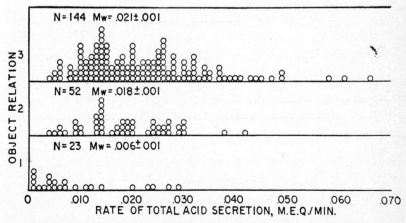

Fig. 10. Rates of total HCl secretion in m.eq./min. and object relations (OR). See Fig. 9 and text for description of symbols and significance of results.

$N=23$) is significantly less than during OR2 and OR3 ($P<$0.001). The mean rates for OR2 and OR3 were .018±.001 and .021±.001 m. eq./min., respectively, a difference not statistically significant at the 5% level (t=1.82; P=0.05—0.1).

SLEEP (Fig. 11)

The rate of secretion of total hydrochloric acid was significantly less during sleep than during any wakeful state except during Depression

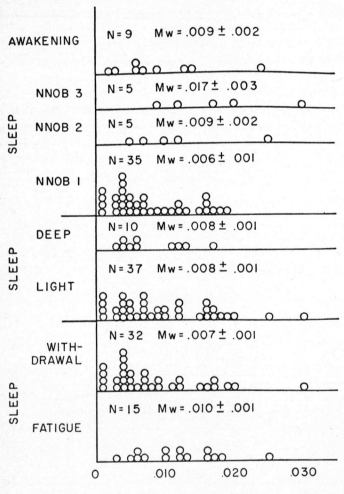

RATE OF TOTAL ACID SECRETION, M.EQ./MIN

Fig. 11. Rates of total hydrochloric acid secretion during sleep. See text and Fig. 9 for description of symbols and for significance of results.

and Object Relation 1. There was no difference in secretion rates during light sleep and deep sleep. The secretion rate was less during sleep coming on during the Depressed-Withdrawal state (.007±.001 m. eq./min.) than during sleep coming on as part of the pattern of fatigue (0.010± .001 m. eq./min.), but this difference is not statistically significant (P<0.1). Since much higher rates of secretion generally preceded Sleep-Fatigue, in comparison with Sleep-Withdrawal, this difference may merely reflect a lag.

When we classified sleep specimens according to the amount of Non-Nutritional Oral Behavior during the sleep, we found a highly significant difference (P<0.001) between hydrochloric acid secretion rates during periods of active sucking (Sleep-NNOB3 = .017±.001 m. eq./min.) in comparison with those with no sucking (Sleep-NNOB1 = .006±.001 m. eq./min.). This was already illustrated in Figs. 6 and 7.

In two experiments we were able to secure a continuous record of intragastric pH by placing within the stomach a glass electrode and a salt bridge extension of the calomel electrode. The pH was recorded on a Photovolt pH meter. As illustrated in Fig. 12, when the baby fell asleep

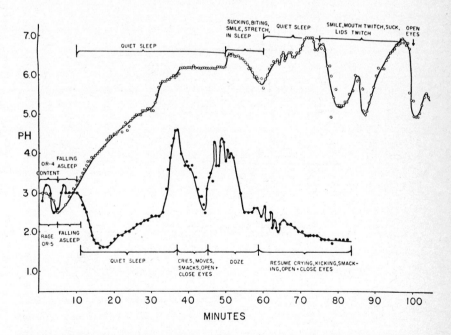

Fig. 12. Intragastric pH changes as measured by a glass electrode placed directly in the stomach. See text for description. It should be noted that pH is not charted on a semi-logarithmic scale and hence the fluctuations at the higher pH levels are relatively exaggerated.

there was a fairly rapid rise in pH, after a lag of 10–20 minutes, corresponding to the affect preceding sleep. Then with sucking and other activity during sleep there were rapid decreases in pH, such fluctuations occurring until the baby awakened.

HISTAMINE

Histamine diphosphate, in doses of 0.1 mg. per 10 Kg. body weight, was administered subcutaneously on nine different occasions. A striking correlation was found between the amount of acid secreted in response to this drug and the behavioral state of the infant. As illustrated in Fig. 13, when the baby was outgoing and relating actively to the experimenter, pleasurably or unpleasurably, the stomach secreted large amounts of hydrochloric acid in the 55 minutes after histamine administration, the total secretion ranging from 1.52–2.39 m. eq. On the other hand, when she was depressed, withdrawn, or asleep, the same quantities of histamine were noted to have little or no effect. Total secretions were 0.16–0.68 m. eq. in 55 minutes, values which did not differ from those obtained in comparable behavioral states without histamine. The high rates, on the other hand, were considerably greater than those observed during comparable behavioral situations without histamine.

TABLE 2. TOTAL HCl — RATES OF SECRETION, MEQ./MIN.

Bottle	.039 ± .003	Depression-Unpleasure	0.14 ± .003
Sham Feeding	.035 ± .004	Sleep-Fatigue	.010 ± .001
Rage	.027 ± .003	Sleep-NNOB2	.009 ± .002
Object Relation 3	.021 ± .001	Sleep-Light	.008 ± .001
Cry 2	.021 ± .002	Sleep-Deep	.008 ± .001
Joy	.019 ± .001	Depression	.007 ± .001
Contentment	.018 ± .001	Sleep-Withdrawal	.007 ± .001
Irritation	.018 ± .002	Awakening	.007 ± .002
Object Relation 2	.018 ± .001	Object Relation 1	.006 ± .001
Cry	.017 ± .001	Sleep-NNOB1	.006 ± .001
Sleep-NNOB3	.017 ± .001	Depression-Sleep	.003 ± .001

RANGE OF TOTAL HYDROCHLORIC ACID SECRETION RATES

Table 2 illustrates the mean fasting secretion rates of hydrochloric acid during the conditions so far analyzed. The highest mean rates occurred during sham feeding (0.035±.003 m. eq./min.) and feeding with the bottle of formula that she did not taste (0.039±.004 m. eq./min.).

It is noteworthy that individual specimens with higher secretion rates than those observed during sham feeding or feeding with the bottle occasionally occurred during Rage, Irritation, Contentment, Joy and OR3. In these four affect categories there were 19 specimens (out of 172) in

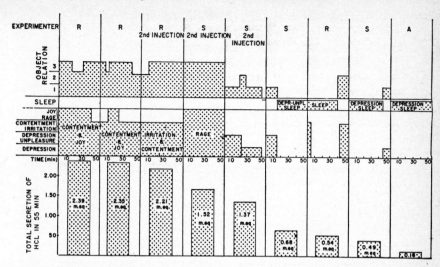

Fig. 13. Effect of histamine: Secretion is recorded as the output of total HCl in m.eq. in the 55 minutes after the histamine administration. When arranged in order of decreasing amounts, secretion is greatest in the outgoing states and least in the withdrawn states.

which secretion rates ranged from .035 to .066 m. eq./min. In OR3 there were 18 specimens out of 144 in which secretion rates were in excess of 0.035 m. eq./min. In other words, the rates of secretion were consistently high in response to sham feeding and the bottle; however, sustained, active outgoing states were occasionally accompanied by secretion rates of a comparable order.

The lowest secretion rates occurred during the depressed, withdrawn state and during sleep. Rates of less than 0.001 m. eq./min. occurred occasionally during the sleep of the Depression-Withdrawal reaction, representing for all practical purposes a cessation of gastric secretion.

The table clearly indicates that when rates of gastric secretion are listed from the highest to the lowest, the corresponding behavioral processes fall from the most active and outgoing to the most withdrawn and inactive.

Discussion

We are aware that it is both tempting and hazardous to generalize from the study of a single infant. The detailed study of the single subject provides valuable information on the laws governing biological processes within that individual, but a different design is necessary to establish the range of variability of the same processes within a population. In this study we deal with a relatively unique individual, a baby born without continuity between mouth and stomach, who was fed for the first two years of her life through an opening in the abdominal wall. Food taken by mouth leaked out of an esophageal fistula in the neck. It is evident that this infant differs in a number of ways from infants without such a defect and that these differences in original endowment and in life experience resulting therefrom must be significant factors in her general development. In this sense she is a member of a population of infants who share the same defects and who may be studied as a group. On the other hand, she also shares many more qualities with infants not so afflicted and, therefore, can be viewed as part of the population of human infants. In discussing the findings of this investigation, the most reliable interpretations will be those that apply only to this one infant. Yet we will call attention to ways in which the data for this infant conform with, as well as differ from, data and concepts obtained from other sources, infant and adult. It remains for future study to establish their general validity.

Although many factors not investigated in this study undoubtedly influenced the rate of secretion of hydrochloric acid by the stomach in the fasting state (this is indicated by the wide spread of values in each behavioral category), it is nonetheless evident that gastric secretion was intimately integrated with the total behavioral activity of this infant. When the child withdrew and her activity was low, as during the Depression-Withdrawal state and sleep, there was marked reduction, at times almost cessation, of hydrochloric acid production. When she related actively to the experimenter, be it with pleasure or anger, the rate of hydrochloric acid secretion rose. The *highest* mean secretion rate occurred during Rage, during which state she related most actively to the object in the environment and during which she appeared to have the least control over instinctual drives. Another situation that regularly evoked very active secretion was reunion with the favored experimenter after a period with a stranger. Under these circumstances hydrochloric acid secretion rates were sometimes as high as those during sham feeding. Even in sleep, during which the rate of acid secretion regularly diminished, sucking and other oral activity were accompanied by a highly significant increase in secretion. We interpret this behavior during sleep as expressing a returning contact with the outside world or its mental representations, that is, either awakening or dreaming.

These data suggest that in this infant, at the level of development at which she was studied, the processes whereby relationships with objects in the external world are established include a general intaking, assimilative organization in which the stomach participates as if the intention is also to take objects into it. In other words, along with other behavioral activities, such as reaching, touching, grasping, looking, hitting, pushing, kicking, all of which take very active cognizance of the object in the environment, the stomach also behaves as though preparing for food, as if that which is in external world is literally to be ingested and digested.

We also regard these findings as evidence that the oral phase of development in the infant, as postulated by Freud, is indeed accompanied by corresponding physiologic activity of the stomach. Further, it would seem that such an oral phase represents not a behavioral organization that is necessarily dependent on the continuity of the connection between mouth and stomach, but rather a total assimilative pattern that includes activities in the service of feeding and the organs associated therewith. From this it appears that the genesis of early object relations includes an assimilative process, largely orally organized. The processes concerned in establishing mental representations of objects and their libidinal and/or aggressive cathexes involve an essentially oral, intaking model. In Monica the secretion rates of hydrochloric acid paralleled in a highly significant way the other behavioral expressions of object cathexes, libidinal or aggressive. Such a finding was predicted from the discoveries of psychoanalysis; whether this is a general phenomenon remains to be established from the study of a series of infants within the first year of life. Theoretically we would predict that this close correlation between gastric secretion and behavioral processes would diminish with further development of the mental apparatus. Whether regression to the oral phase in later life would also involve the corresponding physiological regression, a suggestion by Alexander for the pathogenesis of peptic ulcer, remains to be demonstrated experimentally. (6)

Whether the increased gastric secretion may be merely part of a general increase in the physiological activity of the body and not have the specific meaning we have proposed cannot be settled from a consideration of the data of this study. There is evidence, however, that vigorous muscular activity is usually associated with a decrease rather than an increase in acid secretion. (7) Further clarification may be obtained by studying gastric secretion at a later level of development and by studying other physiological systems not directly involved in intaking, assimilative processes.

The results indicate also that at the level of development of this infant affect may be regarded as the behavioral expression of instinct. In the relatively undeveloped ego one is able to see undisguised the attempts at discharge, e.g. instinct gratification. Here one might distinguish between attempts at tension reduction related to external objects and their mental representations (contentment, joy, irritation and rage), which are accompanied by patterned motor activity and augmented gas-

tric secretion; and attempts at tension reduction of a narcissistic type
(the Depression-Withdrawal reaction and sleep), in which muscular
hypotonia, inactivity, and reduction of gastric secretion predominate.
Other physiologic systems were not studied, but it was certainly established that the stomach participated in a major way in instinct expression, a phenomenon also predicted by psychoanalytic theory.

No less interesting than the data indicating that the oral phase has
its physiological counterpart, is the indication of the existence of a relatively objectless, narcissistic phase in which secretory activity of the
stomach largely ceases. In the Depression-Withdrawal reaction, as described above, there is a profound withdrawal of interest and activity
in relation to the external world. This invariably occurred when the
baby was confronted with a stranger. A more detailed consideration of
the genetic dynamic background of this reaction will be published elsewhere. (4) Suffice it to say we believe that this reaction developed out of
significant disturbances in the mother-child relationship in the first year
of life, interfering seriously with the baby's capacity to tolerate object
loss. As described in the history, she suffered two depressions in the first
15 months, variants of what Spitz has called "anaclitic depression." (8)
Both occurred in response to attenuations of the mother-child relationship and were alleviated by the establishment of more secure and satisfying object relationships in the hospital. Thereafter Monica responded,
when confronted by a stranger, with the same mechanisms used in the
earlier anaclitic depressions, withdrawing cathexes from the external
world and from the systems concerned with it. The end result was a
state of sleep, a narcissistic withdrawal with a reinstatement of the
heightened stimulus barrier of the neonatal or fetal state. During this
situation, as well as during natural sleep, secretion of acid by the stomach greatly diminished.

We interpret this to mean that when cathexes are withdrawn from
the external world, when the child no longer seeks contact with persons
in the environment and withdraws interest, not only does she abandon
use of the motor system, as evidenced by the hypotonia and immobility,
but also she behaves as if nothing is to be taken into the stomach. This
is in contrast to the observation in the outgoing affective states described
above. However, the last statement should not be interpreted to mean
that the baby now decides nothing is to be taken into the stomach, an
adultomorphic interpretation, but rather that a state of organismic organization exists, in which things are not taken into the stomach, a
pre-oral organization. Such a state, of course, existed during fetal life,
when nutrition was achieved passively through the umbilical circulation, and it perhaps is perpetuated to varying degrees in the biological
withdrawals of sleep, even in the adult. Greene has suggested the term

"umbilical stage." (9) As one of us has developed elsewhere, biologic process, and action precede the development of mental representations thereof, and therefore these data mainly point to the biologic anlage of processes that may later have psychologic expression. (10)

Clinical and theoretical considerations have also led us to suggest that what we are calling the Depression-Withdrawal reaction represents an early developmental phase of depression, the anlage, so to speak, for depressive patterns of later life. Originating in a setting of helplessness unduly prolonged and accentuated by disturbances in the mother-child symbiosis, the reaction is reprovoked with exquisite regularity when the infant is threatened, through object loss, with a reactivation of the original shock state of helplessness. This fits well with the concepts of primal depression. The clinical manifestations are those concordant with the development of this child. Later libido and ego developments and the formation of superego add important features to adult depressions, not to be expected in infantile depression. (4)

Finally, we wish to call attention to the remarkable reduction in the response to histamine in the Depression-Withdrawal reaction and in sleep. This suggests an alteration in physiological mechanisms and may provide an opportunity to elucidate some physiological processes in narcissistic states. This matter is now under investigation in our laboratory.

SUMMARY AND CONCLUSIONS

1. Gastric secretory, psychological, and behavioral observations were carried out in 59 experiments in an infant (with a gastric fistula) from the age of 15 to 20 months. Of a number of observed physiological variables, only the total hydrochloric acid secretion rate is considered in this paper.

2. The total hydrochloric acid secretion rate was intimately integrated with the total behavioral activity of the infant.

3. Outgoing affective states, be they libidinal or aggressive, were associated with rising rates of hydrochloric acid secretion.

4. During the Depression-Withdrawal reaction, characterized by sad facies, muscular flaccidity, inactivity, and withdrawal from the outside world, progressing into sleep in the more severe instances, there was a marked decrease in or even cessation of hydrochloric acid secretion.

5. The more active transactions with the environment were associated with rising hydrochloric acid secretion rates.

6. Histamine effect on gastric secretion during the Depression-Withdrawal state was slight or absent, whereas during outgoing states histamine proved to be a potent stimulant of hydrochloric acid secretion. This suggests the possibility of an altered organization at the cellular level under these two conditions.

7. These results support the psychoanalytic concept that, at this level of development, the establishment of object representations involves an oral, intaking model. Our study lends support to the concept of an oral stage of development: as the infant related outgoingly to an experimenter, be it aggressively or libidinally, her gastric glands reacted as if introjection of the cathected object was to take place. We want to emphasize that *our conclusions apply to this particular infant at this particular stage of development* and that generalizations should be made only with caution.

8. The Depression-Withdrawal reaction appeared to be a particular mode of the infant to object loss, the pattern for which had been established by her previous depressions as observed on two admissions to the hospital. The genetic dynamic background of this reaction, which may represent a regression to a preoral stage of development, will be considered extensively in a separate communication. (4)

REFERENCES

1. Wolf, S., and Wolff, H. G. *Human Gastric Function.* New York, Oxford University Press, 1943.

2. Margolin, S. G. The Behavior of the stomach during psychoanalysis. *Psychoanalyt. Quart.* 20: 349, 1951.

3. Wolf, S., and Wolff, H. G. See references above.

4. Engel, G. L., and Reichsman, F. Spontaneous and experimentally induced depressions in an infant with a gastric fistula: A contribution to the problem of depression. *Am. J. Psychoanalysis* 4, 1956.

5. Darwin, C. The Expression of Emotions in *Man and Animals.* 1872 (New Edition, Philosophical Library, New York, 1955).

6. Alexander, F. The influence of psychologic factors upon gastrointestinal disturbances: A symposium I. General principles, objectives, and preliminary results. *Psychoanalyt. Quart.* 3: 501, 1934.

7. Hammar, S., and Obrink, K. J. The inhibitory effect of muscular exercise on gastric secretion. *Acta physiol. Scandinav.* 28: 152, 1953.

8. Spitz, R. Anaclitic depression. *Psychoanalyt. Study of Child* 2: 313, 1946.

9. Greene, W. A., Jr. Process in psychosomatic disorders. *Psychosom. Med.* 18: 150, 1956.

10. Engel, G. L. Homeostasis, Behavioral Adjustment and the Concept of Health and Disease in Grinker, R. *Mid-Century Psychiatry.* Springfield, Ill., Charles C Thomas, 1953.

7

THE MAMMAL AND HIS ENVIRONMENT

D. O. HEBB, Ph.D.
Montreal, Canada

The original intention in this paper was to discuss the significance of neurophysiological theory for psychiatry and psychology, and to show, by citing the work done by some of my colleagues, that the attempt to get at the neural mechanisms of behavior can stimulate and clarify purely behavioral — that is, psychiatric and psychological — thinking. The research to be described has, I think, a clear relevance to clinical problems; but its origin lay in efforts to learn how the functioning of individual neurons and synapses relates to the functions of the whole brain, and to understand the physiological nature of learning, emotion, thinking, or intelligence.

In the end, however, my paper has simply become a review of the research referred to, dealing with the relation of the mammal to his environment. The question concerns the normal variability of the sensory environment and this has been studied from two points of view. First, one may ask what the significance of perceptual activity is during growth; for this purpose one can rear an animal with a considerable degree of restriction, and see what effects there are upon mental development. Secondly, in normal animals whose development is complete, one can remove a good deal of the supporting action of the normal environment, to discover how far the animal continues to be dependent on it even after maturity.

THE ROLE OF THE ENVIRONMENT DURING GROWTH

The immediate background of our present research on the intelligence and personality of the dog is the work of Hymovitch (6) on the intelligence of rats. He reared laboratory rats in 2 ways: (a) in a psychologically restricted environment, a small cage, with food and water always at hand and plenty of opportunity for exercise (in an activity wheel), but with no problems to solve, no need of getting on with others, no pain; and (b) in a "free" environment, a large box with obstacles to pass, blind alleys to avoid, other rats to get on with, and thus ample opportunity for problem-solving and great need for learning during

From *The American Journal of Psychiatry*, 11:826, 1955.

growth. Result: the rats brought up in a psychologically restricted (but biologically adequate) environment have a lasting inferiority in problem-solving. This does not mean, of course, that environment is everything, heredity nothing: here heredity was held constant, which prevents it from affecting the results. When the reverse experiment is done we find problem-solving varying with heredity instead. The *same* capacity for problem-solving is fully dependent on both variables for its development.

To take this further, Thompson and others have been applying similar methods to dogs (9). The same intellectual effect of an impoverished environment is found again, perhaps more marked in the higher species. But another kind of effect can be seen in dogs, which have clearly marked personalities. Personality — by which I mean complex individual differences of emotion and motivation — is again strongly affected by the infant environment. These effects, however, are hard to analyze, and I cannot at present give any rounded picture of them.

First, observations during the rearing itself are significant. A Scottish terrier is reared in a small cage, in isolation from other Scotties and from the human staff. Our animal man, William Ponman, is a dog lover and undertook the experiment with misgivings, which quickly disappeared. In a cage 30 by 30 inches, the dogs are "happy as larks," eat more than normally reared dogs, grow well, are physically vigorous: as Ponman says, "I never saw such healthy dogs — they're like bulls." If you put a normally-reared dog into such a cage, shut off from everything, his misery is unmistakable, and we have not been able to bring ourselves to continue such experiments. Not so the dog that has known nothing else. Ponman showed some of these at a dog show of national standing, winning first-prize ribbons with them.

Observations by Dr. Ronald Melzack on pain are extremely interesting. He reared 2 dogs, after early weaning, in complete isolation, taking care that there was little opportunity for experience of pain (unless the dog bit himself). At maturity, when the dogs were first taken out for study, they were extraordinarily excited, with random, rapid movement. As a result they got their tails or paws stepped on repeatedly — but paid no attention to an event that would elicit howls from a normally reared dog. After a few days, when their movements were calmer, they were tested with an object that gave electric shock, and paid little attention to it. Through 5 testing periods, one dog repeatedly thrust his nose into a lighted match; and months later, did the same thing several times with a lighted cigar.

A year and a half after coming out of restriction they are still hyperactive. Clipping and trimming one of them is a 2-man job; if the normal dog does not stand still, a cuff on the ear will remind him of his duty;

but cuffing the experimental dog "has as much effect as if you patted him — except he pays no attention to it." It seems certain, especially in view of the related results reported by Nissen, Chow, and Semmes (7) for a chimpanzee, that the adult's perception of pain is essentially a function of pain experience during growth — and that what we call pain is not a single sensory quale but a complex mixture of a particular kind of synthesis with past learning and emotional disturbance.

Nothing bores the dogs reared in restriction. At an "open house," we put 2 restricted dogs in one enclosure, 2 normal ones in another, and asked the public to tell us which were the normal. Without exception, they picked out the 2 alert, lively, interested animals — not the lackadaisical pair lying in the corner, paying no attention to the visitors. The alert pair, actually, were the restricted; the normal dogs had seen all they wanted to see of the crowd in the first 2 minutes, and then went to sleep, thoroughly bored. The restricted dogs, so to speak, haven't the brains to be bored.

Emotionally, the dogs are "immature," but not in the human or clinical sense. They are little bothered by imaginative fears. Dogs suffer from irrational fears, like horses, porpoises, elephants, chimpanzees, and man; but it appears that this is a product of intellectual development, characteristic of the brighter, not the duller animal. Our dogs in restriction are not smart enough to fear strange objects. Things that cause fear in normal dogs produce only a generalized, undirected excitement in the restricted. If both normal and restricted dogs are exposed to the same noninjurious but exciting stimulus repeatedly, fear gradually develops in the restricted; but the normals, at first afraid, have by this time gone on to show a playful aggression instead. On the street, the restricted dogs "lead well," not bothered by what goes on around them, while those reared normally vary greatly in this respect. Analysis has a long way to go in these cases, but we can say now that dogs reared in isolation are not like ordinary dogs. They are both stupid and peculiar.

Such results clearly support the clinical evidence, and the animal experiments of others (1), showing that early environment has a lasting effect on the form of adjustment at maturity. We do not have a great body of evidence yet, and before we generalize too much it will be particularly important to repeat these observations with animals of different heredity. But I have been very surprised, personally, by the lack of evidence of emotional instability, neurotic tendency, or the like, when the dogs are suddenly plunged into a normal world. There is, in fact, just the opposite effect. This suggests caution in interpreting data with human children, such as those of Spitz (8) or Bowlby (3). Perceptual restriction in infancy certainly produces a low level of intelligence, but it may not, by itself, produce emotional disorder. The observed results seem to mean, not that the stimulus of another attentive organism (the mother) is necessary from the first but that it may become necessary only as psychological *dependence* on the mother develops. However, our limited data certainly cannot prove anything for man, though they may suggest other interpretations besides those that have been made.

THE ENVIRONMENT AT MATURITY

Another approach to the relation between the mammal and his environment is possible: that is, one can take the normally reared mammal and cut him off at maturity from his usual contact with the world. It seems clear that thought and personality characteristics develop as a function of the environment. Once developed, are they independent of it? This experiment is too cruel to do with animals, but not with college students. The first stage of the work was done by Bexton, Heron, and Scott (2). It follows up some work by Mackworth on the effects of monotony, in which he found extraordinary lapses of attention. Heron and his coworkers set out to make the monotony more prolonged and more complete.

The subject is paid to do nothing 24 hours a day. He lies on a comfortable bed in a small closed cubicle, is fed on request, goes to the toilet on request. Otherwise he does nothing. He wears frosted glass goggles that admit light but do not allow pattern vision. His ears are covered by a sponge-rubber pillow in which are embedded small speakers by which he can be communicated with, and a microphone hangs near to enable him to answer. His hands are covered with gloves, and cardboard cuffs extend from the upper forearm beyond his fingertips, permitting free joint movement but with little tactual perception.

The results are dramatic. During the stay in the cubicle, the experimental subject shows extensive loss, statistically significant, in solving simple problems. He complains subjectively that he cannot concentrate; his boredom is such that he looks forward eagerly to the next problem, but when it is presented he finds himself unwilling to make the effort to solve it.

On emergence from the cubicle the subject is given the same kind of intelligence tests as before entering, and shows significant loss. There is disturbance of motor control. Visual perception is changed in a way difficult to describe; it is as if the object looked at was exceptionally vivid, but impaired in its relation to other objects and the background —a disturbance perhaps of the larger organization of perception. This condition may last up to 12 or 24 hours.

Subjects reported some remarkable hallucinatory activity, some which resembled the effects of mescal, or the results produced by Grey Walter with flickering light. These hallucinations were primarily visual, perhaps only because the experimenters were able to control visual perception most effectively; however, some auditory and somesthetic hallucinations have been observed as well.

The nature of these phenomena is best conveyed by quoting one subject who reported over the microphone that he had just been asleep and had a very vivid dream and although he was awake, the dream was continuing. The study of dreams has a long history, and is clearly important theoretically, but is hampered by the impossibility of knowing how much the subject's report is distorted by memory. In many ways the hallucinatory activity of the present experiments is indistinguishable from what we know about dreams; if it is in essence the same process, but going on while the subject can describe it (not merely hot but still on the griddle), we have a new source of information, a means of direct attack, on the nature of the dream.

In its early stages the activity as it occurs in the experiment is probably not dreamlike. The course of development is fairly consistent. First, when the eyes are closed the visual field is light rather than dark. Next there are reports of dots of light, lines, or simple geometrical patterns, so vivid that they are described as being a new experience. Nearly all experimental subjects reported such activity. (Many of course could not tolerate the experimental conditions very long, and left before the full course of development was seen.) The next stage is the occurrence of repetitive patterns, like a wallpaper design, reported by three-quarters of the subjects; next, the appearance of isolated objects, without background, seen by half the subjects; and finally, integrated scenes, involving action, usually containing dreamlike distortions, and apparently with all the vividness of an animated cartoon, seen by about a quarter of the subjects. In general, these amused the subject, relieving his boredom, as he watched to see what the movie program would produce next. The subjects reported that the scenes seemed to be out in front of them. A few could, apparently, "look at" different parts of the scene in central vision, as one could with a movie; and up to a point could change its content by "trying." It was not, however, well under control. Usually, it would disappear if the subject were given an interesting task, but not when the subject described it, nor if he did physical exercises. Its persistence and vividness interfered with sleep for some subjects, and at this stage was irritating.

In their later stages the hallucinations were elaborated into everything from a peaceful rural scene to naked women diving and swimming in a woodland pool to prehistoric animals plunging through tropical forests. One man saw a pair of spectacles, which were then joined by a dozen more, without wearers, fixed intently on him; faces sometimes appeared behind the glasses, but with no eyes visible. The glasses sometimes moved in unison, as if marching in procession. Another man saw a field onto which a bathtub rolled: it moved slowly on rubber-tired wheels, with chrome hub caps. In it was seated an old man wearing a battle helmet. Another subject was highly entertained at seeing a row of squirrels marching single file across a snowy field, wearing snowshoes and carrying little bags over their shoulders.

Some of the scenes were in 3 dimensions, most in 2 (that is, as if projected on a screen). A most interesting feature was that some of the images were persistently tilted from the vertical, and a few reports were given of inverted scenes, completely upside down.

There were a few reports of auditory phenomena — one subject heard the people in his hallucination talking. There was also some somesthetic imagery, as when one saw a doorknob before him, and as he touched it felt an electric shock; or when another saw a miniature rocket ship maneuvering around him, and discharging pellets that he felt hitting his arm. But the most interesting of these phenomena the subject, apparently, lacked words to describe adequately. There were references to a feeling of "otherness," or bodily "strangeness." One said that his mind was like a ball of cottonwool floating in the air above him. Two independently reported that they perceived a second body, or second person, in the cubicle. One subject reported that he could not tell which of the 2 bodies was his own, and described the 2 bodies as overlapping in space — not like Siamese twins, but 2 complete bodies with an arm, shoulder, and side of each occupying the same space.

Theoretical Significance

The theoretical interest of these results for us extends in 2 directions. On the one hand, they interlock with work using more physiological methods, of brain stimulation and recording, and especially much of the recent work on the relation of the brain stem to cortical "arousal." Points of correspondence between behavioral theory and knowledge of neural function are increasing, and each new point of correspondence provides both a corrective for theory and a stimulation for further research. A theory of thought and of consciousness in physiologically intelligible terms need no longer be completely fantastic.

On the other hand, the psychological data cast new light on the relation of man to his environment, including his social environment, and it is this that I should like to discuss a little further. To do so I must

go back for a moment to some earlier experiments on chimpanzee emotion. They indicate that the higher mammal may be psychologically at
the mercy of his environment to a much greater degree than we have
been accustomed to think.

Studies in our laboratory of the role of the environment during infancy and a large body of work reviewed recently by Beach and Jaynes
(1) make it clear that psychological development is fully dependent
on stimulation from the environment. Without it, intelligence does not
develop normally, and the personality is grossly atypical. The experiment with college students shows that a short period — even a day or
so — of deprivation of a normal sensory input produces personality
changes and a clear loss of capacity to solve problems. Even at maturity, then, the organism is still essentially dependent on a normal sensory
environment for the maintenance of its psychological integrity.

The following data show yet another way in which the organism appears psychologically vulnerable. It has long been known that the chimpanzee may be frightened by representations of animals, such as a small
toy donkey. An accidental observation of my own extended this to include representations of the chimpanzee himself, of man, and of parts
of the chimpanzee or human body. A model of a chimpanzee head, in
clay, produced terror in the colony of the Yerkes Laboratories, as did
a lifelike representation of a human head, and a number of related objects such as an actual chimpanzee head, preserved in formalin, or a
colored representation of a human eye and eyebrow. A deeply anesthetized chimpanzee, "dead" as far as the others were concerned, aroused
fear in some animals and vicious attacks by others (4).

I shall not deal with this theoretically. What matters for our present
purposes is the conclusion, rather well supported by the animal evidence, that the greater the development of intelligence the greater the
vulnerability to emotional breakdown. The price of high intelligence
is susceptibility to imaginative fears and unreasoning suspicion and
other emotional weaknesses. The conclusion is not only supported by
the animal data, but also agrees with the course of development in children, growing intelligence being accompanied by increased frequency
and strength of emotional problems — up to the age of 5 years.

Then, apparently, the trend is reversed. Adult man, more intelligent
than chimpanzee or 5-year-old child, seems not more subject to emotional disturbances but less. Does this then disprove the conclusion?
It seemed a pity to abandon a principle that made sense of so many
data that had not made sense before, and the kind of theory I was
working with — neurophysiologically oriented — also pointed in the
same direction. The question then was, is it possible that something is
concealing the adult human being's emotional weaknesses?

From this point of view it became evident that the concealing agency is man's culture, which acts as a protective cocoon. There are many indications that our emotional stability depends more on our successful avoidance of emotional provocation than on our essential character-istics: that urbanity depends on an urbane social and physical envi-ronment. Dr. Thompson and I (5) reviewed the evidence, and came to the conclusion that the development of what is called "civilization" is the progressive elimination of sources of acute fear, disgust, and anger; and that civilized man may not be less, but more, susceptible to such disturbance because of his success in protecting himself from disturb-ing situations so much of the time.

We may fool ourselves thoroughly in this matter. We are surprised that children are afraid of the dark, or afraid of being left alone, and congratulate ourselves on having got over such weakness. Ask anyone you know whether he is afraid of the dark, and he will either laugh at you or be insulted. This attitude is easy to maintain in a well-lighted, well-behaved suburb. But try being alone in complete darkness in the streets of a strange city, or alone at night in the deep woods, and see if you still feel the same way.

We read incredulously of the taboo rules of primitive societies; we laugh at the superstitious fear of the dead in primitive people. What is there about a dead body to produce disturbance? Sensible, educated people are not so affected. One can easily show that they are, however, and that we have developed an extraordinarily complete taboo system — not just moral prohibition, but full-fledged ambivalent taboo — to deal with the dead body. I took a poll of an undergraduate class of 198 per-sons, including some nurses and veterans, to see how many had en-countered a dead body. Thirty-seven had never seen a dead body in any circumstances, and 91 had seen one only after an undertaker had prepared it for burial; making a total of 65% who had never seen a dead body in, so to speak, its natural state. It is quite clear that for some reason we protect society against sight of, contact with, the dead body. Why?

Again, the effect of moral education, and training in the rules of courtesy, and the compulsion to dress, talk and act as others do, adds up to ensuring that the individual member of society will not act in a way that is a provocation to others — will not, that is, be a source of strong emotional disturbance, except in highly ritualized circumstances approved by society. The social behavior of a group of civilized persons, then, makes up that protective cocoon which allows us to think of our-selves as being less emotional than the explosive 4-year-old or the equally explosive chimpanzee.

The well-adjusted adult therefore is not intrinsically less subject to emotional disturbance: he is well-adjusted, relatively unemotional, as long as he is in his cocoon. The problem of moral education, from this point of view, is not simply to produce a stable individual, but to produce an individual that will (a) be stable in the existing social environment, and (b) contribute to its protective uniformity. We think of some persons as being emotionally dependent, others not; but it looks as though we are all completely dependent on the environment in a way and to a degree that we have not suspected.

REFERENCES

1. Beach, F. A., and Jaynes, J. *Psychol. Bull.*, 51: 239, 1954.
2. Bexton, W. H., Heron, W., and Scott, T. H. *Canad. J. Psychol.*, 8: 70, 1954.
3. Bowlby, J. Maternal Care and Mental Health. Geneva: *WHO Monogr.* #2, 1951.
4. Hebb, D. O. *Psychol. Rev.*, 53: 259, 1946.
5. Hebb, D. O., and Thompson, W. R. In Lindzey, G. (Ed.), *Handbook of Social Psychology*. Cambridge: Addison-Wesley, 1954.
6. Hymovitch, B. *J. Comp. Physiol. Psychol.*, 45: 313, 1952.
7. Nissen, H. W., Chow, R. L., and Semmes, Josephine. *Am. J. Psychol.*, 64: 485, 1951.
8. Spitz, R. A. *Psychoanalytic Study of the Child*, 2: 113, 1946.
9. Thompson, W. R., and Heron, W. *Canad. J. Psychol.*, 8: 17, 1954.

THE EFFECTS OF EXPERIMENTAL VARIATIONS ON PROBLEM SOLVING IN THE RAT

BERNARD HYMOVITCH

University of Michigan

The problem of early learning has been one of increasing interest to psychologists in recent years. It has become clear that investigation of the effects of early experience is essential for a comprehensive understanding of adult behavior.

Numerous experimental studies have demonstrated a relationship between early experience and adult behavior. It was shown by Hunt (9) that rats suffering feeding frustration during infancy tended to display more hoarding behavior after periods of starvation at maturity than rats that had not been so deprived during early life. A similar phenomenon occurred as a result of a lack of satisfaction of sucking needs in puppies (10). In later life these puppies displayed a "perverted" type of continual sucking and oral behavior. The experiments of Lorenz (11) have shown that certain responses of some birds to their parents may be elicited in early life by human beings or specific moving objects. He maintains that there is an innate organization (Angeborene Schema) for these responses. Once established, however, they can be elicited only by the original releaser (Ausloser), whether it be parent bird, moving object, or man. The responses cannot be established for the first time in later life.

Investigations of the effects of rearing rats (2)[1] and particularly chimpanzees (12) in darkness have shown that early experience is required for the development of efficient visual responsiveness. The comprehensive review of patients operated upon for congenital cataract (13) provides similar evidence. A review by Hebb (5) of a number of cases of early and late brain injury in human beings led him to suggest that the effect of brain damage in infancy is less selective and more generalized than such damage sustained in later life.

The exploratory investigation which was directly responsible for the work to be reported here was carried out by Hebb (6). In a first experi-

From *The Journal of Comparative and Physiological Psychology*, August 1952.

[1] In this report Hebb (2) neglected an effect of learning on the rat's perception of pattern. He has, however, modified his interpretation in a later discussion (7).

ment one group of rats was blinded in infancy and another at maturity. Both groups were tested subsequently by a rat "intelligence test" (8). In a second experiment, one group was reared in the usual small cages, another as "pets" in a much wider environment. In both cases, the greater infant experience led to a higher level of intelligence at maturity.

These preliminary experiments were done with small groups and without precise controls. The purpose of the present experiments, accordingly, was to determine whether Hebb's results would obtain with a larger number of animals studied under more carefully controlled conditions and to make further analyses of these effects if they are found.

GENERAL METHODS

The general method of the present experiments was to give different groups of male hooded rats varied kinds of experience during early life. At maturity the problem-solving ability of the animals was tested. The two general techniques of varying early experience were blinding at different ages and rearing in different types of environments.

Blinding

Optic enucleation was performed on one group of rats within 36 hr. after their eyes opened. These rats were then 17 or 18 days old. Rats of the other group were not blinded until they were between 78 and 80 days of age.

Rearing

Normal cages. One type of environment, in which the rats had relatively limited visual and motor experience, was the normal cage. These cages were 12 in. long, 10 in. wide, and 8 in. high with solid sides and back, ½-in. grill top, and a 4-by-4-in. door of wire mesh.

Free-environment box. This apparatus provided extensive opportunity for experience. It was 6 ft. long, 4 ft. wide, and 6 in. high, and its cover was wire mesh. Distributed throughout the box were a number of blind alleys, inclined runways, small enclosed areas, apertures, etc.

Mesh cages. A third environment was the mesh cage, which restricted the space in which the rats could move freely but allowed considerable visual experience. The cages were constructed entirely of wire mesh and were cylindrical in shape. They were 8 in. in diameter and only 6 in. high.

Enclosed activity wheels. These were employed in order to restrict the space of free movement while increasing the opportunity for physical exercise. The wheels were totally enclosed in solid metal structures in order to restrict visual experience. Attached to the door were a food chamber and a water bottle. Fins on the outside of the wheels ensured proper ventilation.

Stovepipe cages. In order to restrict the total experience of the animals, stovepipe cages were constructed. They consisted of covered metal cylinders 8 in. in diameter and 16 in. high. Several holes were placed above and below the animals' field of vision to allow free entry of air and light. A water bottle and a food chamber were suspended on the outside of each cage.

Training and Testing

The problem-solving ability of the rats was measured by the closed-field test developed by Hebb and Williams (8) and modified by Hebb (6). This apparatus consisted of an enclosed field with the entrance and food box constant in position and with barriers varying in number and position in the field. The barriers and walls were painted black in contrast with the gray-white plywood floor and unpainted entrance and food boxes. Painted red lines divided the floor into 36 5-in. squares. These ensured reliable placement of barriers and aided in the scoring procedure. For each subtest various areas of the field other than the path of correct solution were demarcated as error zones. Six training problems and 24 regular subtests were used. The regular subtests were evenly divided into two series, each starting with relatively simple problems and becoming more difficult.

The training problems were presented one per day, and the whole series was repeated until the animals reached the predetermined criterion of completing nine out of ten consecutive runs in 1 min. from the time of entry until a bite of food was taken. It was felt that when a rat's performance met this requirement, neither timidity nor exploration could be a significant factor in determining its behavior in the subsequent test situation.

Each animal made ten runs in each subtest. The rats were tested with one problem per day for 24 days in Experiment I and with two problems per day for 12 days in Experiments II and III. A record was kept of the number of error zones entered by each rat on each run. A rat's score on the total test was the number of error zones it entered during its 240 runs.

The correlations obtained between error scores on the first 12 tests and the second 12 tests ranged between .68 and .88. The Spearman-Brown estimate of the reliability coefficient for the total test ranged between .81 and .94.

Experiment I

Procedure

Nineteen rats were blinded in infancy and 21 at maturity. Eight of the early-blinded and 11 of the late-blinded rats were reared in the normal cages throughout the first 78 days of life. The other 11 early-blinded and 10 late-blinded animals were reared in the same cages but were given added opportunity for experience in the free-environment box. They were first placed in the box at 21 to 27 days of age and subsequently were allowed the free-environment experience for an average of $2\frac{1}{2}$ hr. a day for 46 to 49 days. Training was begun when the animals were 80 days old and completed when they were 125 days old. Thus, there were four groups: Group 1, late-blinded with free-environment experience; Group 2, early-blinded with free-environment experience; Group 3, late-blinded with normal cage restriction; and Group 4, early-blinded with normal cage restriction.

Results

Table 1 shows the mean error scores of the four experimental groups on the closed-field test. The results of an analysis of the raw data are found in Table 2. The data of one rat of the late-blinded restricted group are not included. Its behavior was so different from that of any other animal ever tested that it was assumed the animal was not functioning normally.

TABLE 1. MEAN ERROR SCORES ON THE CLOSED-FIELD TEST (EXPERIMENT I)

Measures	Group 1	Group 2	Group 3	Group 4
N	10	11	11	8
M	495.7	568.0	664.0	793.3
SD	144.7	129.5	166.6	218.4

TABLE 2. P-VALUES OF MEAN DIFFERENCE BETWEEN GROUPS (EXPERIMENT I)

Group	Group				
	2	3	4	2 + 4	3 + 4
1	.270	.033	.004		
2		.172	.011		
3			.188		
1 + 3				.198	
1 + 2					.001

The rats that had received the free-environment experience were superior on the closed-field test to those that had been restricted to the normal cages. The relative effects of late blinding as opposed to early blinding were not as clear. Although the mean error score of each late-blinded group is lower that that of the corresponding early-blinded group, the differences do not attain statistical significance. The mean error score of all experimental groups improved when the second sub-test series is compared with the first, but no group improved significantly more than any other.

EXPERIMENT II

Procedure

Forty male hooded rats of about 27 days of age were used. Rats were placed individually in six stovepipe cages, eight mesh cages, and six activity wheels. Two rats in the activity wheels died during the research period. The remaining 20 rats were put in the free-environment box. No group was handled during rearing.

Six of the eight mesh cages were placed in specific regions of the free-environment box and the other two in different positions in the laboratory. Thus, there were eight locations, serially numbered, for the mesh cages. Each day these cages were advanced to the locations of the next higher numbers.

Recordings were taken of the number of revolutions made by animals in the activity wheels. The recordings were compared with those of two control groups in order to determine whether or not the restricted visual environment had reduced the animals' activity. No significant difference was found. The four experimental groups were: Group 1, rats reared in the free-environment box; Group 2, rats restricted to the mesh cages during early life; Group 3, rats restricted to stovepipe cages during early life; and Group 4, rats restricted to the activity wheels during early life.

The experimental animals were weighed before testing. The mean body weight of Groups 1, 2, and 3 was approximately equal, but that of Group 4 was significantly less.

Preliminary training in the closed-field test was begun when the rats were 79 days old, and testing was completed 21 days later. To determine how much the rats would be disturbed by changing the position of the testing apparatus, each animal, after completing the 24 test items, was given a number of runs in the closed-field test with all barriers removed. Training continued until each animal achieved three successive direct runs to the food box. The testing apparatus was then rotated 90° counterclockwise, and each rat was given seven runs in the new position. The next day the rats were again given a number of runs with the apparatus in its usual position and with barriers. After all rats had achieved two successive correct runs, the apparatus was rotated 90° clockwise, and each rat was given seven runs. Errors were counted on the basis of zones entered, locomotion away from the goal, hesitancy or refusal to enter the food box, "sniffing" in the previous location of the goal, and return to the entry box, and these yielded a disturbance score.

To determine whether or not the variations in early experience would differentially affect the rote-learning ability of the different groups, the rats were first trained to run an inclosed alley to reach food and then allowed a maximum of eight runs in an inclosed ten-unit T maze. The runs were given one per day for two days and then two per day for two or three days. Any rat that made no errors, including retracing errors, on the third day was not run on the fourth day.

Results

The mean error scores of the rats of the four experimental groups on the closed-field test are presented in Table 3.

Both the free-environment group (Group 1) and the mesh-cage group (Group 2) were clearly superior ($P = <.001$) to the stovepipe group (Group 3) and the activity-wheel group (Group 4). There was no discernible difference between the mean error scores of Groups 1 and 2 or of Groups 3 and 4. No group improved significantly more than any other group on the second 12 tests.

Most of the animals were disturbed to some extent by the rotation of the apparatus. The mean disturbance scores of Groups 1 and 2 were significantly ($P = .05$) greater than the mean score of the other two groups combined (Table 4).

On the alley maze, no group obtained a mean error score significantly different from that of any other group (Table 5).

TABLE 3. MEAN ERROR SCORES ON THE CLOSED-FIELD TEST (EXPERIMENT II)

Measure	Group 1	Group 2	Group 3	Group 4
N	20	8	6	4
M	137.3	140.1	233.1	235.0
SD	18.6	10.7	29.1	28.8

TABLE 4. DISORIENTATION SCORES AFTER ROTATION OF THE CLOSED-FIELD TEST (EXPERIMENT II)

Measure	Group 1	Group 2	Groups 3 + 4
N	20	8	10
M	53.0	57.2	30.1
SD	24.0	30.8	10.2

TABLE 5. MEAN ERROR SCORES ON MAZE (EXPERIMENT II)

Measure	Group 1	Group 2	Group 3	Group 4
N	20	8	6	4
M	24.1	18.1	19.26	30.5
SD	11.3	10.0	7.4	12.2

EXPERIMENT III

Procedure

The purpose of this experiment was to determine whether particular experiences in the later part of the growth period would have effects similar to the same experiences during the early part of the growth period.

Two groups, each containing six male hooded rats, were used. The first group of six rats was reared in normal cages but was placed in the free-environment box for 3-hr. periods on 39 occasions between 30 and 75 days of age. The second group was reared in the six stovepipe cages from the age of 30 to 75 days. One animal developed inner-ear disease and was destroyed.

From Day 75 to Day 85 both groups were restricted to their normal cages. The treatment of the two groups was reversed for the ensuing 45 days. The animals that had had the free-environment experience in early life were now put in the stovepipe cages. Those that had been restricted to the stovepipe cages in early life were allotted free-environment experience equivalent in both amount and distribution to that of the former group. The animals were 130 days old when this procedure was completed.

Four other animals were restricted throughout the first 130 days of life to normal cages. Another three were restricted to the normal cages throughout that time, but were given free-environment experience with *both* of the first two groups.

The four experimental groups were: Group 1, rats with early free-environment experience and late stovepipe cage restrictions; Group 2, rats with late free-environment experience and early stovepipe cage restrictions; Group 3, rats with both early and late free-environment experience; and Group 4, those with continual restriction to normal cages.

Results

Table 6 presents the test results obtained with these four groups. The animals that had the free-environment experience in early life (Group 1) were decidedly superior to those that had this experience later ($P = <.001$). The effect of the late free-environment experience upon test scores was negligible. The group with both early and late free-environment experience (Group 3) displayed no significant advantage over the group that had only early free-environmental experience (Group 4).

TABLE 6. Mean Error Scores on Closed-Field Test (Experiment III)

Measure	Group 1	Group 2	Group 3	Group 4
N	6	5	3	4
M	161.3	248.8	152.6	221.5
SD	17.2	26.1	27.2	26.3

The mean error score of the rats that never had the wider environment (Group 4) was not significantly lower that that of the late free-environment group (Group 2).

These results can be compared with those of Experiment II. The rats reared in the stovepipe cages during early life (Group 3, Experiment II) were not inferior to those that were, in addition, given late free-environment experience (Group 2, Experiment III). Thus the late free-environment experience had no effects on the test results.

Discussion

In general, Hebb's preliminary findings (6) have been confirmed even though the early- and late-blinding experiment did not yield clear-cut results. This investigation has fully confirmed the conclusions concerning the effect of widened experience upon problem solving.

How can we account for these results? It might be suggested that the superior performance of certain groups was motivational in origin. For example, the free-environment group of Experiment I received extra handling in being placed in and removed from the free-environment box. Thus, it might be contended that these animals were tamer than the others and that, therefore, they performed more efficiently on the closed-field test. But a number of facts make this explanation untenable. In Experiment I the restricted animals also had considerable handling during early life. Second, it had been previously shown that prolonged training did not affect test results (6). Third, the use of the "criterion of readiness for testing" should have minimized the influence of motivational factors on test performance. Finally, in Experiment II no group received any handling during the rearing period.

On the other hand it might be postulated that the early experience in the free-environment box provided training in dealing with specific situations which were also present in the test situation. That is, there were identical elements in the two environments, such as being confronted by barriers, and the early experience provided for a simple transfer of the learned stimulus-response habits. The numerous differences between the free-environment box and the method of testing make this explanation unlikely. The fact that the late-blinded rats were superior to the early-blinded is further evidence against an explanation in terms of simple transfer, for any *visual* stimulus-response relationships that may have been acquired during early life could not have been operative in the late-blinded rats. Then again, if simple transfer of specific learning, such as learning not to enter blinds, had produced the effects, one would have expected the same transfer to have occurred in the alley maze. But the wider-environment animals were not superior in that situation. Finally, the performance of the mesh-cage group makes the argument for simple transfer completely indefensible, for the animals reared in these cages had little opportunity to learn specific reactions.

It might be hypothesized that the differences between the free-environment and the restricted groups can be explained on the basis of differential opportunities for muscular exercise. This explanation is also inadequate inasmuch as the rats reared in the activity wheels were not superior to those reared in stovepipe cages. Similarly, the free-environment group was not superior to the mesh-cage group in spite of the reduced muscular exercise of the latter.

Thus, it appears that the differential effects did not result from motivation, the acquisition of specific stimulus-response habits, or purely motor factors in early life. It would appear that the differential opportunities presented the various groups for *perceptual learning* were responsible for the results. The significant role of visual perception was particularly established by the mesh-cage group. Nonvisual perceptual learning was also effective. The early-blinded group that had the free-environment experience scored fewer errors than the early-blinded group with the restricted experience.

It has also been demonstrated that the wider experience must occur early in the life of the animals to result in a more highly developed perceptual organization at maturity. The results of Experiments I and II demonstrated that the effects of early experience were maintained on the second as well as the first series of subtests. It was shown, therefore, that when the rats were given the same intensive training and testing experience at maturity, the differences between groups were not eliminated. In Experiment III changes produced in the problem-solving ability of the rats during the first 75 days of life were still present 75 days later. Furthermore, the superiority of the wider-environment group was not erased by the group which was deprived in early life, despite an adequate opportunity for experience during later life. Hence, the effects seem to be relatively permanent and possibly irreversible.

Because the free-environment and the mesh-cage groups were significantly more disturbed by rotation of the testing apparatus than the restricted groups, it is assumed that the wider-environment animals used cues beyond the problem box to a greater extent than the restricted groups did. It appears that the problem-solving behavior of the superior rat is more dependent than that of the inferior rat upon a "wider sensory environment"(1, 3, 4). The added early experience may have made possible the acquisition of rather broad "cognitive maps" (14).

Finally, it is to be noted that the differences between groups were not evident in their performance on the alley maze. Thus, it seems that the rote-learning ability of the animals was not affected.

SUMMARY

1. In Experiment 1, groups of rats were blinded in early life or at maturity and reared either in a free environment or in normal cages. Results on a closed-field test at maturity decisively indicated that the free-environment rats were superior to the normal-cage groups. Differences between early-blinded and late-blinded groups were not significant.

2. In Experiment II, groups of rats were reared in individual stovepipe cages, in mesh cages, in enclosed activity wheels, or in the free-environment box. At maturity the animals were tested on the closed-field apparatus and on a ten-unit inclosed T maze. The mesh-cage and the free-environment groups were clearly superior to the stovepipe and the activity-wheel groups on the closed-field test, but differences between the mesh-cage and free-environment groups and between the stovepipe cage and the activity-wheel groups were not significant. The groups did not differ significantly in performance on the inclosed T maze.

3. In Experiment III, one group was given free-environment experi-

ence during early life and restricted to stovepipe cages later, and another group was restricted to the stovepipe cages in early life and given free-environment experience later. The first group was conclusively superior to the second group.

4. The effects were not attributable to motivation, specific stimulus-response habits, or purely motor factors. The differential opportunity presented the various groups for perceptual learning was responsible for the results. The effects appear to be relatively permanent and possibly irreversible.

REFERENCES

1. Carr, H. A. Maze studies with the white rat. I. Normal animals. *J. Anim. Behav.*, 1917, 7: 259–275.
2. Hebb, D. O. The innate organization of visual activity. I. Perception of figures by rats reared in total darkness. *J. genet. Psychol.*, 1937, 51: 101–126.
3. Hebb, D. O. Studies of the organization of behavior. I. Behavior of the rat in a field orientation. *J. comp. Psychol.*, 1938, 25: 333–352.
4. Hebb, D. O. Studies of the organization of behavior. II. Changes in the field orientation of the rat after cortical destruction. *J. comp. Psychol.*, 1938, 26: 427–442.
5. Hebb, D. O. The effect of early and late brain injury upon test scores and the nature of normal adult intelligence. *Proc. Amer. phil. Soc.*, 1942, 85: 275–292.
6. Hebb, D. O. The effects of early experience on problem-solving at maturity. *Amer. Psychologist*, 1947, 2: 306–307.
7. Hebb, D. O. *The organization of behavior.* New York: Wiley, 1949.
8. Hebb, D. O., and Williams, K. A method of rating animal intelligence. *J. gen. Psychol.*, 1946, 34: 59–65.
9. Hunt, J. McV. The effects of infant feeding-frustration upon hoarding in the albino rat. *J. abnorm. soc. Psychol.*, 1941, 36: 338–360.
10. Levy, D. M. The hostile act. In T. M. Newcomb and E. L. Hartley (Eds.), *Readings in social psychology.* New York: Holt, 1947.
11. Lorenz, K. Der Kumpan in der Umwelt des Vogels. *J. Orn., Lpz.*, 1935, 83: 137–213, 289–413.
12. Riesen, A. H. Visual discriminations by chimpanzees after rearing in darkness. *Amer. Psychologist*, 1947, 2: 299.
13. Senden, M. v. *Raum- und Gestaltauffassung bei operierten Blindgeborenen vor und nach der Operation.* Leipzig: Barth, 1932.
14. Tolman, E. C. Cognitive maps in rats and men. *Psychol. Rev.*, 1948, 55: 189–208.

9

EARLY VISUAL AND MOTOR EXPERIENCE AS DETERMINERS OF COMPLEX MAZE-LEARNING ABILITY UNDER RICH AND REDUCED STIMULATION

RONALD H. FORGUS

University of Pennsylvania

In a recent paper (2) the writer reported evidence which he interpreted as indicating that early experience can be a hindrance or an aid to problem solving depending on the nature of the experience and its relationship to the problem. This interpretation is an extension of the theory of Hebb since in the work published so far by Hebb (3) and his collaborators, Forgays (1) and Hymovitch (5), they have stated that the "freer" the early experience of an animal is, the better it will be in solving a variety of problems. Up to now, however, most of the studies of these psychologists have dealt with performance on the Hebb-Williams intelligence test for rats.

In the paper referred to above we reported, among other facts, that a group of rats which had had extensive visual experience with inanimate objects learned to discriminate visual forms faster than another group of rats which also had had extensive visual experience with the same objects, but which had also been permitted to explore these objects physically. This result appears, at first sight, to be contradictory to Hebb's theory. However, it must be remembered that Hebb has dealt only with the gross aspects of perceptual experience and has not, as yet, dealt with the effect of varying the complexity of experience in different sensory channels. We have hypothesized that animals which had a varied experience, both visually and physically, with inanimate objects, would attempt various methods of solving the problem; e.g., they would respond to position and response cues as well as to visual cues. The animals whose motor experience with inanimate objects was relatively restricted as compared with complex visual experience with the same objects should have a greater probability of responding exclusively to the visual cues, earlier, and therefore should learn to discriminate visual forms more quickly. The longer learning time taken by the first group can be attributed to the time it takes these animals to abolish their wrong responses to the "irrelevant" cues. This "explanation" seems all the more plausible since there was no difference in form generalization after both groups had learned the discrimination. This hypothesis is consistent with Witkin's (7) inference from his study that rats appear to display rather stable "reaction sets" when attempting to solve a problem.

The present study was performed to test further the hypothesis which was offered, viz., that whether a group of animals with more varied early experience will be superior in problem solving to a group with less varied early experience depends on the relationship of the experience to the requirements of the problem. We are arguing that the group of animals whose early experience was qualitatively more complex would be superior in solving a problem when external stimuli are reduced, i.e., they are able to change their reaction sets more readily when the solution requires such a change. We therefore specifically tested the following hypothesis: *If two groups of animals, one reared in a complex visual and motor environment and the other reared in a complex visual but relatively simple motor environment were to learn, partially, a complex open maze with visual cues present and were then tested for complete learning with the visual cues greatly reduced, then the first group would be superior in performance on the second test.*

METHOD

Rearing

Two groups of male hooded rats were reared under two different conditions from the age of 25 days until they were 85 days old. There were 16 rats in each group. The rearing conditions were almost identical with those reported in the author's previous study (2). The cage which housed group 1 was 5 ft. long, 5 ft. wide, and 15 in. high. The walls were painted a flat black, and the white objects were within 15 in. from the wall all around the sides of the cage. Group 1 was called the complex visual-motor group since the animals had complex visual as well as complex motor experience with the inanimate objects in their cage. They learned to explore and climb over the objects quite easily.

The cage which housed group 2 had the same dimensions as those of the cage that housed group 1, and the white objects were in the same relative position. However, these animals were permitted to live only in the inner 900 sq. in. of their cage. This was accomplished by inserting a plastic cage, 30 in. long, 30 in. wide, and 15 in. high inside a large box, identical with that of group 1. Thus, these animals could only see the inanimate objects but were never permitted to traverse them. For this reason group 2 was called the complex visual but relatively simple motor group. Food and water were in the same relative positions in both cages. Both cages had very good lighting during the day.

Before we continue with the procedure we should point out certain limitations of this design. Because of the practical limitations imposed on us by the amount of laboratory space, cages, etc., we had to rear these animals in groups. Thus, it is incorrect to say that the animals of group 2 had restricted kinesthetic experience as such. Any differences in maze learning found between these groups cannot be attributed to differences in "kinesthetic learning" per se. The kinesthetic experience which the animals in group 2 derived from playing with their cage mates was probably comparable to the kinesthetic experience of the animals in group 1. The animals in both groups should have been equally good in reacting to internal postural, sequential stimuli. There is also no reason to believe that the visual learning of the two groups was significantly different, especially since the objects in the second cage were well within the rat's field of clear vision.

The experiences of the two groups were very different in one important respect, however. The animals in group 1, living in a complex, object-filled environment, had much motor experience in learning to negotiate elevated platforms, alleys, and blinds, etc. This kind of experience should improve their ability to solve complex mazes when visual cues are reduced since they had ample experience in exploring these kinds of environments in the dark.

In spite of the limitations of the design, it seems justifiable to state two things about the rearing conditions: First, the two groups were reared under similar conditions, especially with respect to visual experiences with inanimate objects. Second, the greatest difference in the rearing conditions was that the animals in group 1 had more opportunity for motor experience in negotiating a complex physical environment.

Procedure

When the rats were 85 days old they were transferred to smaller wire mesh laboratory cages, 21 in. long, 18 in. wide, and 10 in. high. At this stage of the experiment the rats of both groups were mixed so that they could have the experience of living together socially with members of the other group. We used four cages, each cage housing eight rats. There were four rats from each group in each cage. The animals were housed in these cages until the experiment was completed.

For the next seven days the animals were placed on a $23\frac{1}{2}$-hr. food-deprivation schedule and were handled extensively. They were fed Purina Dog Chow and lettuce for $\frac{1}{2}$ hr. every day. At the end of this week the following test was begun: The animals were run in a large open room having very good lighting and many objects around the sides of the room. The maze consisted of an elevated 11-unit T maze. The units were painted a flat black. The height of the maze from the floor was 30 in., and each arm measured 15 in. The sequence of correct turns was: R *L L* R R *L L* R *L* R *L* R R *L* R *L* R *L L* R R (the italicized letters refer to forced turns). On any one trial there was a maximum of 11 possible errors. The animals were given one trial per day after being deprived of food for $23\frac{1}{2}$ hr. After they made the eleventh correct choice there were allowed to nibble at some Purina Dog Chow at the goal. At the end of the daily run the animals were fed Purina Dog Chow and lettuce for $\frac{1}{2}$ hr. They were never deprived of water. An animal was run under these conditions until it reached the criterion of making one error or less per trial on two consecutive trials.

When this preliminary criterion was reached, the second and critical test was started. In this critical test the visual cues were greatly diminished by turning out all the lights. The room was almost completely dark while the animal ran the trial. The E was able to follow the rat, which had a luminescent ring around its neck. The critical test ended when the animal reached the criterion of 5 out of 6 consecutive errorless trials.

We used a lenient criterion in the first test so that the second test would begin before the "chain" responses, suggested by Ritchie *et al.* (6), were formed. Ritchie *et al.* theorized that, in an open maze, a rat initially learns to avoid incorrect turns by utilizing visual cues primarily. After the correct turns have been repeated many times, however, a chain response (presumably of kinesthetic stimulus-response bonds) is formed. When this chain response of correct choices becomes well established, the rat utilizes visual cues progressively less and performs primarily on the basis of kinesthetic cues. Assuming that this theory is correct, we wanted to be relatively sure that we started the test in the dark before the rat reached the chain response stage of learning; otherwise, the reduction of visual stimulation would have made little difference.

During both the preliminary test and the critical test olfactory cues were held constant by randomly interchanging the units from day to day. Since there were no constant sounds localized in any fixed position we may assume that auditory cues were also eliminated. If we accept Honzik's (4) conclusions that a rat learns almost nothing when visual, auditory, olfactory, and kinesthetic cues are all removed, then we must deduce that during the first test the animals were learning primarily on the basis of visual and kinesthetic cues while during the critical test they were completing learning primarily on the basis of kinesthetic cues.

Before the experiment was completed one rat in each group died, leaving us with 15 rats per group.

RESULTS

Error and time scores were recorded for performance on both the preliminary and the critical test.

We will report the results of the preliminary test first. The mean number of trials to reach the preliminary criterion and the standard deviation were computed for each group. The mean for group 1 was 11, SD 2.33, and the corresponding values for group 2 were 7.20 and 1.60. The t of the difference between the means is significant beyond the .001 level. Now it was found that although the animals in group 1 took longer to reach the preliminary criterion, they were faster runners than the animals in group 2. The mean number of seconds per trial for group 1 was 162.5, SD 46.5, and for group 2, 240.3 with an SD of 119. The t of the difference in means is significant beyond the .001 level. When we take these two sets of results together, it is quite clear that the animals in group 1 made more errors but were faster runners than group 2 animals on the preliminary test carried out in the light with many cues (especially visual) present.

In contrast with the preliminary test findings, group 1 performed better than group 2 on the critical test taken in the dark. The mean number of trials for group 1 to reach the critical test criterion was 7.50, SD 1.59, and the corresponding values for group 2 were 13 and 2.36. The t of 7.27 is highly significant ($p < .001$). From this we may conclude with confidence that group 1 was very superior to group 2 in complex maze learning under conditions of reduced visual cues. Figure 1 contains a graph which strikingly illustrates this point.

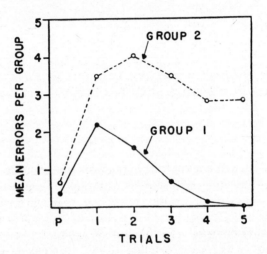

Fig. 1. Graph showing the mean number of errors per trial for both groups beginning at the trial when each animal met the preliminary test criterion (P) and continuing for five subsequent trials in the dark.

The graph begins with the last preliminary criterion trial (P). We notice that the errors increased for both groups when the lights were turned off. However, the animals in group 1 quickly readjusted to the changed conditions and rapidly decreased their errors to zero while most of the animals in group 2 were still making many errors.

An analysis of the time scores showed that, in the dark, the animals of group 1 were also faster runners than the animals in group 2. The mean number of seconds per trial during the critical test was 67.3 (SD, 20.6) for group 1, 91.4 (SD, 23.9) for group 2. The t is significant for 28 df ($p < .01$). So we see that, in addition to making fewer errors to reach the critical test criterion, group 1 animals were also faster runners.

Now, it might be argued that the reason group 1 was superior to group 2 on the critical test was the fact that group 1 had more preliminary experience with the maze than group 2, since the former took longer to reach the preliminary criterion. To equalize the groups with respect to this uncontrolled factor, we performed an analysis of covariance of the data. The results of the analysis of covariance gave us a within-groups correlation of only .008. We conclude that the effect of the preliminary training on the critical test is negligible. The obtained F ratio of 40.52 ($df = 1,27$) is highly significant ($p < .001$). The conclusions already drawn with respect to the differences in performance between group 1 and group 2 on the critical test in the dark are therefore considered to be valid.

Finally, in an attempt to find out the relationship between errors and time, we calculated a Pearson product-moment correlation coefficient between these two sets of scores for the preliminary test and obtained an r of $-.25$. This low negative correlation indicates that the fast animals were not making fewer errors. As a matter of fact, an inspection of the raw data revealed that a few fast animals were making most of the errors.

Discussion

First, we may conclude that the hypothesis we set out to test has been confirmed. In this study the animals of group 1 were reared in a cage which afforded much opportunity for visual experience with inanimate objects and which also permitted physical exploration of this complex, object-filled environment. The animals of group 2 were reared under similar conditions with respect to breadth of visual experience but were not permitted physical exploration of the complex, object-filled environment which they saw. The problem is to explain why group 1 was poorer on the preliminary test but superior on the critical test. To interpret this fact, we will discuss three alternative explanations which immediately seem possible.

The first explanation is based on the assumption that the two groups had different emotional reactions to the task situation. Thus it might be argued that the group 2 animals, having little experience with elevated objects, are more frightened when they have to turn around after entering a blind on the elevated maze. Consequently they are more cautious not to re-enter the blinds, and thus avoid making errors more quickly in the preliminary test performed in the light. Furthermore, the animals in group 1 were quite used to falling off, climbing up, and turning around on elevated platforms since they presumably had much of this kind of experience in their living cage during the night when the lights were turned out. Group 2 animals were not. Thus it could be said that the group 2 animals were much more emotionally disturbed by the necessity of finding their way around a strange place, like the elevated maze, in the dark. This disturbance would account for their poorer performance in the dark. There are two reasons why this interpretation is not very plausible. The first is that we previously found no difference between two similar groups when we tested their emotionality on an elevated maze by using fairly standard emotionality tests (2, pp. 332–333). Second, it seems difficult to believe that darkness per se would produce such startling differences since rats are normally dark adapted. We might add that the group 2 animals did not exhibit such disturbances. For example, there was not an obvious increase in defecation when the rats ran the maze in the dark. Moreover, no animal in either group ever fell off the maze.

The second alternative would assume that the animals in group 1 developed greater exploratory tendencies because of dealing with more varied inanimate objects. This greater exploratory behavior masks their learning in the preliminary test. But since they explored the maze more fully, they knew more about it. Thus they were better able to cope with the problem presented in the dark. This possibility is more appealing than the first, but again there is evidence which casts doubt on its validity. In our previous study (2, pp. 332–333) we also found no differences in variability of behavior between two groups which were similar to the ones used in this study. Exploratory tendencies are usually revealed in variability of behavior.

We thus feel that the first two explanations taken alone are not adequate. We would like to suggest a more general type of explanation which probably includes aspects of the first two alternatives. This interpretation is based on the obvious fact that the animals in group 1 were more familiar with traversing elevated platforms. Thus they were less cautious when they ran on the elevated maze. This is supported by the fact that they ran much faster than group 2 animals. One of the reasons that the group 2 animals took a longer time per trial was the fact that they hesitated more at the bifurcation points on the maze. Now the arms of the maze were very short (15 in.) and the next T could vaguely be seen from the bifurcation point. Since the group 2 animals hesitated more frequently, they eliminated errors earlier and thus performed better during the preliminary test. We mentioned earlier that Ritchie et al. (6) consider that the initial stage of maze learning is based primarily on visual cues. Because group 1 animals ran so much faster, they were not utilizing these cues as well as the animals in group 2. When the lights were turned out, however, both groups were forced to rely on nonvisual cues. Since group 1 animals had much experience in this kind of situation in their living cage, they were better able to negotiate the maze during the critical test.

In conclusion we wish to stress what we said in the introduction: In examining the effects of early experience on adult problem-solving behavior it seems to be the relationship between the kind of early experience and the demands of the problem task which is the important factor.

Summary

This paper reported a study which investigated the influence of early visual and motor experience on the maze-learning ability of adult rats. Two groups of rats were reared under different conditions from weaning until they were 85 days old. Group 1 was reared in a large complex environment which offered much opportunity for visual and motor experience whereas the environment of group 2 offered much opportunity for visual experience but relatively little opportunity for motor experience with inanimate objects. As adults these rats were tested for maze-learning ability under conditions of rich and reduced visual cues. Group 2 was superior when many cues were present whereas group 1 was superior when the visual cues were reduced. Three alternative explanations of the results were considered. It was concluded that results such as these point to the fact that the important theoretical issue in these developmental studies seems to be the relationship between the quality of early experience and the nature of task to be solved. Only in this light will we arrive at a clear idea of the effect of early experience on adult problem-solving ability.

References

1. Forgays, D. G., & Forgays, Janet W. The nature of the effect of free-environmental experience in the rat. *J. comp. physiol. Psychol.*, 1952, 45: 302–312.

2. Forgus, R. H. The effect of early perceptual learning on the behavioral organization of adult rats. *J. comp. physiol. Psychol.*, 1954, 47: 331–336.

3. Hebb, D. O. *The organization of behavior.* New York: Wiley, 1949.

4. Honzik, C. H. The sensory basis of maze learning in rats. *Comp. Psychol. Monogr.*, 1936, 13: No. 64.

5. Hymovitch, B. The effects of experimental variation on problem solving in the rat. *J. comp. physiol. Psychol.*, 1952, 45: 313–326.

6. Ritchie, B. F., Aeschliman, B., & Peirce, P. Studies in spatial learning: VIII. Place performance and the acquisition of place dispositions. *J. comp. physiol. Psychol.*, 1950, 43: 73–85.

7. Witkin, H. A. "Hypotheses" in rats: an experimental critique: II. The displacement of responses and behavior variability in linear situations. *J. comp. Psychol.*, 1941, 31: 303–336.

10

LEARNING BEHAVIOR IN GUINEA PIGS SUBJECTED TO ASPHYXIA AT BIRTH

R. FREDERICK BECKER AND WILLIAM DONNELL

Department of Anatomy, Duke University School of Medicine

In 1938, Schreiber (8, 9), a pediatrician, reported that 70 per cent of a large group of children with neurological disorders that he had encountered in his practice had histories of marked apnea at birth. Among this group were convulsives, spastic paralytics, and mentally retarded children. He suggested that these functional disturbances were related directly to the ravages of anoxia upon the central nervous system. The birth records all bore evidence of oversedation of the mother in the administration of obstetrical drugs during labor.

Schreiber's observations received support in a significant study by Darke (3). From hospital records of children with histories of severe apnea at birth, this investigator culled out a group, still living, whose sibs had uncomplicated birth histories. To as many of them as he could find, he administered the Terman revision of the Binet test. In all instances, the intelligence quotient of the asphyxiated child measured significantly lower than that of its normal-born sib.

Neurologists have had their attention directed toward manifestations of cerebral pathology in human infants as long ago as 1862, when Little described spastic paralysis (Little's Disease) as "due to abnormal parturition, difficult labours, premature birth and asphyxia neonatorum" (7, p. 304). It is also well known that cytological changes in the adult brain follow anoxia induced by breathing atmospheres low in oxygen content, or after arrest of cerebral circulation (2, 4, 11). Even lesser degrees of oxygen deficiency, provided they are of frequent occurrence, likewise can result in permanent brain damage (5, 10). But, aside from the suggestive evidence of Schreiber and Darke, there is no real experimental evidence that anoxia at birth can terminate with such residual effects as paralyses, convulsions, sensory disorders, and disturbances in intellectual development. It should be possible to subject this latter hypothesis to an experimental test in a controlled situation.

From *The Journal of Comparative and Physiological Psychology*, April 1952.

METHOD

The abdomens of pregnant guinea pigs near term were anesthetized locally with procaine hydrochloride to avoid embarrassment of the fetal respiratory center with general anesthesia. The belly wall was incised and the uterus secured. One fetus was delivered at once by Caesarean section to serve as a littermate control. The remaining fetuses were asphyxiated in utero by clamping the uterine vessels. Intrauterine anoxia was induced in this way in 103 litters.

The guinea pig was selected as the test animal for several reasons. (a) The estrous cycle is well established so that matings can be timed with fair exactitude. (b) Gestation is reasonably brief. (c) Multiple litters were essential. Although the monkey might have been preferred, multiple births are rare in this species. (d) Placentation in the guinea pig is quite comparable to that in man. (e) Survival time under anoxia at term is shorter than in many other species. In this respect, the guinea pig at birth resembles the human newborn. (f) Its central nervous system, however, is more highly developed than the human being's at birth. It might be anticipated, then, that the effects of anoxia upon this highly organized nervous system could be observed with ease and readily described.

Normally, intrauterine respiratory-like efforts do not occur during gestation (12, 15). But, the respiratory center can be induced to discharge, even early in fetal life, under anoxic duress. The experimental animals were asphyxiated to the point where intrauterine respiratory-like movements were initiated. When this stage was reached, the experimental procedure followed one of two courses. Either the fetuses were delivered at the last intrauterine gasp and were allowed to establish their air-breathing existence spontaneously, or delivery was delayed until all signs of an intrauterine respiratory-like rhythm had ceased and a heart beat was no longer palpable.

The "spontaneous recovery group" consisted of 58 litters. Such animals were apneic for only a few minutes after delivery. They soon established a viable respiratory rhythm, but often not without some difficulty. The remaining 48 litters, constituting the "delayed recovery group," were totally atonic and apneic and required artificial respiration. The skin was cold and pale. Blood had shifted from the periphery to deeper capillary beds, and circulation was obviously stagnant. These animals were truly in a state of asphyxia pallida. Resuscitation was accomplished by inserting a fine hypodermic needle into the trachea through a skin incision in the neck. The needle was attached to a small Douglas gas-bag containing either oxygen, or 10 per cent carbon dioxide in oxygen. The lungs were insufflated gently under light positive pressure until a spontaneous respiratory rhythm was established.

In marked contrast to either of the experimental groups, Caesarean-delivered controls breathed at once, righted immediately, and were soon actively engaged nursing on a foster mother. No experimental animal was able to right and assume normal activity until several hours, or, more frequently, several days after delivery.

The respiratory, cardiac, and neurological aspects of recovery, as well as the pathology encountered in the central nervous system, have been discussed in other articles (14, 16). This report is concerned primarily with the subsequent behavioral changes after recovery and, especially, with the learning and retention of a simple problem scaled to the ability of a guinea pig. The literature covering the general topic of learning ability in the guinea pig has been reviewed in another paper (1).

Thirty-eight litters (a control and an experimental animal in each case) were allowed to survive long enough (8 to 10 weeks) to test learning ability in a specially designed problem box. This combined some of the aspects of a visual discrimination apparatus with the running of a simple alternating maze pattern. For want of a more descriptive term, we shall call the testing apparatus a "problem box." It contained a starting pen, an activity chamber with blind alleys and electric grids, and two goal-boxes.

Actually, two types of problem box were used. In a preliminary experiment, 18 litters, including 6 from the spontaneous recovery group and 12 from the delayed recovery group, were tested in the box shown in Figure 1. This box was also used to train a large group of animals born normally in our colony, and a group of Caesarean deliveries from singleton litters. An analysis of these data suggested that this problem box was not a highly reliable measuring instrument for evaluating small group differences. It did, however, point up certain definite trends. It was felt that the addition of another blind alley would increase the difficulty of the problem sufficiently to highlight any real intergroup differences that might exist. Hence, the problem box was modified to the type shown in Figure 2. Twenty new litters from the delayed recovery group were trained in this box and retested two weeks after initial learning. It is, chiefly, with the performance of this group that this report is concerned.

Animals entered the box from a starting pen, the door of which was opened by remote control. A grid on the floor of the pen was connected to an Enivolt stimulator. It was used to coax recalcitrant animals into the activity chamber. After a few initial trials, shocking through the feet was seldom necessary to move an animal out. Animals ran promptly as soon as the door was opened.

Twenty inches from the pen door, a removable L-shaped partition formed the first blind alley. Twenty inches behind it (Fig. 2) a second, similar piece formed another blind on the opposite wall. These partitions could be flipped over to the opposite walls with ease so that the zigzag path an animal had to traverse to a goal-box could be reversed at will. The entrance to the goal-boxes was narrowed by a fixed T-shaped partition. By closing down a glass panel, one goal-box alley was converted into an additional blind. The two removable partitions, when in place (Fig. 2), extended well beyond the mid-line of the activity chamber, leaving only narrow passageways between their side walls and the opposite retaining walls of the activity chamber. This relationship may not be too well represented in the freehand drawings. It is, probably, best illustrated in Figure 1. When, therefore, an animal emerged into the activity chamber, its view of the second blind was cut off by the first blind, and, similarly, the second blind hid the open goal-box directly behind it. Partitions were also high enough to prevent sighting over the top, even when animals stood on their hind legs. Hence, the zigzag path to the goal-box was, actually, much more acute than the figures may suggest.

Electric grids crossed the floors of all blind alleys and also extended across adjacent open runways. Animals were shocked mildly through the feet if they entered a blind, but never when they traversed open runways.

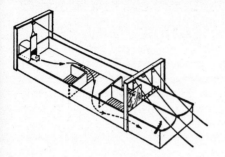
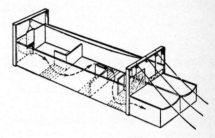

Fig. 1. Simple problem box.   Fig. 2. More complex problem box.

Initial training consisted of 15 trials in the problem box with the removable partitions lifted away, and with both goal-boxes open. A reward of lettuce was available within the darkened interior of the goal-box. In the actual learning situation which followed, the food reward did not seem to enhance motivation. Animals very rarely nibbled at the lettuce between trials. Only when left alone for a period at the end of a day's run did they consume the food. During any given trial, the main objectives seemed to be to avoid as much punishment as possible and to reach a safe, dark haven as quickly as possible.

Preliminary experiments indicated that the learning period had to be presented in three stages. Stage 1 consisted of learning to run to the right-hand goal with partitions in place as in Figure 2. In stage 2, the position of the partitions and the goal-box was reversed to a left-hand pattern. In stage 3, right- and left-hand patterns alternated in random order but with the same sequence maintained for each animal. As a rule, 20 trials at each stage proved sufficient to establish criteria of 5 successive, errorless trials for stages 1 and 2, and 10 successive, errorless, trials for stage 3. If animals were introduced to the chance-alternation sequence (stage 3) from the start, it took well over one hundred trials before they were able to meet even the lowest criterion of perfection. Largely in the interest of time economy, it proved best to proceed in this stepwise fashion to the chance-alternation series. Moreover, the 60-trial sequence conveniently allowed comparison of performance on the basis of an equal number of trials.

Entering a blind (even with two feet) was counted an error, and the animal was shocked for it. In the final problem-box it was possible to commit three separate errors per trial — one in each blind alley. Repetition of errors per blind per trial was counted separately as a perseveration score. Total error and perseveration scores provided the best comparison data. Running time did not give reliable estimates of the establishment of learning. There was, of course, a general reduction in time scores as learning progressed, but it was still possible for a slow runner to make fewer, or more, errors than a fast runner. Similarly, the number of trials necessary to attain a criterion of perfection bore little relationship to the number of errors committed in the process. Animals that reached a criterion early might make many more errors than those that reached it late by slipping up once every other trial or so.

Only the 20 litters tested in the second problem box were given a retest. This consisted of 20 trials directly on the chance-alternation series. The retest came two weeks after initial learning.

All tests were run in a softly lighted, completely soundproofed room to eliminate glare and extraneous noise. Manipulation of doors and the shocking device was carried out from a distance, the progress of the animals being watched in a large, overhanging mirror.

RESULTS

Performance of Caesarean-Delivered Animals and of the Animals with Normal Birth Histories

Twenty-one males and 21 females were selected at random from those born normally in our colony and were trained in the simpler problem box (Fig. 1). Training was begun in the sixth week of life for 26 animals and in the twelfth week for 16 animals. No significant sex differences were observed in the mean total error and perseveration scores, or in the mean scores for the initial 20 trials of learning. Fisher's method to test the reliability of the differences between means yielded P-values ranging from .60 to .90 for the various stages of the learning process. A similar range of P-values was obtained when the performance scores of the animals trained at 6 weeks were compared with those of the animals trained at 12 weeks.

Thirty-two Caesarean-delivered animals performed as well as, or better than, those of normal birth. The means for these groups were almost identical: 41.50 errors total for the normal group, 43.47 for the Caesarean group. Apparently, Caesarean birth alone does not alter performance significantly from the normal values.

Performance of Asphyxiated Animals

Eighteen experimental litters were trained in preliminary experiments, 6 from the spontaneous recovery group and 12 from delayed recovery group. There was no significant difference in total performance when the mean scores of all asphyxiated animals were compared with those for the total control group. Similarly, no significant difference appeared in the mean scores between experimental and control members of the spontaneous recovery group. In the delayed recovery group, however, the difference between experimental and control performance approached significance at the 5 per cent level (Table 1).

Such findings led us to doubt the effectiveness of the simple form of the problem box. For, in many respects, the behavior of the asphyxiated animals differed markedly from that of the controls. Their very method of attack on the problem was different. Selection of the correct pathways seemed purely random in that there was no definite pattern in their running responses. They eliminated incorrect responses purely on a trial-and-error basis. An error in one blind would be repeated in later trials. Controls, on the other hand, would eliminate the first blind alley early, and then eliminate the other blinds in turn. They were never caught making the same error again once a particular blind had been eliminated from the running pattern.

TABLE 1. Differences between Caesarean-Delivered Controls and Their Asphyxiated Littermates in Learning a Simple Problem

Measure	Control	Asphyxiated	P*
Mean total errors			
Delayed recovery†	40.25	55.95	.05
Spontaneous recovery†	31.33	28.83	<.50
Total	36.33	39.27	<.40
Mean perseveration			
Delayed recovery	14.08	16.50	<.40
Spontaneous recovery	8.17	4.68	<.20
Total	12.17	12.56	<.90

* P-values are calculated for t based on the differences in means of related measures (6).
† The delayed recovery group comprised 12 litters; the spontaneous recovery group, 6 litters.

A much more noticeable difference was the assurance demonstrated by a control once incorrect responses had been overcome. By midway in the learning process, controls would emerge from the pen, glance quickly right and left, and, apparently, taking a cue from the setting of the first blind, they would run a swift, unerring, zigzag course to the correct goal-box. Few asphyxiated animals ever developed this certainty of response. Instead, their errorless trials were marked by hesitancy before one blind or another. They seemed impelled to peek in for assurance, even if they did not enter.

Table 2 indicates that although the total number of correct responses in 60 trials was about equal for control and experimental groups, the number of correct responses that were hesitant was approximately twice as great in the experimental groups. The differences in this respect are highly significant. Even the behavior of the spontaneous re-

covery group falls in line in this respect, although Table I shows them
making slightly fewer errors than their controls.

It was largely from this evidence that we felt that even a slight
stiffening of the difficulty of the problem would convert hesitancy
into frank error. A real background of confusion seemed to exist

TABLE 2. EVALUATION OF HESITANCY OF RESPONSE IN ASPHYXIATED ANIMALS
AND IN LITTERMATE CONTROLS

Group	Mean for Asphyxiates	Mean for Controls	P*
Total Number of Correct Responses in 60 Trials			
Delayed recovery †	37.42	39.67	< .30
Spontaneous recovery †	41.67	41.67	1.0
Total	38.28	40.33	< .30
Number of Correct, but Hesitant, Responses in 60 Trials			
Delayed recovery	21.00	10.80	< .01
Spontaneous recovery	21.00	9.80	.02
Total	21.00	10.50	< .01
Per Cent Hesitancy in 60 Trials			
Delayed recovery	56.1	27.2	< .01
Spontaneous recovery	50.3	23.5	< .05
Total	54.8	26.0	< .01

* P-values are calculated for t based on the differences in means of related measures (6).
† The delayed recovery group comprised 12 litters; the spontaneous recovery group, 6 litters.

among the experimental group. The problem box was modified (Fig.
2) to include an additional blind alley. By this time there were only
20 litters surviving, and these were all from the delayed recovery
group. These animals were trained in the second problem box when
they were 8 weeks old, and they were retested two weeks after initial
learning was completed. Table 3 presents the data from this experiment. It is evident that the controls were significantly superior at
every stage of the learning process and on the retest.

During retest, all asphyxiated animals required retraining; 11 controls did not, but ran the 20 trials of the chance-alternation sequence
without error. The remaining controls made fewer than 3 errors, and
repeated none of them. Errors in the asphyxiated group ranged from
3 to 32 with an average of 12.7. Ten asphyxiated animals made 10
or more errors. The range of repeated errors in the experimental group
was from 1 to 14 with an average of 3. At first, we felt that the performance of the control animal, after a lapse of two weeks time, was
somewhat amazing. But we have since discovered in other experiments
(effects of chronic exposure to high altitude, and effects of concussion)

that many control animals will retest perfectly even after a lapse of 8-weeks time.

Other Behavioral Patterns Peculiar to the Asphyxiated Animal

There was a marked difference, both in exposure time to intrauterine asphyxiation and in the length of the apneic period after delivery, between spontaneous and delayed recovery groups. On the average, the delayed recovery group was asphyxiated for 15.5 min., and was apneic for 43 min. The spontaneous recovery group suffered only 7 min. of anoxia in utero, and was apneic about 8 min. at most. Yet postoperative behavior was remarkably similar in the two groups. Regardless of the severity of the anoxic bout, all experimental animals reacted much more sluggishly than the controls. They sat quietly in their cages, and displayed none of the scurrying and inquisitive exploring common to the normal animals. This reduction in spontaneous activity level lasted for weeks. The experimental animals did not move when reached for in the cage, and they were limp and relaxed when held. They submitted to stroking without blinking or shudder-

TABLE 3. DIFFERENCES BETWEEN CAESAREAN-DELIVERED CONTROLS AND THEIR ASPHYXIATED LITTERMATES IN LEARNING A MORE COMPLICATED PROBLEM

Measure	N	Stage 1 (20 Trials Right)		Stage 2 (20 Trials Left)		Stage 3 (20 Trials Chance-Alternate)		60 Trials Total	
		Mean	P	Mean	P	Mean	P	Mean	P
Initial Learning									
Errors									
Experimental	20	41.75		19.75		7.75		69.25	
			< .01		< .01		< .01		< .01
Control	20	19.10		9.30		2.05		31.45	
Perseveration									
Experimental	20	15.80		6.45		1.50		23.75	
			< .01		< .01		< .30		< .01
Control	20	6.70		1.75		0.10		8.55	
Retest									
Errors									
Experimental	19					12.68			
							< .01		
Control	19					0.70			
Perseveration									
Experimental	19					3.05			
							< .01		
Control	19					0.			

P-values are calculated for t based on the differences in means of related measures (6).

ing. This was quite a contrast to the attempt to capture a scurrying, alert and elusive, normal animal. Even when held, controls were tense, fearful, and ready to escape when released.

There was a marked contrast in reactivity to shock in the activity chamber. Probably many of the errors committed by controls were due to frantic scurrying as a fear response in a novel situation. Shock-. ing merely enhanced the initial wild running, and it was responsible for driving the animal into some blind alleys it might otherwise have avoided. Controls often expressed anger by teeth gnashing, vocifera- tion, and biting at the partitions. Or they would "freeze" in a corner, urinate, and defecate. Asphyxiated animals displayed none of these emotional signs. When shocked for error, they shuffled slowly out of the blind, and like as not would amiably back in. The random run- ning pattern and the degree of hesitancy among experimental animals has been mentioned.

DISCUSSION

Recovery after experimental asphyxia was marked by severe neurological sequelae in all experimental animals regardless of the degree of anoxia suffered or the length of the apneic period. Some members of the spontaneous recovery group were as severely affected as some of the worst cases among the delayed recovery group. Each of the neurological disturbances reported by Schreiber in his children was seen in one or another of these animals. The detailed neurological findings have been reported elsewhere (14).

Suffice to say here, all of the following motor aberrations were observed: spastic paralysis in greatest frequency; flaccid paralysis (and hypalgesia of the lower extremities along with cord bladders) in a few cases; delayed and impaired righting in all; ataxias; body and head tremors; facial, pharyngeal, and hypoglossal paralyses; convul- sive and choreiform twitching; hyperactive running movements and propulsive lunging.

On the sensory side, there was a lack of startle response in many, hypalgesia in some, and visual disturbances in a few. Some animals were remarkably somnolent.

Neuronal damage was widespread throughout the brain and brain- stem. The cord suffered extensive damage only in the case of the few flaccid paralytics. The cerebellum and basal ganglia were remarkably free of pathology despite the neurological evidence of cerebellar and striatal symptoms of motor injury.

Cell loss was extensive in the lateral hypothalamic area, the ven- trolateral nuclei of the thalamus, and the geniculate bodies of several animals. This would account for the somnolence and the sensory disturbances encountered.

Recovery from sensory loss took longer than recovery from motor disability. Motor coordination was as good as that in the control animal by the end of a month, though startle was absent at eight to ten weeks. But, only in those animals dying at the time of motor difficulties, was there any evidence of chromatolytic changes in the motor cortex and in the various brainstem motor nuclei. Motor centers in animals which survived were as free of pathology as the same centers in the control brains. But, the small associational neurons in various areas of the cortex, and the tegmental nuclei of the brain stem, were extensively destroyed in all experimental animals. Apparently, although some cells are permanently damaged under anoxia, others, like the motor neurons, are more resistant and undergo phases of partial chromatalysis from which they recover if the animal survives. It should be noted that human children are not likely to recover from their motor disorders as rapidly, or as completely, as did these animals.

When our learning data and the postoperative changes in "personality" are coupled with these neurological and pathological findings, our study lends strong support to the previous report of Schreiber and Darke (8, 9, 3). Obviously, the present study does not buttress Schreiber's main contention that obstetrical drugs administered in massive dosages to women in labor, are the prime factor in inducing neonatal asphyxia and its sequelae. But, certainly, volatile anesthetics and, especially, the barbiturate derivatives, which cross the placental barrier readily, can be every bit as effective in embarrassing the fetal respiratory system as our more direct methods of clamping the maternal uterine vessels (13). The warning to expectant mothers is obvious: It is not wise to insist on being "snowed under" at delivery. A little pain at childbirth, mollified by light sedation, may prevent extreme sorrow later.

SUMMARY

Guinea pigs were asphyxiated in utero by clamping the maternal uterine vessels after one animal in each litter, near term, had been delivered as a nonasphyxiated control. One group was freed from the uterus at the time of the last intrauterine respiratory-like gasp. These began to breathe air spontaneously after a brief apneic period. A second group was asphyxiated until they were comatose, totally apneic, and atonic. These were artificially revived with gas mixtures. All asphyxiated animals exhibited a wide variety of neurological symptoms on recovery. All motor symptoms disappeared by the end of four weeks.

Eighteen litters with their controls were subjected to a learning situation in a specially constructed problem box. Preliminary experiments had indicated that there were no sex or age differences between 6- and 12-week groups, and no difference between normal-born and Caesarean-delivered animals in the mastery of this simple problem. Animals from the delayed recovery group made more errors and were significantly more hesitant in their correct responses than their littermate controls. Members of the spontaneous recovery group were merely more hesitant.

The difficulty of the problem was increased, and 20 more litters were trained in the modified problem box when they were eight weeks old. At every stage of the learning process, these animals made more errors and repeated the same errors far more than their littermate controls. Differences were significant at the .01 level. At a retest two weeks after initial learning, all experimental animals required extensive retraining. The majority of the controls performed perfectly, and the rest made fewer than three errors. Again, differences between error and perseveration scores were highly significant.

Other pertinent differences in behavior between the asphyxiated animals and their Caesarean-delivered littermates are discussed. The neurological findings on recovery and the cerebral pathology at death are similar to those observed in children with histories of apnea at birth induced by oversedation of the mother with volatile anesthetics or barbiturate derivatives. Mental retardation has been reported as a common finding in children with such birth histories.

REFERENCES

1. Becker, R. F. Some observations on learning ability in the guinea pig. *Quart. Bull. Northwestern Univ. med. Sch.*, 1946, 20: 318–328.

2. Courville, C. B. Asphyxia as a consequence of nitrous oxide anesthesia. *Medicine*, 1936, 15: 129–245.

3. Darke, R. A. Late effects of severe asphyxia neonatorum. *J. Pediat.*, 1944, 24: 148–158.

4. Gildea, E. F., and Cobb, S. The effects of anemia on the cerebral cortex of the cat. *Arch. Neurol. Psychiat.*, Chicago, 1930, 23: 876–903.

5. Jensen, A. V., Becker, R. F., and Windle, W. F. Changes in brain structure and memory after intermittent exposure to simulated altitude of 30,000 feet. *Arch. Neurol. Psychiat.*, Chicago, 1949, 60: 221–239.

6. Lindquist, E. F. *Statistical analysis in educational research.* Boston: Houghton Mifflin, 1940.

7. Little, W. J. On the influence of abnormal parturitions, difficult labours, and asphyxia neonatorum on the mental and physical conditions of the child, especially in relation to deformities. *Trans. Obstet. Soc.*, Lond., 1862, 3: 293–344.

8. Schreiber, F. Apnea of the newborn and associated cerebral injury. *J. Amer. med. Ass.*, 1938, 111: 1263–1269.

9. Schreiber, F., and Gates, N. Cerebral injury in newborn due to anoxia at birth. *J. Mich. med. Soc.*, 1938, 37: 145–150.

10. Thorner, M. W., and Lewy, F. H. The effects of repeated anoxia on the brain. *J. Amer. med. Ass.*, 1940, 115: 1595–1600.

11. Tureen, L. L. Effect of experimental temporary vascular occlusion on the spinal cord. I. Correlation between structural and functional changes. *Arch. Neurol. Psychiat.*, Chicago, 1936, 35: 789–807.

12. Windle, W. F., and Becker, R. F. Relation of anoxemia to early activity in the fetal nervous system. *Arch. Neurol. Psychiat.*, Chicago, 1940, 43: 90–101.

13. Windle, W. F., and Becker, R. F. Role of carbon dioxide in resuscitation at birth after asphyxia and after nembutal anesthesia. *Amer. J. Obstet. Gynec.*, 1941, 42: 852–858.

14. Windle, W. F., and Becker, R. F. Asphyxia neonatorum. *Amer. J. Obstet. Gynec.*, 1943, 45: 183–200.

15. Windle, W. F., Becker, R. F., Barth, E. E., and Schulz, M.D. Aspiration of amniotic fluid by the fetus. *Surg. Gynec. Obstet.*, 1939, 69: 705–712.

16. Windle, W. F., Becker, R. F., and Weil, A. Alterations in brain structures after asphyxia at birth. *J. Neuropath. exp. Neurol.*, 1944, 3: 224–237.

Part II

PSYCHOSOMATIC DISORDERS AND NEUROSIS

11

STRESS AND DISEASE

HANS SELYE

Institute of Experimental Medicine and Surgery, University of Montreal

Almost two decades have passed now since the publication of a short note on "A syndrome produced by diverse nocuous agents" (*1*). Since that time, the relationships between this "general-adaptation syndrome" or "stress syndrome," and virtually every branch of physiology and clinical medicine have been subjected to study. Those who seek detailed information concerning certain aspects of the stress problem will find a key to the world literature in the monographs (*2–10*) and yearbooks (*11–14*) that are especially devoted to this topic. Hence there is no need to burden this text with numerous references. It may be opportune, however, to take stock now in the form of a brief synopsis surveying the most fundamental facts that we have learned about the relationships between stress and disease. This will give us an opportunity also to outline what we would consider to be the principal scope and the limitations of this new approach to problems of medicine (*15*).

Ever since man first used the word *disease,* he has had some inkling of the stress concept. The very fact that this single term has been used to denote a great variety of manifestly distinct maladies clearly indicates that they have been recognized as having something in common. They possess, as we would now say, some "nonspecific disease features" (the feeling of being ill, loss of appetite and vigor, aches and pains, loss of weight, and so forth), that permit human beings to distinguish illness from the condition of health. Yet, precisely because these manifestations are not characteristic of any one disease, they have received little attention in comparison with the specific ones. They were thought to be of lesser interest to the physician, for, unlike the specific symptoms and signs, they did not help him to recognize the "eliciting pathogen" or to prescribe an appropriate specific cure. Whenever it was impossible to determine precisely what the cause of the trouble was, therapy had to be limited to such general measures as the recommendation of rest, an easily digestible and yet nutritious

From *Science,* 122:625, 1955.

diet, protection against great variations in the surrounding temperature, or the use of salicylates to stop pain.

Experience had likewise shown long ago that what we now call nonspecific stress can also have certain remarkable curative properties under certain conditions. Nonspecific therapy was consciously or unconsciously based on this principle. In the Middle Ages, flogging of the insane was practiced to "drive the evil spirit out of them." This procedure was subsequently replaced by the more humane fever therapy, Metrazol shock, insulin shock, electroshock, and numerous other measures, but all of these have in common the property of producing a state of systemic, nonspecific stress. Such practices as bloodletting, fasting, or the parenteral administration of milk, blood, and colloidal metals may serve as additional examples of nonspecific procedures, which undoubtedly can produce beneficial results in patients afflicted by a variety of diseases. These measures were, and some of them still are, widely used for lack of more effective and less traumatic means of therapy. However, the mechanism of their action remained obscure, and therefore scientifically minded physicians were always reluctant to use them, for they recognized that these treatments were actually stabs in the dark whose consequences could never be accurately foretold.

Perhaps the most fundamental difference between medieval and modern medicine is that the former was primarily based on pure empiricism and directed by mysticism and intuition, whereas the latter attempts to understand the mechanisms of disease — through an objective scientific analysis — and to treat it by influencing well-defined points along the pathways of its development. Up to the present time, the greatest progress that has been made along these lines has resulted in specific therapeutic procedures that are designed to eliminate in each case the particular primary cause — the eliciting pathogen of a disease — for instance, by chemotherapeutic measures or with the surgeon's knife.

By contrast, throughout the centuries, we have learned virtually nothing about rational, scientifically well-founded procedures that would help the body in its own natural efforts to maintain health quite apart from the attacks on the pathogen. Yet, often, the causative agent cannot be recognized or is not amenable to any therapeutic procedures directed specifically against it. Besides, elimination of the causative agent frequently does not cure, because the effects of the disease producer may greatly outlast its actual presence in the body. Let us remember that it is not the microbe, the poison, or the allergen but our reactions to these agents that we experience as disease. A man may die from a single exposure to ionizing rays, a rheumatic heart, or an infectious nephritis long after the original cause of his illness is no longer present in his body.

Whenever the available procedures of specific therapy are imperfect, the physician is forced to say that he has done what he could and "nature will do the rest." The fact is that very often nature actually does the rest, but unfortunately not always. Indeed, we may say that the leitmotiv of our work on stress was the question: "How does nature do 'the rest' and, when nature fails in this, could we not help if we learned more about natural methods?"

When we were first confronted with the "alarm reaction," the idea that presented itself most vividly was that the very tangible and accurately measurable morphologic characteristics of this first stage of the stress response might give us a key to the objective scientific analysis of systemic, nonspecific reactions. The enlargement of the adrenal cortex and the atrophy of the thymus and lymph nodes, for example, were changes that could be expressed in strictly quantitative terms, and they were certainly not specific, since any agent that caused systemic damage or stress elicited them.

A multitude of questions presented themselves immediately. Which among the manifestations of this alarm reaction are useful for the maintenance of health and which are merely signs of damage? How does an injury to a limited area of the body reach the various internal organs that are eventually affected during the alarm reaction? For instance, how does a trauma to one limb eventually influence such distant structures as the adrenal cortex or the thymus? Which organ change is the cause and which the consequence of another structural alteration? For instance, does the disintegrating thymus tissue liberate substances that stimulate the adrenals or does the enlarged adrenal cortex secrete hormones that affect the thymus?

It was quite evident, of course, that to answer these questions would take much time and probably long series of often monotonous stereotypic experiments, using various stressors on various species of animals. Nevertheless, a general blueprint for the dissection and clinical utilization of the stress syndrome presented itself immediately. In particular, we asked ourselves five questions, which we thought would now be amenable to experimental analysis: (i) What are the changes characteristic of stress as such? (ii) How does the stress response evolve in time? (iii) What are the pathways through which stress reaches various organs? (iv) Are there "diseases of adaptation," that is, maladies principally the result of errors in the adaptation syndrome? (v) To what extent are the animal experiments on stress applicable to clinical medicine?

None of these questions has been fully answered and, indeed, the complete clarification of biologic problems is hardly an attainable aim. However, partial answers have been obtained to all of these basic questions, and — most important of all — it appears that they have been so formulated that further progress is now largely a matter of time.

We have learned, for instance, that acute involution of the lymphatic organs, diminution of the blood eosinophiles, enlargement and increased secretory activity of the adrenal cortex, and a variety of changes in the chemical constitution of the blood and tissues are truly nonspecific and characteristic of stress as such. It has also become evident that they represent a syndrome, in that they are closely correlated with one another, both in time and in intensity. Whenever disassociations among them tend to occur, it can usually be shown that these are attributable to one of the following two reasons: (i) either the specific actions of the evocative agent are superimposed upon the stress syndrome and thus obscure some of the nonspecific manifestations (for example, if insulin is used as a stressor, the glycemic response is masked by the hypoglycemic effect of the hormone); or (ii) one of the pathways through which stress acts in the organism is deranged (for example, stress causes no thymus involution after adrenalectomy).

No agent produces only stress. Hence, in actual experimentation, the stress response is invariably complicated by certain superimposed specific changes, and in every species — indeed, in every individual — one or the other pathway is more or less functional than the rest. These factors tend to mask or deform the typical stress response, and failure to recognize them was undoubtedly the principal handicap to clear characterization of the stress response in the past. Let us now return to our five basic problems and enumerate at least the most important facts about them that have come to light during these 20 years of research on stress.

CHANGES CHARACTERISTIC OF STRESS

In attempting to answer the question, "What are the changes characteristic of stress as such?" the first problem was, of course, to define *stress*, at least as accurately as definitions can be formulated in biology. The word, especially when it is used with its mate *strain*, has long been in everyday usage, but its significance in biology had never been defined. The layman speaks, for instance, of *eyestrain*, or *mental stress* in referring to rather specific complaints. Cannon, the great student of homeostasis, also used the terms *stresses* and *strains* in connection with specific reactions. He emphasized, for instance, that the stresses and strains of oxygen lack, hemorrhage, and starvation elicit totally different and specific homeostatic reactions. Conversely, it is a characteristic of the stress syndrome, as we understand it, that it is always the same, no matter what happens to elicit it. For over-all responses, which include specific and nonspecific features — and this is even more true of purely specific responses — the term now used would be *reaction* (not *stress*) and the the eliciting agent would be called a *stimulus* (not a *stressor* or *alarming stimulus*). Such specific reactions are precisely the part of the over-all response that we must subtract to arrive at our stress syndrome.

To make this distinction clear, we always used the term *nonspecific stress* in our early publications. Later, unfortunately, it became customary to omit the adjective, for brevity's sake. To avoid confusion, we then pointed out that in the sense in which we use the term, stress may be defined as a nonspecific deviation from the normal resting state; it is caused by function or damage and it stimulates repair.

Here, the nonspecific causation of the change has been selected as its most characteristic feature. However, even the term *specific* had been used somewhat loosely in medicine; we therefore defined a nonspecific change as one that can be produced by many or all agents, as opposed to a specific change, which is elicited only by one or few agents. Correspondingly, a nonspecific agent acts on many targets, a specific one acts on few targets, and a stressor is an agent that causes stress.

Of course, we realized from the outset that these, like all biologic definitions, are imperfect, but trying to formulate them helped us to impart precision to our own concepts of *stimulus, stressor, stress, specific,* and *nonspecific.* Among other things, these considerations brought out with particular clarity the fact that stress is not necessarily the result of damage but can be caused by physiologic function and that it is not merely the result of a nonspecific action but also comprises the defense against it. These are cardinal facts, as we shall see later when we consider the relationship between stress and disease.

In our efforts to identify the characteristics of stress, our main problem was to eliminate all specific manifestations that are typical either of the agent or of the reacting organism. Hence, a large number of animal species had to be studied, following exposure to a great variety of essentially different stimuli, to compare the resulting structural, chemical, and functional changes. This made it possible to determine which are the responses common to all types of exposure, and only these could be considered to be truly nonspecific — that is, the result of stress as such. The residue that remained after subtraction of all the specific changes is the general-adaptation syndrome.

In this response, every part of the body is involved, but the two great integrators of activity, the hormonal and the nervous systems, are especially important. The facts known today may lead us to believe that the anterior pituitary and the adrenal cortex play the cardinal roles in coordinating the defense of the organism during stress. This view is probably distorted by the fact that the syndrome has been studied primarily by endocrinologists, and investigations concerning the participation of the nervous system are handicapped by the greater complexity of the required techniques. It is considerably easier to remove an endocrine gland and to substitute for its hormones by the injection of extracts than it is to destroy minute individual nervous centers selectively and then restore their function to determine the role they may play during stress.

Stress Response in Time

To establish the evolution of the stress response in time, animals had to be repeatedly exposed to stressors (cold, forced muscular exercise, bloodletting, and drugs) of a constant intensity over long periods of time. It was found that, after a while, the same agent does not continue to produce the same nonspecific response. For instance, treatment with a drug that initially causes discharge of adrenocortical lipid granules will later actually promote accumulation of lipids in the adrenal cortex, after the animals have become more resistant to the damaging effects of the agent. Upon still more continued exposure, sooner or later, this acquired adaptation is invariably lost; then the animals again show signs of damage, and their adrenal cortices again discharge their lipid granules.

These adrenal changes are taken as only one example among the many characteristics of the general-adaptation syndrome that show such a triphasic pattern (for example, glycemia, chloremia, and body weight). In fact the whole syndrome is essentially triphasics; thus its manifestations depend as much on the stressor effect of the eliciting agent as on the time elapsed since the organism was first exposed to it.

The three stages of the stress syndrome are (i) the alarm reaction, in which adaptation has not yet been acquired; (ii) the stage of resistance, in which adaptation is optimum; and (iii) the stage of exhaustion, in which the acquired adaptation is lost again.

The physicochemical basis of the curious terminal loss of acquired adaptation is still quite obscure. Exhaustion cannot be fully compensated, either by changes in the caloric intake or by any known hormonal substitution therapy. The term *adaptation energy* has been suggested to designate the adaptability that is gradually consumed during exposure, but despite much research we have learned nothing about the nature of this "energy."

Many of the changes characteristic of the stage of exhaustion are strikingly similar to those of senility. It is tempting to view the general-adaptation syndrome as a kind of accelerated aging. It appears as though, because of the greater intensity of stress, the three major periods of life — infancy (in which adaptation has not yet been acquired), adulthood (in which adaptation has been acquired to the usual stresses of life), and senility (in which the acquired adaptation is lost again) — are here telescoped into a short space of time.

However, these will remain sterile speculations until some ingenious mind can devise new experimental procedures with which to analyze them in quantitative terms. It is only to stimulate thought along these lines that I venture even to mention these problems here. I hope that some talented young mind, still sufficiently uninhibited by textbook knowledge to see a new approach, will follow this trail. To me it seems more promising of truly great progress in the understanding of life and adaptability than any other aspect of stress research.

PATHWAYS OF STRESS

To clarify the pathways through which stress reaches various organs, it was merely necessary to use the classic procedures of experimental medicine — namely, the destruction of suspected relay stations and, wherever possible, their restoration (for example, removal of an endocrine gland and substitution therapy with extracts containing its hormones). Figure 1 helps to summarize the principal data that have come to light in this respect.

All agents that act on the body or any of its parts exert dual effects: (i) specific actions, with which we are not concerned in this review, except insofar as they modify the nonspecific actions of the same agents and (ii) nonspecific or stressor effects, whose principal pathways (as far as we know them today) are illustrated in Fig. 1. The stressor acts on the target (the body or some part of it) directly (thick arrow) and indirectly by way of the pituitary and the adrenal. Through some unknown pathway (labeled by a question mark), the "first mediator" travels from the directly injured target area to the anterior pituitary. It notifies the latter that a condition of stress exists and thus induces it to discharge adrenocorticotrophic hormone (ACTH).

It is quite possible that this first mediator of hormonal defense is not always the same. In some instances, it may be an adrenaline discharge, in others a liberation of histaminelike toxic tissue metabolites, a nervous impulse, or even a sudden deficiency in some vitally important body constituent (such as glucose or an enzyme). During stress it is rarely the lack of adrenal corticoids that stimulates ACTH secretion, through a self-regulating "feed-back" mechanism.

ACTH, alone or in cooperation with other hormones, stimulates the adrenal cortex to discharge corticoids. Some of the cortical hormones, the mineralocorticoids, also known as prophlogistic corticoids

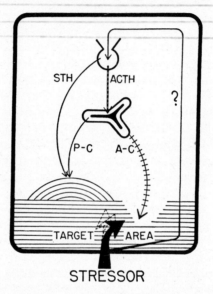

Fig. 1. Diagram illustrating the principal pathways of the stress response. After Selye (3).

(P-Cs), stimulate the proliferative ability and reactivity of connective tissue; they enhance the "inflammatory potential." Thus, they help to put up a strong barricade of connective tissue through which the body is protected against further invasion by the pathogenic stressor agent (examples are desoxycorticosterone and aldosterone).

However, under ordinary conditions, ACTH stimulates the adrenal much more effectively to secrete glucocorticoids, also known as antiphlogistic corticoids (A-Cs). These inhibit the ability of the body to put up granulomatous barricades in the path of the invader; in fact, they tend to cause involution of connective tissue with a pronounced depression of the inflammatory potential. Thus they can suppress inflammation, but, by this same token, they open the way to the spreading of infection (examples are cortisol and cortisone).

Certain recent experiments suggest that, depending on the conditions,

ACTH may cause a predominant secretion of one or the other type of corticoid. However, be this as it may, the "growth hormone," or somatotrophic hormone (STH), of the pituitary increases the inflammatory potential of connective tissue very much as the prophlogistic corticoids do; hence, it can sensitize the target area to the actions of the prophlogistic corticoids.

It is possible that the hypophysis also secretes some special corticotrophin that induces the adrenal to elaborate predominantly prophlogistic corticoids; indeed, STH itself may possess such effects, but this has not yet been proved. Probably the electrolyte content of the blood can also regulate mineralocorticoid production. In any event, even if ACTH were the only corticotrophin, the actions of the corticoids produced under its influence can be vastly different, depending on "conditioning factors" (such as STH) that specifically sensitize the target area for one or the other type of corticoid action. Actually, conditioning factors could even alter the response to ACTH of the adrenal cortex itself, so that its cells would produce more antiphlogistic or prophlogistic corticoids. Thus, during stress, one or the other type of effect can predominate.

As work along these lines progressed, it became increasingly more evident that the actions of all the "adaptive hormones" (corticoids, ACTH, STH) are so largely dependent on conditioning factors that the latter must be considered to be equally as important, in determining the final outcome of a reaction to stress, as the hormones themselves. It will be rewarding, therefore, to discuss this topic thoroughly.

Conditioning of hormone actions. Heredity, age, previous exposure to stress, nervous stimuli, the nutritional state, and many other factors can affect both the production of the adaptive hormones and their effect on individual target organs. The action of mineralocorticoids on most of their target tissues is augmented, and that of glucocorticoids is diminished, by an excess of dietary sodium. However, stress during the secretion of adaptive hormones is perhaps the most effective and most common factor capable of conditioning their actions. Thus systemic stress augments the antiphlogistic, lympholytic, catabolic, and hyperglycemic actions of antiphlogistic corticoids. Furthermore, one of the salient effects of the adaptive hormones, that of modifying the course of inflammation, naturally cannot manifest itself unless some "topical stressor" (for example, a nonspecific irritant acting on a circumscribed tissue region) first elicits an inflammatory response.

A few words about the recently introduced concept of the "permissive actions" of corticoids may be in order here. This hypothesis assumes that the corticoids do not themselves affect the targets of stress but merely permit stressors to act on them. Thus the presence or absence of corticoids could only allow or disallow a stress reaction but could not vary its intensity. To illustrate this concept, one might compare the production of light by an electric lamp to the biologic reaction and the switch to the permissive factor. The switch cannot produce light or regulate the degree of its intensity, but unless it is turned on the lamp will not function. Correspondingly, the functional signs — generally considered to be characteristic of overproduction of corticoids during stress — would result not from any actual increase in corticoid secretion but from the extra-adrenal actions of the stressors themselves. The presence of corticoids would be necessary only in a "supporting capacity" to maintain the vitality and reactivity of tissues (*16*).

Actually, it is precisely in the specific and not in the nonspecific (stress) reactions that the corticoids play a purely permissive role of this type. Here they are necessary only to prevent stress and collapse, thus keeping the tissues responsive. For instance, adrenalectomized rats will not respond to injected STH with somatic growth or to sexual stimulation with mating without a minimal-maintenance corticoid treatment. However, these are specific reactions; they are not characteristic either of stress or of the corticoids and could not be duplicated in the absence of the specific stimulus (STH and sexual stimulation), even with the highest doses of corticoids.

The characteristics of antiphlogistic corticoid overproduction that we see in the alarm reaction (for example, atrophy of the lymphatic organs, catabolism, and inhibition of inflammation) are also impeded by adrenalectomy; they are also restored even by mere maintenance doses of antiphlogistic corticoids in the presence of stress, because the latter sensitizes, or conditions, the tissues to them. The fundamental difference is, however, that — unlike specific actions — these nonspecific effects can be duplicated, even in the absence of any stressor, if large doses of antiphlogistic corticoids are given.

The importance of such conditioning influences is particularly striking in the regulation of stress reactions, because, in the final analysis, they are the factors that can actually determine whether exposure to a stressor will be met by a physiologic adaptation syndrome or cause "diseases of adaptation." Furthermore, in the latter instance, these conditioning factors can even determine the selective breakdown of one or the other organ. We are led to believe that differences in predisposition, caused by such factors, might explain why the same kind of stressor can cause diverse types of diseases of adaptation in different individuals.

"Buffering action" of the adrenals. It has long been noted that it

is much more difficult to obtain overdosage with either glucocorticoids or mineralocorticoids in the presence than in the absence of the adrenals. Thus, for instance, cortisol exerts its typical actions (for example, on inflammation, body weight, and the thymicolymphatic organs) at much higher dose levels in intact rats than it does in adrenalectomized rats. This is largely, if not entirely, the result of the absence of mineralocorticoids, for it proved possible to restore the glucocorticoid resistance of the adrenalectomized rat to normal by treatment with small doses of mineralocorticoids (desoxycorticosterone and aldosterone). Even a mere excess of dietary sodium can, at least partially, substitute for the adrenal in such experiments; hence it is reasonable to assume that here the mineralocorticoids antagonize the glucocorticoids, as a direct result of their effect upon mineral metabolism.

These experiments definitely disproved the so-called "unitarian theory" of adrenocortical function, which was still held by some of the most distinguished adrenal physiologists a short while ago. It is clear not only that the cortex produces more than one kind of corticoid but that the mineralocorticoids and the glucocorticoids are mutually antagonistic in many respects, as postulated by the "corticoid balance theory."

However, several observations still did not seem to be consonant with our concept of corticoid antagonism. For instance, in the presence of the adrenals, both in experimental animals and in man, it proved extremely difficult to stimulate inflammatory reactions much above normal, even with very large doses of mineralocorticoids. On the other hand, glucocorticoids always succeed in overcoming the buffering action of an intact adrenal, as long as the dosage is sufficiently high.

It is only quite recently that the cause of this apparent exception to the concept of adrenal hormone antagonism has been clarified by the demonstration that the corticoids act in accordance with the "law of intersecting dose-effect curves."

Law of intersecting dose-effect curves. When a solution containing fixed proportions of cortisol acetate and desoxycorticosterone acetate (DCA) is administered to adrenalectomized rats, the cortisol action (catabolism, thymolysis, and inhibition of inflammation) predominates at high, and the opposite, desoxycorticosterone type of activity, predominates at low dose levels. This was ascribed to the fact that the DCA activity rises rapidly to its optimum level, but then a "ceiling" is reached, and raising the dose further will not increase the effect. The cortisol type of activity, on the other hand, rises more slowly but does not flatten out until it far exceeds the ceiling of its antagonist (Fig. 2).

The relationship between the two types of corticoids explains why it is readily possible to overcome the adrenal buffer with appropriate doses of cortisol-like hormones, whereas even the highest doses of DCA cannot inhibit this effect. In the presence of the adrenals the normal level of mineralocorticoid production is usually already at its optimum of efficacy. This may also explain the frequently made observation that in adrenalectomized animals and man — where the starting

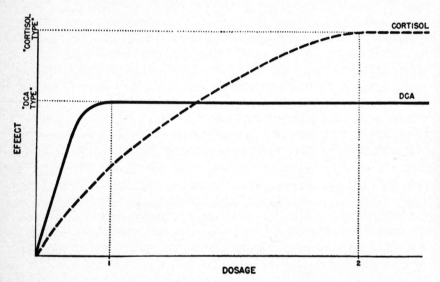

Fig. 2. Effect of varying the dose while the cortisol/desoxycorticosterone quotient is kept constant. Difference in the slopes results in intersecting dose-effect curves. After Selye and Bois (18).

point is below the mineralocorticoid ceiling — desoxycorticosterone stimulates inflammatory phenomena (for example, arthritis), and this can be antagonized by concurrent treatment with cortisol.

However, in certain respects, the desoxycorticosterone action does not appear to have a definite ceiling. Thus, in the rat, the production of renal damage by desoxycorticosterone is quite proportional to the amount given, with a very wide dose range.

Exceptional position of the kidney among the targets of corticoid activity. Numerous observations show that there exists a rather special relationship between the corticoids and the kidney, a relationship that clearly distinguishes renal tissue from other targets of corticoid activity.

Thus, the renal damage (nephrosclerosis) produced with high doses of desoxycorticosterone, in the rat, is not antagonized but is actually aggravated by concurrent treatment with cortisol. In other words, here there is no mineralocorticoid-glucocorticoid antagonism.

Furthermore, the kidney-damaging effect of various agents (for example, cold, foreign proteins, large doses of STH-preparations, and methylandrostenediol) can be prevented by adrenalectomy, while their extrarenal effects (including, for instance, the influence of STH and methylandrostenediol upon inflammation) are not markedly affected.

The cause of this exceptional reactivity of renal tissue to corticoids is not yet known. However, two factors undoubtedly play an important role here: (i) glucocorticoids and mineralocorticoids are not strictly antagonistic (and may even be synergistic) in their actions on the kidney; (ii) the inability of mineralocorticoids to produce more than a limited effect on extra-adrenal tissues (no matter how much the dose is raised) does not apply to the kidney.

In the preceding discussion we have just barely mentioned the "topical stressors," but now we shall have to consider these a little more carefully before we turn our attention to the diseases of adaptation.

Concept of the local-adaptation syndrome. In Fig. 1 we have indicated that nonspecific damage to a limited tissue area can influence the pituitary-adrenal system and consequently initiate systemic reactions to stress. It has long been known, furthermore, that many local responses to injury are nonspecific; it has been observed, for instance, that a variety of topical stressors (burns, microbes, drugs) share the power of producing local nonspecific tissue damage and/or inflammation. However, it is only recently that the close relationship between the systemic and local types of nonspecific reactions has been more clearly established. While the characteristic response of the body to systemic stress is the general-adaptation syndrome, which is characterized by manifold morphologic and functional changes throughout the organism, topical stress elicits a local adaptation syndrome, the principal repercussions of which are confined to the immediate vicinity of the eliciting injury. Local reactions consist, on the one hand, of degeneration, atrophy, and necrosis and, on the other hand, of inflammation, hypertrophy, hyperplasia, and, under certain conditions, even of neoplasia.

At first sight, there appears to be no striking similarity between the systemic and the local reaction types. A patient in traumatic shock furnishes a characteristic example of the general-adaptation syndrome and, in particular, of its earliest stage, the shock phase of the general alarm reaction. On the other hand, an abscess formed around a splinter of wood represents a typical example of the local-adaptation syndrome and, in particular, of its stage of resistance, during which the defensive inflammatory phenomena predominate. On the surface, these two instances of disease reveal no striking similarities; yet more careful study shows them to be closely related: (i) both are nonspecific reactions, comprising damage and defense; (ii) both are triphasic (with systemic or local alarm, resistance, and exhaustion); (iii) both are singularly sensitive to the adaptive hormones (ACTH, STH, and corticoids); (iv) if the two reactions develop simultaneously in the same individual, they greatly influence each other — that is, systemic stress markedly alters tissue reactivity to local stress and vice versa.

The fundamental reaction pattern to topical stressors is a local-adaptation syndrome; to systemic stressors the fundamental reaction pattern is the general-adaptation syndrome. Various modifications of these two basic responses constitute the essence of most of the diseases known today.

ARE THERE DISEASES OF ADAPTATION

By diseases of adaptation, we mean maladies that are caused principally by errors in the adaptation syndrome. Thus we arrived at the conclusion that the pathogenicity of many systemic and local stressors depends largely on the function of the hypophysis-adrenocortical system. The latter may either enhance or mitigate the body's defense reactions against stressors. We think that derailments of this adaptive mechanism are the principal factors in the production of certain maladies, which we consider, therefore, to be essentially diseases of adaptation (17).

It must be kept in mind that such diseases of adaptation do not necessarily become manifest during exposure to stress. This is clearly demonstrated by the observation that temporary overdosage with desoxycorticosterone can initiate a self-sustaining hypertension, which eventually leads to death, long after hormone administration has been discontinued. Here, we speak of "metacorticoid" lesions. The possibility that a temporary excess of endogenous mineralocorticoids could induce similar delayed maladies deserves serious consideration.

Among the derailments of the general-adaptation syndrome that may cause disease, the following are particularly important: (i) the absolute excess or deficiency in the amount of adaptive hormones (for example, corticoids, ACTH, and STH) produced during stress; (ii) an absolute excess or deficiency in the amount of adaptive hormones retained (or "fixed") by their peripheral target organs during stress; (iii) a disproportion in the relative secretion (or fixation) during stress of various antagonistic adaptive hormones (for example, ACTH and antiphlogistic corticoids, on the one hand, and STH and prophlogistic corticoids, on the other hand); (iv) the production by stress of metabolic derangements, which abnormally alter the target organ's response to adaptive hormones (through the phenomenon of "conditioning"); and (v) finally, we must not forget that, although the hypophysis-adrenal mechanism plays a prominent role in the general-adaptation syndrome, other organs that participate in the latter (for example, nervous system, liver, and kidney) may also respond abnormally and become the cause of disease during adaptation to stress.

With this in mind it may be convenient for investigative purposes to classify as "diseases of adaptation" those maladies in which an inadequacy of the adaptation syndrome plays a particularly important role. This means that the term should be used only when the maladaptation factor appears to be more important than the eliciting pathogen itself. No disease is purely a disease of adaptation, any more than it could be purely a disease of the heart or an infectious disease, without overlap with other nosologic groups. Conversely, there is no disease in which adaptive phenomena play no part.

It is undoubtedly useful to realize, however, that some agents are virtually "unconditional pathogens," in that their influence on the tissues is so great that they cause damage almost irrespective of any sensitizing or adaptive factors (for example, immediate effect of x-rays or of several thermal and mechanical injuries, and the actions of certain micro-organisms to which everybody is susceptible).

Most disease-producing agents, however, are to a greater or lesser extent "conditionally acting pathogens"; that is, their ability to produce illness is largely dependent on our adaptive reactions to them. Here, correct adaptation may prevent disease (for instance, a focus of tuberculosis perfectly held in check by an appropriate inflammatory barricade), but insufficient or excessive adaptive reactions may themselves be what we experience as illness (excessive and unnecessary inflammation around an otherwise harmless allergen).

APPLICATION OF ANIMAL EXPERIMENTS TO CLINICAL MEDICINE

Since most of the fundamental work on stress had been performed on laboratory animals, it was reasonable to question its applicability to problems of clinical medicine. It may now be said, however, that although there are certain differences in the stress response of every species, the general pattern of reaction is essentially the same in the various kinds of experimental animals and in man. Furthermore, a good deal of evidence has accumulated in support of the view that the experimental similes of spontaneous diseases produced in animals by exposure to stress, or by overdosage with certain adaptive hormones, are closely related to the corresponding maladies of man.

Let us merely mention a few of the most striking similarities in the responses to stress and to adaptive hormones which occur in animals and man.

Morphologic and functional adrenocortical changes during stress. There can be no doubt that, during intense stress (for example, severe mechanical or thermal injuries and massive infections), the adrenal cortex of man, just as that of laboratory animals, shows morphologic changes characteristic of hyperactivity. At the same time, there is a demonstrable increase in the blood concentration and urinary excretion of corticoids and their metabolites. The other manifestations (morphologic, functional, and chemical) of the stress syndrome also failed to exhibit any fundamental dissimilarity in the reaction patterns of animals and man.

Corticoid requirements during stress. During stress, the corticoid requirements of all mammals are far above normal. After destruction of the adrenals by disease (as after their surgical removal), the daily dose of corticoids, necessary for the maintenance of well-being at rest, is comparatively small, but it rises sharply during stress (for example, cold, intercurrent infections, and hemorrhage), both in experimental animals and in man.

Anti-inflammatory effects of corticoids. The same antiphlogistic corticoids (cortisone and cortisol) that were shown to inhibit various types of experimental inflammations in laboratory animals exert similar effects in a human being afflicted by inflammatory diseases (for example, rheumatoid arthritis, rheumatic fever, and allergic inflammations).

Sensitivity to infection after treatment with antiphlogistic corticoids. In experimental animals, the suppression of inflammation by antiphlogistic hormones is frequently accompanied by an increased sensitivity to infection, presumably because the encapsulation of microbial foci is less effective and perhaps partly also because serologic defense is diminished. Thus, even a species naturally resistant to the human type of tuberculosis, such as the rat, can contract this disease during overdosage with ACTH or cortisone. Similarly, in patients undergoing intense treatment with antiphlogistic hormones (for example, for rheumatoid arthritis), a previously latent tuberculosis focus may suddenly spread. It is a well-known fact that in patients suffering from tuberculosis the disease is especially readily aggravated by exposure to any kind of stress situation. Rest cures have long been practiced in view of this. It is perhaps not too farfetched to consider the possibility that an increased ACTH and cortisol secretion during

stress may play an important part in the development of clinical tuberculosis.

Sensitization to mineralocorticoids by sodium and the buffering effect of the adrenals. In experimental animals, mineralocorticoids tend to raise the blood pressure and to cause vascular and renal damage (nephrosis and nephrosclerosis) often with edema. The effect is aggravated by simultaneous treatment with sodium chloride and becomes particularly severe after adrenalectomy. Similarly, in man on a high sodium intake, and especially after adrenalectomy, otherwise nontoxic doses of desoxycorticosterone will produce hypertension and edema. Apparently, in man as in the laboratory animal, sodium acts as a conditioning factor for mineralocorticoids, while the adrenal exerts a buffering effect.

This may also explain why, in many cases of clinical hypertension, bilateral adrenalectomy exerts a beneficial effect, as long as only cortisone or cortisol is used for substitution therapy, while treatment with desoxycorticosterone restores or further aggravates the hypertensive disease. Apparently, the adrenals of these patients produce some desoxycorticosteronelike factor that plays at least an adjuvant role in the pathogenesis of hypertension.

In patients suffering from rheumatoid arthritis, adrenalectomy has also been reported to exert a beneficial influence if only glucocorticoids are used for maintenance. Furthermore desoxycorticosterone tends to elicit arthritic changes only in the adrenal-deficient but not in the intact patient. The effect of desoxycorticosterone is, in turn, corrected by simultaneous cortisone treatment.

Finally, let us point out that, both in man and in animals, the various characteristic effects of cortisone are also obtained at especially low dose levels after adrenalectomy.

Psychological and psychiatric effects of corticoid overdosage. Considerable attention has been given of late to the possible mental effects of stress and of the adaptive hormones. It would be beyond the scope of this article (and certainly outside my competence) to discuss these in detail, but a few remarks based on our experimental observations may be in order.

It has long been noted that various steroids — including desoxycorticosterone, cortisone, progesterone, and many others — can produce in a variety of animal species (even in primates such as the rhesus monkey) a state of great excitation followed by deep anesthesia. It has more recently been shown that such steroid anesthesia can also be produced in man, and, of course, the marked emotional changes (sometimes bordering on psychosis) that may occur in predisposed individuals during treatment with ACTH, cortisone and cortisol are well known. Several laboratories reported furthermore that the electro-shock threshold of experimental animals and their sensitivity to anes-thetics can be affected by corticoids.

Thus, it appears very probable that corticoids secreted during stress also have an important influence on nervous and emotional reactions. Conversely, it is now definitely established that nervous stressors (pain and emotions) are particularly conducive to the development of the so-matic manifestations of the stress syndrome; thus stress can both cause and be caused by mental reactions.

In conclusion, let us reemphasize that no illness is exclusively a disease of adaptation, but considerable evidence has accumulated in favor of the view that stress, and particularly the adaptive hormones produced during stress, exert an important regulating influence on the development of numerous maladies.

It is virtually certain that our concepts concerning the role of pit-uitary and corticoid hormones in the pathogenesis of certain diseases of adaptation will have to undergo modifications as more facts become known. However this is true with every theory. The same was true, for instance, of the original theory that related diabetes to a simple hypoinsulinism, when the role of the anterior pituitary was discovered. Yet, the realization of some pathogenic relationship between insulin and diabetes was an almost indispensable step in the subsequent devel-opment of this field.

The best theory is that which necessitates the minimum number of assumptions to unite the maximum number of facts, since such a theory is most likely to possess the power of assimilating new facts from the unknown without damage to its own structure. Our facts must be correct; our theories need not be if they help us to discover new facts, even if these discoveries necessitate some changes in the structure of the theory.

Meanwhile, the stress theory, as outlined in this article, permits us to correlate the known facts and furnishes a concrete plan for the sys-tematic development of this field through planned investigation rather than through the mere empirical collection of chance observations.

OUTLOOK

Pasteur, Koch, and their contemporaries introduced the concept of specificity into medicine, a concept that has proved to be of the greatest heuristic value up to the present time. Each individual, well-defined disease, they held, has its own specific cause. It has been claimed by many that Pasteur failed to recognize the importance of the "terrain," because he was too preoccupied with the pathogen (microorganism) itself. His work on induced immunity shows that this is incorrect. Indeed, at the end of his life he allegedly said, "Le microbe n'est rien, le terrain est tout."

The theory that directed the most fruitful investigations of Pasteur and his followers was that the organism can develop specific adaptive reactions against individual pathogens and that by imitating and complementing these, whenever they are short of optimal, we can treat many of the diseases that are caused by specific pathogens.

To my mind, the general-adaptation syndrome represents, in a sense, the negative counterpart, or mirror image, of this concept. It holds that many diseases have no single cause, no specific pathogen, but are largely due to nonspecific stress and to pathogenic situations that result from inappropriate responses to such nonspecific stress.

Our blueprint of the pathways through which stress acts may be partly incorrect; it is certainly quite incomplete. But in it we have a basis for the objective scientific dissection of such time-honored, but hitherto rather vague, concepts as the role of "reactivity," "constitution and resistance," or "nonspecific therapy," in the genesis and treatment of disease.

If I may venture a prediction, I would like to reiterate my opinion that research on stress will be most fruitful if it is guided by the principle that we must learn to imitate — and if necessary to correct and complement — the body's own autopharmacologic efforts to combat the stress factor in disease.

REFERENCES

1. H. Selye *Nature* 138: 32 (1936).
2. ―――― *Stress. The Physiology and Pathology of Exposure to Stress* (Acta, Montreal, 1950).
3. ―――― *The Story of the Adaptation Syndome* (Acta, Montreal, 1952).
4. H. G. Wolff *Stress and Disease* (Thomas, Springfield, Ill., 1953).
5. H. G. Wolff, S. G. Wolff, C. C. Hare, Eds. Life Stress and Bodily Disease, *Research Publs. Assoc. Research Nervous Mental Disease* 29 (1950).
6. United States Army Medical Service Graduate School and Division of Medical Sciences, National Research Council (Sponsors), Symposium on Stress, Walter Reed Army Medical Center, Washington, D.C., March 16th–18th (1953).
7. H. Ogilvie and W. A. R. Thomson, Eds. Stress, *The Practitioner* 172: No. 1027 (1954).
8. R. Q. Pasqualini *Stress*. Enfermedades de Adaptacion. ACTH y Cortisona (Libreria El Ateneo, Buenos Aires, 1952).
9. I. Galdston, Ed. *Beyond the Germ Theory* (N.Y. Acad. Med. Health Education Council, New York, 1954).
10. J. Jensen *Modern Concepts in Medicine* (Mosby, St. Louis, Mo., 1953).
11. H. Selye *First Annual Report on Stress* (Acta, Montreal, 1951).

12. H. Selye and A. Horava *Second Annual Report on Stress* (Acta, Montreal, 1952).

13. ——— *Third Annual Report on Stress* (Acta, Montreal, 1953).

14. H. Selye and G. Heuser *Fourth Annual Report on Stress* (Acta, Montreal, 1954).

15. The major part of the investigations upon which this article is based was subsidized in part by a consolidated grant from the National Research Council of Canada and in part by the Medical Research Board, Office of the Surgeon General, Department of the Army, contract DA-49-007-MD-186.

16. D. J. Ingle, in *Recent Progress in Hormone Research* (Academic Press, New York, 1951), vol. 6, p. 159.

17. H. Selye *J. Clin. Endocrinol.* 6: 117 (1946).

18. H. Selye and P. Bois, in *Fourth Annual Report on Stress*, H. Selye and G. Heuser, Eds. (Acta, Montreal, 1954), pp. 533–552.

12

DUODENAL ULCER IN ONE OF IDENTICAL TWINS

MARTIN L. PILOT, M.D., L. DOUGLAS LENKOSKI, M.D.,
HOWARD M. SPIRO, M.D., AND ROY SCHAFER, PH.D.

Yale University School of Medicine, New Haven

The study of illness in identical twins has been used by many investigators as a method of identifying genetic factors in the pathogenesis of disease. Twin methods may also be used to shed light on the differential effect of environment in the development of personality and illness. The study of a patient with a peptic ulcer and his identical twin affords an opportunity to clarify some basic concepts concerning the etiology of this condition.

Many authors have investigated schizophrenia both by the individual-case-study method and the prevalence approach in mass survey. Manic depressive psychosis, epilepsy, mental deficiency, and criminality have also received considerable attention (9, 10, 19).

However, few reports of twin cases are available in the psychosomatic field. Flynn, Kennedy, and Wolf (5) studied hypertension discordant in identical twins, pointing to low birth weight and infantile illness (empyema) as possible causes for the development of personality difference and illness in the affected twin.

A review of the literature up to 1955 shows that 15 cases of peptic ulcer concordant in identical twins have been reported (2, 4, 6, 7, 8, 11, 12, 15–18). None of the patients studied was investigated psychologically. Three reports are of special interest. Freedman (6) describes a pair of 30-year-old RAF members, one of whom died of acute hemorrhage 6 weeks after discharge from service; within 3 weeks the brother appeared, acutely depressed over his brother's death, and with ulcer symptoms of 6 weeks' duration, also dating from time of discharge. Reicher (16) describes a pair of young women, the first developing an ulcer at age 18, 4 weeks after the delivery of her first child, and the twin, 2 years later, developing an ulcer 4 months after the delivery of her first living child. Camerer (3) collected 7 pairs of identical twins. In one pair both twins had peptic ulcers, but the other 6 were discordant with respect to the illness. He also found 7 pairs of

From *Psychosomatic Medicine*, May–June 1957. © 1957 by American Psychosomatic Society, Inc.

fraternal twins with concordance of ulcer in one set only. From this and other genetic work, he concluded that predisposition for ulcer is hereditary, but that it will manifest itself in only a small number of cases, probably due to the intervention of exogenous factors.

The twins in this study are 46-year-old, male, semiskilled workers of German-English parentage, one of whom, John, has a duodenal ulcer of 8 years' duration with a history of one episode of bleeding. The brother, Fred, has no history of gastrointestinal difficulty. Their appearance is strikingly identical and it has always been assumed that they were identical twins.

METHOD

Each twin was interviewed by two psychiatrists and a gastroenterologist. The patient, John, was seen for a total of 25 hours and the normal twin, Fred, for 6 hours. X-rays of the stomach were studied, blood pepsin levels as a reflection of gastric secretion were determined. Simple gene traits as recommended by Sorsby (20) were investigated. Psychological tests (Wechsler Adult Intelligence Scale, Rorschach, and TAT) were administered blind by one psychologist and interpreted blind by a second psychologist.

FAMILY HISTORY

The subjects were born in Cuba, the sixth and seventh of eight siblings. Fred was born 5 minutes before John. The father was an unsuccessful and chronically alcoholic son of a well-to-do New England manufacturer who had gone to Cuba to make his fortune, failed there as a farmer, also failed in Florida where the family had moved when the boys were 4, and eventually returned to New England to live with the twins' maternal grandmother.

Between the ages of 6 and 15, there was little parental supervision — the twins did poorly in school, engaged in many escapades, such as boxing at smokers and hopping freight cars.

Manifest differences in childhood are described by the twins as follows: Fred was "always" a little taller and heavier than John (the ulcer patient), and Fred has been able to "take things easier." They did not consider that they had been reared differently or treated differently by their parents and the available information does not indicate gross differences in attitudes or treatment. Since adolescence they have both been "worriers." They did little dating until the time of Fred's engagement at age 25, preferring to "hang around" with a group of young men.

They have remained in the same community since returning to New England as children. The patients remember little of their first 5 years, but characterize the next ten years, up to their father's death when they were 15, as being extremely difficult for them. John, in particular, emphasizes the cruel, demanding behavior of his father, and the economic deprivation resulting from his father's poor work record. The father was a heavy drinker and abusive toward all the siblings, except an older sister, who was recognized as the favorite. The mother is described as being impartial, industrious, and long-suffering. She apparently accepted her husband's behavior without expressing much dissatisfaction, and was, for the most part, responsible for rearing the children. She left the disciplining of the children to her husband, however, whose word was accepted by the entire family. John considers that the only good thing that his father ever did was to buy a house when he inherited some money. At age 10 they moved to a more acceptable neighborhood and the patients remember beginning to take some interest in their schooling. Prior to this, they had attended school rather sporadically and spent more of their time doing odd jobs, to earn money. In reflecting on his various family members, John often expresses the feeling that only he and his brother consistently helped their mother, and as the years passed she came to depend on them to maintain the household.

After the father died the twins left school having completed the eighth grade and went to work in the same factory. They made only one shift in employment and have worked at identical jobs for over 20 years.

The twins both are shy in the interview situation. Deferent and respectful to physicians, they are always apologetic about something, usually the way they look, dress or speak. Remarkably similar in style of speech and emotional reaction, they appear to be relatively passive people with open and dependent attitudes. With each new interviewer they are initially reserved. As time goes by they warm up, drop a good deal of the deference and show feelings unreservedly in a rough, good-natured way.

JOHN M.

Up to age 25 the twins were inseparable, but at this time Fred met a girl whom he soon married. John remembers that his mother did not object to his brother marrying, ostensibly because she still had John to count on for support, but when John met his future wife two years later, his mother opposed his marriage. He married at 28 despite her objection, and moved into his own home. John had rarely dated before meeting his wife, and showed little interest in sexual affairs. His wife, who is twelve years his junior, had just been graduated from high school when they married. Mrs. M. has been in psychiatric treatment intermittently between 1950–1955, and her record was available to us. She married, at least in part, to escape from a difficult home situation, in which her stepfather sought to molest her sexually. She is described as quite masculine in appearance and dissatisfied with her lot as a woman in many ways.

John considers that the first six or seven years of his marriage were quite happy. They had a son during their third year of marriage (1944), and a daughter four years later (1948). Following the birth of the second child, his wife became extremely irritable and abusive, and had frequent episodes of uncontrollable rage, when she would threaten to kill the children. He describes graphically how she "threw the children around" and how frightened and angry he became. When at work, he worried constantly about what was happening at home.

Following the birth of a third child in 1949, an unplanned event, his wife became even more seriously disturbed. The patient learned from his wife in 1949, that she had been carrying on an affair with a well-to-do older man. She had told the patient only after she had been rejected by her suitor and then goaded him into seeing the man. For the first time, he blew up at his wife, struck her on one occasion and then visited the other man. He acknowledges getting quite angry with him, but quickly rationalized that it certainly was not the other man's fault. He is not sure whether he noticed symptoms before or after learning of his wife's infidelity, but during this period (1948–1949) the patient first developed gastrointestinal symptoms suggestive of peptic ulcer. He was first seen at the Grace-New Haven Hospital, December 22, 1950, with a severe exacerbation of symptoms he had been experiencing for approximately two years. The recurrence of symptoms which brought him to the hospital began two weeks after his wife entered treatment at the psychiatric clinic.

Over the past five years (1950–1955), she has become much easier to live with. She began and completed teachers' college, and is currently a schoolteacher. During this period, he has had several exacerbations of ulcer symptoms, including one bleeding episode in August, 1954, and a severe exacerbation of symptoms in September, 1955, requiring hospitalization. The latter occurred the week that school opened and his wife went to teach for the first time.

Following the bleeding episode, Mrs. M. asked to have a psychiatrist see him, because she felt his symptoms were due to his troubles at home with her. He was willing to talk to a psychiatrist and was seen for approximately seven hours. He expressed a feeling of desperation, saying that though his wife was not as troublesome as previously, that he had been unable to forgive her. He felt trapped in an unacceptable life situation because he would have to continue to live with his wife for the sake of the children, but he could live with her only if he did not care about anything that she did.

He was seen again in 1955 by a psychiatrist while he was hospitalized. During this brief contact, he denied that he had anything that he wanted to talk about, and attributed his exacerbation of symptoms to the poor performance of his favorite major league baseball team.

Following discharge, he was seen in the gastrointestinal clinic and remained asymptomatic for several months. He returned to the psychiatric clinic again only because he wanted to do anything he could "for science," i.e., help in the study, but he seemed rather disappointed when this contact was terminated. He felt that he did not need continuous treatment, and seemed pleased to know that he could return to the clinic if he should feel the need.

John M.'s Medical History

When first seen he complained of two years' duration of well localized epigastric pain relieved by food and antacids. The pain was completely relieved by an ulcer regimen. Upper GI series in January of 1951 was completely normal. However, during the next six months, his epigastric pain returned, and was only partially relieved by a medical regimen. X-ray studies on December 31, 1951, showed a constant ulcer crater on the lesser curvature aspect of the duodenum. His complaints disappeared on a stringent ulcer regimen. He was not seen again until August, 1954, when he began to have anorexia and weakness and had passed black stools for several days. His hematocrit on admission was 15 and his stool showed a 4+ guaiac test. After seven transfusions his hematocrit rose to 37. A duodenal ulcer with marked deformity and a small niche in the prepyloric region along the lesser curvature was seen by x-ray. Thereafter, the patient was followed in the gastrointestinal clinic. A repeat x-ray in June, 1955, showed a persistent deformity of the duodenal bulb and a small, prepyloric ulcer which was now believed to be in the pyloric channel, almost completely healed. The patient did well until September, 1955. At this time he again developed severe, gnawing, epigastric pain which, for the first time, awakened him at night. He developed anorexia, nausea, and was again admitted to the hospital.

According to the patient, his mother had pernicious anemia and his father died at age 53 of tuberculosis of the stomach. One brother had died of septicemia; six siblings were living and well.

X-ray studies on September 23, 1955, showed deformity of the duodenal bulb and elongation of the pyloric stem with marked scarring from the old pyloric stem ulcer. He was discharged from the hospital on an ulcer regimen, and since that time he has continued to do very well. Blood pepsin level was 730 units.

FRED M.

Fred's recollections of family life during childhood are similar to John's. He too emphasizes the economic deprivation, but seems to carry less animosity toward his father. His memory of the father's death is in terms of how much worse things become for the family.

His attitude toward his mother is more forgiving than his brother's. John had told us that their mother had inherited over one hundred thousand dollars about ten years ago, and gives both of them small gifts on Christmas and on their birthdays, while supporting their younger sister. Whereas John has been disappointed in not receiving more financial help from her during difficult times, Fred feels she has been quite generous.

Fred, who describes himself as self-conscious and a worrier, suggests that rather than John, he should have the ulcer, as he has been married three years longer. He describes his wife as a good cook and mother, who has always taken care of the family finances and made the major decisions. She always tells him not to worry, reassuring him that they will meet their debts, and then somehow in a manner beyond his understanding, they do. She has returned to work to enable them to buy a new home. An eldest child who helped raise her 4 siblings from an early age, she is regarded by them as their mother.

Fred has two children, one of whom has a scholarship at an "ivy league" university. He speaks of his children with pride, whereas John mentions his children only when asked about them, and in fact, speaks with more feeling regarding Fred's son.

At work, Fred is the "good one" and the "quiet one," John the "bad one" and the "noisy one"; John gets into more arguments and trouble, whereas Fred walks away from irritating situations.

While Fred describes himself as a worrier, concerned about finances and the possibility that his wife might become pregnant again, there seems to be little pressure behind his stated concerns.

Fred M.'s Medical History

Fred had no complaints. He seemed in good health and was examined only for the purpose of the study. On direct questioning his only complaint concerned his heart. Four or five months before the examination he began to suffer from palpitations when he exerted himself too much. He could not climb more than four or five flights of stairs without getting somewhat short of breath. When shovelling heavy snow a week prior to examination he felt that he had strained his heart. He continued to have mild soreness in his anterior chest for the next day or two.

A past medical history was completely unremarkable. He had black stools for two or three days, four months prior to admission, but these had been examined by his local physician, who said that it was something he had eaten; apparently there had been no blood in the stool.

Physical examination was within normal limits. X-rays of the stomach were completely normal. Blood pepsin level was 680 units.

PSYCHOLOGICAL TEST REPORT OF THE TWINS

While John and Fred both manifest a marked authoritarian orientation, putting themselves in the submissive position for the most part, John appears to be significantly more shut-in emotionally, more rigid, defensive, bitter, querulous, grim in outlook, and intolerant of others as well as of his own impulses and feelings. Fred tends more toward greater self-awareness and greater tolerance of others, and shows capacity for warmth, spontaneity, tenderness and hopefulness. He appears to expend less energy in repression and suppression. Fred shows a clearer and more ego-syntonic feminine trend that appears to be part of his greater emotional security and freedom and of his less assertive, more maternal approach to others. In Fred's greater self-awareness there is room for feeling guilt, dejection, deprivation and also anger and "disgust," but not at the expense of positive and tender feelings and impulses. In contrast, John appears to tend more toward a one-sided negative and contentious position with masochistic, projective, competitive and opportunistic features. While both are conspicuously defensive with respect to such fantasy and behavior as would evoke their own aggression and guilt, John leans more toward "an underdog" self-righteous aggressiveness and complaintiveness, while Fred leans toward denial and minimization of conflict and freer acceptance of blame even in ambiguous situations. John works hard to keep a brighter view of himself and others than is his spontaneous inclination, but the results appear relatively superficial and very likely are unconvincing to others. John seems less firmly adaptive in orientation than Fred; and more stubbornly and negativistically determined to "survive"; Fred appears to be more easy-going and self-disparaging in his approach to problems and people, and less threatened by feelings of shame, inferiority and dependency. Fred, however, might be better described as somewhat fluid in his emotional position than as flexibly integrated.

Both John and Fred significantly emphasize oral themes in their test responses but the total context of results strongly indicates that John reacts more easily and intensely with anxiety, anger, feelings of disappointment and deprivation than Fred; Fred, within the limits of his submissive, self-abasing, and somewhat emotionally fluid, feminine and conflict-denying position, is likely to be more easily gratified in interpersonal relationships and to be more at peace with himself. In view of his less ambivalent conformity and greater tolerance, Fred appears to be the "better" family man and man in the community and at work; he also appears less disturbed by problems of dominance and competition in the twin relationship. Both John and Fred show adequately maintained reality testing; the problems of ego integration that are evident do not suggest psychotic trends in them. Intellectually, the twins are quite similar, John obtaining a Total IQ of 105 and Fred a Total IQ of 101; the difference in the IQ's is not great enough to suggest a significant difference in their intellectual potential or presently usable assets. Knowing that one of the twins has an ulcer, it seems reasonable to assume from current concepts concerning the personality of ulcer patients, that John is the patient.[1]

TESTS OF GENETIC SIMILARITY

As mentioned above the twins are remarkably identical in appearance. The ability to taste phenylthiourea (P.T.C.) was present in both at a concentration of 2.5 mg./liter. Hair follicles on the second phalanges of the fingers were found to be absent in each subject. Iris color and hair color are the same.

[1] Dr. Margaret Thaler, reviewing the Rorschach protocols of the subjects, blind, also chose the patient correctly and her conception of the differences between the twins is substantially in agreement with Dr. Schafer's.

Blood Type Investigation

Fred M.	*John M.*
Type O, Rh Positive	Type O, Rh Positive
Rh D-pos	Rh D-pos
C-neg	C-neg
E-neg	E-neg
c-pos	c-pos
e-pos	e-pos
Kell-neg	Kell-neg
Duffy-neg	Duffy-neg
M-pos	M-pos
N-pos	N-pos

DISCUSSION

Heredity and childhood experience seem to have given this pair of twins a passively oriented anxious approach to existence as well as providing them with the gastric hypersecretion represented by high blood pepsin levels.

Mirsky has suggested that individuals who have high rates of pepsin secretion may develop peptic ulcers more frequently, even though they may do so under fairly specific emotional circumstances. Mirsky and Reiser (13) have shown that ulcers occur in newly inducted soldiers whose blood pepsin levels are elevated; they have ascribed this to the stress of separation from home and induction into the army. Eighty per cent of normal individuals have levels between 200 and 450 units by our method. (21) The range of gastric hypersecretion, and therefore by inference, the "ulcer range" is above 450 units in about 80 per cent of all ulcer patients; in patients under the age of 40 almost 100 per cent of ulcer patients show levels above 450. The levels of the patients discussed in this study are 730 units and 680 units; the difference between them is not significant. We have studied a few pairs of identical twins and found parallel blood pepsin levels.

The existence of large groups of people with personality structures apparently similar to those observed in patients with peptic ulcer, yet who never develop the illness, has puzzled investigators. (14)

The present study calls attention to the importance of three factors pertinent to this observation: the presence of hypersecretion, the nuances in the character development of individuals, and the occurrence of acute stress.

John's illness began when his marriage was disintegrating. It appears that even though his own needs were not gratified by the marriage, he would not dissolve it. He became embittered and angered, but sought to repress or isolate the sources of his unhappiness. It was during this frustrating and embittering period when he had to assume the major responsibility for the children, that he developed his ulcer.

We might conjecture that the choice of wives was determined by the personality of each twin and that the differences between individuals which determine object choice and manner of living have pertinence to the general problem of genesis of illness. We will attempt to develop a speculative conception of the way in which the twins came to their present position.

The mother was apparently a fairly good mother; the deprivations, including the economic ones, emerge much more clearly in relation to their father. His decline in social status may have raised problems of self-esteem in the whole family. His harshness and negligence must have interfered with the development of secure masculine identification and thereby with the integration under masculine primacy of dependent and feminine trends. He ultimately fell back on the protection of a maternal figure providing a model of defeated, dependent invalided manhood to the boys. By his failure and death, he prematurely precipitated the twins into the joint role of father-surrogate through having to support the family and being the mother's stand-bys. This deprived them of education and the time to grow into manhood, and also quite likely put on them a special burden of anxiety and guilt related to Oedipal problems, as their limited dating may suggest. Through his drinking and abusiveness, he provided a model of "badness" that probably was held up to them as what not to be and thus probably created serious superego and ego ideal problems as to how to live out their impulse life safely and with self-esteem. The material available suggests that the model of their mother pervades a lot of their behavior, especially submissiveness before authority. We must not underestimate the influence of the father in determining aspects of their identity and through his unsuitability as a model leaving them no course but to relate themselves to the mother. Fred would seem to have identified more with her maternal warmth, and John, more with what must have been a streak of bitter masochism in her, which he then seems to have repeated in his own marriage. Twins often tend to divide up "roles" or identifications offered by the family in a complementary way, as well as developing similar trends; both features are suggested by this material.

Fred, who otherwise developed less rigid defenses against his needs, including his dependency needs, was able to marry a woman more capable of giving and intimacy; because of less ambivalence toward the mother, he actually found a suitable mate. Fred seems trusting of his wife while John does not and probably was not, even before the overt difficulty began. Their attitudes toward work and co-workers would support the idea of more generalized mistrust, defensiveness and unadaptiveness in John.

This case study supports the hypothesis that the level of blood pepsin is determined early in life, perhaps genetically, and that the occurrence of ulcer depends upon the presence of gastric hypersecretion plus a special combination of circumstances. We find support for Alexander's conception of ulcer occurring in a personality distinguished by conflict over passive-dependent needs, when the nurturance of these needs is compromised. (1) Our findings neither support nor contradict the hypothesis that oral deprivation in early childhood is a necessary prerequisite for the development of peptic ulcer. They do emphasize the importance of analyzing the total family configuration, with its history and future, its place in the community and its divisions and overlapping of roles.

Summary

A case of peptic ulcer in one 46-year-old male identical twin has been presented. Both subjects have strikingly similar backgrounds and character structure; passive, shy, dependent, anxious, semiskilled workers. The twin with the ulcer began to have symptoms during a near-psychotic breakdown in his wife when she was having an affair with another man and threatened to kill their children. The patient's difficulty with his wife, though somewhat diminished, has persisted since the onset of illness and so have the ulcer symptoms. In contrast, is his brother's marriage to a motherly woman who dependably manages the family affairs. Both patients have high blood pepsin levels, but show on interview and psychological testing, modest but real differences in their responses to stressful circumstances.

This paper serves as a demonstration of the use of identical twins in the study of psychosomatic disorders, and illustrates techniques of examining hypotheses concerning these disorders in this unusual setting.

References

1. Alexander, F. *Psychosomatic Medicine*. New York, Norton, 1950, p. 103.

2. Bauer, J. Bemerkungen zur prinzipielle bedeutung des studiums der physiologie und pathologie einiger zwillinge. *Klin. Wchnschr.*, 32: 1222, 1924.

3. Camerer, Y. W. Die bedeutung der erblichkeit für die entstehung des magen und zwölffingergeschwürs. *Ztschr. f. Konstitutionslehre*, 19: 416, 1935.

4. Dell 'Acqua, G. L'importanza della eredopatologia nella medicina clinica. *Minerva Med.*, 2: 45, 1949.

5. Flynn, J., Kennedy, M., and Wolf, S. Essential hypertension in one of identical twins. *Res. Pub. A. Res. Nerv. & Ment. Dis.*, 29: 954, 1950.

6. Freedman, A. G. Peptic ulceration in identical twins. *British Medical Journal*, 1: 765, 1947.

7. Goodrich, J. P., and Gregory, P. O. Duodenal ulcers occurring in twins. *Maine M.A.J.*, 41: 29, 1950.

8. Ivy, A. C., and Flood, F. T. Is susceptibility to peptic ulcer inherited?: Occurrence of ulcer in identical twins. *Gastroenterology*, 14: 375, 1950.

9. Kallmann, F. J. *The Genetics of Schizophrenia*. New York, J. J. Augustin, 1938.

10. Kallman, F. J. *Heredity in Health and Mental Disorder*. New York, Norton, 1953.

11. Leorat, M., Wegelin, and Madona. The hereditary factor in gastroduodenal ulcer: A case in twins. *Arch. Mal. app. digest.*, 40: 1239, 1951.

12. McHardy, G., and Browne, D. C. Duodenal ulcer concomitant in identical twins. *J.A.M.A.*, 124: 503, 1944.

13. Mirsky, I. A., and Reiser, M. Paper delivered at the meeting of The American Psychosomatic Society, March 1956.

14. Mirsky, I. A. Personal communication.

15. Ramos, A. Duodenal ulcer in univitelline twin brothers. *Rev. clin. españ.*, 42: 44, 1951.

16. Reicher, H. H. Peptic ulceration in identical twins. *Ann. Int. Med.*, 24: 878, 1946.

17. Robinson, H. M. Duodenal ulcer (with hyperthyroidism) concomitant in identical twins. *Rev. Gastroenterol.*, 14: 489, 1947.

18. Schindler, E. Perforated gastric ulcer in identical twins. *Chirurg.*, 7: 327, 1935.

19. Slater, E. *Psychotic and Neurotic Illnesses in Twins*. London, H. M. Stationery Office, 1953.

20. Sorsby, A. *Clinical Genetics*. London, Butterworth, 1953.

21. Spiro, H., Ryan, A., and Jones, C. The utility of the blood pepsin assay in clinical medicine. *New England J. Med.*, 253: 261, 1955.

13

AN EXPERIMENTAL INVESTIGATION OF THE ROLE OF PSYCHOLOGICAL FACTORS IN THE PRODUCTION OF GASTRIC ULCERS IN RATS

WILLIAM L. SAWREY, JOHN J. CONGER AND EUGENE S. TURRELL

University of Colorado School of Medicine

In a recent publication Sawrey and Weisz (5) have shown that it is possible to produce gastric ulcers in hooded rats, using a conflict situation in which approach responses based on hunger and thirst drives are in competition with avoidance responses based on electric shock (3).

In their study, two groups of hooded rats were used, an experimental and a control group. The experimental animals were placed in a box with a wired grid floor and put on 47-hr. hunger and thirst drives. A food cup was placed at one end of the box, water at the other end. The sections of the grid adjacent to the food and water were continuously charged, while the center part was not charged. The result was that if an animal approached either the food or the water, it was shocked. The animals lived in this box throughout the 30-day course of the experiment. The shock was turned off for 1 hr. after 47 hr. of deprivation, and the animals were allowed to eat and drink freely during this period.

The control animals were simply placed on 47-hr. hunger and thirst drives for 30 days. The experimental animals developed gastric ulcers, while the control animals did not.

While these results are of considerable interest and represent successful experimental production of gastric ulcers through presumably psychological means, there were not enough experimental groups to permit full interpretation of the results. The present study represents an attempt to correct these omissions, while employing similar methodology.

In interpreting the results of the Sawrey and Weisz study, it is clear that the combination of [1]shock, [2]hunger, [3]thirst, and [4]conflict is sufficient to produce ulcers, but hunger and thirst alone are not sufficient. This is as much as can be safely stated on the basis of the

From *The Journal of Comparative and Physiological Psychology*, October 1956.

results. However, by adding a number of other groups, additional conclusions should become possible.

The aim of the present study is to separate out, as much as possible, the relative contributions of the shock, hunger and thirst, and conflict per se to the production of ulcers in the situation described by Sawrey and Weisz (5).

METHOD

Apparatus

The apparatus used in the present experiment consisted of 12 experimental boxes with grid floors formed of brass rods $\frac{3}{32}$ in. in diameter and spaced $\frac{1}{2}$ in. apart. Each box was approximately 36 in. long, 18 in. high, and 12 in. wide. Four boxes (Group 1) were similar to the box used by Sawrey and Weisz (5) for their experimental group. Each contained a food platform at one end and a water bottle at the other. The sections of the grid adjacent to the food and water receptacles were continuously charged, using a constant-current, variable-resistance shocking apparatus of a type described by Muenzinger and Walz (4). The center portion of the grid was not charged. Thus, an animal placed in the center of one of these boxes was shocked only if it approached food or water. Each of four other boxes (groups 2, 3, 5, and 8; see Table 1) had its entire grid floor wired in series with the corresponding group 1 box. Thus, an animal in any of these boxes was involuntarily shocked the same amount and according to the same schedule as an animal in a group 1 box. In other words, every time a group 1 animal approached food or water and shocked itself, it also similarly shocked a group 2, 3, 5, or 8 animal. The remaining boxes (groups 4, 6, 7, and 9) did not have their grid floors electrically charged.

All boxes had water bottles at one end and food cups at the other. Whether or not the water and food in these receptacles were accessible to the animal, or whether they were sealed off by means of clear plastic covers, was, however, a function of the particular experimental condition involved.

Subjects and Procedure

One hundred and forty naive, Sprague-Dawley albino rats 100 to 160 days of age served as Ss. These animals were randomly distributed among the nine experimental conditions shown in Table 1.

Each replication of this experimental design necessarily involved only one animal in each box. Therefore, it required ten entire replications to obtain 10 animals each in groups 2 through 9. Because of the greater number of group 1 animals required for each replication, this design produced 40 animals in group 1.

In addition to the 120 animals required by this basic design, 20 additional animals (10 group 1 animals and 10 paired group 2 animals) were run later, in order to increase the statistical power of group 1–group 2 comparisons. Thus, from the basic study and this additional investigation a total of 20 group 1 animals and 20 group 2 animals (paired for exact amount of shock, hunger, and thirst with group 2 animals) was obtained. As Table 1 indicates, these additions increased the total number of group 1 animals studied to 50, and the total group 2 animals to 20.

The aim of the above experimental conditions was successively to eliminate various factors involved in Sawrey and Weisz's original ulcer-producing situation.

Group 1 was simply a duplication of this situation.

In group 2, the animals were under the same conditions of hunger and thirst drives as group 1 animals. They were also shocked when a group 1 animal shocked itself, since the grid floor of their box was wired in series with the group 1 box. They were not, however, faced with the approach-avoidance conflict faced by group 1 animals. It was the investigator's expectation that tension resulting from group 1's being presented with a continuing choice situation (i.e., whether to try to get food and water or to avoid shock) would be a crucial factor in the ulcer production. While it was believed the group 2 animals might very well become fearful as a result of occasional shocks over which they had no voluntary control, it was thought that the ulcer-contributing effects of any such fear would be slight compared with the effects of the continuous approach-avoidance conflict of group 1.

In group 3, animals received the same hunger drive and shock as group 1 and 2 animals, but had water freely available, and hence were not under thirst drive. Differences between group 2 and 3 animals in any of the physiological measures must therefore be attributed to the differential presence of thirst drive in group 2.

Groups 4 and 5 were similar to group 3, except that in group 4 hunger and thirst were present and shock was absent. In group 5, thirst and shock were present, but animals were allowed to eat freely and hunger was absent.

Animals in groups 6, 7, and 8 were under conditions, respectively, of hunger drive alone without thirst drive or shock; thirst drive alone without hunger drive or shock; and shock alone without hunger or thirst drive.

Animals in group 9 were simply control animals living in the same physical surroundings as all other groups. They had food and water freely available and received no shock.

An analysis of the differences in ulcer production among the above groups should help to separate out the relative effects of each of the four variables of shock, hunger, thirst, and conflict.

It obviously was not possible to isolate completely the individual and interaction effects of these variables since the variables are not independent; hence, all the 16 logically possible combinations of these variables which would be necessary for a complete analysis were not practically feasible. For example, it was obviously not possible actually to have a condition of conflict which would be comparable to the conflict in group 1 with no hunger or thirst drives and no shock.

As a result, there are a number of statements which cannot be made on the basis of the present experiment, regardless of the actual findings. It will not be possible, for example, to say that conflict per se is a necessary and sufficient cause of gastric ulcers in the absence of food and water deprivation and in the absence of shock. Many other statements, tending to pin down etiological factors or combinations of factors should, however, be possible.

Exploratory Work

In pilot work, using the above design, a number of important findings were made. Foremost among these was that there appeared to be significant strain differences in the susceptibility of rats to ulcer formation. In Sawrey and Weisz's study (5) Nebraska hooded rats over 90 days of age were employed. Under the group 1 condition, these animals, when placed on 47-hr. hunger and thirst drive, developed ulcers in approximately 30 days. In the exploratory phase of the present research, Nebraska hooded rats were not available, and Sprague-Dawley albinos of comparable age were employed. These animals soon proved unable to stand the same feeding schedule as the hooded rats. They tended to lose weight rapidly and to become ill and die. Although many of them tended to develop ulcers, often within a very few days, consistent differences between groups did not emerge clearly — largely, in the opinion of the investigators, because their regimen was too severe, permitting the operation of too many extraneous factors, such as intercurrent illness and, in the case of group 1 animals which did not develop ulcers, because of constriction which tended to keep food in the stomach, thus apparently serving as a protection against the effects of stomach acid (1, 2).

While strain differences appeared important in producing different effects in the hooded and albino groups, the effects of the differences were confounded with the possible social effects of the presence or absence of other animals in the experimental situation. In Sawrey and Weisz's original research, animals were tested in groups of three. Because of the demands of the present experimental situation, only one animal at a time could be tested. It is conceivable that the stress of the testing situation may be reduced by the presence of other animals. At any rate, for purposes of the present research, it appeared advisable, before beginning the experiment proper, to permit all animals to adapt by living in the experimental boxes for five days with free access to food and water.

One further modification of Sawrey and Weisz's original procedure was also made. Rather than waiting an arbitrary period of time before autopsying the animals in order to examine for ulcers, the Es decided to operate on a group when it appeared that one one of the group might not survive for another 24 hr. In this way, the problem of attempting to operate on deceased animals, with its consequent complications, was avoided.

The results reported here have incorporated all three of these modifications.

RESULTS

At autopsy, the number of clearly observable ulcers was determined for each animal. All these ulcers were located in the rumen of the stomach. In addition, areas of hemorrhage as described by Shay et al. (7) were frequently noted in the body of the stomachs of ulcerated animals, but these could not be quantified by present techniques. Figure 1 shows a characteristic ulcerated stomach obtained in the present study, as well as microscopic sections of lesions from both the upper and lower portions of the stomach. The incidence of ulcers for each of the various experimental conditions is shown in Table 1.

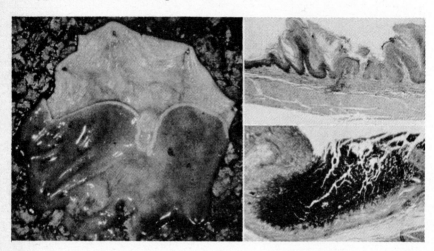

Fig. 1. Left, stomach of group 1 animal, showing numerous ulcers. Top right, microscopic section of ulcer in rumen of stomach of group 1 animal. Lower right, microscopic section of ulcer in body of stomach of group 1 animal.

It will be noted that only the total number of ulcers occurring in each group is reported. Actually ulcers were also classified as to size (i.e., under 1 mm., 1 to 2 mm., and over 2 mm.). However, since analyses of each of these subgroups revealed the same general distribution as the total number of ulcers, these analyses are not reported here.

As may be seen from Table 1, the greatest number of ulcers occurred in group 1 animals, which had been subjected to conflict, as well as to the conditions of hunger, thirst, and shock. When only hunger, shock, and thirst were present, as in group 2, a lesser number of ulcers occurred. A statistically significant difference between these two groups would indicate that conflict itself is at least a contributory factor in the production of ulcers. A Wilcoxon signed-rank test for paired observations (9) was computed for the significance of the difference in the mean number of ulcers between the 20 group 2 animals and *the 20 group 1 animals which had been wired in series with the group 2 animals*. A value of 39 was obtained, which is significant at the .02 level of confidence.

The difference in the over-all percentage of animals in groups 1 and

TABLE 1. INCIDENCE OF ULCERS OCCURRING UNDER VARIOUS
EXPERIMENTAL CONDITIONS

Group Number	Experimental Condition	Number of Animals in Group	Percentage of Animals Developing Ulcers	Number of Ulcers	Average Weight Loss in Grams
1	C H S T*	50	76	434	99.5
2	NC H S T	20	30	44	79.8
3	NC H S NT	10	40	26	75.1
4	NC H NS T	10	0	0	54.7
5	NC NH S T	10	0	0	42.9
6	NC H NS NT	10	20	4	54.6
7	NC NH NS T	10	0	0	25.4
8	NC NH S NT	10	0	0	10.7
9	NC NH NS NT	10	0	0	29.2†

* Code — S = Shock; NS = Not Shocked; T = Thirst; NT = Not Thirsty; H = Hunger; NH = Not Hungry; C = Conflict; NC = No Conflict.
† This group gained weight.

2 developing ulcers (76 and 30 per cent, respectively) is also highly suggestive. A chi-square test of the significance of the difference in the number of animals in the two groups developing ulcers yielded a value of 12.94, which is significant at the .001 level of confidence.

Thus it appears that conflict itself contributes significantly to ulcer formation in these animals. However as Table 1 suggests, other factors may also play an important role. If the variables of hunger, shock, and thirst are considered separately from the conflict variable, they form a complete $2 \times 2 \times 2$ factorial design, which ideally should be analyzed by analysis of variance. However, in this instance it is obvious that the underlying assumptions of this technique are violated since many of the groups had a zero incidence of ulcers. Consequently, separate 2×2 tables had to be constructed for each of the variables, hunger, shock, and thirst (see Table 2).

These tables were then analyzed by the chi-square technique. In the case of the hunger variable, a chi-square value of 12.75, which is significant at the .001 level of confidence, was obtained. For the shock variable, a chi-square of 5.16 was obtained. This value is significant at the .05 level of confidence. The corresponding chi-square value for the thirst variable is obviously not significant. Thus, it appears that hunger and shock both make significant contributions to the production of ulcers in these animals. However, as inspection of Table 1 makes readily apparent, it is the interaction of hunger and shock

TABLE 2. NUMBER OF ANIMALS DEVELOPING ULCERS UNDER
DIFFERENT CONDITIONS

	Hunger		Thirst		Shock	
	Hungry	Not Hungry	Thirsty	Not Thirsty	Shocked	Not Shocked
Ulcer	11	0	5	6	9	2
Non-Ulcer	29	40	35	34	31	38

which accounts for this significance, rather than either variable operating independently.

Selye (6) has discussed the role of various stress factors in ulcer formation. Among the intervening variables which may be playing a role in determining the stressful effects of the conflict, hunger, and shock conditions in the present experiment, weight loss is a potentially important consideration, as Table 1 indicates. For this reason, a *t* test was made of the difference in the mean weight losses between the 20 group 2 animals and the 20 group 1 animals which had been wired in series with the group 2 animals. A *t* of 2.67 was obtained, which is significant at the .02 level for 19 *df*. Thus, it appeared possible that weight loss alone might account for the differences in ulcer formation obtained between groups 1 and 2.

In order to determine whether there was a difference in ulcer formation between the two groups, above and beyond any difference which might be attributed to weight loss, a covariance type of analysis as described by Walker and Lev (8) was employed. After adjusting the weight loss of group 2 animals to equal the weight loss of group 1 animals, a *t* test of the resulting differences was performed. This test yielded a value of 1.81, which, based on 36 *df*, is significant at better than the .05 level of confidence for a one-tailed test. It is, of course, true that *t* tests assume normal distribution of the underlying variables, and that the present data may not entirely fulfill this requirement. However, it appears improbable that the significant results obtained in the above analysis could be attributed simply to possible non-normality of the data, especially since any non-normality would be as likely to decrease as to increase the statistical power of the test employed. Thus, while the findings are not completely conclusive, they strongly suggest that weight loss per se cannot be viewed as accounting for all the difference in ulcer formation obtained between groups 1 and 2. In addition, an analysis of variance was computed for weight loss in groups 2 through 9, employing a $2 \times 2 \times 2$ factorial design. The results of this analysis indicate that the hunger, shock, and thirst conditions were each significantly associated with weight loss. However, in the case of hunger and thirst, the significance was due to an interactive effect, rather than to either variable alone. It should be noted that the weight loss in these cases was not directly related to ulcer formation.

DISCUSSION

The present study demonstrated that conflict and the interaction of hunger and shock contributed significantly to the production of gastric ulcer in these animals, while thirst, and hunger and shock operating independently, did not. Further, it appears that weight loss as such cannot be considered to account for these results. Perhaps the most important experimental finding is that psychological conflict per se may contribute to ulcer formation.

The present study, however, leaves a number of interesting questions unanswered. For one thing, there appear to be strain (and possibly sex differences) in the ulcer susceptibility of rats. There also appear to be observable pre-experimental emotional differences within strains which are related to ulcer susceptibility. Further, it appears that an animal's social experience, both in early life and in the testing situation, may affect its ulcer susceptibility. A beginning has been made in investigating these factors systematically, although no results are yet available. Additional investigation of various physiological changes associated with ulcer formation under the present experimental conditions is also indicated. Finally, the applicability of the present methodology and findings to species other than the rat can only be determined through further research.

SUMMARY

A pilot study (5) has shown that it is possible to produce gastric ulcers in rats by means of a conflict situation in which approach responses based on hunger and thirst drives are in competition with avoidance responses based on electric shock.

The aims of the present study were to vary experimental conditions systematically in order to evaluate the relative contributions of the electric shock, hunger and thirst drives, and the approach-avoidance conflict itself in the production of gastric ulcers.

The results indicate: (a) that conflict per se contributes significantly to ulcer formation, (b) that hunger and shock also contribute significantly, but only in interaction, (c) that thirst does not contribute significantly, (d) that weight loss alone cannot account for the differences in ulcer formation between conflict and nonconflict groups, and (e) that weight loss is significantly related to the variables of shock, hunger, and thirst, though in the case of the latter two, only through interaction. However, the weight loss in these cases is not directly related to ulcer formation. Areas needing further research are discussed.

REFERENCES

1. Mahl, G. F. The effect of chronic fear on the gastric secretions of HCl in dogs. *Psychosom. Med.*, 1949, 11: 30–44.

2. Mahl, G. F. Anxiety, HCl secretion and peptic ulcer etiology. *Psychosom. Med.*, 1950, 12: 140–169.

3. Miller, N. E. Experimental studies in conflict, in J. McV. Hunt (Ed.), *Personality and the behavior disorders.* New York: Ronald, 1944. Vol. I. Pp. 431–465.

4. Muenzinger, K. F., & Walz, F. C. An examination of electrical current stabilizing devices for psychological experiments. *J. gen. Psychol.*, 1934, 10: 447–482.

5. Sawrey, W. L., & Weisz, J. D. An experimental method of producing gastric ulcers. *J. comp. physiol. Psychol.*, 1956, 49: 269–270.

6. Selye, H. *The physiology and pathology of exposure to stress.* Montreal: Acta, Inc., 1950.

7. Shay, H., Komorov, S. A., Fels, S. S., Meranze, D., Gruenstein, M., and Siplet, H. A simple method for the formation of gastric ulcerations in the rat. *Gastroenterology*, 1945, 5: 43–61.

8. Walker, H. M., & Lev, J. *Statistical inference.* New York: Holt, 1953.

9. Wilcoxon, F. *Some rapid approximate statistical procedures.* New York: American Cyanamid Co., 1949.

14

REPRODUCIBLE PSYCHOGENIC ATTACKS OF ASTHMA
A Laboratory Study

E. DEKKER, M.D., AND J. GROEN, M.D.

INTRODUCTION

The histories obtained from patients with asthma often contain examples of asthmatic attacks following emotional events. Most of these observations, as recorded in the literature, are of an anecdotal character (Dunbar, 1938). Clinical observations (Miller, 1950, 1953; Bastiaans, 1954; Huet, 1953), the investigation of patients by means of psychoanalysis (French, 1951), or the method of biographical anamnesis (Bastiaans, 1954; Groen, 1950) also reveal striking examples of psychogenic asthmatic attacks. Clinical material like this is undoubtedly valuable, but it can never constitute a definite proof of the etiology of the attacks. Most of the evidence is reconstructed from case histories, and many of the recorded observations are incidental and not reproducible. We felt therefore that additional insight might be gained if it were possible to produce, study, and register psychogenic asthmatic attacks under laboratory conditions.

METHODS

The experiments concerning the significance of the psychogenic factors in asthma were combined with an investigation into the role of allergic factors. Skin and inhalation-sensitivity tests were carried out on thirty-one patients, using ten commonly used inhalants. The inhalation tests were carried out by the technique of Herxheimer (1951 and 1952) as modified by Orie and Ten Cate (1953 and 1954). In this method the vital capacity of the patient is registered spirographically every 4 min. The allergens are nebulized in an atomizer by means of a constant flow of oxygen. The aerosol is administered to the patient through rubber tubing and a glass-tube mouthpiece. The inhalation test is considered positive when the vital capacity decreases by more than 10 per cent, and if the curve registering this decrease has a regular course in the succeeding determinations.

From the Second Medical Service of the Wilhelmina Gasthuis in Amsterdam, and published in the *Journal of Psychosomatic Research*, 1:58, 1956.

The investigation of the effect of psychological stimuli was made with twelve of these thirty-one patients. In these experiments we also used the vital capacity as the parameter of the patient's condition. It is admitted that the registration of vital capacity as a yardstick of asthma is not ideal, but it has the advantage of simplicity; moreover, by using the same measurement technique during the tests with allergological and psychological stimuli, it made the results of the psychological and the allergic tests comparable.

A base line was obtained by observing the patients, and registering the vital capacity every 4 min for a period of time without the application of stimuli. Then the patients were exposed to a certain emotional stress. During the whole experiment the vital capacity was determined every 4 min; only occasionally a single determination had to be omitted when a too-severe attack followed the stimulus. The psychogenic provocation test, like the inhalation test, was considered positive if it was followed by a reduction in vital capacity of more than 10 per cent of the mean of the base-line values, providing the curve recording this decrease had a regular course in succeeding determinations.

The emotional stimulus used in these tests was selected from the history.

When asthma patients are questioned about the causes of their attacks, most of them give a history pointing to heterogeneous causative factors; e.g., inhalation or ingestion of certain substances, the weather, circumstances connected with the patient's occupation, the season of the year, or the time of day. In addition, various emotional states may be blamed. Most patients volunteer this information upon superficial inquiry without any inhibition. This does not apply to situations of a somewhat bizarre character, about which the patients express themselves only if the physician inquires after these without signs of prejudice. The following enumeration gives some of the statements obtained from our patients after they were encouraged to talk freely about the cause of their attacks:

A female patient *A* gets a sense of constriction merely by *looking* at dust, but only during the hay-fever season.

One asthmatic boy *B* becomes dyspnoeic when the sun shines into his room; he then sees the dust particles float in the sunlight. When there is no sunshine, he has no symptoms in the same room.

Another female patient *C* becomes dyspnoeic when listening to radio speeches by a certain highly-placed political person or to the broadcast of a children's choir, or when she heard the national anthem.

Patient *D* gets a sense of constriction when her back gets cold at about waist level. Rubbing of her back by her husband causes her attack to disappear.

Two ladies *E F* told of becoming nervous when knitting; they would start knitting faster and faster until they had to put down their work on account of an oncoming attack of dyspnoea. *F* also gets an attack when something catches her interest, e.g., a waterfall or a bicycle-race.

A jewellery salesman *G* frequently becomes dyspnoeic when lifting his sample bag.

A female patient *H* gets an attack of asthma whenever she uses an elevator.

A young woman *J* feels "suffocated" when she visits her father's grave, but only when her mother is there too.

Another female patient *K* stated that she was so hypersensitive to aspirin that merely watching someone else swallowing an aspirin tablet gave her a feeling of suffocation. The noise of the sheet-iron workshop below her flat had the same effect.

Two other patients *L M* stated that looking at a goldfish in a bowl caused an asthmatic attack. Both these patients reacted in a similar way when watching a bird in a cage, one of them *L* also when she saw a prison-van.

Patient *N* gets asthma when she smells a certain perfume, sees a picture of a horse, or reads stories of cruelty or disaster in the papers. She has also had attacks when someone touched her neck, or when she had a fear of height.

Hearing her mother use the front-door key, entering the street where she had once lived with her now-divorced husband, seeing a picture of an asthmatic child, others interfering with her running the household, caused attacks in patients *L, O, P,* and *Q* respectively.

Patient *R* got an attack whenever she *wanted* to go to the town of Enschede in the Netherlands.

The occurrence of these and similar data in the history is not exceptional. The above list was obtained from eighteen out of twenty-four consecutive patients, who were encouraged to tell their own observations freely.

These anamnestic data formed the starting-point for the observations reported in this paper, for a number of the situations described above lent themselves to reproduction under laboratory conditions.

This was done in twelve of these eighteen patients. All patients had either been admitted to the Second Medical Service of the Wilhelmina-Gasthuis, or had been referred to us for allergological examination. All had bronchial asthma to serious degree.

RESULTS

The results of the psychological provocation tests can be classified in three groups:

Group 1 (six patients) did not react at all when exposed to the artificial limitation of the "asthmatogenic" situation.

Group 2 (three cases) showed a transient decrease of vital capacity accompanied by minor symptoms and signs.

In group 3 (three patients) frank asthmatic attacks occurred together with a considerable decrease in vital capacity.

Group 1 (Patients A, B, C, D, E, G)

Showing a well-sealed glass container with thick flakes of dust to patient A, blowing an aerosol of physiologic saline and house-dust extract in a strong beam of light into the view of the boy B, and reproducing on a gramophone a speech of the politician who used to

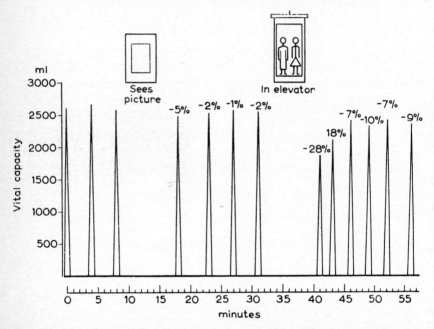

Fig. 1. Patient H. No effect on looking at a picture with emotional contents. Drop in vital capacity after going up and down in an elevator for a few minutes.

bring patient C into an emotional state, had no effect on the vital capacity or the clinical status of these patients. Patient D was not influenced by placing an icebag on her back. In patient E the baseline vital capacity was too irregular to allow estimation of the influence of knitting. No attack of dyspnoea was observed when she was asked to knit before us. Neither was there a reaction when patient G handled his jewellery samples in the laboratory.

Group 2 (Patient H, I, K)

Patient *H* had told us that she had asthmatic attacks when she used an elevator. Figs. 1 and 2 illustrate the reactions of the vital capacity during the experiments. First she was shown the picture of an asthmatic child which had produced an asthmatic attack in patient *P*. It had no influence on her. She agreed to make a short trip in an elevator. This caused a transient reduction of the vital capacity, with slight dyspnoea, which could be reproduced. Walking from the laboratory to the elevator and back had no influence, nor was there any reaction when she stayed in a dark cupboard. Allergens in the air of the elevator could not be held responsible for this

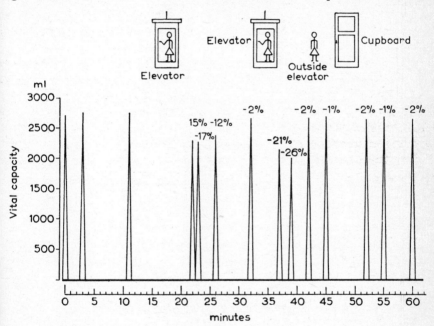

Fig. 2. Patient H. Reproducible drop in vital capacity after staying a few minutes in an elevator between two floors. No effect when standing before the open elevator or in a closed cupboard.

effect, because on the next occasion there was no reaction when she sat on a chair in the elevator which did not move. During these experiments the patient spontaneously recounted emotional stories, a dream, and how she used to be locked up in a cupboard by her mother.

Patient *I* showed a transient decrease of vital capacity of 17 per cent after being shown a picture, of a man mourning at a grave, which reminded her of her father's death. She then told us about the emotional events connected with his death and burial. At that time she had had a very severe attack of asthma.

Patient *K* got a transient but reproducible decrease of vital capacity up to 21 per cent when she saw the experimenter swallow a tablet of calcium lactate from a wrapping of aspirin.

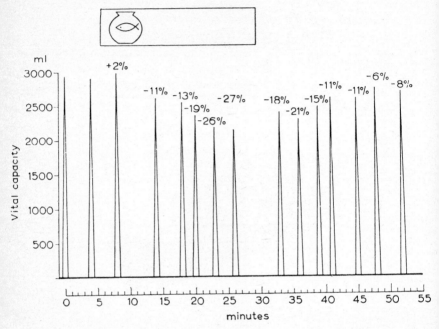

Fig. 3. Patient L. Severe attack of asthma with fall in vital capacity after looking at goldfish in bowl. Disappearance of symptoms and signs after removal of the object.

Group 3 (*Patients L, M, N*)

In this group the decrease in vital capacity after emotional stimuli was more pronounced and prolonged, and accompanied by a clinically clear-cut asthmatic attack.

Patient *L* had told us that she got an asthmatic attack from looking at a goldfish. After a baseline had been obtained, a goldfish in a bowl was brought into the room (Fig. 3). Under our eyes she developed a severe asthmatic attack with loud wheezing, followed by a gradual remission after the goldfish had been taken from the room. During the next experiment the goldfish was replaced by a plastic toy which was easily recognized by the patient as such (Fig. A.), but a fierce attack resulted (Fig 4). Upon this she told the investigator the following dream, which she had had after the preceding investigation.

In her home stood a big goldfish bowl. On a shelf high up near the window were her books. In one of them she wanted to read why goldfish cause asthma. She climbed on a chair and reached for the

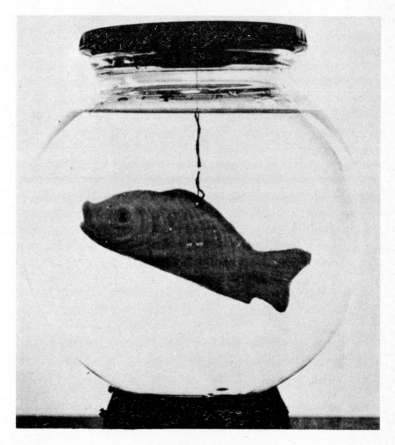

Fig. A.

book, but it was too high. She lost her balance and fell into the goldfish bowl. She gasped for breath behind the glass. The fishes swam around her. Her neck was caught in a streak of water weed. She awoke with an attack of asthma. She also remembered suddenly how when she was a child her mother threw away her bowl of goldfish, which she loved so much. The patient had saved her pocket-money to buy them. Mother threw the fishes into the water closet and flushed them through.

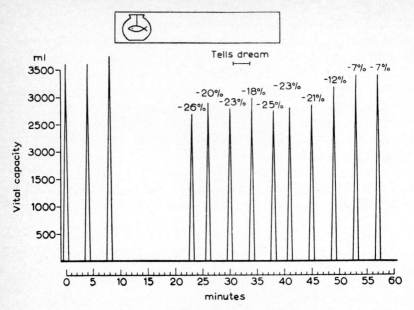

Fig. 4. Patient L. Attack of asthma with decrease in vital capacity, on looking at the toy goldfish in the bowl. Followed by recovery.

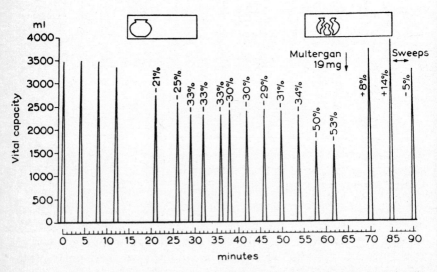

Fig. 5. Patient L. Severe attack on looking at the empty bowl, increasing in severity after the investigator shatters the bowl in pieces on the floor. Prompt reaction of this attack to thiacinamine.

During a third experiment (Fig. 5) even looking at the empty bowl was followed by a severe asthmatic attack. This time there was no remission after the bowl was taken from the room. The investigator in an attempt to break through the patient's reaction threw the bowl into pieces on the floor. "That is exactly what my mother did," she exclaimed, "she threw the bowl into pieces into the dustbin." The dyspnoea increased still further, so that it became necessary to interrupt the attack by an injection. The patient insisted on sweeping the pieces together herself. After she had done this, the vital capacity was again decreased.

This observation could be almost duplicated in patient *M*. Fig. 6 shows the effect of the first exposure to the sight of the goldfish. During the base-line period this patient began to talk about one

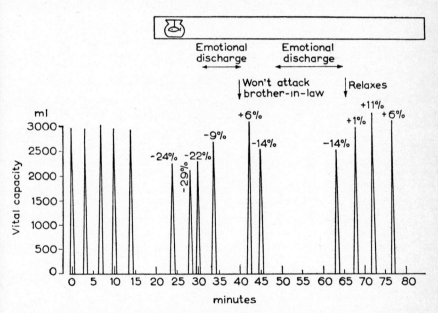

Fig. 6. Patient M. No effect on vital capacity of discussion on emotional subject. Severe attack of asthma with marked decrease in vital capacity on looking at goldfish in bowl.

of her greatest actual difficulties, viz., her son's homosexuality. She showed great emotion, and wept between and even during the vital-capacity measurements, which gave them a somewhat irregular value; however, there was no progressive drop. After changing the topic, a more regular base-line was obtained and the bowl with the goldfish was brought in. Within a few minutes the patient developed an excited behaviour, reproaching the doctor for keeping the poor creature imprisoned in a bowl. She could not get away from the idea that the creature was suffocating and gasping for breath behind the glass.

In our presence she developed a severe attack of typical asthmatic dyspnoea with loud wheezing. During the exposure to this situation she suddenly recalled her first attack of asthma which had occurred eight years earlier than she had hitherto remembered. It started when her husband, a butcher, had made her mop up the blood of a slaughtered calf from the floor, just after her marriage. Upon this a violent emotional discharge followed, accompanied by an increase in dyspnoea with severe cyanosis. After the bowl was taken away and the patient reassured, the vital capacity returned to its base-line level.

The exposure to the plastic toy goldfish (Fig. 7) left her slightly amused for about three minutes. But eight minutes later the vital capacity had dropped to 29 per cent and she was in a severe attack

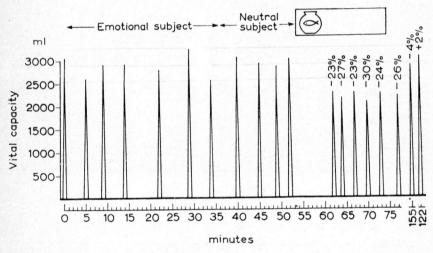

Fig. 7. Patient M. Severe attack of asthma followed by emotional discharge after looking at the toy goldfish in the bowl.

of asthma, during which she expressed strong self-reproach: "Fancy my choking because of that silly toy thing. It isn't even alive." She managed to draw herself together somewhat, and suddenly remarked that she was now sure she would not attack her brother-in-law, who had approached her sexually. After this the attack stopped. She then told the emotional story of her struggle against her family to keep the butcher's shop going after her husband had become an invalid, and after his death. After having unburdened herself about this, she recovered completely, the vital capacity increased above baseline value, while the bowl was still standing in front of her.

The third patient in this group, *N*, reacted in a similar though somewhat less violent way when asked to look at the picture of a horse (Fig. B) and at two sensational reports of a different nature in a well-known illustrated periodical. While wheezing, she produced strong emotional discharges and told traumatic life experiences, which

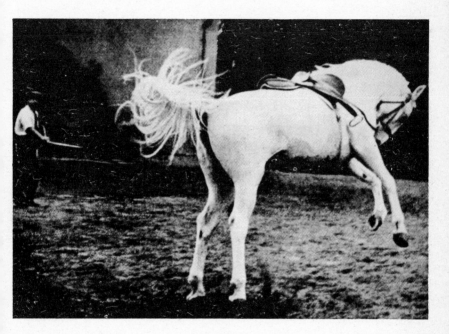

Fig. B.

up to this moment she had never revealed to anyone. Similar emotional discharges followed after she was exposed to the smell of the perfume to which she regarded herself as hypersensitive, after she looked down the staircase from the second floor, and after feeling hands being laid around her neck. But from these stimuli she got no asthmatic attacks.

DISCUSSION

In the course of these experiments it was possible to register a decrease in vital capacity, associated in some cases with attacks of typical asthmatic dyspnoea, after the exposure of asthmatic patients to certain emotional environmental stimuli which were chosen from

their history. The interpretation of the results as examples of psychogenic attacks rests not only upon the exclusion of other causes, but
also on the marked emotional response that was elicited by the
exposure. Consequent to the provocation tests these patients related
traumatic life experiences, emotional phantasies, and disturbing
dreams. No attempt will be made to give a psychiatric interpretation
of these observations, but in a number of instances it was quite obvious that the environmental asthmatogenic stimulus was associatively
related to former traumatic life experiences.

The clinical picture of the patients during these psychogenic attacks
was indistinguishable from "spontaneous" attacks or from attacks
provoked by the inhalation of allergens. They could be aborted by
the administration of thiacinamine or isoprenaline.

The positive results were reproducible in five out of six patients who
reacted. The positive response in the sixth patient I was not controlled
for reproducibility for psychological reasons; it was felt that showing
this patient the picture of the graveyard for a second time was not
justified from a medical ethical standpoint.

The six failures to obtain a psychogenic response are of some
interest. The patients A, B, C, and D volunteered the information
that the experimental condition did not resemble closely enough the
circumstances under which their attacks had "naturally" occurred.
Patient E was quite surprised that she got no attack after knitting
for an hour in the laboratory. The attacks of the jewellery salesman G
on handling his sample-bags may well have been connected with a
greater amount of physical effort during his actual work, or with more
emotional tension while visiting his customers.

In a similar series of provocation tests where patients were tested
for their reactions to the inhalation of allergens, positive reactions
were obtained in about an equal percentage, viz., in nine out of thirty-
one cases. These percentages of positive and negative provocation
tests naturally do not allow an estimate about the relative importance
of psychological or allergic factors in the production of the attacks
occurring naturally in asthmatic patients.

Of particular importance seems the observation that a high intensity
of emotion in itself was not sufficient to produce an attack in these
patients. Patient M for example was markedly emotional when she
discussed the difficulties she had with her homosexual son. However,
this gave her no asthma, whereas looking at a goldfish produced a
severe attack. Patient N was emotionally very upset when exposed
to the smell of a certain perfume, when she felt the hands round her
neck, and when she felt afraid of height. She told about traumatic
episodes connected with these stimuli, but her vital capacity did not

react. Looking at a picture of a horse and at a sensational newspaper report caused no greater display of emotion, but after each of these stimuli an asthmatic attack followed. It was repeatedly observed during these and other studies that the sympathetic discussion of traumatic experiences with a doctor, although often producing emotional reactions, seldom caused a decrease in vital capacity. It seems as if the emotional setting must not only have a certain intensity to produce an attack, but must also be of a more or less specific quality. Our observations so far are too limited in number to allow a more precise definition of this specific quality involved.

The exposure to these asthmatogenic situations was often followed by the reproduction of much more abundant factual and other pertinent information than could have been obtained in the same time during an ordinary interview. It is possible that this way of obtaining information and producing emotional discharge opens up new perspectives for psychotherapeutic efforts along this line.

When we modified the experimental situation we were especially impressed by the fact that, in some of the experiments, the conscious knowledge of the artificiality of the experimental situation did not prevent the onset of an asthmatic attack. Patients L and M had a severe attack of asthmatic dyspnoea on looking at a toy goldfish, much to their own astonishment. Later they felt self-reproach and powerlessness. In another series of experiments, to be reported elsewhere (Dekker, in preparation), we observed the same inability to prevent an attack by a conscious effort of will, even when it was provoked by a stimulus which was obviously innocuous and without "organic" or "logical" significance so far as the patient could judge. We are inclined therefore to bring the phenomena described in this paper in line with the process of acquired conditioning (Noelpp, 1952). Experiments to investigate this problem further are now in progress.

Our results also seem to shed some light on the question as to whether asthmatic patients can be classified into an "allergic" and a "psychic" category (Pollnow, 1929; Wittkower, 1932). Two patients in this series, who had shown a positive response to psychogenic stimuli, reacted also to the inhalation of one or more extracts of allergens. Patient L got asthmatic attacks and a decrease in vital capacity after the inhalation of extracts of moulds and house-dust, patient I after pollen extract. Control experiments ruled out the possibility of psychological factors in these observations. In this, as in other work (Bastiaans, 1954), it has been possible therefore to demonstrate that in at least some asthmatic patients attacks can be provoked both by the inhalation of allergens and by psychic stimuli.

For this reason our experiences do not seem to make it likely that such a classification is justified, and another explanation for the partly psychological, partly allergic genesis of asthma will have to be looked for (Bastiaans, 1954).

REFERENCES

Dunbar, Flanders H. (1938) *Emotions and Bodily Changes.* (New York).

Miller, H., and Baruch, D. W. (1950) Emotional traumata preceding the onset of allergic symptoms in a group of children. *Ann. Allergy,* 8: 100.

Miller, H., and Baruch, D. W. (1953) Psychotherapy in acute attacks of bronchial asthma. *Ann. Allergy,* 11: 438.

Bastiaans, J., and Groen, J. (1954) Psychogenesis and psychotherapy of bronchial asthma. In: *Modern Trends in Psychosomatic Medicine.* Edited by Desmond O'Neill, London, p. 242.

Huet, G. J. (1953) Psychosomatiek en clinische symptomen bij het asthma van kinderen. In: *Psyche en Allergische Ziekte,* Leiden, p. 43.

French, T. M., and Alexander, F. (1941) Psychogenic factors in bronchial asthma. *Psychosomatic Medicine,* monograph, 4.

Groen, J. (1950) *Asthma bronchiale seu nervosum.* Amsterdam.

Herxheimer, H. G. (1951) Induced asthma in man. *Lancet,* 1: 1337.

Herxheimer, H. G. (1952) *The Management of Bronchial Asthma.* London.

Ten Cate, H. J., and Orie, N. G. M. (1953) Intracutane reacties bij asthmalijders vergeleken met de resultaten van inhalatie van allergeenextracten. *Ned. Tijdschr. v. Geneesk.,* 97: 598.

Ten Cate, H. J. (1954) Onderzoek bij asthmapatiënten naar overgevoeligheid voor verstoven allergeenextracten, *Proefschrift,* Groningen.

Dekker, E., Pelser, H. E., and Groen, J. The role of conditioning in the production of asthmatic attacks (in preparation).

Noelpp, B., and Noelpp-Eschenhagen, I. (1952) Experimental asthma in the guinea pig. *Int. Arch Allergy,* 3: 108.

Pollnow, H., Petow, H., and Wittkower, E. (1929) Zur Psychotherapie des Asthma Bronchiale. *Z. Klin. Med.,* 110: 701.

Wittkower, E., and Petow, H. (1932) Zur Psychogenese des Asthma Bronchiale. *Z. Klin. Med.,* 119: 293.

15

THE PHYSIOLOGY OF FEAR AND ANGER

DANIEL H. FUNKENSTEIN

Harvard Medical School

When the late Walter B. Cannon, by his historic experiments nearly half a century ago, showed a connection between emotions and certain physiological changes in the body, he opened a new frontier for psychology and medicine. His work, coupled with that of Sigmund Freud, led to psychosomatic medicine. It also made the emotions accessible to laboratory measurement and analysis. Within the last few years there has been a keen revival of interest in this research because of some important new discoveries which have sharpened our understanding of specific emotions·and their bodily expressions. It has been learned for instance, that anger and fear produce different physiological reactions and can be distinguished from each other. The findings have given us a fresh outlook from which to study mental illnesses.

The best way to begin the account of this recent work is to start with Cannon's own summary of what he learned. Cannon found that when an animal was confronted with a situation which evoked pain, rage or fear, it responded with a set of physiological reactions which prepared it to meet the threat with "fight" or "flight." These reactions, said Cannon, were mobilized by the secretion of adrenalin: when the cortex of the brain perceived the threat, it sent a stimulus down the sympathetic branch of the autonomic nervous system to the adrenal glands and they secreted the hormone. Cannon graphically described the results as follows:

"Respiration deepens; the heart beats more rapidly; the arterial pressure rises; the blood is shifted away from the stomach and intestines to the heart and central nervous system and the muscles; the processes in the alimentary canal cease; sugar is freed from the reserves in the liver; the spleen contracts and discharges its content of concentrated corpuscles, and adrenin is secreted from the adrenal medulla. The key to these marvelous transformations in the body is found in relating them to the natural accompaniments of fear and rage — running away in order to escape from danger, and attacking in order to be dominant. Whichever the action, a life-or-death struggle may ensue.

From *Scientific American*, 192:74, 1955.

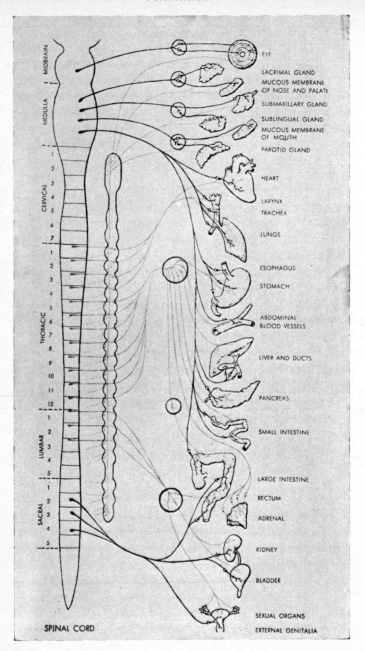

Fig. 1. The autonomic nervous system is represented by this diagram. The parasympathetic branches, arising from the brain and sacral vertebrae, are indicated in black; the sympathetic branches, arising from the thoracic and lumbar vertebrae, are in color.

"The emotional responses just listed may reasonably be regarded as preparatory for struggle. They are adjustments which, so far as possible, put the organism in readiness for meeting the demands which will be made upon it. The secreted adrenin cooperates with sympathetic nerve impulses in calling forth stored glycogen from the liver, thus flooding the blood with sugar for the use of laboring muscles; it helps in distributing the blood in abundance to the heart, the brain, and the limbs (*i.e.*, to the parts essential for intense physical effort) while taking it away from the inhibited organs in the abdomen; it quickly abolishes the effects of muscular fatigue so that the organism which can muster adrenin in the blood can restore to its tired muscles the same readiness to act which they had when fresh; and it renders the blood more rapidly coagulable. The increased respiration, the redistributed blood running at high pressure, and the more numerous red corpuscles set free from the spleen provide for essential oxygen and for riddance of acid waste, and make a setting for instantaneous and supreme action. In short, all these changes are directly serviceable in rendering the organism more effective in the violent display of energy which fear or rage may involve."

Cannon recognized that among all these physiological changes there were a few which could not be ascribed directly to the action of adrenalin. He therefore postulated that the hormone was supplemented by two additional substances from the sympathetic nerves. An active agent, distinguishable from adrenalin, was eventually identified in 1948, when B. F. Tullar and M. L. Tainter at length succeeded in preparing the optically active form of the substance. It proved to be a second hormone secreted by the adrenal medulla. Called nor-adrenalin, it differs markedly from adrenalin in its physiological effects. Whereas adrenalin elicits profound physiological changes in almost every system in the body, nor-adrenalin apparently has only one important primary effect; namely, it stimulates the contraction of small blood vessels and increase the resistance to the flow of blood.

An animal exhibits only two major emotions in response to a threatening situation: namely, rage and fear. A man, however, may experience three: ①anger directed outward (the counterpart of rage), ②anger directed toward himself (depression)③and anxiety, or fear. In studies of physiological changes accompanying various emotional states among patients at the New York Hospital, H. C. Wolff and his co-workers noticed that anger produced effects quite different from those of depression or fear. For example, when a subject was angry, the stomach lining became red and there was an increase in its rhythmic contractions and in the secretion of hydrochloric acid. When the same subject was depressed or frightened, the stomach lining was pale in color and there was a decrease in peristaltic movements and in the hydrochloric acid secretion.

The experiments of Wolff, the evidence that the adrenal medulla secreted two substances rather than one and certain clinical observations led our group at the Harvard Medical School to investigate whether adrenalin and nor-adrenalin might be specific indicators which distinguish one emotion from another. The clinical observations had to do with the effects of a drug, mecholyl, on psychotic patients. We had been studying their blood-pressure responses to injections of adrenalin, which acts on the sympathetic nervous system, and mecholyl, which stimulates the parasympathetic system. On the basis of their blood-pressure reactions, psychotic patients could be classified into seven groups [see Fig. 4]. This test had proved of value in predicting patients' responses to psychiatric treatments, such as electric shock and insulin: certain groups responded better to the treatments than others. But more interesting was the fact that psychotic patients with high blood pressure reacted to the injection of mecholyl in two distinctly different ways. In one group there was only a small drop in the blood pressure after the injection, and the pressure returned to the usually high level within three to eight minutes. In the other group the blood pressure dropped markedly after the injection and remained below the pre-injection level even after 25 minutes. Not only were the physiological reactions different, but the two groups of patients also differed in personality and in response to treatment. Thirtynine of 42 patients whose blood pressure was sharply lowered by mecholyl improved with electric shock treatment, whereas only three of 21 in the other group improved with the same treatment. Further, the two groups showed distinctly different results in projective psychological tests such as the Rorschach.

All this suggested that the two groups of patients might be differentiated on the basis of emotions. Most psychotic patients in emotional turmoil express the same emotion constantly over a period of days, weeks or months. Psychiatrists determined the predominant emotion expressed by each of 63 patients who had been tested with mecholyl, without knowing in which physiological group they had been classified. When the subjects' emotional and physiological ratings were compared, it turned out that almost all of the patients who were generally angry at other people fell in Group N (a small, temporary reduction of blood pressure by mecholyl), while almost all those who were usually depressed or frightened were in Group E (sharp responses to mecholyl). In other words, the physiological reactions were significantly related to the emotional content of the patients' psychoses.

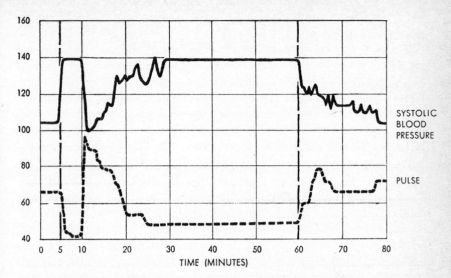

Fig. 2. Effect of nor-adrenalin was observed by administering an infusion of the hormone for 60 minutes. After 5 minutes the blood pressure of the subject rose. After 10 minutes mecholyl was injected and the blood pressure fell. Then it rose in a Type N response.

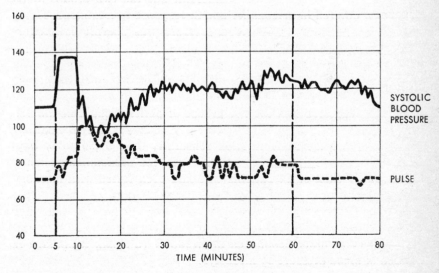

Fig. 3. Effect of adrenalin was observed by the same procedure. After the injection of mecholyl the systolic blood pressure of the subject remained depressed in a Type E response.

The next step was to find out whether the same test could distinguish emotions in normal, healthy people, using medical students as subjects. They were studied at a time when they were under stress — while they were awaiting the decisions of hospitals on their applications for internships. As the competition among the students for the hospitals of their choice is keen, the period just prior to such announcements is a time of emotional turmoil for the men. A group of students who responded to this situation with elevated blood pressure was given the standard dose of mecholyl. The results were the same as for the psychotic patients: students who were angry at others for the situation in which they found themselves had a Type N physiological reaction; those who felt depressed (angry at themselves) or anxious showed a Type E physiological reaction. The reaction was related only to their temporary emotional state; after the internships were settled and their blood pressures had returned to pre-stress levels, all the students reacted the same way to the injection of mecholyl.

It was at this point that we undertook to investigate the comparative effects of adrenalin and nor-adrenalin. A group of workers at the Presbyterian Hospital in New York had shown that injections of nor-adrenalin and adrenalin produced two different types of rise in blood pressure, one due to contraction of blood vessels and the other to faster pumping of the heart. Upon learning of this work, we designed experiments to test the hypothesis that the two types of elevated blood pressure, differentiated by us on the basis of mecholyl tests, indicated in one instance excessive secretion of nor-adrenalin and in the other excessive secretion of adrenalin. Healthy college students were first given a series of intravenous injections of salt water to accustom them to the procedure so that it would not disturb them. Then each subject was tested in the following way. He was given an injection of nor-adrenalin sufficient to raise his blood pressure by 25 per cent. Then, while his blood pressure was elevated, he received the standard dose of mecholyl, and its effects on the blood pressure were noted. The next day the subject was put through the same procedure except that adrenalin was given instead of nor-adrenalin to raise the blood pressure.

Ten students were studied in this way, and in every instance the effect of nor-adrenalin was different from that of adrenalin [see Fig. 5]. When the blood pressure was elevated by nor-adrenalin, mecholyl produced only a small drop in pressure, with a return to the previous level in seven to 10 minutes. This reaction was similar to the Type N response in psychotic patients and healthy students under stress. In contrast, when the blood pressure was elevated by adrenalin, mecholyl produced the Type E response: the pressure dropped markedly and did not return to the previous level during the 25-minute observation period.

These results suggested, in the light of the earlier experiments, that anger directed outward was associated with secretion of nor-adrenalin, while depression and anxiety were associated with secretion of adrenalin. To check this hypothesis, another series of experiments was carried out.

A group of 125 college students were subjected to stress-inducing situations in the laboratory. The situations, involving frustration, were contrived to bring out each student's habitual reaction to stresses in real life; that the reactions actually were characteristic of the subjects' usual responses was confirmed by interviews with their college roommates. While the subjects were under stress, observers recorded their emotional reactions and certain physiological changes — in the blood pressure, the pulse and the so-called IJ waves stemming from the action of the heart. This test showed that students who responded to the stress with anger directed outward had physiological reactions similar to those produced by injection of nor-adrenalin, while students who responded with depression or anxiety had physiological reactions like those to adrenalin.

There remained the question: Does the same individual secrete unusual amounts of nor-adrenalin when angry and of adrenalin when frightened? Albert F. Ax, working in another laboratory in our hospital, designed experiments to study this question. He contrived laboratory stressful situations which were successful in producing on one occasion anger and on another occasion fear in the same subjects. His results showed that when a subject was angry at others, the physiological reactions were like those induced by the injection of nor-adrenalin; when the same subject was frightened, the reactions were like those to adrenalin. This indicated that the physiology was specific for the emotion rather than for the person.

In all these experiments the evidence for excessive secretion of nor-adrenalin and adrenalin was based on the physiological changes being similar to those which can be produced by the intravenous injection of nor-adrenalin and adrenalin. Since the substances involved have not been identified chemically, and the evidence is entirely physiological, at the present time we prefer to limit ourselves to the statement that the reactions are *like* those to the two hormones. However, nothing in our experiments would contradict the hypothesis that these substances are actually adrenalin and nor-adrenalin.

What is the neurophysiological mechanism whereby different emotions evoke different adrenal secretions? Although no conclusive work in this area is yet available, some recent investigations suggest a pos-

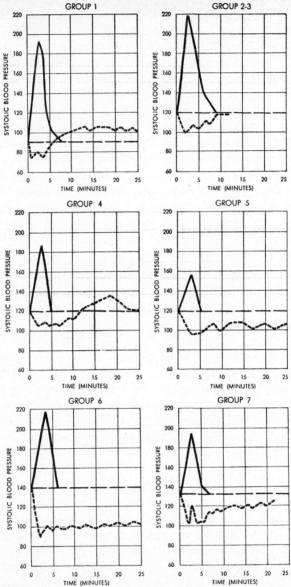

Fig. 4. Seven groups of psychotic patients were distinguished on the basis of their blood pressure after injection with adrenalin or mecholyl. In these six charts the basal systolic blood pressure of the patients is indicated by the broken horizontal line. The solid curve shows their response to adrenalin; the broken curve, their response to mecholyl. Groups 2 and 3 are combined because the difference between them is too slight to show in the graph. The mecholyl response for Group 7 is incomplete because of experimental difficulties.

sible answer. U. S. von Euler in Sweden found that stimulation of certain areas of the hypothalamus caused the adrenal gland to secrete nor-adrenalin, whereas stimulation of other areas caused it to secrete adrenalin. These areas may correspond to those which the Nobel prize winner, W. R. Hess of Zurich stimulated to produce aggressive behavior and flight, respectively, in animals. The experiments suggest that anger and fear may activate different areas in the hypothalamus, leading to production of nor-adrenalin in the first case and adrenalin in the second. Until more experiments are made, these possibilities must remain suppositions.

Some of the most intriguing work in this field was recently reported by von Euler. He compared adrenal secretions found in a number of different animals. The research material was supplied by a friend who flew to Africa to obtain the adrenal medullae of wild animals. Interpreting his findings, J. Ruesch pointed out that aggressive animals such as the lion had a relatively high amount of nor-adrenalin, while in animals such as the rabbit, which depend for survival primarily on flight, adrenalin predominated. Domestic animals, and wild animals that live very social lives (e.g., the baboon), also have a high ratio of adrenalin to nor-adrenalin.

These provocative findings suggest the theory that man is born with the capacity to react with a variety of emotions (has within him the lion and the rabbit), and that his early childhood experiences largely determine in which of these ways he will react under stress. Stated in another way, the evolutional process of man's emotional development is completed in the bosom of the family. We have found in other studies that individuals' habitual emotional reactions have a high correlation with their perceptions of psychological factors in their families.

This entire series of experiments yielded data which can be understood in the frame of reference of psychoanalytical observations. According to theory, anger directed outward is characteristic of an earlier stage of childhood than is anger directed toward the self or anxiety (conflicts over hostility). The latter two emotions are the result of the acculturation of the child. If the physiological development of the child parallels its psychological development, then we should expect to find that the ratio of nor-adrenalin to adrenalin is higher in infants than in older children. Bernt Hokfelt and G. B. West established that this is indeed the case: at an early age the adrenal medulla has more nor-adrenalin, but later adrenalin becomes dominant.

Paranoid patients show a greater degree of regression to infantile behavior than do patients with depression or anxiety neurosis. And it will be recalled that in our tests paranoid patients showed signs of

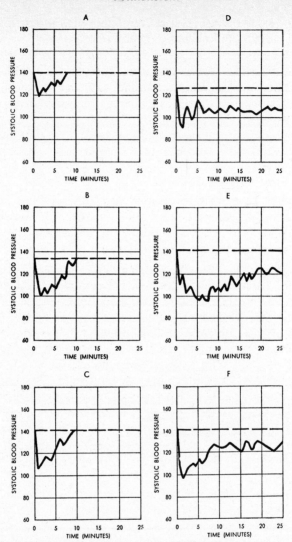

Fig. 5. Type N response to the injection of mecholyl is traced by the heavy line. The broken line represents the basal blood pressure. The response is shown for three kinds of subject: (A) healthy individuals under stress who respond with anger toward others, (B) healthy individuals whose blood pressure has been elevated with nor-adrenalin and (C) psychotic individuals with elevated blood pressure and anger toward others.

Type E response to the injection of mecholyl is similarly traced by the heavy line. In these charts the response is shown for three different kinds of subject: (D) healthy individuals under stress who respond with anger directed inward, or depression, (E) healthy individuals whose blood pressure has been elevated with adrenalin and (F) psychotic individuals with elevated blood pressure and depression.

excessive secretion or nor-adrenalin, while depressed and anxious patients exhibited symptoms of adrenalin secretion.

These parallels between psychological and physiological development suggests further studies and some theories for testing. Standing on the shoulders of Cannon and Freud, we have extended our view of human behavior and discovered fertile new fields for exploration.

16

ON THE PHENOMENON OF SUDDEN DEATH
IN ANIMALS AND MAN

CURT P. RICHTER, Ph.D.

Johns Hopkins Medical School, Baltimore

"Voodoo" Death — that is the title of a paper published in 1942 by Walter Cannon. (1) It contains many instances of mysterious, sudden, apparently psychogenic death, from all parts of the world. A Brazilian Indian condemned and sentenced by a so-called medicine man, is helpless against his own emotional response to this pronouncement — and dies within hours. In Africa a young Negro unknowingly eats the inviolably banned wild hen. On discovery of his "crime" he trembles, is overcome by fear, and dies in 24 hours. In New Zealand a Maori woman eats fruit that she only later learns has come from a tabooed place. Her chief has been profaned. By noon of the next day she is dead. In Australia a witch doctor points a bone at a man. Believing that nothing can save him, the man rapidly sinks in spirits and prepares to die. He is saved only at the last moment when the witch doctor is forced to remove the charm. R. Herbert Basedow in his book *The Australian Aboriginal* (2) wrote in 1925:

The man who discovers that he is being boned by an enemy is, indeed, a pitiable sight. He stands aghast with his eyes staring at the treacherous pointer, and with his hands lifted to ward off the lethal medium, which he imagines is pouring into his body. His cheeks blanch, and his eyes become glassy, and the expression of his face becomes horribly distorted. He attempts to shriek but usually the sound chokes in his throat, and all that one might see is froth at his mouth. His body begins to tremble and his muscles twitch involuntarily. He sways backward and falls to the ground, and after a short time appears to be in a swoon. He finally composes himself, goes to his hut and there frets to death.

Cannon made a thorough search of reports from many primitive societies before he convinced himself of the existence of voodoo deaths. He concluded:

. . . the phenomenon is characteristically noted among aborigines — among human beings so primitive, so superstitious, so ignorant, that they feel them-

From *Psychosomatic Medicine*, May–June 1957. © 1957 by American Psychosomatic Society, Inc.

selves bewildered strangers in a hostile world. Instead of knowledge, they have fertile and unrestricted imaginations which fill their environment with all manner of evil spirits capable of affecting their lives disastrously . . .

Having, after a painstaking search of the literature, convinced himself of the reality of this phenomenon, Cannon next addressed himself to the question "How can an ominous and persistent state of fear end the life of man?" To answer this question he had recourse to his experimental observations on rage and fear in cats. He believed that while rage is associated with the instinct to attack and fear with the instinct to flee, these two emotions have similar effects on the body. Thus, when either of these instincts is aroused the same elemental parts of the nervous system and endocrine apparatus are brought into action, the sympathicoadrenal system.

If these powerful emotions prevail, and the bodily forces are fully mobilized for action, and if this state of extreme perturbation continues in uncontrolled possession of the organism for any considerable period, without the occurrence of action, dire results may ensue.

Thus, according to Cannon, death would result as a consequence of the state of shock produced by the continuous outpouring of adrenalin. Voodooed individuals would, therefore, be expected to breathe very rapidly, have a rapid pulse, and show a hemoconcentration resulting from loss of fluids from the blood to the tissues. The heart would beat faster and faster, gradually leading to a state of constant contraction and, ultimately, to death in systole.

Cannon expressed the hope that anyone having the opportunity to observe an individual in the throes of voodoo influence would make observations on respiratory and pulse rates, concentration of the blood, etc., to test this theory.

I bring this up here not because I have had opportunity to examine human victims — I have not — but because I have observed what may be a similar phenomenon in rats and because our studies may throw light on the underlying mechanisms of sudden unexplained death in man, not only in voodoo cultures. We are still actively at work on the problem and consequently this communication must be considered simply as a report of work in progress.

As so often happens, this phenomenon was discovered accidentally, as it were, during the course of other experiments. The first observation was made with Dr. Gordon Kennedy in 1953 while studying the sodium metabolism of rats on very high salt diets. To determine the amount of sodium excreted, three animals on a diet containing 35 per cent NaCl were kept in metabolism cages over large glass funnels.

The urine was collected in a cylinder. To prevent contamination of the urine with this salt-rich food, the food-cup in each cage was placed at the end of a passageway, as far as possible from the neck of the funnel; however, despite our precautions, food was still dragged over the funnel, apparently on the whiskers or hair of the snout. In a further attempt to prevent this contamination the whiskers and hair were trimmed away with electric clippers. One of the three rats at once began to behave in a very peculiar manner, incessantly pushing its snout into the corners of the cage or into the food-cup with a cork-screw motion. Although before the clipping procedure it had seemed entirely normal, eight hours afterwards it was dead.

This observation was recalled a year or two later, while we were studying differences in the response to stress of wild and domesticated Norway rats. For these studies we measured endurance by means of swimming survival times, using specially designed tanks — glass cylinders 36 inches deep, standing inside glass jars 8 inches in diameter and 30 inches in depth. A jet of water of any desired temperature playing into the center of each cylinder precluded the animal's floating, while the collar of the cylinder itself prevented escape. The study was started with observations on our domesticated rats. Figure 1 shows the relationship between swimming time (drowning) and water temperature.

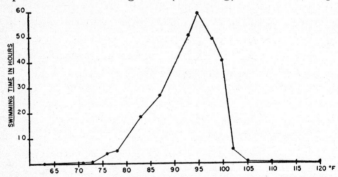

Fig. 1. Curve showing average swimming time (end point, drowning) of unconditioned tame domesticated Norway rats with relation to water temperature. Averages for 7 rats at each point.

The ordinates show average (7 rats at each point) swimming time in hours, and the abscissas water temperature in degrees Fahrenheit. As can be seen, the average survival times were directly related to the temperature of the water; thus, the swimming times ranged from 10–15 minutes at 63–73° F., to 60 hours at 95° F., to 20 minutes at 105°.

The significance of this average curve was greatly reduced by the marked variations in individual swimming times. At all temperatures, a small number of rats died within 5–10 minutes after immersion, while in some instances others apparently no more healthy, swam as long as 81 hours. The elimination of these large variations presented a real problem, which for some time we could not solve. Then the solution came from an unexpected source — the finding of the phenomenon of sudden death, which constitutes the main topic of this communication. On one occasion while I was watching rats swim it occurred to me to investigate the effect of trimming the rat's whiskers on its performance in water. Would a rat swimming without whiskers show the peculiar behavior of the original rat in the metabolism cage?

Our observations were started with twelve, tame, domesticated rats. Using electric clippers, the whiskers and hair of the facial area were trimmed before the animals were placed in water at 95° F., a temperature at which most intact, control rats swim 60 to 80 hours. The first rat swam around excitedly on the surface for a very short time, then dove to the bottom, where it began to swim around nosing its way along the glass wall. Without coming to the surface a single time, it died 2 minutes after entering the tank. Two more of the twelve domesticated rats tested died in much the same way; however, the remaining 9 swam 40 to 60 hours.

Five of 6 hybrid rats, crosses between wild and domesticated rats, similarly treated, died in a very brief time. We then tested 34 clipped wild rats, all recently trapped. These animals are characteristically fierce, aggressive, and suspicious; they are constantly on the alert for any avenue of escape and react very strongly to any form of restraint in captivity. All 34 died in 1–15 minutes after immersion in the jars.

From the results we concluded that trimming the rats' whiskers, destroying possibly their most important means of contact with the outside world, seemed disturbing enough, especially to wild rats, to cause their deaths. However, when we began analyzing the various steps involved in transferring the fierce, wild rats from their cages to the water jars without the use of any anesthetic, it became obvious that a number of other factors had to be taken into account. To evaluate the relative importance of these factors, it became necessary to follow the rats from the time they left their cages until they finally died at the bottom of the swimming jars.

A metal cage was used for the wild rats; the bevelled end contained a hinged door, the flat end a sliding door. A black opaque bag was used for catching and holding the rat. The open end is held over the sliding door at the flat end of the cage. When the sliding door is opened, the rat sees the dark opening — an avenue of escape — and usually within seconds, almost "shoots" in. The instant the rat is out of the cage its retreat is cut off by a rod pressed down across the mouth of the bag. By means of the rod, the rat is then pushed into the end of the bag, where it is firmly but gently prevented from turning. The head is located by palpation and is held between the thumb and fingers, with care not to exert any pressure on the neck, while the body is held in the palm of the hand. Over 2000 rats have been held in this way, and none has ever made an attempt to bite through the bag. The rat is then lifted and the black cloth is peeled back exposing its head and body. Held in this way the rat can neither bite nor escape; its whiskers can be trimmed, it can be injected, or it can be dropped directly into a swimming jar.

Thus, in evaluating the possible causes of the prompt death of the wild rats in this experiment, account must be taken of the following factors:

1. Reaction of the rat to confinement in the holding bag.
2. Reaction to being held in the experimenter's hand, while being prevented from biting or escaping.
3. Peripheral and cerebral vascular reactions to being held in an upright position. (The upright posture is reported to be fatal to wild rabbits.) (3)
4. Peripheral and cerebral vascular reactions to possible unavoidable pressure on the carotid sinus, carotid body, or larynx, exerted by the tips of the forefinger and thumb in holding the rat. (Prolonged pressure on the carotid sinus can produce syncope and even death in man as well as animals through its effect on vascular and respiratory mechanisms.) (4)
5. Reaction to the process of being clipped.
6. Reaction to confinement in swimming jar, with no avenue of escape.
7. Reaction of the clipped rats to a new situation, determined by the loss of stimulation from whiskers.
8. Respiratory reaction to immersion in water. (Diving produces marked slowing in heart rate.) (5)
9. Peripheral and cerebral vascular reactions to immersion in water at a temperature of 95° F. (Immersion in water of this temperature could produce a marked drop in pressure, resulting in cerebral anemia.)
10. Vascular reaction to nearly upright swimming posture. (Similar to, but presumably more marked than in No. 3.)

At present it appears that of all these factors, two are the most important: the restraint involved in holding the wild rats, thus suddenly and finally abolishing all hope of escape; and the confinement in the glass jar, further eliminating all chance of escape and at the same time threatening them with immediate drowning. Some of the wild rats died simply while being held in the hand; some even died when put into the water directly from their living cages, without ever being held. The combination of both maneuvers killed a far higher percentage. When in addition the whiskers were trimmed, all normal wild rats tested so far have died. The trimming of the whiskers thus proved to play a contributory, rather than an essential, role.

What kills these rats? Why do all of the fierce, aggressive, wild rats die promptly on immersion after clipping, and only a small number of the similarly treated tame domesticated rats?

On the basis of Cannon's conclusions and under the influence of the current thinking about the importance of the part played by the adrenals and the sympathetic nervous system in emotional states, and especially under stress, we naturally looked first of all for signs of sympathetic stimulation, especially for tachycardia and death in systole. Accordingly we were first interested in measuring the heart rate.

Electrocardiographic records were taken by means of electrodes consisting of short pieces of sharpened copper wire, each with a very fine insulated wire soldered to the blunt end. The pointed copper wires were dipped into electrode jelly and inserted under the skin of the two hind legs and one foreleg. They were inserted up the legs and the connecting wires were bent back up over the legs. A piece of plastic adhesive tape wrapped around the leg held the electrode and wire in place, insuring that a force exerted on the connecting wire would pull the electrode further under the skin rather than dislodge it. The connecting wires were brought together over the animal's back. In this way the rat could swim without getting itself entangled. Surprisingly, records taken under water were indistinguishable from those taken in air.

Contrary to our expectation, the EKG records indicated that the rats succumbing promptly died with a slowing of the heart rate rather than with an acceleration. Figure 2 shows portions of the underwater EKG record typical of a rat dying promptly after immersion. Terminally, slowing of respiration and lowering of body temperature were also observed. Ultimately the heart stopped in diastole after having shown a steady gradual decrease in rate. As expected, autopsy revealed a large heart distended with blood. These findings indicate that the rats may have died a so-called vagus death, which is the result of overstimulation of the parasympathetic rather than of the sympathicoadrenal system.

It should be pointed out that the first response to stress, whether that of restraint in the hand or confinement in the water jars, was

often an accelerated heart rate; only subsequently, with prolongation
of the stress situation, was this followed by slowing. In some rats the
latter response developed very promptly, in others not for a few
minutes.

The following additional facts are in agreement with such a preliminary formulation: (a) pretreatment with atropine prevented the

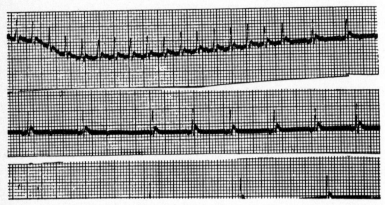

Fig. 2. Part of electrocardiogram on wild rat taken a few minutes after the
rat's immersion in the water jar.

prompt death of 3 out of 25 clipped wild rats. By increasing the dose
or by varying the interval between the injections and the test it might
have been possible to achieve a higher survival rate; (b) domesticated
rats injected with definitely sublethal amounts of cholinergic drugs
(morphine, physostigmine, mecholyl), i.e., of parasympathetic stim-
ulants, died within a few minutes after being put in the swimming jars.
Thus, one-tenth of the LD 50 of morphine sufficed to bring out the sudden death response in these rats, in effect eliminating this distinction
between domesticated and wild rats; (c) so far all the adrenalectomized
wild rats tested still showed sudden-death response, indicating that
the deaths were not due to on overwhelming supply of adrenalin. Thy-
roidectomy likewise did not prevent the appearance of the sudden-
death phenomenon.

The situation of these rats scarcely seems one demanding fight or
flight — it is rather one of hopelessness; whether they are restrained in
the hand or confined in the swimming jar, the rats are in a situation
against which they have no defense. This reaction of hopelessness
is shown by some wild rats very soon after being grasped in the hand
and prevented from moving; they seem literally to "give up."

Support for the assumption that the sudden-death phenomenon depends largely on emotional reactions to restraint or immersion comes

from the observation that after elimination of the hopelessness the rats do not die. This is achieved by repeatedly holding the rats briefly and then freeing them, and by immersing them in water for a few minutes on several occasions. In this way the rats quickly learn that the situation is not actually hopeless; thereafter they again become aggressive, try to escape, and show no signs of giving up. Wild rats so conditioned swim just as long as domesticated rats or longer.

Another observation worthy of record concerns the remarkable speed of recovery of which these animals are capable. Once freed from restraint in the hand or confinement in the glass jars, a rat that quite surely would have died in another minute or two becomes normally active and aggressive in only a few minutes. Thus, in order to measure the maximum swimming time, we now try to free the rats of all emotional reactions to restraint or confinement by successively exposing them to these situations and freeing them several times beforehand. In this way we have succeeded in eliminating most of the individual variations and are now obtaining quite constant, reproducible, endurance records for both domesticated and wild rats.

It is interesting that a few wild rats have also been protected by pretreatment with chlorpromazine, without other "conditioning."

That the wild rats as compared to the domesticated rats seem much more susceptible to this type of death would suggest that they have a higher vagus tone. In agreement with this thought are the well-known observations that vagus tone is higher in healthy, vigorous individuals than in weaker ones; also that vagus tone is higher in wild than in domesticated animals in general. (6)

Other wild animals — rabbits, shrews, and pigeons — as well as some domesticated animals — ewes — are known to show a sudden-death response; whether of the same kind as we have described here is not known at present.

How can these results be applied toward the understanding of the voodoo-death response in man? Apparently the "boned" victim, like the wild rat, is not set for fight or flight, but similarly seems resigned to his fate — his situation seems to him quite hopeless. For this reason we believe that the human victims — like our rats — may well die a parasympathetic rather than a sympathicoadrenal death, as Cannon postulated.

Like the wild rat, primitive man, when freed from voodoo, is said to recover almost instantaneously, even though he had recently seemed more dead than alive. These observations suggest that the sudden-death phenomenon may be a one-time occurrence both in rats and man — in any particular circumstances, ending either in death or in immunity from this particular kind of death. In human beings as well as in rats we see the possibility that hopelessness and death may result from the effects of a combination of reactions, all of which may operate in the same direction, and increase the vagal tone.

There is the further suggestion that the incidence of this response varies inversely as the degree of civilization, or domestication, of the individual, since it occurs more frequently in wild than in domesticated rats and so far certainly has been described chiefly in primitive man, that is to say, in creatures living in precarious situations.

However, some physicians believe that this phenomenon exists also in our culture. Thus, according to Cannon, Dr. J. M. T. Finney, the well-known surgeon at the Johns Hopkins Hospital, apparently believed in it, since he absolutely would not operate on any patient who showed a strong fear of operation. Many instances are at hand of sudden death from fright, sight of blood, hypodermic injections, or from sudden immersion in water.

During the war a considerable number of unaccountable deaths were reported among soldiers in the armed forces in this country. These men died when they apparently were in good health. At autopsy no pathology could be observed. (7)

Of interest here also is that, according to Dr. R. S. Fisher, Coroner of the City of Baltimore, a number of individuals die each year after taking small, definitely sublethal doses of poison, or after inflicting small, nonlethal wounds on themselves; apparently they die as a result of the belief in their doom.

SUMMARY

A phenomenon of sudden death has been described that occurs in man, rats, and many other animals apparently as a result of hopelessness; this seems to involve overactivity primarily of the parasympathetic system. In this instance as in many others, the ideas of Walter Cannon opened up a new area of interesting, exciting research.

REFERENCES

1. Cannon, W. B. "Voodoo" death. *Am. Anthrop.*, 44: 169, 1942.
2. Basedow, H. *The Australian Aboriginal*. Adelaide, Australia, 1925.
3. Best, C. H., and Taylor, N. B. *Physiological Basis of Medical Practice*. (Fifth Ed.) Baltimore, 1950.
4. Weiss, S. Instantaneous "physiologic" death. *New England J. Med.*, 223: 793, 1940.
5. Irving, L. The action of the heart and circulation during diving. *Tr. New York Acad. Sc.*, 5: 11, 1942.
6. Clark, A. S. *Comparative Physiology of the Heart*. London, Cambridge, 1927.
7. Moritz, A. R., and Zamchek, N. Sudden unexpected deaths of young soldiers. *Arch. Path.*, 42: 459, 1946.

17

ELECTROMYOGRAPHIC STUDY OF HYPNOTIC DEAFNESS

ROBERT B. MALMO, THOMAS J. BOAG, AND BERNARD
B. RAGINSKY

Allan Memorial Institute of Psychiatry, and McGill University
Montreal Jewish General Hospital

Freud (4) believed that similar mechanisms were involved, basically, in hysterical and hypnotic phenomena of sensory exclusion. The work of Erickson (2, 3) on hypnotically induced deafness, viewed together with the recent work of Malmo, Davis, and Barza (9) on hysterical deafness, provided some evidence favoring this general point of view. Although Erickson employed pneumatic apparatus in an attempt to record involuntary reactions to sound in his hypnotically deaf subjects, it is rather difficult to compare his data with the physiological study of hysterical deafness. In particular, electromyography is useful in detecting small involuntary reactions, some of which are impossible to detect in any other way. The present study was therefore designed as a comparative one, to investigate the question of similarities and differences between hypnotic deafness and the hysterical phenomena previously reported.

In addition, we hoped to secure objective data which would be useful in enriching our general understanding of hypnosis and in particular to bring data to bear on our working hypothesis: that recorded reactions to loud sound under hypnotically induced deafness will differ significantly from reactions in waking subjects attempting not to react, and also from the reactions in true organic deafness.

METHODS

Using two subjects selected from a much larger group, we repeated the auditory test in the same way in which it had been administered to the hysterical subject in the previous study (9).

Subjects. Both subjects who served in the hypnotic experiments were women, psychiatric nurses. We shall designate them A and B. Ages were 24 and 35 respectively. A third case, of total middle-ear deafness, served as a control subject. The fourth case, Anne, referred to in this

From the *Journal of Clinical and Experimental Hypnosis*, October 1954.

paper is the case of "total" hysterical deafness which was studied previously (9).

Procedure. The two subjects used for the following experiments were chosen after screening a group of some 35 volunteers. This group was made up of trained nurses and post-graduate psychology students. The selection of these two subjects was made on the basis of their marked suggestibility and the ease with which hypnotic deafness was induced during the first trial session. During the following six weeks, each of the subjects was trained to go into a deeper hynotic state. Under these conditions deafness was induced finally by the signal of pressing the left shoulder and hearing re-established by pressing the left wrist. These training periods lasted at first about one hour and a half, but were diminished in time as their efficiency in reaching the desired state increased. The training sessions took place in the room where the final experiments were to be carried out. The subjects were not told beforehand what was expected of them in the experiments nor were they made aware of the object of the investigation.

Both subjects were trained nurses at the Institute and accustomed to the research projects being carried out in the various departments of the hospital. The training period and the experiments themselves required a considerable amount of their free time.

Hypnotic deafness was induced by direct suggestion in Subject A. In the control waking situation, whenever she was left alone for several minutes, she would tend to lapse into a mild hypnotic state. This was difficult to control.

Total deafness could not be produced in Subject B by direct suggestion alone. It was found necessary to have her imagine herself in a complete void. The next step was to have her hallucinate visually a noisy traffic corner. This she was able to do without hearing any of the attending sounds. Total deafness was then suggested and she was able to defend against hearing loud banging noises made close to her ear. This "deafness" never appeared to be as complete as in Subject A.

During the experiment the subject lay on a hospital bed in a sound-shielded room separated from our instrument control room but with a one-way vision window between these two rooms. Muscle potentials were recorded by means of the following standard surface leads (1): chin, sterno-mastoid, and neck. Eye blink was also recorded electrically. The auditory stimuli were 700-cycle tones approximately 90 db. above auditory threshold. There were ten stimulus presentations in the first test ("deaf" state) and ten stimulus presentations in the second test, several days later,[1] in the waking state. Stimuli were presented

---

[1] Dates of testing were as follows: Hypnotic sessions: 13 June 1952, 19 June 1952, and waking control sessions, 17 June 1952 and 24 June 1952, for Subjects A and B respectively.

regularly at intervals of one minute and they were transmitted to the subject through binaural earphones. It should be mentioned that, although duration of tone was three seconds, a constant feature of the stimulus was a sharp "on effect," which gave the impression of a click of very brief duration.

Audograph sound recordings were made during the sessions to provide verbatim accounts of what was said during hypnotic induction and interviews.

Control conditions. Controls were of two kinds, internal or reversible, in which the two subjects, who had previously taken the auditory test under hypnotic conditions, went through the test again under waking conditions. They were asked to try, on a conscious voluntary basis, not to react to stimulation. In this and every way we attempted to satisfy Hull's criteria (7) for adequate internal control conditions. The second kind of control was external, or irreversible, the subject with complete organic deafness.

RESULTS

Subject A

Sensory phenomena, introspective data. The subject, in interview following the hypnotic session, denied hearing any sounds during the period of hypnotic deafness. Motor data, to be described in detail presently, showed clear reaction to the first stimulus, however, without the emotional disturbance with weeping which Anne displayed.[2] It seemed unwise to question the hypnotic subjects following each stimulus, as we had done with the hysterical subject, Anne; but at the end of the session during interview (after the subject had been awakened) we were especially careful to raise questions which might yield a report from Subject A concerning sensations of any kind which may have accompanied her motor reaction to the first stimulus.

Questioning the present subject did bring out the interesting subjective report of brief thermal sensation which she was positive had occurred no more than twice during the session. She said: "I had goose pimples a couple of times, a feeling of cold which came on suddenly; I was aware of it and then it was gone." The feeling was localized to

---

[2] "The first stimulus produced a startle reaction . . . The observer in the room with Anne noted a slight movement at the time of stimulation. This observer also noted trembling which began with the head and spread to the rest of the body. A few seconds following her startle reaction, Anne displayed a marked emotional reaction, with crying. This reaction alarmed the therapist to the extent that he risked spoiling the test by hurrying into the room to give reassurance to the patient.

When asked whether she had heard the sound, Anne replied that she had heard nothing, but that she had felt pain in her head 'as if something hit me on the head.' Later, after the test, she added: 'It felt as if the top of my head were going to blow off' " (9, p. 190 f.).

her bare leg. Although further questioning did not definitely establish that the sensation occurred at the same time as the motor reaction, it appeared possible that the two phenomena were associated. It is of interest to note that this girl is particularly sensitive to stimulation by currents of air (e.g., breezes or drafts striking the body, and especially in the region of the head and neck).

Questioning the subject following the second (waking control) session revealed an element of vagueness in her report which suggested that she may have fallen into a hypnotic state, lasting from stimulus number five to the end of the session. Following the fourth stimulus it was necessary to make some adjustments in the instruments, and there was a delay of several minutes. It appeared to us that during this delay, the subject put herself in a trance. It will be important to keep this possibility in mind as we review the behavioral and physiological data.

Habituation. Hilgard and Marquis (6, p. 105) have defined intrinsic inhibition or adaptation as the reduction in response resulting from continued elicitation of the response itself. Habituation or negative adaptation are terms commonly applied to decremental changes in reflex responses, as a function of its repeated elicitation. Except for the blink component, the startle reflex normally shows this phenomenon of habituation. Examples of habituation in the sternomastoid muscle reaction may be seen in the graphs for the waking reactions of Subject A (and B) shown in Figure 1. Our measure of reaction was the difference between average resting muscle potential and average muscle potential following each stimulation. Mean resting muscle potential was determined by averaging the ten integrator spike values from the one-second period immediately preceding stimulation. Four integrator spike values were averaged to yield a measure for the stimulation period: from 0.2 seconds thru 0.5 seconds following onset of stimulation. The spike for the first 0.1 second of stimulation was regularly omitted from the averaging in order to avoid error due to possible slight deviation from perfect synchronization between integrator and stimulator.

In Figure 1 note the gradual decline in reaction through the first four stimulations in the waking state. Neck muscle reactions, as may have been expected on the basis of the close functional relationship with sternomatoid, also showed progressive decrement through the first four stimulations. Chin muscle reaction, which is functionally dissimilar to neck and sternomastoid will be dealt with separately later on.

Now observe in Figure 1 how, under hypnosis, sternomastoid reaction in this subject dropped from a strong reaction on stimulus one to practically no reaction on stimulus two. This sudden decrement in reaction, unlike the progressive tapering off of reaction observed under waking conditions, exactly resembled our previously reported observations of hysterical deafness (9, Fig. 1, p. 192). As noted before, however, Subject A did not appear to be emotionally disturbed following her obvious reaction to the first stimulus, nor was there any indication of perturbation in her physiological record. In this respect she was decidedly different from the hysterical subject, Anne, who was so disturbed that she wept.

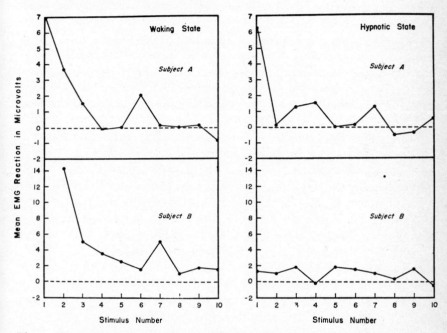

Fig. 1. Sternomastoid reaction to auditory stimulation. In Subject A, compare progressive fall in reaction through first four stimuli in waking session with abrupt fall from first to second stimulus in hypnotic session. Note that Subject B also shows a typical habituation curve in the waking state, but not under hypnosis. In Subject B, the point for stimulus one, waking state, is not plotted, because artifacts interfered with measurement. A lively reaction was obtained, however.

Reliability of differences between hypnotic and waking conditions. The first row of Table 1 presents average microvolt values for reaction. In preparing the data for this part of the table the ten reaction measures for each of the ten stimuli were combined in a single average value. Mean neck muscle reaction under the hypnotic condition was 0.5 microvolts, whereas under the control condition, average reaction was 1.1 microvolts. The table shows further that whereas the mean neck muscle reaction of 1.1 microvolts for the control (waking) session was significantly above zero (reliable below the one per cent level), the value of 0.5 microvolts for the hypnotic session was not reliably above zero. Although the control value for sternomastoid was slightly higher than the value for hypnosis, neither was reliably above zero. Finally, it may be noted that the mean chin muscle reaction of 1.1 microvolts for the hypnotic session was reliable.

TABLE 1.   COMPARISON OF MEAN WAKING REACTION TO AUDITORY STIMULATION WITH MEAN HYPNOTIC REACTION

Mean EMG Reaction to Auditory Stimulation
(Minus values represent fall in EMG with reference to
pre-stimulation level)*

	Neck		Sternomastoid		Chin	
	Hypnosis	Control	Hypnosis	Control	Hypnosis	Control
Subject A						
Mean microvolts	0.5	1.1	1.1	1.4	1.1	−0.5
P	—	<.01	—	—	<.02	—
Subject B						
Mean microvolts**	−0.1	2.2	0.8	4.0	−6.0	0.5
P	—	<.01	<.05	<.01	<.05	<.01

Reliability of Differences between Mean Reaction
under Control and Hypnotic Conditions
(Minus values represent greater mean reaction under hypnosis)

	Neck	Sternomastoid	Chin
Subject A			
Mean microvolts	0.6	0.3	−1.6
P	—	—	<.05
Subject B			
Mean microvolts	2.3	3.2	6.5
P	<.01	<.01	<.02

*Pre-stimulus EMG level was average for one sec. immediately preceding stimulation. The period of reaction measured was from 0.2 sec. thru 0.5 sec., inclusive.
**Based on nine stimuli (number one omitted; see text).

The lower part of Table 1 presents differences between mean reaction under control and hypnotic conditions, together with the statistical reliability of these differences. The values in the first row are simply the differences between mean reactions: control reaction minus the reaction under hypnosis. For example, for the neck muscle the mean values were 1.1 microvolts for the control condition and 0.5 for the hypnotic condition. The difference, shown in the lower half of the table was 0.6 microvolts. This was not a reliable difference nor was the difference for sternomastoid significant. The greater chin muscle reaction under hypnosis than under the "waking" condition was, however, a significant difference. In line with other evidence for change in the subject following the intermission, as possibly produced by spontaneous induction of hypnosis, it may be noted that before intermission there were no instances of fall in chin potentials upon stimulation, whereas after intermission five of six stimulations produced a drop in muscle potentials from the chin.

Blink reaction. The observer, who carefully watched the subject all through the experiment, noted definite eye blink in only three of the ten stimulations under hypnosis: on the first, second, and ninth stimulations. Question marks were entered in the blanks for the third and fourth stimulations, signifying doubt as to whether blink had actually occurred. Sensitive electrical recorders, however, revealed evidence of activity in the blink apparatus with all stimulations.

In the control (waking) session definite blinks were noted with the first four stimulations. Following the intermission for instrumental adjustments, however, with the possible exception of stimulus seven where slight lid movement was noted, no blinks were observed from stimulus five to the end of the session. This observation fits with other evidence that the subject may have fallen into a state of hypnosis during the intermission. But, again, the electrical recorders showed action in the blink apparatus with all stimulations.

Background or resting level of muscle potentials from the chin. In the second part of the control session (after intermission for instrumental adjustments) the subject's background level of muscle potentials from the chin became higher. It were as though the presumed hypnotic state was associated with an increased background level of potentials in the "speech muscles." With this higher background level of potentials the immediate effect of auditory stimulation changed. Now, instead of a sudden increase in potential, the opposite occurred, namely, a sudden drop in muscle tension (when the tone was presented). We shall observe later in the protocols from Subject B that such drops occurred in muscle potential from her chin, under the condition of hypnosis. In both cases, statistical analysis showed significant association between high resting level of chin tension and fall in potential upon stimulation.

Subject B

Sensory phenomena, introspective data. The subject awoke from the hypnotic session saying that she had a "funny feeling" in her head, and presently she said, "I've got a headache." She described the sensation as almost like a boring feeling in the top of her head, immediately below the headpiece for earphones. The sensation was directed inward, a boring in rather than out. The subject was reasonably sure that the sensation came on after the stimulations had commenced, although not immediately following the first time she heard the tone.

"I heard something like a bell a couple of times," she said. The first time she heard the sound it was very loud, but after that much less loud. The experience of hearing was neither startling nor emotionally disturbing, although she distinctly recalled being surprised that she was not startled, "because everything had been quiet up to then." She indicated that her level of awareness was lowered, and that what she heard reminded her of someone striking a gong which resounded for a second or two and then died out.

In interview following the control (waking) session, the subject compared the experience of her waking session, just concluded, with the memory of her hypnotic experience: "Last time I heard only a couple of sounds through the earphones, and I didn't feel at all startled by them. This time it seemed to me a dozen or so because at first I started counting and that seemed to increase the tension, so I tried to forget how many there were, and it seemed to me that at the end I wasn't as tense as I was at first. But I could feel myself reacting to them a certain amount no matter how I tried not to. (Subjects were instructed, in the waking condition, to try not to react to the sound.) I don't know whether I did the last time or not; I may have, but I'm not sure, but this time I was completely aware of it."

The subject was then asked to compare the quality of the sounds in the two sessions. The subject's own words were as follows: "Last time, the times when I heard it, it sounded like a — as though someone had struck a gong, the initial — the onset of the sound was very sharp, and then it faded away. But even at that it had a — oh — I don't know how to describe it. It was generally fuzzier than the sounds were today. They were much clearer today and quite well defined. There was no — I didn't notice any particular fading from the onset of the sound until it ended — today. But last time it just seemed to spin out a bit."

When asked to give further details concerning the fading away, and to give examples of sounds like those she heard, she said: "All I can think of — perhaps you've seen them in the — well, all I can think of is the things they used to have at school. Ring the bell for recess time or something like that and there would just be one twang, and then you could hear the vibration until it died out completely. That's all I can think of. You know the type they hang on the wall with a string hanging down from it; somebody pulls and the clapper hits the bell?"

(Examiner: "Yes. So that you have a fading away.") "Yes. Today it sounded more like the CBS time signals."

When asked to compare the sounds with respect to pitch she replied: "I think it seemed a bit deeper last time. The pitch today seemed a bit higher and sharper."

When asked to contrast the two sessions in other ways she answered: "The last time there was the unawareness of anything else, or anyone else in the room. This time I was aware of other movements, such as coughing, and chair moving, and so on. This time I was aware all the time of the lead attachments, whereas the last time I don't remember that at all." She reported absence of the boring sensation this time and said, "I feel quite relaxed and satisfied, but not quite as relaxed as I did the last time."

Habituation. We have already had occasion to note the subject's gradual decrement in waking reaction, from the second stimulus to the sixth (refer again to data from sternomastoid muscle in Fig. 1). Reaction to the first stimulus was so vigorous that movement artifacts precluded accurate measurement; the downward trend thus began from stimulus one. This, of course, is the normal picture of habituation. Now compare this curve with her curve from data taken during the hypnotic condition. Observe the small fluctuating reactions under hypnosis. Inasmuch as the hypnotic session preceded the waking session, overall habituation (presuming it occurs, to some extent, under hypnosis) should have reduced the latter more than the former. It may be noted that waking and hypnotic reactions from the neck muscle resembled those of sternomastoid.

This subject differed from Subject A and the hysterical subject, Anne, in not showing a strong reaction to stimulus one, in the "deaf" state.

Reliability of differences between hypnotic and waking conditions. Mean neck muscle reaction for the control session was 2.2 microvolts, whereas the corresponding value for the hypnotic session was −0.1. The value for the control session was significantly greater than zero (see Table 1). For the sternomastoid muscle, mean control reaction was 4.0 microvolts (reliable at the one per cent level) compared with 0.8 microvolts for reaction under hypnosis (reliable at the five per cent level of significance).

Muscle potentials from the chin actually dropped significantly with stimulation under hypnosis. The mean drop was −6.0 microvolts, as opposed to a mean rise of 0.5 microvolts under control conditions. Both mean values were significantly different from zero (see Table 1). Figure 2 shows the chin reaction data plotted for each tenth-second period for the first second immediately following stimulation. In the

figure single values from each of the ten stimulations have been averaged. Although the largest drop in chin tension occurred almost immediately after stimulation (second tenth-second), reduced tension
in the chin area continued to persist as long as one second after stimulation (the value for the last tenth-second was significantly lower than
the resting value).

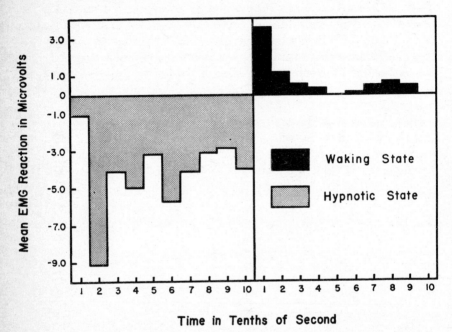

Fig. 2. Comparison of change in muscle potentials from chin under conditions
of waking control versus hypnotic "deafness." Note reversal in direction of
change, from condition to condition. Deviation from zero reaction was
significant for second, third, sixth, and last tenths in the hypnotic state, and
for first and eight tenths in the waking state.

In complete contrast to these minus values (tensional drop) under
hypnosis, the values for the waking state were all positive (increased
muscle potential upon stimulation).

Turning now to the lower portion of Table 1 we find that the two
functionally related muscles, neck and sternomastoid, both showed
significantly greater reaction under the control condition than under
hypnosis. Mean values from the chin muscles were also reliably different from condition to condition, but as we have noted the pronounced fall in chin tension with auditory stimulation under hypnosis
was the most outstanding feature.

Blink reaction. Definite eye blink was noted by the observer (and in the electrical records) with every instance of auditory stimulation, under hypnotic as well as under waking conditions.

Background or resting level of muscle potentials from the chin. Relationship between high resting level and high incidence of negative reaction (fall in muscle potentials with auditory stimulation) previously noted in the protocols for Subject A, was found definitely present in this subject. There were six stimuli, in the hypnotic session which produced a fall in chin electromyogram (EMG) within the first fifth second. Of these six stimuli, five occurred at times when mean resting level, immediately preceding stimulation, was above the median value of 9.3 microvolts.

Control case of middle-ear deafness

This was a woman of 30 who, following a bilateral mastoidectomy at age 5, had been completely deaf. There is little doubt that this is a case of middle-ear deafness. She has not learned much lip reading and her speech is almost incomprehensible. Communication is possible only through writing. She came to the psychiatric clinic because she had become more and more suspicious in recent years and developed delusions that people were talking about her.

This patient took the auditory test under the same conditions as the other "deaf" subjects. Careful scrutiny of her records revealed no reaction to stimulation. No record of blink appeared nor did the observer note any movement or blink during stimulations.

Obtaining valid introspective data was considerably hampered by difficulties in communicating with the patient. When questioned she denied any uncomfortable or disturbing sensations during the test, although there was some indication in her report that she may have experienced some vibratory sensations.

DISCUSSION

Hypnotic and hysterical "deafness": similarities and differences. The most obvious similarity was the absence of complete deafness. Although reaction to strong auditory stimulation was significantly less in hypnotic deafness and in hysterical deafness than in their respective control conditions (waking state and recovery of hearing), the reaction in all these cases was greater than in the control case of middle-ear deafness.

Our findings are in line with those of Kline, Guze, and Haggerty (8) who concluded from their study of delayed feedback that hypnotically induced deafness appeared "to represent a valid alteration of hearing function but not a state akin to organic deafness." Incidentally, they reported that "hypnotically induced deafness was found to produce all loss of startle reflexology" (8, p. 147). In light of our findings such a statement appears hazardous, inasmuch as our sensitive recorders revealed reactions to sound when they could not be detected by careful observation of the subject.

Another important similarity lay in the observation that when motor reaction to sound appeared on the first stimulus, in both hypnosis and hysteria, reaction to the next stimulation was less than would have been predicted on the basis of habituation only.

Although we cannot be certain about the hypnotic subject, it was very clear in the hysterical subject and there was some suggestion in all subjects that somesthetic sensations took the place of auditory ones. There was the suggestion of sensory displacement. For example, when Anne was asked whether she had heard the sound (to which she reacted) she replied that she had heard nothing, but that she had felt pain in her head "as if something hit me on the head." Later, after the test, she added: "It felt as if the top of my head were going to blow off."

As an alternative interpretation to that of sensory displacement we may consider that the actual sensations reported were residual, in the sense of being what was left from total stimulation when the auditory component had been removed. The introspective data from our organic case, while not completely satisfactory because of difficulties in commsunciation, were on the whole opposed to this point of view. Certainly, in the case of middle-ear deafness, there was nothing uncomfortable or disturbing about the stimulations. Furthermore, this case demonstrated that exclusion of the auditory pathways reduced intensity of the total stimulation well below the level for even the slightest startle reaction. It seems safe, therefore, to conclude that all motor phenomena of startle, and the strong, unpleasant sensations associated with startle (certainly in the hysterical case, and possibly in the hypnotic cases) were mediated by auditory pathways.

We must be very cautious in our conclusions concerning the sensory phenomena (e.g., "goose pimples" and "boring feeling") in our hypnotic subjects. It is tempting to suggest that these, like the somesthetic sensations in the hysterical subject, may have been manifestations of sensory displacement from the auditory to other modalities. It does not seem likely that they were residual sensations (resulting from "subtraction" of auditory component from total stimulation). Intensity of stimulation was below the threshold for nonauditory tactual sensation (10, p. 59).

The chief differences between the two states, insofar as present observations are concerned, appeared to be affective in character. There was no apparent emotional reaction when "hypnotic defense against sound" was broken through, in contrast to marked affective disturbance in the penetration of the hysterical defense.

Question of inhibitory mechanisms in hysteria and hypnosis. Comparison of data from waking sessions with data from hypnotic sessions, in the present investigation, leads to the distinction between two quite different inhibitory phenomena. Habituation, which is a special case of reactive inhibition (or adaptation) was clearly demonstrated in the waking state. With repetition of the auditory stimulus, strength of reaction diminished, gradually becoming weaker and weaker from trial to trial, over the first four or five trials. Decrement was chiefly observed in neck and sternomastoid muscles (we have no evidence of habituation of blinking).

In the hypnotic (and hysterical) state, on the other hand, a different phenomenon was seen. Unlike reactive inhibition, there was an immediate (rather than a progressive) effect on motor reaction, and, of course, the loss of conscious auditory sensation. This could conceivably be inhibition by interference, which occurs when two incompatible responses are elicited at the same time. Although almost completely speculative at the present time, we may suppose that a hypnotically induced reaction could block the response pattern of hearing. Some data from the chin leads (which tap activity from the speech muscles) in the present experiment might be adduced to encourage this point of view. We freely admit the highly speculative nature of the following comments; but we feel that it may prove instructive to try to account for these "speech muscle" data by reference to current psychodynamic and neuropsychological concepts.

There was some evidence, though by no means conclusive, that level of tension in these muscles was higher in hypnotic than in waking states. Chin tension level was considerably higher in Subject B under hypnosis than in the waking condition, and when Subject A appeared to put herself into a hypnotic state, there was pronounced rise in chin tension. On the other hand, it should be noted that Subject A's chin tension for the first four stimuli in the control session (when she appeared quite "awake") was slightly higher than it was in her hypnotic session. We must be exceedingly cautious, therefore, to avoid premature conclusions.

Speculations concerning nature of inhibitory mechanism. First, we may view deafness as the result of a defense mechanism which prevents sound from reaching consciousness. We posit further that the mechanism is highly symbolic with a large verbal component. Therefore we should expect to see chin tension reflecting this subvocal verbal activity, building up high when the mechanism is effective in excluding sound, and falling in amplitude when the mechanism is rendered ineffective by intense auditory stimulation.

Restated in terms of neuropsychological theory, phase sequences (5) initiated under the direction of the hypnotist break up the phase sequences essential for report of hearing. These interfering sequences involve central speech mechanisms in large measure, and their activity is reflected in chin tension. These same phase sequences which interfere with hearing are themselves vulnerable to very loud sounds. Correlation is thus observed between high level of chin tension and effective blocking out of hearing, on the one hand, and lowered level of chin tension and decreased effectiveness of the blocking, on the other.

An illustration which may concretize these ideas is taken from observations which were made during early training sessions for inducing hypnotic deafness. At this stage the hypnotist made the suggestion that the subject would become more and more deaf. As part of this procedure the subject was instructed to move hand to face as ability to hear progressively decreased, in such a way that hand resting on face signified absolute deafness and proximity of hand to face at any point in time indicated degree of deafness. In one case particularly, we watched the hand approach the face as the hypnotist tapped his finger very lightly, and saw the hand stop and retreat away from the face as the tapping became louder. Unfortunately, we were not recording muscle potentials during this stage of training. With electromyographic recording we may have expected to see rise in chin tension and approach of hand to face going along together, and also the converse: fall in chin tension accompanying movement of hand away from face, as louder sounds broke through. In closing we wish to remind the reader again how highly speculative this analysis is, and to warn him against accepting these propositions as conclusions from present data. We feel that their usefulness lies in the formulation of questions for further experimental attack on these problems.

SUMMARY AND CONCLUSIONS

The main purpose of the present study was to investigate the question of similarities and differences between hysterical deafness, previously studied, and hypnotically induced deafness. The study was designed to repeat the objective physiological tests previously carried out with a case of "total hysterical deafness." There was also the more general aim of securing objective data to enrich our general understanding of hypnosis.

Similarities between hysteria and hypnosis which we observed may be listed as follows: (a) Significantly reduced motor reaction (exclusive of blink) to strong auditory stimulation in the deaf state. (b) Complete hearing loss in the hysteric and in one of the hypnotic subjects, even with strong auditory stimulation (i.e., denial of any auditory sensation). (c) With elicitation of strong startle reaction to the first stimulus in the deaf state, much smaller reaction to the next stimulus than would have been predicted on the basis of habituation. (d) Suggestion of substitution of somesthetic for auditory sensations in all subjects (although this was much less definite in the hypnotic subjects than the hysteric).

The most outstanding dissimilarity lay in the absence of emotional reaction when "hypnotic defense against sound" was broken through, in contrast to marked affective reaction in the hysterical subject under these conditions.

The question of inhibitory mechanisms in hysteria and hypnosis was discussed.

REFERENCES

1. Davis, J. F. *Manual of surface electromyography*. Montreal: Laboratory for Psychological Studies, Allan Memorial Institute of Psychiatry, 1952.
2. Erickson, M. H. A study of clinical and experimental findings on hypnotic deafness: I. Clinical experimentation and findings. *J. gen. Psychol.*, 1938, 19: 127–150.
3. Erickson, M. H. A study of clinical and experimental findings on hypnotic deafness: II. Experimental findings with a conditioned response technique. *J. gen. Psychol.*, 1938, 19: 151–167.
4. Freud, S. *Collected papers*, Volume II. London: Hogarth, 1950, pp. 105–110.
5. Hebb, D. O. *The organization of behavior*. New York: Wiley, 1949.
6. Hilgard, E. R., and Marquis, D. G. *Conditioning and learning*. New York: D. Appleton-Century, 1940.
7. Hull, C. L. *Hypnosis and suggestibility*. New York: D. Appleton-Century, 1933.
8. Kline, M. V., Guze, H., aud Haggerty, A. D. An experimental study of the nature of hypnotic deafness: effects of delayed speech feedback. *J. clin exp. Hypnosis*, 1954, 2: 145–156.
9. Malmo, R. B., Davis, J. F., and Barza, S. Total hysterical deafness: an experimental case study. *J. Person.*, 1952, 21: 188–204.
10. Stevens, S. S., and Davis, H. *Hearing*. New York: Wiley, 1938.

18

A COGNITIVE THEORY OF DREAM SYMBOLS

CALVIN S. HALL

Department of Psychology, Syracuse University

It is not my intention in this article to discuss theories of symbolism in general, nor even to review the history of thought regarding symbols in dreams. Rather I have set for myself the more modest task of proposing an alternative theory for one which now occupies the center of the stage whenever dreams are mentioned. I refer, of course, to Freud's theory of dream symbolism.

In order to gain some perspective on the psychoanalytic theory of dream symbols, let us consider briefly the origin and history of dream books, a task that H. B. Weiss has made lighter by his interesting and informative article on them (12). We learn from this article that the first dream book was written by an Italian physician, Artemidorus, who lived in the second century A.D. Artemidorus collected reports of dreams in his travels, through correspondence, and by the purchase of manuscripts. From these sources, he compiled a work of five volumes under the title *Oneirocritics*, a word which means the art of interpreting dreams. Following the invention of the printing press in the fifteenth century, Artemidorus's work was widely published, going through numerous editions in various languages. *Oneirocritics* is the Adam of all dream books, past and present. The first American dream book, *The Book of Knowledge*, was published in Boston in 1767. It was followed by a spate of others so that today there is a wide selection available to those who seek help in interpreting their dreams.

A dream book is actually a special type of dictionary, in which the entries are words or phrases descriptive of dream items followed by their meanings; that is, symbols and referents. In a typical dream book, the referent is usually either "good fortune" or "bad fortune," since the dream book exploits the notion that dreams are prophetic and that what most people want to know is what the future holds for them. Dream books also rest on the assumptions that dreams are symbolic and that the symbols of dreams have universal significance. For example, we read in Artemidorus that to dream of *eating cheese* signifies profit and gain to the dreamer. It is not stated that sometimes

From *The Journal of General Psychology*, 48:169, 1953.

this is its meaning, or that it depends upon the state of the dreamer, or upon the context in which this activity appears. The meaning of eating cheese in dreams is *univocal, universal,* and *timeless.* It is this feature of universal symbol-referent connections that accounts for the popularity of dream books. Since they do not make qualifications and exceptions which would require the use of judgment and discrimination, anyone can decode dreams and foretell the future if he has a dream book handy.

Freud borrowed two of the dream books assumptions, dream symbols and the universality of *some* dream symbols, and rejected the third, the prophetic character of dreams. Why are there symbols in dreams? Freud answered that symbols appear in dreams because the referents for which the symbols are surrogates are distasteful to the censor. The dream-work can smuggle reprehensible things into a dream by transforming them into innocuous symbols. One dreams of climbing a tree instead of masturbating because climbing trees (the symbol) is condoned and masturbating (the referent) is condemned. In short, symbols are disguises for referents.[1]

In order to determine what referents are commonly symbolized, a search of the psychoanalytic literature was made by the writer and his students. Although not exhaustive, our search turned up 709 symbols. The two most popular referents are *penis* for which there are 102 symbols, and *vagina* for which there are 95 symbols. Other referents that have a large number of symbols are *death* (62 symbols), *coitus* (55 symbols), *masturbation* (25 symbols), *mother* (15 symbols), *father* (14 symbols), *breasts* (13 symbols), and *castration* (12 symbols). Be it noted, with the possible exception of *death,* all of the referents are concrete things, people, or activities, and similarly all of the symbols, as *gun* for *penis, bag* for *vagina, ploughing* for *coitus, playing the piano*

---

[1] This, of course, is not all that Freud had to say about symbolism. He felt that the subject went beyond dreams. Symbolism is an archaic form of expression, a primordial language which is found in myths and fairy tales, in popular sayings and songs, in colloquialisms and in poetry. Even if there were no censorship in dreams, dreams would be rendered incomprehensible by the use of symbols. The fact remains, however, that Freud believed that symbolism served the purpose of disguise. He writes: "Symbolism, then, is a second and independent factor in dream distortion existing side by side with the censorship. But the conclusion is obvious that it suits the censorship to make use of symbolism, in that both serve the same purpose: that of making the dream strange and incomprehensible" (2, p. 150). "Everything points to the same conclusion, namely, that we need not assume that any special symbolizing activity of the psyche is operative in dream-formation; that on the contrary, the dream makes use of such symbolizations as are to be found ready-made in unconscious thinking, since these, by reason of their ease of representation, and for the most part by reason of their being exempt from the censorship, satisfy more effectively the requirements of dream-formation" (1, p. 368). "Dreams employ this symbolism to give a disguised representation to their latent thoughts" (1, p. 370). Quotations from Freud could be multiplied to show that for him the most important function of symbols in dreams is that of disguise.

for *masturbating,* queen for *mother,* king for *father,* apple for *breast,* etc., are concrete things, people, or activities. In short, something concrete, the symbol, is substituted for something else concrete, the referent.

If one adopts Freud's theory of symbolism, an essential feature of dream interpretation consists of finding a referent for each symbol. Since the meaning of numerous symbols has been set forth by psychoanalysts it is fairly simple for anyone to decode his dreams by using a modern psychoanalytic dream book, for instance, Gutheil's *Language of the Dream* (3). The following dream reported by a young woman can be readily deciphered.

I was in a big room talking to one of my friends. She said she was going riding and I decided to join her. I waited for her to come back for me; when she did return, she said she had already ploughed the field and that the horse was upstairs. I said that I'd probably have trouble getting it down the stairs, and she told me one of the men had helped her down. However, I decided against riding.

Later we were all sitting around in the room and I looked up and saw a friend of mine who was in New Orleans. He came over and we were talking until everyone was handed an enormous gun and we all started shooting out of the windows. I recall loading and reloading the gun.

In psychoanalytic dream language this dream is a versatile portrayal of sexuality. *Riding, ploughing a field, climbing stairs,* and *shooting* symbolize masturbation or coitus. *Gun, horse,* and *plough* are phallic symbols, room and windows are vaginal symbols. *Being handed an enormous gun* = being given a penis. Apparently the dreamer's wish is to be a man.

According to Freud, how does a symbol become a symbol? How does it happen that one object or activity becomes a stand-in for another object or activity. Freud draws upon the laws of association, particularly the law of resemblance, to explain the formation of symbol-referent connections. Some of the ways in which association by resemblance operates are as follows:

(1). Association by resemblance in shape. All circular objects and containers = vagina, and all oblong objects = penis.

(2). Association by resemblance in function. All objects that are capable of extruding something, e.g., gun, fountain pen, bottle = penis.

(3). Association by resemblance in action. Any act that separates a part from a whole, e.g., beheading, losing a tooth, an arm or a leg, having a wheel come off an automobile = castration. By the same token, dancing, climbing stairs, riding horseback, going up and down in an elevator = coitus.

(4). Association by resemblance in color. Chocolate = feces, yellow = urine, milky substance = semen.

(5). Association by resemblance in value. Gold = feces, jewelry = female genitals.

(6). Association by resemblance in number. Three = penis and testicles.

(7). Association by resemblance in sound. The blaring of a trumpet or bugle or the sound of a wind instrument = flatulence.

(8). Association by resemblance in quality. Wild animal = sexual passion, horse = virility.

(9). Association by resemblance in personal quality. Policeman, army officer, teacher = father, nurse = mother.

(10). Association by resemblance in physical position. Basement = the unconscious mind.

(11). Association by resemblance in status. King = father, queen = mother.

In addition to association by resemblance, there are several other ways in which two items may become paired as symbol and referent.

(12). Association by contiguity. Church = virtue, night club = sensuality, bathtub = cleanliness.

(13). Association of part with whole. A specific accident = difficulties of life, a school test = a test of fitness for life.

(14). Association by contrast. Crowd = being alone, clothed = naked, to die = to live. Freud wrote that "inversion or transformation into the opposite is one of the most favored and most versatile methods of representation which the dream-work has at its disposal" (1, p. 352), thereby acknowledging one of the oldest maxims of dream lore "that dreams go by contraries."

My skepticism regarding Freud's theory of symbols-as-disguises began with a simple question for which I could find no satisfactory answer within the framework of Freud's theory. Having read hundreds of dream series in the past few years, I noticed that within the same series outspoken dreams occurred along with "symbolized" dreams. It is fairly common for one to dream of sexual activities in the frankest terms one night and in disguised terms the next night. Open incest dreams alternate with camouflaged incest dreams. Parricide and fratricide are sometimes overt, sometimes concealed. I wondered what was the sense of preparing an elaborate deception in one dream when it was discarded in a subsequent dream. To this question I could not find a convincing answer.

Another flaw in the Freudian theory appeared. In collecting dreams, I often ask a person to give his interpretation of the reported dream. I found that many people have real talent for dream interpretation although some of these have little or no information about Freudian symbolism. Why should one bother to deceive oneself by dreaming in symbols when they can be translated so readily by the dreamer himself? Again I could not find a plausible answer within the context of the Freudian formulation.

While thinking about the lay person's ability to translate his dreams, it occurred to me that people have been using a consciously contrived form of symbolism in their daily speech for centuries. It is called slang. Although there are slang expressions for many things, much of it is sexual in character. In order to get evidence concerning the relation of slang to dream symbols, I went through Partridge's *A Dictionary of Slang and Unconventional English* (8) noting every slang expression for penis, vagina, and coitus. There were 200 expressions for penis, 330 for vagina and 212 for coitus. The results of this study will be published elsewhere; suffice it to say here that many of the dream symbols for the sex organs and for sexual intercourse are identical with those found in Partridge. Many of these slang words have been in the English language for centuries.

If slang and dream symbols coincide as closely as they do and if the referents of slang are as well known as they are, how can these same expressions (or vizualizations of them) function effectively as disguises in dreams? It would be absurd for a dreamer to deceive himself with symbols during sleep when these same symbols are used so self-consciously during waking life. This is not the place to discuss the motives for the development of slang; at another time we intend to show that the same principles govern slang formation as govern dream symbol formation. Both spring from man's disposition to express his ideas in concrete form; slang uses figures of speech and dreams use images.

These explorations in the world of slang led me to consider the psychological significance of figures of speech or *tropes*, of which four principal varieties have been delineated: (*a*) *synecdoche*, (*b*) *metonymy*, (*c*) *metaphor*, and (*d*) *irony*. Synecdoche is a figure of speech in which a part is used for a whole, a whole for a part, the cause for the effect, the effect for the cause, the name of the material for the thing made, the species for the genus and so on. Metonymy is a figure in which the name of one thing is changed for that of another to which it is related by association and close relationship. A metaphor is a figure which consists in the transference to one object of an attribute or name which strictly and literally is not applicable to it, but only figuratively and by analogy. Irony is a figure whose intended implication is just the opposite of that which is stated. One associates figures of speech with poetry, although they are used more or less widely in all forms of writing and speaking. Modern literary criticism and research have become aware of the importance of trope analysis in shedding light upon the intrinsic meaning of a literary creation *and* upon the personality dynamics of the creator. Noteworthy among those who have analyzed writings and writers by paying attention to figures of speech is Caroline Spurgeon, whose exegesis of Shakespeare is a remarkable *tour de force* (11) although wanting in the insights that dynamic psychology might have provided. Another example of this approach is found in Mark Schorer's *Fiction and the "Matrix of Analogy"* (10) in which he scrutinizes Jane Austen, Emily Bronte, and George Eliot through their metaphors.

The relation of tropes to slang and of both to dream symbols is one of psychological identity. Slang expressions are figures of speech; they are an idiom by which the person tries to communicate his conceptions. It is the thesis of this paper that dream symbols belong to the same idiom; a dream symbol or any symbol, for that matter, reveals thought rather than conceals it.

Before developing this thesis, two other flaws in Freud's theory of dream symbols will be mentioned. We have seen that a multitude of symbols can stand for the same referent. Why is it necessary to have so many disguises for the genitals, for sexual intercourse, and for masturbation? Psychoanalysis has not given this question proper attention.[2] If one hypothesizes that dream symbols are the embodiments of conceptions, then the reason for the multiplicity of symbols for a single referent becomes clear. People have many different conceptions of the same object; thus they need a versatile idiom for conveying the precise shade of meaning for each idea.

Finally, a critique of Freud's position regarding dream symbols should take note of an assumption that is implicit in his theory, namely, that the mind works in a very complex manner during sleep. To assert that part of the work done by the mind in forming a dream consists of transforming referents into symbols for the purpose of veiling the referents is to ascribe to the sleeping mind a heavier responsibility than seems warranted. Since we usually think of sleep as a period of reduced mental activity, would it not be better to formulate a theory of dream symbolism that makes symbolizing dependent upon simpler processes?

[2] Freud did suggest an answer in the following passage. "Wherever he has the choice of several symbols for the representation of a dream-content, he will decide in favor of that symbol which is in addition objectively related to his other thought-material; that is to say, he will employ an individual motivation besides the typically valid one" (1, p. 370). Had Freud developed the thought of this passage, he might have come to the conclusion that we have reached, namely, that a particular symbol is chosen because it expresses better than any other symbol would the precise conception in the mind of the person.

These questions prompted me to reexamine the whole structure of Freud's theory of dreams. Upon undertaking this task I discovered that Freud had proposed two reasons why symbols appear in dreams, one is the necessity to smuggle contraband psychic material past the border separating the unconscious from the conscious and the other is what Freud called *regard for representability*. The latter formulation states that in order for such abstract and impalpable mental contents as thoughts, feelings, attitudes, and impulses to appear in dreams, they must be converted into sensible, palpable forms. These forms are usually pictorial in character, so that it may be said that the pictures of a dream are symbols of mental states. For example, conscience may be symbolized by a church, chastity by a lily, the sex impulse by fire, feelings of inferiority by nudity, and remembering the past by walking through a series of rooms.[3]

When one compares Freud's two hypotheses regarding the function of dream symbols, it is evident that they are diametrically opposed to one another. In one, a symbol conceals the referent, in the other, a symbol reveals the referent. Preferring the simplicity of a single hypothesis to the complexity of two separate and incompatible hypotheses, I decided to explore the possibility of abandoning the disguise theory and let *regard for representability* carry the whole burden of explaining dream symbols.

This enterprise led to the formulation of a cognitive theory of dreams which is presented in another paper (5). In that paper, I set forth the view that a dream is a perceptible embodiment of a dreamer's conceptions (ideas). Dreaming is pictorialized thinking; the conceptual is made perceptual. I now intend to show how this view leads directly to the formulation of a theory of dream symbols. Both theories represent extensions of Freud's concept of *regard for representability* in dreams.

A dream symbol is an image, usually a visual image, of an object, activity, or scene; the referent for the symbol is a conception. The function of the symbol is to express as clearly as possible the particular conception that the dreamer has in mind. For example, a dreamer who conceives of his mother as a nurturant person may represent her in a dream as a cow. Or a young woman who conceives of sexuality as a powerful, alien, and criminal force which she is unable to control might have the following dream, as one of our subjects did.

[3] Had Freud himself not commented upon regard for representability we might still have deduced it from our collection of symbol-referent pairs. It is obvious that some of the referents are objects which might be represented directly were it not for censorship while others are mental states, which require pictorialization if they are to appear as dream images.

I was the warden at a very inefficient prison for criminals. All at once the gates to the prison opened and all of the criminals tried to escape. They tried to beat me up and trample on me and I was left standing there completely helpless.

A young man conceiving of his phallus as a dangerous weapon might picture it as a gun or sword in his dreams. A woman who thought that her marriage was going on the rocks dreamed that she was looking for her wedding dress and when she found it, it was dirty and torn. In these examples, the visualization is an expression of, not a disguise for, an idea.

An object, activity, or scene is selected to serve as a symbol because the dreamer's conception of the object, activity, or scene is congruent with his conception of the *referent object*.[4] A nurturant mother appears as a cow because the dreamer conceives of cows as nurturant animals. If the dreamer thought cows were dangerous, a cow could not serve as a mother-symbol unless at the same time he conceived of his mother as dangerous. Occasionally, a change of conceptions can be detected as in the following dream.

I dreamed that an old man was coming towards me with a gun. I become frightened and put my glasses on to see him better. Then I noticed that he was not holding a gun but a bottle of whisky.

The young woman's first conception of the man is that he is dangerous, but this idea gives way to the contradictory one that he is harmless. The change in conceptions is symbolized by the act of putting on her glasses; the better view follows this act.

In some cases, a symbol may represent several ideas concurrently. In psychoanalytic writings, such a symbol is said to be *over-determined*. This term is not a happy choice since no phenomenon is ever *over*-determined; it is always *just* determined, never too little or too much. I prefer to call such symbols *condensed*. The moon, for example, may be thought of as a condensed symbol for woman. The monthly phases of the moon resemble the menstrual cycle, a resemblance that has support from etymology since the words *moon* and *menses* are derived from the same Latin word. The filling out of the moon from new to full simulates the rounding out of the woman during pregnancy. The moon is inferior to the sun, a male symbol. The moon is changeable like a fickle woman while the sun is constant. The moon sheds a weak light, which embodies the idea of female frailty. The moon controls

[4] The term *referent* will be used to denote the dreamer's conception and the term *referent object* will be used to denote the object, person, or activity about which the dreamer has a conception. Thus, the referent object of cow is mother, and the referent is the conception of the mother as a nurturant person.

the ebb and flow of the tide, which is another likeness to the female rhythm. Rhythm, change, fruitfulness, weakness, and submissiveness, all of which are conventional conceptions of the female are compressed into a single visible object. As Susanne Langer observes, the choice of moon as a symbol of woman is determined by the many ways in which lunar characteristics are congruent with popular conceptions of the female. Mrs. Langer reminds us that the conceptions develop first, followed by the selection of a symbol which will best represent all of the conceptions.[5]

When one analyzes a series of dreams from a person, various symbols for the same referent object may be found. As we have seen, the male member may be symbolized in no less than 102 different ways. According to our theory of dream symbols, since the referent is not an object, person, or activity but a conception, the 102 different phallic symbols represent 102 different ways of conceiving of the male genitals.[6] Thus in a dream series, one may find multiple conceptions of the same phenomenon because the dreamer conceives of it in diverse ways at different times. A father may be represented as a teacher, a policeman, a king, and an army officer in order to depict the multiple conceptions of a wise, guiding father, a punitive father, an exalted, remote father and a disciplining father.

To recapitulate, regard for representability explains why symbols are found in dreams. Dream symbols are visible representations of conceptions. In order for an object, activity, or scene to serve as a symbol, it is necessary that the dreamer's conception of that object, activity, or scene be identical with his conception of the referent object.

It is now time to say how we would limit the use of the term, *dream symbol*. Since dream images *are* images and not perceptions of reality, it could be argued that all images are symbols. One might even go further and assert that everything mental, whether perceptions, memories, or images, is really symbolic since the mental is not the real world but only a representation of the real world. We prefer, however, to restrict the definition of a dream symbol to an image that does not embody the referent object directly. If one dreams of his mother, the image of the mother in the dream does not qualify as a dream symbol. If one dreams of a cow and the image of the cow stands for the mother,

[5] My great intellectual debt to Mrs. Langer will be apparent to those who have read her book, *Philosophy in a New Key* (7).

[6] Although no two symbols probably express exactly the same idea, subtle nuances may be ignored for the sake of reducing the many particulars to a relatively few general classes. For example, we found that a large number of the 200 slang expressions for penis could be categorized under the following headings: (1) projecting or protruding objects, (2) insertive objects, (3) extruding objects, (4) suspended objects, (5) burrowing objects or animals, (6) oblong objects, (7) tools, (8) weapons, and (9) body extremities.

then the cow is said to be a dream symbol. According to this view, symbolizing in dreams consists of transforming one object (the referent object) into another object (the symbol), and this transformation is made in order to convey the dreamer's conception of the referent object. *Cow* is substituted for *mother* because the dreamer's conception of his mother is that of a cow-like person, i.e., one who is nurturant. Similarly *gun* symbolizes the dreamer's conception of the phallus as a dangerous, powerful weapon. Slang and metaphor may be explained in like manner; they are used to convey one's conceptions of referent objects. If one speaks of sexual intercourse as *grinding one's tool,* it is clear that the speaker conceives of coitus as a mechanical operation performed by a mechanical tool, the penis. Quite different but no less revealing conceptions of intercourse are conveyed by the slang expressions *stab in the thigh, playing at horses and mares,* and *doing the naughty.*

Symbols raise hob with dream interpretation since one must not only translate symbols into referent objects, e.g., *cow* into *mother, gun* into *penis, playing the piano* into *masturbating,* but one must also discover the dreamer's conception of the symbol. If one dreamed only of referent objects it would be relatively simple to discover the dreamer's conceptions of these objects by observing the context in which they appear. That is, if one dreamed of his mother performing nurturant acts it would be apparent that he conceived of his mother as a nurturant person. If she appears as a cow it is necessary to decipher cow into mother and then decide upon the dreamer's conception of cows in order to determine his conception of mother.

There are several lines of evidence that tell us when it is necessary to decipher a dream and how the deciphering should proceed. This evidence is of two kinds, internal and external. Internal evidence is that which is found in the dream itself or which is furnished by other dreams of the same dreamer. External evidence is secured from information external to the dream.

The following dream reported by a young woman illustrates the way in which a symbol is detected from internal evidence.

I was riding a horse with a saddle and everything was fine. All of a sudden the saddle and reins fell off except for one rein. The horse was a large, powerful horse. The horse told me that he was going to try and throw me off. I told him that I would stay on no matter what happened. He kicked and ran between trees as fast as he could. I stayed on him and then woke up.

The presence of a symbol is suggested by the "talking horse." One may converse with a horse, but save in fairy tales the horses do not talk back; only other humans do that. Accordingly, we feel that it is justified to translate *horse* into *human*. Since the horse is referred to by the masculine pronoun, it is assumed to be male. The description of the horse as large and powerful suggests that the male is an adult. The identity of the man, whether father, brother, boy friend, or someone else cannot be determined from the dream. It is possible, however, to interpret the dream as one that reveals the girl's conception of her relationship with an adult male.

A second kind of internal evidence is that which is obtained from other dreams of a series. For example, if other dreams of the girl who had the "talking horse" dream disclosed that she was having a conflict over her relationship with her father, that she felt he was trying to get rid of her, this knowledge would support the equation, horse = father. Then the looks and actions of the horse would divulge the dreamer's conception of her father.

This second line of internal evidence may be illustrated by the dream of a young married woman. She dreamed that it was her first wedding anniversary and that they had planned to reenact the ceremony. She could not find her wedding gown and searched for it frantically.

Finally when I found the gown it was dirty and torn. With tears of disappointment in my eyes I snatched up the gown and hurried to the church. Upon my arrival my husband inquired why I had brought the gown with me. I was confused and bewildered and felt strange and alone.

A literal interpretation of this dream might be that the dreamer is unhappy because her dress is dirty and torn and because her husband asks her why she has brought it to the church. Suppose we assume, however, that the state of the wedding dress symbolizes the dreamer's conception of her marriage, and muster what evidence we can to support this assumption. It might be argued that her emotional reactions are out of proportion to the stimuli of a dirty wedding dress and a husband's question, that the intense feelings which these conditions produce are appropriate to something more vital, such as an unhappy marriage. If the reader remains unconvinced by the evidence from a single dream, other dreams of this young woman can be summoned to give their testimony. Here are themes of some of them.

(1). She dreams about a recently married girl who is getting a divorce.

(2). She dreams that she is riding on a streetcar with her husband through a poor section of the city.

(3). She dreams that she is waiting for her husband but he does not appear. She learns that he has tuberculosis.

(4). She dreams that the diamond in her engagement ring is missing.

(5). She dreams that her girl friend who is getting married receives a lot of useless bric-a-brac for wedding presents.

(6). She dreams that she is shopping and has to wait a long time to be served. She worries about getting home to her husband on time. She loses her way, falls on the sidewalk, and is delayed by a train.

These dreams indicate that the dreamer conceives of her marriage as an unhappy one and corroborate the hypothesis that the torn and dirty wedding dress is a concrete embodiment of this idea.

The analysis of a dream series provides, in our opinion, the best evidence for the validity of symbol translation. Since many dream series contain unsymbolized versions of the dreamer's conceptions, one may use these bareface dreams as a check on one's interpretation of dreams freighted with symbolism.[7]

External evidence as to the meaning of symbols may be secured from several sources. The traditional method is to ask a person to "free associate" to the various dream items. The free association method of deciphering dream symbols is a valuable one, but as Walter Reis has shown (9) the dream series method yields almost as clear and as complete a picture of the dreamer's personality as do dreams plus free associations. A practical drawback to free association is that it is time consuming. Although this may not be a limitation when dreams are being interpreted during therapy, it is when one is doing research on dreams. For the latter purpose, the dream series method is more feasible.

The identification and meaning of dream symbols may be determined by the "acting out" that occurs during nocturnal emission dreams. The writer has collected a number of such dreams and the outcome of an emission often proves unequivocally the meaning of the symbols occurring in the dream. The following dream reported by a young man demonstrates the equivalence of "opening a door" with "sexual intercourse."

My sister's girl friend came in the front door and smiled at me. She continued on through the living room and I arose from my chair and followed her. She walked through a hallway and into the bathroom of our home and closed the door. As I opened the door I had an emission.

Another nocturnal emission dream in the writer's collection validates the sexual significance of a number of dream symbols.

I and four or five companions of the same age got out of our car at some place that was like Mentor Park. It was winter and the place was abandoned. Ice was all over the ground. We walked across an open area and as we passed through some passageways we found ourselves threading our way down a sunny mountain trail looking for gold. We noticed small animals resembling pigs running around. As we got into the jungle proper which was very light and sunny we saw all sorts of wild life, lions, giraffes, pythons standing out in my mind. For safety we decided to climb trees. I first climbed a small tree but found it was not safe enough so I came down and began to climb a larger tent pole which I had not noticed before. As I did so, I had a nocturnal emission.

The outcome of a sexual ejaculation suggests that the climatic change from cold to warm, the change in setting from an icy, abandoned park to a light, sunny jungle, the searching for gold, the passageways, the entrance into the jungle, the animals, and the trees and tent pole are objective representations of the dreamer's conception of sexuality. Lacking the outcome of an emission, one might have inferred that this dream is replete with sexual symbols; with the outcome the meaning of the symbols in the dream is more firmly established.

Finally, external evidence for the meaning of dream symbols is found in such diverse material as slang, figures of speech, myths, fairy tales, the visual arts, and word origins. Since these sources have been exploited fully by psychoanalytic investigators, they will not be discussed in this paper. The writer has found them, particularly slang and etymology, a great help in recognizing and deciphering dream symbols. Although evidence secured from such sources is suggestive rather than definitive, a suggestion often puts one on the track of an inference that can be verified by other evidence.

Now let us see how the dream symbol theory as it has been formulated on the basis of *regard for representability* meets the criticisms that we made of Freud's symbol-as-disguise theory. In the first place, we criticised the latter theory because it does not account for unsymbolized dreams appearing in the midst of symbolized ones. Our theory states that symbols do not serve as masks; consequently, the presence of symbols and referent objects in the same dream series is not paradoxical. In fact, it is to be expected if one holds a cognitive theory of dreams. Since dreams are representations of conceptions, a dreamer may convey his ideas either by having a referent object behave in a certain manner or by symbolizing the referent object, in which case the symbol chosen conveys the dreamer's conception. In either case, the dream is a series of images that embody the ideas of the dreamer. In waking life, symbols and referent objects are used interchangeably to communicate ideas; it has never been suggested that the object of using symbols in waking life is to hide one's thoughts. On the contrary, symbols are often thought to be more expressive than referent objects.[8]

Since dream symbols are ways of expressing conceptions, it is not surprising that some people can decipher their own dreams. On the other hand, we would not expect all people to have this ability since many people are not aware of their conceptions. Probably a great deal of thinking, which we define as the forming of conceptions, is unconscious.

The present theory integrates dream symbols with other symbolic forms of expression, such as slang and figures of speech, and provides thereby the basis for a general theory of symbolism. The task of formulating a general theory of symbolism has already been done by Susanne Langer (7), and our special theory of dream symbolism is congruent with this larger formulation.

With respect to multiple symbols for the same referent, it is asserted here that the same referent object, not the same referent, may be symbolized in various ways. The referent is always a conception of a referent object; thus, the versatility with which a referent object may be symbolized is restricted only by the number of ideas that can be developed regarding a given object.

Finally our theory does not rest on the assumption that during sleep one performs complex mental operations such as is assumed when one sees the dream as an elaborate subterfuge. We believe that dreaming is a simple form of thinking in which one uses the language of pictures instead of a more abstract mode of expression. We agree with Freud that dreaming is a regressive and archaic mental process.

What takes place in a hallucinatory dream we can describe in no other way than by saying that the excitation follows a retrogressive course. It communicates itself not to the motor end of the apparatus, but to the sen-

---

[8] Dr. Dwight W. Miles, who read this paper in manuscript, has raised the question as to why symbols are used on some occasions and why referent objects are used on other occasions. To this important question, I would give the following answer, realizing as I do so that it leaves much to be desired. One uses symbols for reasons of economy; they are a form of shorthand, by which complex ideas can be rendered simply. A figure of speech in a poem may be freighted with meaning; indeed we find that the interpretation of a poetic phrase often requires a lengthy discourse. Much meaning can be compressed within a symbol. For example, a dreamer may represent his mother as performing nurturant acts or he may sum up his conception by saying in effect "My mother is a cow." In order to convey the full significance of the latter statement by having the mother act out the dreamer's conception might require a very lengthy dream. Why should he choose a more difficult task when a simple substitution of cow for mother does just as well? For less complex ideas, it may be just as easy to use the referent object directly. To sum up, we would say that referent objects appear in dreams when the conceptions of these objects are relatively uncomplicated and may be readily conveyed by the behavior or appearance of the referent objects, and that symbols appear in dreams when the dreamer's conceptions are complex, and are not easily portrayed by actions and appearances of referent objects.

sory end, and finally reaches the system of perception. If we call the direction which the psychic process follows from the unconscious into the waking state *progressive,* we may then speak of the dream as having a *regressive* character (1, p. 492).

. . . *primitive* modes of operations that are suppressed during the day play a part in the formation of dreams (1, p. 527).

. . . dreaming is on the whole an act of regression to the earliest relationships of the dreamer, a resuscitation of his childhood, of the impulses which were then dominant and the modes of expression which were then available (1, p. 497).

Evidence obtained from studies of children, primitive people, psychotics, and brain injury cases suggests that their modes of thought bear some resemblance to the characteristics of dreaming.

Having introduced this paper with a discussion of dream books, let us bring it to a conclusion on the same theme. Is it possible to develop a dream book on the basis of the ideas presented in this paper? This is tantamount to asking whether there are any universal symbol-conception connections. In order to establish universality it would necessitate collecting a representative sample of dreams from the world's population. Obviously, such an undertaking would present difficulties of such magnitude that it is hardly worth considering. About the most that could be done would be to investigate whether there are *common* symbol-conception associations in a given culture or subculture. Since no such studies have been done, we can only speculate about what might be found. Having read thousands of dreams, it would not surprise the writer if some fairly common symbols for conceptions of referent objects exist. We have been struck by the prevalence of guns and other weapons in dreams, and how often they seem to stand for the conception of the penis as a dangerous weapon. Similarly, pocketbook or purse are fairly common dream objects and appear to symbolize a conception of the female genitals as a place where valuables are stored. It seems to me, after studying a large number of dreams of normal people, that many of the symbol-referent linkages discovered by psychoanalysis are valid. However, I would warn against any mechanical decoding of dreams using a psychoanalytic dream book for two reasons: first, because more proof is needed of the fixed connection between symbol and referent, and second, because it is the conception in the mind of the dreamer and not the referent object that needs to be discovered.

I suspect that many condensed symbols exist in dreams, symbols that express a variety of conceptions like the example of moon mentioned earlier in this paper. It may very well be that there are types of condensed symbols which correspond to the types of ambiguities discussed by Kaplan and Kris in a penetrating article on esthetic ambiguity (6). They distinguish four main types of ambiguities: (*a*) *disjunctive*, when the separate meanings are alternatives, excluding and inhibiting one another, (*b*) *additive*, when the separate meanings are not fully exclusive but are to some extent included in each other, (*c*) *conjunctive*, when the meanings are linked, and (*d*) *integrative*, when the meanings form a unified, coherent system.

To speak the language of Gestalt, in disjunctive ambiguity there are several distinct and unconnected fields; additive ambiguity consists in a restructuring of a single field to reveal more or fewer details; in conjunctive ambiguity several fields are connected though remaining distinct; with integrative ambiguity, they are fully reconstituted — integrated, in short, into one complex meaning (6, p. 420).

If there are such types of condensed symbols in dreams, then the task of constructing a dependable and useful dream book is made more difficult.

Until more evidence is made available concerning the prevalence of fixed symbol-conception linkages in dreams, it would be well for the dream interpreter to be wary about depending upon short-cuts as dream books provide. We believe that dream interpretation can best be accomplished by working on a series of dreams and by setting as one's goal the development of an internally and externally consistent formulation of the person's conceptions.

Summary

Freud's theory of dream symbols as disguises for reprehensible referents has been examined and found wanting in several respects: (*a*) it does not explain why censurable referents appear in some dreams in their naked form and in other dreams as symbols, (*b*) it does not explain why some people are able to decipher their own dream symbols with facility, (*c*) it does not take into account the self-conscious and intentional use of slang and figures of speech for referent objects which are symbolized in dreams, (*d*) it does not deal adequately with the question why there should be multiple symbols for the same referent object, and (*e*) it assumes that the mind during sleep is capable of performing exceedingly complex operations.

Starting from Freud's other hypothesis regarding dream symbols, that which he called *regard for representability*, the following theory of dream symbols has been formulated: (*a*) the referent of a dream symbol is the dreamer's conception (idea) of a referent object, (*b*) a dream symbol is substituted for a referent object in order to express clearly and economically the conception that the dreamer has in mind,

(c) symbols are employed because conceptions are abstract and must be represented by visible embodiments if they (conceptions) are to appear in dreams, and (d) a symbol is selected because the dreamer's conception of the symbol is identical with his conception of the referent object.

Dream symbols may be decomposed into conceptions by making use of various clues: (a) clues that are present within the context of the dream itself, (b) clues from other dreams of the person, (c) free association, (d) acting out as exemplified by dreams that terminate in nocturnal emissions, and (e) evidence from slang, figures of speech, myths, fairy tales, etymology, and the visual arts.

The theory presented in this paper has been called a *cognitive* theory of dream symbols because it assumes that the process of symbolizing is a function of the cognitive system of the ego.

REFERENCES

1. Freud, S. *The Basic Writings of Sigmund Freud.* New York: Modern Library, 1938.
2. ———. *A General Introduction to Psychoanalysis.* Garden City: Garden City Publishing, 1948.
3. Gutheil, E. A. *The Language of the Dream.* New York: Macmillan, 1939.
4. Hall, C. S. Diagnosing personality by the analysis of dreams. *J. Abn. & Soc. Psychol.,* 1947, 42: 68–79.
5. ———. A cognitive theory of dreams. *J. Gen, Psychol.,* (in press).
6. Kaplan, A., & Kris, E. Esthetic ambiguity. *Phil. & phenomenol. Res.,* 1948, 8: 415–435.
7. Langer, S. K. *Philosophy in a New Key.* New York: Penguin Books, 1948.
8. Partridge, E. *A Dictionary of Slang and Unconventional English.* (Third edition.) London: Routledge & Kegan Paul, 1949.
9. Reis, W. A comparison of personality variables derived from dream series with and without free associations. (Unpublished Ph.D. thesis on file at Western Reserve University Library, 1951.)
10. Schorer, M. Fiction and the "matrix of analogy." *Kenyon Rev.,* 1949, 11: 539–560.
11. Spurgeon, C. *Shakespeare's Imagery and What It Tells Us.* New York: Macmillan, 1935.
12. Weiss, H. B. Oneirocritica Americana. *Bull., N. Y. Publ. Libr.,* 1944, 48: 519–541.

19

USE OF CONDITIONED AUTONOMIC RESPONSES IN THE STUDY OF ANXIETY

JOHN I. LACEY, Ph.D., ROBERT L. SMITH, B.A., AND
ARNOLD GREEN, B.A.

Fels Institute for the Study of Human Development, Yellow Springs, Ohio

Experimental studies of "complex guiding processes . . . formed, retained, and used without the person's being aware of the process at any step," to quote Leeper, are relatively few, and are limited mainly to studies of hypnosis or of concept formation. Simple Pavlovian conditioning, however, with its impressive accumulation of quantitative findings and principles upon which special investigations may be based, may prove to be a more rigorous and efficient tool for the experimental demonstration and study of such unconscious processes. It has been known for many years that the conditioning process in human subjects is responsive to the subjects' cognitions of and attitudes towards the experimental situation. (7) Rather than viewing these facts as obstacles to the study of "pure" laws of conditioning, we are exploring the utility of the conditioning experiment as a tool for (*a*) objectively demonstrating unconscious emotional processes; (*b*) studying the difference it makes whether a cognitive and emotional process is conscious or not; and (*c*) developing experimentally derived principles and generalizations about unconscious affect.

We have undertaken the study of unconscious anxiety using a conditioning procedure which is an adaptation of a method first described by Diven. Our procedure is described in full in an earlier report. (9)

PROCEDURE

To the subject, who is a male freshman at Antioch College, it appears that he is participating in a study of the physiological cost of mental-motor coordination. He is seated comfortably in an armchair with his eyes closed. Over a loudspeaker he hears a word, perhaps the word "copper." This is the signal to him to begin a combined mental-motor performance: he must produce aloud as many single-word associations to the word "copper" as he can and at the same time he must tap

From *Psychosomatic Medicine*, May–June 1955. © 1955 by American Psychosomatic Society, Inc.

a telegraph key at as even a rate as possible. He continues this combined performance until he hears the word "stop" over the loudspeaker. He then "relaxes" and waits for the next word, again with eyes closed.

From time to time he receives an electric shock on his left upper arm, which produces a violent muscular spasm. The shock burns and stabs, but he is more disturbed by the muscular cramp and by his lack of control of an important part of his body. He has accepted the experimenter's explanation that the purpose of the shock is to stimulate the muscles he uses in tapping. He wonders how many shocks he is going to get, and he is aware that he is rather tense and anxious about them. He tries to ignore this concern, the better to get on with the difficult job of producing an even tapping performance and a long list of associations.

He soon becomes aware that shock is never administered until he hears the word "stop," but that shock does not conclude each association-tapping episode. He wonders if he gets shocked when his tapping performance has been erratic, or when he produces too few associations. But the pressure of events is too much for him and he has no time to think clearly about these and other possibilities; he must tap and associate, associate and tap.

He can discover no rationale to the shocks. He is aware that "there are an awful lot of farm words," and that "some words are repeated a lot." Why, oh why, did he let himself in for this? It is on the whole a rather unpleasant experience.

The experimenter, of course, perceives the situation differently. The subject is chain-associating for 15 seconds each to a phonographically recorded list of 40 stimulus words, at intervals of 45 seconds. Four words are repeated six times each. Two of the words, "cow" and "paper," are critical words. The members of one group of subjects — the cow-shock subjects — will be shocked each of the six times they complete chain-associating to the word "cow"; the members of a second group of subjects — the paper-shock subjects — will be shocked each of six times they complete chain-associating to the word "paper."

The shock is of constant current (13 ma.) and constant wave shape and frequency, and is delivered to a motor point of the upper arm, in the region of the musculospiral nerve, so as to produce violent flexion at wrist and elbow, with rigid extension and adduction of the fingers. For the entire hour of the experiment, three physiologic variables are being simultaneously and continually recorded. These variables are plantar skin resistance, digital blood flow, and heart rate.

In the word list there are also 8 words with obvious rural meaning (plow, corn, chicken, haystack, grain, sheep, tractor, and farmer), and 8 words with no specifically rural connotations (clock, book, soft, gray, copper, blue, smooth, and yellow). These rural and nonrural words, and the words "cow" and "paper" appear in temporally counter-balanced positions throughout the word list.

After the conditioning session, the subject will be carefully interviewed. An extinction session will follow immediately, in which, unknown to the subject in advance, no shocks will be administered as the subject responds to the same list of 40 words.

RESULTS

1. Unconscious Conditioning and Generalization

As conditioned word and shock were repeatedly paired, evidence appeared of discrimination between the words "cow" and "paper." Cow-shock subjects came to exhibit greater autonomic changes upon hearing and responding to the word "cow" than they did to the word "paper." Paper-shock subjects did the reverse. The degree of autonomic discrimination increased with increased numbers of reinforcements (the electric shock following association to "cow" or "paper").

This differential reaction appeared *in anticipation* of the disturbing shock, i.e. in the 15-second interval between the presentation of the word and the shock. These physiologic changes that follow a signal of future painful stimulation constitute an operational description of an elementary state of anxiety. This anxiety is unconscious in the sense that the subject never "knew" when the shock was coming. Despite intensive questioning and prodding in the interview following the conditioning session, they could not verbalize the association between word-signal and shock. This unawareness was found in 22 of 31 subjects.

This unconscious anxiety was not limited to the conditioned words themselves. It spread to other symbols. Both cow-shock and paper-shock subjects developed autonomic discrimination between rural and nonrural words. Cow-shock subjects came to react more to rural words than to nonrural words, whereas paper-shock subjects developed the reverse reaction. This generalized response was also a function of the number of reinforcements and, indeed, was stronger and more reliable than the primary anxiety response.

These phenomena were represented and analyzed in detail in our first report. (9) Let us turn now to the results of further analyses.

2. Conscious and Unconscious Conditioning Compared

First, what are the differences between conscious and unconscious anxiety? To answer this question, we compare the responses of our unaware group with those secured from a group of 20 "informed aware" subjects. These latter subjects were treated exactly as the unaware subjects, with the single exception that at the beginning of the experiment they were specifically told after which word they were to be shocked. Ten members of this group were shocked after associating to the word "cow," ten after the word "paper." Figure 1 shows the results for heart rate response, which is the only physiologic variable we have exhaustively analyzed to date.

On the X-axis are plotted trials in moving blocks of three. This technique was adopted to smooth out temporal irregularities. The first

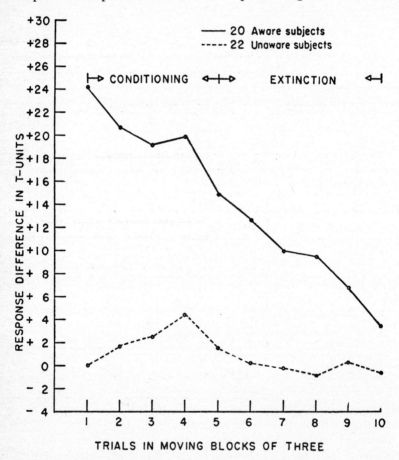

Fig. 1. Comparison of the acquisition and loss of conscious and unconscious anxiety, in moving blocks of three trials; i.e., the first block of trials includes the first, second, and third trials; the second block includes the second, third, and fourth trials, and so on. A positive response difference indicates greater heart rate reaction to the conditioned word than to the control word (see text).

block of trials compares the average of the first three reactions to the word "cow" with the average of the first three reactions to the word "paper"; the second block compares the second, third, and fourth set of responses; the third block compares the third, fourth, and fifth reactions; and so on.

On the Y-axis are plotted the *response-differences, i.e.*, the average response to "cow" minus the average response to "paper" for cow-shock subjects, and the reverse for paper-shock subjects. A positive response-difference, then, signifies greater response to the conditioned word-stimulus than to the control word-stimulus.

These response-differences are expressed in an abstract system of measurement rather than in beats per minute. The abstract unit of measurement, the intrasubject autonomic lability score, simultaneously compensates for individual differences in over-all cardiac reactivity, and for varying "resting" levels of heart rate, and is fully described in our earlier report.

The solid line shows the results for the 20 aware subjects; the broken line for 22 unaware subjects. Of the latter, 10 are cow-shock subjects and 12 are paper-shock subjects.

A dramatic quantitative and qualitative difference is seen in this figure. Informed aware subjects instantly show a tremendous over-reaction to the conditioned word-stimulus. For the first block of three trials, their average reaction to the critical word is 24 T-units (2.4 standard deviations) greater than to the control word-stimulus. This overreaction slowly but consistently exhibits adaptation, but persists throughout the period of observation. Having verbally forewarned the subject that one word was a signal of a forthcoming painful and unpleasant experience, a strong emergency response was immediately induced, which did not grow as a function of repeated reinforcements, but instead showed steady and gradual adaptation.[1]

This conscious anxiety response was not eliminated easily; even repeated omission of the reinforcing shock did not destroy the subject's apprehension and anxiety. The curve exhibits no sharp break during the extinction session. The apparent linearity of the curve makes it difficult to say whether the extinction procedure itself was effective, or whether the continued decline is to be attributed only to a continued process of adaptation.

The results for the unconsciously formed anxiety responses are

[1] Cook and Harris have reported similar results for aware conditioning of the galvanic skin response to a light stimulus. The significance of these findings, and the obstacle they present to easy application of modern behavior theory have been ignored. Response strength grows as a function of repeated reinforcements only under certain conditions not yet completely specified. The cognitive variable is obviously an important one.

radically different. Note, in the first place, that the autonomic discrimination is considerably less. The data of Table 1, which summarizes the performance, block by block, of the aware and unaware subjects, show that this quantitative difference is statistically significant throughout the experimental session until the final block of extinction trials. In the second place, a typical conditioning curve is found. The unconscious anxiety response, unlike the conscious one, grew as a function of repeated nonreinforced trials.[2]

TABLE 1. COMPARISON OF THE FORMATION AND EXTINCTION OF CONDITIONED HEART-RATE DISCRIMINATION BETWEEN A CRITICAL AND NONCRITICAL WORD FOR 22 UNAWARE SUBJECTS AND 20 AWARE SUBJECTS

	Means		Medians		Ranges		
Trials	Aware subjects	Unaware subjects	Aware subjects	Unaware subjects	Aware subjects	Unaware subjects	p[a]
1, 2, 3	24.1	0.0	23.0	− 0.5	+ 4.3 to + 50.0	− 15.3 to + 16.3	< .01
2, 3, 4	20.7	1.7	20.0	0.0	0.0 to + 41.3	− 18.7 to + 20.7	< .01
3, 4, 5	19.2	2.5	17.6	2.2	− 1.0 to + 44.0	− 8.3 to + 23.0	< .01
4, 5, 6	19.9	4.4	20.5	3.6	+ 2.0 to + 38.7	− 4.7 to + 25.0	< .01
5, 6, 7	14.9	1.5	17.3	0.8	− 11.3 to + 41.0	− 10.0 to + 13.3	< .01
6, 7, 8	12.7	0.2	14.2	0.2	− 6.3 to + 36.0	− 13.0 to + 15.7	< .01
7, 8, 9	10.0	− 0.2	11.0	1.2	− 6.3 to + 31.3	− 12.0 to + 10.3	< .01
8, 9, 10	9.5	− 0.9	10.7	− 0.6	− 4.0 to + 22.0	− 17.7 to + 15.0	< .01
9, 10, 11	6.8	0.3	6.2	− 0.8	− 6.7 to + 23.3	− 10.0 to + 26.0	.01 < p < .05
10, 11, 12	3.4	− 0.6	2.8	− 0.2	− 15.0 to + 22.3	− 10.6 to + 15.0	.05 < p < .10

Entries are response-differences: heart-rate response in T-score form to the conditioned word minus response to the control word. Conditioning is reflected in Trials 1 through 7, extinction in Trials 8 through 12. Between Trials 6 and 7, the session was interrupted for an interview, which produced a decrement in the conditioned response.
[a] Confidence levels computed by a nonparametric test, the Wilcoxon-White unpaired replicates test, (18) which, for the N's involved, does not give accurate estimates of the .001 level. The first eight p's are considerably below the .01 level.

3. Conscious and Unconscious Generalization Compared

We turn now to a consideration of the effect of awareness-unawareness upon semantic generalization as indicated by heart-rate responses. By the term "semantic generalization" we refer to the phenomenon that the primary conditioned response is not limited to the conditioned word-stimulus itself, but spreads to other word-symbols meaningfully related to the conditioned word. (12, 13)

In Figs. 2A and 2B, the results for 10 informed aware cow-shock subjects are shown by the solid line, and those for 10 unaware cow-shock subjects by the broken line. Results are not presented for paper-shock subjects because no conclusive evidence was secured in

[2] The drop in the curve, before any extinction trial, from Block 4 to Block 5, between which a rest period and the interview occurred, is analyzed in our first report of these experiments. (9)

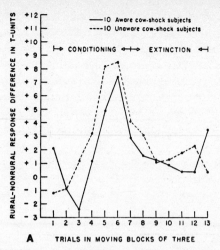

Fig. 2A. Comparison of the acquisition and loss of generalized anxiety in aware and unaware subjects. A positive response-difference means greater heart rate response to rural words, excluding the conditioned word "cow," than to nonrural words. The first block of trials compares reactions to the first rural and nonrural words; the second block compares reactions to the second, third, and fourth rural words with reactions to the second, third, and fourth nonrural words, and so on.

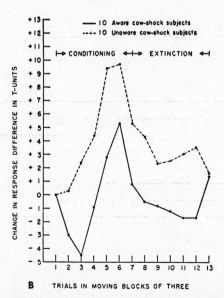

Fig. 2B. Data of Fig. 2A when the initial response-differences of the two groups are equated and set equal to zero.

our first analyses (9) that they exhibited generalization, although it was conclusively shown that their results differed significantly from those for cow-shock subjects.

Figure 2A shows the obtained results in their original form. To make the differences between the two groups more explicit, Figure 2B shows the results when the initial response-differences shown by the two groups in the first block of trials (response to first three rural words minus response to first three nonrural words) are equated and set equal to zero. Unaware subjects, it can be seen, developed progressively greater response to rural words than to nonrural words. The extent of the autonomic discrimination between the two classes of words grew as a function of repeated reinforcements of the word "cow," and then declined under the influence of an extinction procedure. Aware subjects, despite the greater precision of their conscious understanding, nevertheless also show generalization. Their discrimination between which symbols are "dangerous" and which are not, however, is somewhat better than that of the unaware subjects. This is seen in the less regular development of a generalized response exhibited by the aware subjects, and in the fact that quantitatively they show less generalization than the unaware subjects.

Statistical analyses of these differences were performed using the data of Table 2, where we compare (a) the rural-nonrural response-difference to the words "book" and "corn," before the first reinforce-

TABLE 2. RESPONSE-DIFFERENCES IN T-UNITS BETWEEN HEART-RATE REACTIONS TO RURAL AND NONRURAL WORDS FOR 10 AWARE COW-SHOCK SUBJECTS AND 10 UNAWARE COW-SHOCK SUBJECTS

	Aware subjects			Unaware subjects		
Subject	Zero preceding reinforcements	Five preceding reinforcements	Five preceding extinctions	Zero preceding reinforcements	Five preceding reinforcements	Five preceding extinctions
A	+ 1	+ 2	− 15	+ 6	+ 11	+ 12
B	+ 2	+ 23	− 13	− 16	+ 8	+ 29
C	− 1	+ 11	0	0	+ 15	+ 13
D	+ 13	+ 20	− 19	− 18	+ 12	− 10
E	− 2	+ 18	− 13	− 8	+ 8	− 13
F	− 6	− 6	+ 17	0	+ 17	− 3
G	− 8	+ 32	+ 28	− 5	+ 9	− 8
H	+ 11	+ 14	+ 15	− 6	+ 16	− 8
I	+ 25	+ 13	+ 7	0	+ 14	− 6
J	+ 8	+ 14	+ 2	− 40	+ 8	+ 12
Average	+ 4.3	+ 14.1	+ 0.9	− 8.7	+ 11.8	+ 1.8
Median	+ 1.5	+ 14.0	+ 1.0	− 5.5	+ 11.5	− 4.5
Range	− 8 to + 25	− 6 to + 32	− 19 to + 28	− 40 to + 6	+ 8 to + 17	− 10 to + 29

Reaction to a nonrural word is subtracted from reaction to a rural word. The words compared are as follows: no preceding reinforcements, book and corn; five preceding reinforced or non-reinforced trials, smooth and tractor.

ment of "cow" occurred; (b) the rural-nonrural response-difference to the words "smooth" and "tractor," after the subject has been given five shocks following "cow"; and (c) the response-difference to the words "smooth" and "tractor" in the second session, after the subject has had five non-reinforced trials on the word "cow." These words are selected for the sake of uniformity with the mode of analysis used in our first report (9) and because in that report we show that the change in autonomic discrimination for these words is indeed a function of the experimental procedure, and not of the words themselves.

It can be seen by comparing the second and third columns in Table 2 that 8 of the 10 aware subjects showed larger response-differences in favor of rural words after five preceding reinforcements than they did before "cow" and shock were paired. Ten out of 10 unaware subjects developed this generalized response. By a nonparametric test, the Wilcoxon paired replicates test, (19) the trend is significant at better than the 5 per cent level of confidence for aware subjects, and at better than the 1 per cent level for unaware subjects. The increase is, on the average, larger for the unaware subjects. This difference between aware and unaware subjects is significant at the 5 per cent level, by Wilcoxon's unpaired replicates test. (19)

It might appear from Table 2 that, although unaware subjects show greater *change* in the rural-nonrural response-difference from zero to five preceding reinforcements, they show less actual discrimination between rural and nonrural words. For zero preceding reinforcements, the average response-difference is $+4.3$ for aware subjects and -8.7 for unaware subjects. This difference is significant at between the 5 per cent and 2 per cent levels of confidence, by the Wilcoxon test. After five preceding reinforcements, the aware subjects are still showing a greater average response-difference than the unaware subjects, the figures being $+14.1$ and $+11.8$ respectively. This small difference, however, is not statistically significant. As Figure 2A shows, moreover, when we use the more reliable procedure of comparing responses to three rural words with responses to three nonrural words, the amount of generalization becomes and remains quantitatively greater for unaware subjects after the second block of trials. Unfortunately, these differences, too, are not statistically significant, and this particular quantitative issue is left for future experimentation to answer. The data taken as a whole suggest that the verbal forewarning given the aware subjects induced some semantic generalization prior to reinforcement. Repeated reinforcements, however, did not cause the generalized response to increase as regularly and dramatically as it did in unaware subjects, and unaware subjects soon came to show greater generalization than aware subjects.

In extinction, too, the aware and unaware groups differ. After five preceding extinction trials, eight out of ten aware subjects show either a loss of relative overreaction to a rural word or develop overreaction to a nonrural word, as compared with the results after five preceding reinforcements. The trend is significant at the 5 per cent level of confidence. Of the unaware subjects, seven show a loss of the generalized response, but the extinction trend is not significant.

4. Effect of Chronic Anxiety Level

Our freshmen subjects had been administered [3] a battery of psychological tests upon entrance to Antioch. The Taylor Manifest Anxiety Scale, (17) which several experiments have shown to be related to ease of conditioning and extinction (1, 6, 14–16) was a part of this battery. We scored only 35 "nonsomatic" items, omitting those items of this questionnaire inventory that deal with somatic complaints of headache, gastrointestinal upsets, ease of blushing, and the like. Those scoring in the upper and lower thirds of the entering freshman class in the frequency of complaints such as sleep disturbance, frightening dreams, feelings of worry, tension, unhappiness, restlessness, irrational fears, and inability to concentrate were classified as high anxiety and low anxiety respectively. The range of scores for the high anxiety group was from 13 to 29; for the low anxiety group from 0 to 7. Half of each of the experimental groups were high anxiety, and half low anxiety.

We wanted to determine the effect of such psychometrically identified anxiety levels upon the acquisition and spread of new anxiety responses, and to determine whether the relationship held for both consciously and unconsciously conditioned anxiety.

The results are shown in Fig. 3. While none of the differences obtained meets the criteria of statistical significance, they are worth presenting because the results show a consistent pattern, and have biological and psychological importance. We are, moreover, continuing the investigation of the problem in a new series of experiments.

The first two sets of the bar graphs in the figure show that for both the first and last presentations of the critical word-signals, the low anxiety aware subjects exhibit a larger response-difference than the high anxiety aware subjects. As can be seen in the third set of bar graphs the unaware subjects show the same effect, at the characteristically diminished level of autonomic discrimination and activity. For these unaware subjects, too, the effect is made clear only by

[3] We are indebted to Mrs. Ruth Churchill, Antioch College Examiner, for the administration and scoring of these tests.

averaging the last three conditioning trials, because of the previously mentioned temporal irregularities in conditioning.

The final two sets of bar graphs show an apparent reversal. Both for aware and unaware subjects, the low anxiety subjects show less generalization.

Low anxiety subjects, then, seem to condition better but generalize less.

The two sets of findings point to a common interpretation: low anxiety subjects make more accurate discriminations than high anxiety subjects. In the first place, low anxiety subjects, during conditioning, respond accurately; the dangerous signal (the conditioned word-stimulus) brings forth an appropriately larger emergency response than the nondangerous signal (the control word). In the second place, the low anxiety subjects limit their emergency responses to the appropriate stimulus more than high anxiety subjects, and therefore do not show as much generalization. These differences in accuracy and precision, in appropriateness of response, hold for both conscious and unconscious conditioned anticipation of shock.

Conclusions and Discussion

First of all, it is clear that situational anxiety can be easily induced by the conditioning process at an unconscious level. We have been impressed with the rapidity with which such anxiety responses are formed. Two or three reinforcements suffice to produce observable changes. Anxiety responses in rats, as others have noted (2, 5, 8, 11), require many fewer pairings of conditioned and unconditioned stimuli than other responses. The human organism, too, seems extremely sensitive to danger even in the slight degree employed in our experiments. We are anxiety-prone.

Secondly, this situational anxiety is not limited to the truly dangerous symbol. It spreads to meaningfully related symbols at both the conscious and unconscious levels. Unlike other studies of generalization, we find that the generalized response was of greater magnitude than the primary response.

Third, the role of conscious understanding in enabling more accurate, appropriate, and reality-bound responses is given quantitative expression in both conditioning and generalization curves.

Fourth, it appears that the chronic anxiety level of the individual may be a factor in the ease with which he acquires and generalizes new anxiety responses.

These results, and the current developments of the basic technique in our laboratory, lead us to the belief that the conditioning procedure,

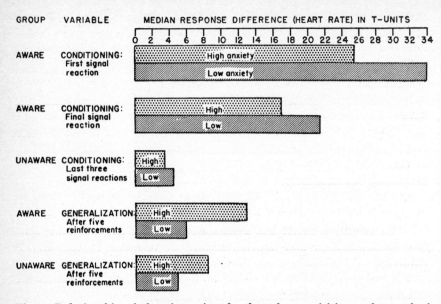

Fig. 3. Relationship of chronic anxiety level to the acquisition and spread of new anxiety responses. High and low anxiety subjects were identified by the Taylor Manifest Anxiety Scale (see text).

with its simplicity, objectivity, and possibility for experimental manipulation and quantification, is a valuable experimental tool for the analysis of elementary forms of unconscious and conscious anxiety. When used with due regard for the realities of the enormously more complex and more subtle anxiety processes with which we deal clinically, it may provide greatly increased precision of our clinical tools and concepts.

SUMMARY

In the experiments reported in this paper, the subject chain-associates for 15 seconds to each of a list of 40 stimulus words. After each of six presentations of one of these words, electric shock is administered. Although the subject is unaware of the relationship between word-signal and shock, as determined by intensive interview subsequent to the conditioning session, the subject's autonomic responses in the 15 second interval between hearing the stimulus word and receiving the shock reveal the existence of unconscious anticipation of shock. This unconscious anxiety is not limited to the conditioned word-stimulus itself but spreads to other words meaningfully related to the conditioned word. Subjects shocked after the word "cow" develop relative overreaction to other words with rural connotations. The development of such responses is very rapid, revealing the anxiety-proneness of humans.

The conditioning curves of aware and unaware subjects differ sharply. Aware subjects immediately develop a strong emergency response that does not grow as a function of the number of reinforcements, but instead shows gradual adaptation. Unaware subjects show typical conditioning curves at a much lower level of autonomic activity and discrimination.

The spread of anxiety as seen in curves of generalization seems greater at the unconscious than at the conscious level.

The chronic anxiety level of the subject may be related to the ease of acquisition and spread of new anxiety responses. Low anxiety subjects condition better but generalize less. This implies more accurate discrimination and appropriateness of response in low anxiety subjects.

The possibilities of using conditioning in the study of unconscious emotional processes are thus seen to be considerable.

REFERENCES

1. Bitterman, M. E., and Holtzman, W. H. Conditioning and extinction of the galvanic skin response as a function of anxiety. *J. Abnorm. & Social Psychol.*, 47: 615, 1952.

2. Brown, J. S., Kalish, H. I., and Farber, I. E. Conditioned fear as revealed by magnitude of startle response to an auditory stimulus. *J. Exper. Psychol.*, 41: 317, 1951.

3. Cook, S. W., and Harris, R. E. The verbal conditioning of the galvanic skin reflex. *J. Exper. Psychol.*, 21: 202, 1937.

4. Diven, K. Certain determinants in the conditioning of anxiety reactions. *J. Psychol.*, 3: 291, 1937.

5. Gwinn, G. T. Resistance to extinction of learned fear-drives. *J. Exper. Psychol.*, 42: 6, 1951.

6. Hilgard, E. R., Jones, L. V., and Kaplan, S. J. Conditioned discrimination as related to anxiety. *J. Exper. Psychol.*, 42: 94, 1951.

7. Hilgard, E. R., and Marquis, D. G. *Conditioning and Learning*, New York, Appleton-Century-Crofts, 1940.

8. Kalish, H. I. Strength of fear as a function of the number of acquisition and extinction trials. *J. Exper. Psychol.*, 47: 1, 1954.

9. Lacey, J. I., and Smith, R. L. Conditioning and generalization of unconscious anxiety. *Science*, 120: 1045, 1954.

10. Leeper, R. "Cognitive processes." In Stevens, S. S. (ed.): *Handbook of Experimental Psychology*, New York, Wiley, 1951.

11. Miller, N. E. "Learnable drives and rewards." In Stevens, S. S. (ed.): *Handbook of Experimental Psychology*, New York, Wiley, 1951.

12. Osgood, C. E. *Method and Theory in Experimental Psychology*, New York, Oxford, 1953.

13. Razran, G. Stimulus generalization of conditioned responses. *Psychol. Bull.*, 46: 337, 1949.

14. Spence, K. W., and Farber, I. E. Conditioning and extinction as a function of anxiety. *J. Exper. Psychol.*, 45: 116, 1953.

15. Spence, K. W., and Taylor, Janet A. Anxiety and strength of the UCS as determiners of the amount of eyelid conditioning. *J. Exper. Psychol.*, 42: 183, 1951.

16. Taylor, Janet A. The relationship of anxiety to the conditioned eyelid response. *J. Exper. Psychol.*, 41: 81, 1951.

17. Taylor, Janet A. A personality scale of manifest anxiety. *J. Abnorm. & Social Psychol.*, 48: 285, 1953.

18. White, C. The use of ranks in a test of significance for comparing two treatments. *Biometrics*, 8: 33, 1952.

19. Wilcoxon, F. *Some Rapid Approximate Statistical Procedures*, Stamford Conn., American Cyanamid Co., 1949.

20

SEDATION THRESHOLD

A Neurophysiological Tool for Psychosomatic Research

CHARLES SHAGASS, M.D.

Allan Memorial Institute of Psychiatry, McGill University, Quebec

Several recent neurophysiological advances, such as the elucidation of reticular system functions (12, 13) seem highly relevant to the understanding of brain mechanisms involved in psychological disorders. Most of this information has come from the animal laboratory or from patients subjected to surgical operations. Pertinent methods for neurophysiological study of the *intact human subject* are needed to provide closer links between the data of the psychiatric clinic and the neurophysiology laboratory. This paper deals with one such method, the sedation threshold.

The sedation threshold is an objective pharmacological determination, which depends upon the electroencephalographic (EEG) and speech changes produced by intravenous Sodium Amytal. (19) Starting from the common clinical impression that effective sedative dosage is correlated with the degree of tension, the method was originally developed to measure tension or manifest anxiety. After the realization of this initial aim, continued research revealed additional psychological correlates of the sedation threshold. The results indicated that the method has important potentialities as a tool in psychiatric and psychosomatic research.

The purpose of this paper is to present the evidence which supports the statement that the sedation threshold is a valid clinical neurophysiological approach to the investigation of psychopathological problems.

METHOD

Test Procedure

Sodium Amytal is injected intravenously at the rate of 0.5 mg./Kg. body weight every 40 seconds. The EEG is recorded continuously. The injection solution is made up so that 1 cc. contains .05 mg./Kg.;

From *Psychosomatic Medicine*, September–October 1956. © 1956 by American Psychosomatic Society, Inc.

1 cc. is given as rapidly as possible at the beginning of every 40-second interval. Twenty-five seconds after each injection the subject is asked to repeat sibilants, such as 567, 77, etc. The Sodium Amytal generally produces marked increase of the EEG fast frequency activity (15- to 30-cps). This effect is greatest in the frontal areas and is best recorded from bifrontal electrodes. Since the bifrontal recording is particularly subject to contamination by muscle artifact, a record from sagittal frontocentral electrodes is also taken routinely. The latter usually contains less muscle artifact and is measured if the bifrontal tracing is obscured. The left-hand side of Fig. 1 shows the effect of Sodium Amytal on the bifrontal tracing. The amplitude of the 15- to 30-cps activity is measured, and a dosage-response curve is plotted. The right-hand side of Fig. 1 shows a typical curve. Usually the curve is S-shaped and contains a fairly clear inflection point, preceding which the amplitude rises quite sharply, and following which the curve tends to plateau. This inflection point usually coincides with the onset of slurred speech. The sedation threshold is defined as the amount of Sodium Amytal, in mg./Kg., which is required to produce the inflection point in the amplitude curve of frontal 15- to 30-cps activity; the inflection point must occur within 80 seconds of the clinical observation of slurred speech. The slurred speech is thus used as a rough guide to the threshold and the EEG change as a precise guide.

Technical Data

More than 700 tests on about 600 subjects have been carried out to date. All data have not yet been fully analyzed; much of the present material comes from a full analysis of the first 340 technically valid tests on 320 subjects. Somewhat less than 1 in 10 tests is invalid for technical reasons.

The effects of age, sex, and previous intake of sedatives were assessed by determining whether there was any correlation between these factors and the threshold. No significant correlations were found. It was surprising to find that the threshold was unaffected by previous sedative consumption. However, this conclusion must be qualified, since addicts, alcoholics, and patients receiving exceptionally heavy doses of sedatives were not included in these studies.

Body surface was calculated in 60 patients and the threshold worked out in terms of milligrams per square meter. The correlation between thresholds based upon body weight and those based upon body surface was 0.91. This indicates that little would be gained if body surface were to replace body weight as a base for calculating the threshold. As regards repeatability, the correlation between initial and repeat determinations, carried out after time intervals, averaging 30 days and as great as 15 months, was 0.91 in a group of 20 subjects. Ninety per cent of repeat determinations were within 0.5 mg./Kg. of the initial threshold.

Measurement of the EEG has so far been done on samples by a precise hand method. This yields results comparable to those obtained with an automatic frequency analyzer, (19) but is laborious. An electronic device, incorporating the analyzer principle, but much smaller, is now giving promising initial results, and may replace the hand method.

Clinical Criteria

These have included numerical ratings of tension based upon specially directed interviews, the Saslow Screening Test (18) in control subjects, and assessments based upon conventional psychiatric diagnostic interviews and hospital case records. It has been our impression that the most reliable criterion available to us was obtained by combining the diagnostic interviews of at least two psychiatrists with the hospital record of the course and outcome of a hospital stay averaging 5 weeks in duration.

Results

Anxiety

The following results bear upon the correlation between the sedation threshold and degree of manifest anxiety.[1]

1. If the threshold is correlated with the degree of manifest anxiety, it should be significantly higher in a group of psychoneurotics than in a nonpatient control group. The mean threshold of 121 psychoneurotic patients was 4.15 mg./Kg., as compared with the mean of 3.09 mg./Kg. in 45 control subjects. (22) The difference was highly significant statistically.

2. Sixty-five nonpsychotic patients were rated by two psychiatrists on a 5-point scale for degree of "tension," which, as defined, was equivalent to what we now call "manifest anxiety." (19) The correlation between the sedation threshold and the average tension rating was 0.72. This coefficient was almost as high as that for agreement between the two raters, which was 0.78.

3. Clinically, one would expect the different psychoneuroses to differ

[1] It is difficult to select a completely acceptable term for the phenomena here called "manifest anxiety." Originally it was thought that "tension" would be suitable. However, psychotic depressives, who appeared very tense clinically, were later found to have low sedation thresholds. The qualifying term "manifest," is used here to avoid confusion with concepts of "unconscious anxiety."

in degree of manifest anxiety. The greatest amount of anxiety would be expected in anxiety states and the least in conversion hysterics; mixed neuroses should be intermediate. Sedation thresholds of the different neurotic groups were found to conform to clinical expectation. A sample of 121 psychoneurotics was classified according to fairly definite clinical criteria. (22) Mean thresholds in the diagnostic groups were as follows: anxiety state, 5.4; neurotic depression, 4.6; obsessive compulsive; 4.3; anxiety hysteria, 4.0; mixed neurosis, 3.7; conversion hysteria and hysterical personality, 2.9. Most of the intergroup differences were statistically significant, indicating that the threshold differentiated well between these groups.

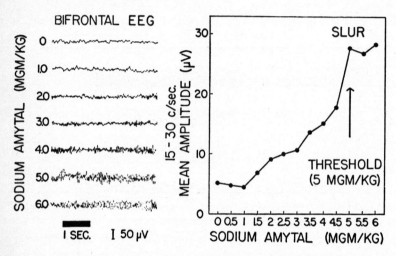

Fig. 1. Illustrates effect of Sodium Amytal on bifrontal EEG. Note progressive increase of the fast-frequency amplitude. Arrow points to inflection point in the amplitude curve which indicates sedation threshold.

4. A nonpatient control group, containing 45 subjects, was interviewed clinically and given the Saslow Screening Inventory prior to sedation threshold determination. (22) Significant correlations were found between the sedation threshold and the number of anxiety symptoms elicited during interview and in the inventory.

These data lead to the conclusion that the sedation threshold is highly correlated with degree of manifest anxiety in psychoneurotic patients and in nonpatient control subjects. Studies of psychotic patients did not give similar results. The only statistically significant relationship between the threshold and anxiety in psychotics was found in a group of chronic ambulatory schizophrenics. (23) A probable explanation for the results in psychotics will be considered in a following section.

Hysterical-Obsessional Personality Traits

In the study of psychoneurotic patients, it became evident that the sedation threshold was correlated not only with degree of manifest anxiety but with related personality manifestations. The thresholds of hysterical patients, either with conversion symptoms or hysterical personalities, or both, were almost invariably in the lower half of the scale, while those of patients with obsessional personalities were almost always high. Patients with both obsessional and hysterical personality characteristics were most often diagnosed as having a mixed neurosis, and their thresholds usually fell into the intermediate range.

Figure 2 shows the proportion of high and low thresholds in four diagnostic groups which were selected because they represent well-

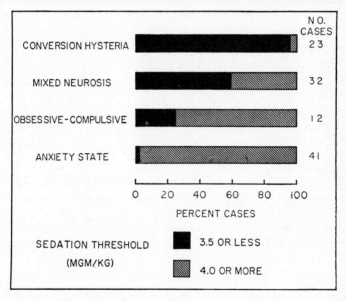

Fig. 2. Relationship between sedation threshold and predominance of hysterical or obsessional characteristics.

defined points on the hysterical-obsessional continuum. All 23 conversion hysterias had major somatosensory conversion symptoms. The 12 obsessive-compulsives all had rituals or constant ruminations, or both. The 41 anxiety states presented severe anxiety and nearly all had obsessional personalities, although they were not true obsessive-compulsives. These data show that the more obsessive the personality, the higher the sedation threshold. However, average thresholds of the true obsessive-compulsives were actually lower than those of the anxiety states. This suggests that in the presence of frank obsessive-compulsive symptoms, there may be less anxiety than when such symptoms do not develop in the obsessional. This would be in accord with the postulated "anxiety-binding" function of compulsions and obsessions.

Impairment of Ego Functioning

There were 11 schizophrenics in the experimental population of the first sedation threshold study. (19) The threshold was not significantly correlated with degree of tension in this group, but it was noted that the recent and acute cases had lower thresholds than equally tense chronic ones. This difference between acute and chronic schizophrenics provided a clue to a factor, other than degree of anxiety, which might influence the sedation threshold. In acute psychoses, ego functions are thought to be more impaired than in nondeteriorated psychoses of long duration, in which reparative processes have taken place. This concept led to the hypothesis that the sedation threshold was negatively correlated with degree of impairment of ego functions. According to this hypothesis, the greater the degree of ego impairment, the lower the threshold.

Since adequate methods of measuring ego impairment are not available, it was not possible to test this hypothesis directly. However, certain predictions, based on the hypothesis, could be checked. Two such predictions were tested in one study. (23) The first was that the thresholds of chronic schizophrenics, who were ambulatory and did not show significant evidence of personality deterioration, should be significantly higher than those of acute schizophrenics or agitated depressions, who were equally tense but whose psychosis was of brief duration. The second prediction concerned the organic psychoses. The cardinal signs of organic psychosis are gross impairments of such ego functions as memory, judgment, and attention. Since ego functions are impaired to the greatest extent in organic psychoses, it was predicted that the thresholds of these patients should be lower than those of all other subjects. The results confirmed both predictions.

The data for organic psychoses, acute and chronic schizophrenias, and agitated depressions, shown in Fig. 3, are those of the original study on ego impairment, supplemented by additional cases. Thresholds of the chronic schizophrenics were significantly higher than those of the acute "functional" psychoses; thresholds of the latter groups were, in turn, significantly higher than those of the organic psychoses.

Figure 3 also contains data for a group of "borderline states." Patients in this group generally presented neurotic symptoms, but were found to have one or two of the following symptoms: ideas of reference, depersonalization, derealization, distortion of the body percept, paranoid trend. These patients probably would fall into the pseudoneurotic schizophrenia classification of Hoch and Polatin. This group was included here to test a third prediction from the ego-impairment hypothesis. Of the various psychotic groups in Fig 3, the borderline schizo-

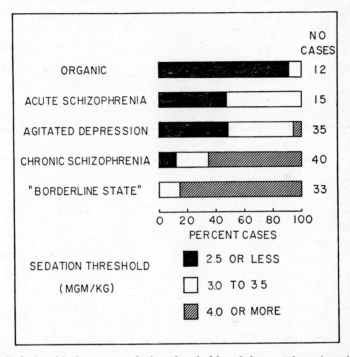

Fig. 3. Relationship between sedation threshold and degree of ego impairment, as represented by different psychotic groups, ranging from greatest impairment in organic psychoses to least in "borderline" psychoses.

phrenic group would be considered to have the least degree of ego impairment; consequently their sedation thresholds should be highest. The data verified this prediction. The mean threshold of the borderline group was 4.9 compared with 4.1 for the chronic schizophrenic group. This difference was significant at the 1 per cent level of confidence.

These data indicate that gross impairment of ego functions lowers the sedation threshold, while manifest anxiety raises it.

Differential Diagnosis of Depression

Differentiation between psychotic and neurotic depressive reactions is often difficult, particularly if a rapid decision is needed. From the factors related to the sedation threshold, it would follow that psychotic depressions should have low thresholds, whereas neurotic depressions, providing they do not occur in severe hysterics, should have high ones. Figure 4 shows the distribution of sedation thresholds above and below

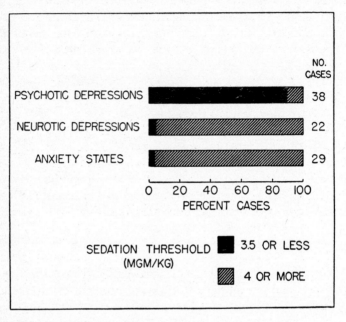

Fig. 4. Differentiation of psychotic depressions from neurotic depressions and anxiety states by the sedation threshold.

the patient median in all the psychotic depressions, neurotic depressions, and anxiety states, among the first 275 patients tested. It is clear that the threshold differentiated between psychotic depressions and neurotic depressions or anxiety states with a very high degree of accuracy. This finding has proved of considerable practical clinical value.

Discussion

The preceding results show that the sedation threshold is meaningfully related to several important psychopathological phenomena. It may therefore be regarded as a valid clinical neurophysiological approach to study of these phenomena. Some practical and theoretical implications of the data will be considered under the following headings: clinical and research applications, neurophysiological aspects, and relation to personality theory.

Clinical Applications

The sedation threshold is now used as a routine clinical test at Allan Memorial Institute. Like any test, it gives information which is meaningful only in a context of clinical differential diagnosis. It is most frequently employed to help distinguish between neurotic and psychotic depression and to estimate degree of anxiety. In connection with the latter application, a low threshold in an apparently severe anxiety state may lead to a fruitful review of the communicative, hysterical aspects of the case. An example has been cited elsewhere. (22) Another cause for an unexpectedly low threshold in an apparent anxiety state may be an oncoming psychotic episode.

An extremely low threshold may point to an organic mental state. The Amytal test for organic brain disease, developed by Weinstein *et al.*, may be combined with the sedation threshold as a further diagnostic measure in such cases. When a high threshold is found in an apparently acute schizophrenic patient, recheck of the history usually reveals that the illness has been of a considerably long duration.

Research Applications

The sedation threshold holds a number of possibilities for application to psychiatric and psychosomatic research problems. A few investigations utilizing it have already been undertaken at this Institute. The test has been used to select subjects at the low and high extremes of the anxiety scale for electromyographic studies (3). Investigations are in progress on the effect of certain drugs, electroconvulsive therapy, and brief psychotherapy on the threshold. Practically no work has been done with the classical psychosomatic syndromes, except for study of a small number of hyperthyroid cases. In these the thresholds were generally high and tended to decrease when thyroid function was normalized.

It seems likely that the sedation threshold could provide objective data relevant to some hypotheses concerning psychosomatic disorders. Suppose the thresholds of adequate samples of patients suffering from different disorders were determined. Would the distributions resemble those of a normal group or a neurotic group? Would the distributions be similar for all disorders, or would they differ from one to the other? If they differed, would the differences agree with prevailing concepts about associated emotional state and personality patterns? For example, certain conditions, such as arterial hypertension (8) and Raynaud's disease (14) have been associated with obsessional personality traits or compared with anxiety attacks. Other conditions, notably certain skin disorders, have been regarded as depressive equivalents or as hysterical symptoms. (1, 17) One would expect high thresholds in the former cases and low thresholds in the latter.

Neurophysiological Aspects

Since Sodium Amytal is a central nervous system depressant, which should quantitatively counteract excitatory processes, the sedation threshold may be regarded as a measure of cerebral excitability. This view is reinforced by evidence obtained by Gastaut and his co-workers in a study of the cortical excitability cycle. They showed that barbiturates diminish the amplitude of cortical responsiveness to photic stimuli, and lengthen the time it takes to recover normal excitability of the cortex.

Anxiety, associated with a high sedation threshold, probably reflects increased cerebral excitability. In psychotic depression, associated with a low threshold, the neural processes seem to be different from those involved in anxiety. Some of the main clinical features of depression suggest that it involves inhibitory processes. (2) This is supported by studies in progress on the effect of electroconvulsive therapy on the sedation threshold. Results so far indicate that this treatment, in relieving depression, also increases the threshold. Additional evidence that anxiety and depression are neurophysiologically different was obtained in two recent studies of the EEG response to intermittent photic stimulation, which showed that these affects were associated with different response characteristics. (20, 21)

Rothballer has recently found that a component of the reticular system responds to epinephrine by producing arousal. He found this adrenergic component to be particularly sensitive to barbiturates and to other depressants. Indeed, it was more sensitive than other parts of the reticular system which, as a whole, is especially sensitive to barbiturates. (6) These facts, in conjunction with present data, suggest that excessive excitatory activity of the adrenergic component of the reticular system may be a key mechanism in the mediation of anxiety.

The capacity to attend to external stimuli, which is essential for adequate ego functioning, depends upon intact reticular system function. (12) Barbiturates in sufficient dosage impair ego functioning. When they are used for daytime sedation one attempts to find a dose which will reduce anxiety without impairing ego functions. The fact that this can frequently be done favors the concept that the reticular system contains a number of functional components. It also suggests that different components are involved in anxiety and in the maintenance of ego functioning.

Relation to Personality Theory

The relationship of the sedation threshold to relative predominance of hysterical or obsessional personality traits suggests the possibility that the threshold may reflect some basic neurophysiological aspect of personality organization. Since significant personality factors must be consistent over long periods of time, such a hypothesis would be supported by evidence that the threshold is a relatively enduring biological characteristic of the individual. This is not yet proved, but is in agreement with available data. These data include the high test-retest reliability, and the fact that relatively quick changes in the threshold have so far been produced only by such major agents as severe toxicity and electroconvulsive therapy; even these changes are apparently temporary. The data relating the threshold to symptomatic variables, like anxiety, can easily be fitted into the personality context, since proneness to certain kinds of symptoms may be regarded as a personality characteristic.

Several personality typologies of the past have been based on a concept similar to the hysterical obsessional continuum. Eysenck (4) provided strong experimental support for the validity of this concept. He factor-analyzed several kinds of objective data on large groups of subjects and derived three dimensions of personality. One of these, the introversion-extraversion dimension, is equivalent to the hysterical-obsessional continuum. The hysteric is the extreme extravert, the obsessional or dysthymic, the extreme introvert. No direct studies have so far been done, which correlate the sedation threshold with measured introversion-extraversion, but there is strong indirect evidence that they may be closely related. This evidence comes from a study by one of Eysenck's students, Hildebrand, who measured introversion-extraversion by means of six psychometric tests and a body index. Subjects were a group of psychoneurotics who were classified in much the same way as those studied here. The introversion-extraversion scores arranged the various neuroses in an order which was almost the same as that in which they were arranged by the sedation threshold.

There is another point in favor of assuming a close relationship between the sedation threshold and Eysenck's introversion-extraversion dimension. Eysenck (5) has recently proposed a theory of anxiety and hysteria, in which he distinguishes between hysterics and dysthymics in terms of differences in reactive inhibition. Reactive inhibition is a term borrowed from Hull, but Eysenck's theory has its origin in Pavlov's attempt to classify the nervous systems of experimentally neurotic dogs according to predominance of excitatory or inhibitory process. According to Eysenck's theory, hysterics should generate reactive inhibition more quickly and strongly than dysthymics, and should dissipate it more slowly. He also postulated that brain injury should increase reactive inhibition and extraversion, and drew attention to the extraverting effects of inhibitory drugs like alcohol and Sodium Amytal. If one follows Eysenck in equating reactive inhibition with the inhibitory effects of Sodium Amytal, one would predict lower sedation thresholds in hysterics and organic psychotics than in dysthymics, a prediction in accord with the results. Thus, not only the order but also the direction of sedation threshold differences agrees with Eysenck's data and theory on introversion-extraversion.

In another approach to personality investigation, that of Sheldon and Stevens, high resistance to alcohol is listed as one of the criteria for the cerebrotonic temperament. This would lead one to expect high sedation thresholds in cerebrotonics. Since cerebrotonics seem very similar to obsessionals or dysthymics, this expectation also agrees with present results. It is unusual and encouraging to find such apparent agreement between results of personality investigations which differ widely in method and theoretical orientation. The various methods appear to be tapping different aspects of some process common to all.

The foregoing discussion implies that the sedation threshold measures neural processes which may be important determinants of personality. These processes could be considered to influence proneness toward development of one or another kind of character trait or neurotic symptom. Although it is easy to think of such processes as constitutional factors, there is no evidence which would allow one to speculate about the relative importance of heredity or environment in their development. However, it should be technically feasible to obtain data on this point, e.g., by determining the sedation thresholds of identical twins.

SUMMARY

1. The sedation threshold is an objective pharmacological determination which represents the amount of intravenous Sodium Amytal required to elicit certain EEG and speech changes. The purpose of this paper was to present the evidence which bears on the validity of this method as a clinical neurophysiological approach to investigation of psychopathological problems.

2. Data were drawn from tests on over 500 psychiatric patients and 45 nonpatient controls. The following general results were obtained: (a) The sedation threshold was positively correlated with degree of manifest anxiety in nonpsychotic subjects. The greater the manifest anxiety in psychoneurotics or control subjects, the higher the threshold. (b) Obsessional personality characteristics tended to be associated with

a high threshold, hysterical characteristics with a low threshold. (c) The sedation threshold was negatively correlated with degree of gross impairment of ego functioning in psychotics. The greater the ego impairment, the lower the threshold. (d) The threshold differentiated between neurotic and psychotic depressions with a high degree of accuracy. Thresholds were low in psychotic depressions and high in neurotic depressions.

3. It was concluded that the sedation threshold was meaningfully related to several important psychopathological phenomena, and that the results supported its validity as an investigative approach. The findings were discussed from the following standpoints: clinical and research applications; some neurophysiological aspects of anxiety, depression, and ego functioning; and relation to personality theory, with special emphasis upon Eysenck's theory.

REFERENCES

1. Alexander, F. *Psychosomatic Medicine*. New York, Norton, 1950, p. 164.
2. Cameron, D. E. Some relationships between excitement, depression and anxiety. *Am. J. Psychiat.*, 102: 385, 1945.
3. Davis, J. F., Malmo, R. B., and Shagass, C. Electromyographic reaction to strong auditory stimulation in psychiatric patients. *Canad. J. Psychol.*, 8: 177, 1954.
4. Eysenck, H. J. *Dimensions of Personality*, London, Routledge, 1947.
5. Eysenck, H. J. A dynamic theory of anxiety and hysteria. *J. Ment. Sci.*, 101: 28, 1955.
6. French, J. D., Verzeano, M., and Magoun, H. W. A neural basis of the anesthetic state. *A.M.A. Arch. Neurol. & Psychiat.*, 69: 519, 1953.
7. Gastaut, H., *et al.* Etude électrographiques du cycle d'excitabilité cortical. *Electroencephalog. & Clin. Neurophysiol.*, 3: 401, 1951.
8. Gressel, G. C., *et al.* Personality factors in arterial hypertension. *J.A.M.A.*, 140: 265, 1949.
9. Hildebrand, H. P. Cited by Eysenck (1955). A factorial study of introversion-extraversion by means of objective tests. Ph.D. thesis. London, 1953.
10. Hoch, P., and Polatin, P. Pseudoneurotic forms of schizophrenia. *Psychiatric Quart.*, 23: 248, 1949.
11. Hull, C. L. *Principles of Behavior*, New York, Appleton, 1943.
12. Jasper, H. Diffuse projection systems: The integrative action of the thalamic reticular system. *Electroencephalog. & Clin. Neurophysiol.*, 1: 405, 1949.
13. Magoun, H. W. Caudal and cephalic influences on the brainstem reticular formation. *Physiol. Rev.*, 30: 459, 1950.
14. Millet, J. A. P., Lief, H., and Mittelmann, B. Raynaud's disease. Psychogenic factors and psychotherapy. *Psychosom. Med.*, 15: 61, 1953.
15. Pavlov, I. P. *Conditioned Reflexes*, London, Oxford, 1927.
16. Rothballer, A. B. The adrenergic component of the reticular activating system. *Proc. Res. Conf. Psychopharmacol.*, Mar. 26, 1955. Abstracted in *Bull. Canad. Psychiatric Assn.*, 3: 12, 1955.

17. Rothenberg, S. Depressions in psychosomatic disorders. *Psychosom. Med.*, 16: 231, 1954.

18. Saslow, G., Counts, R. M., and Dubois, P. H. Evaluation of a new psychiatric screening test. *Psychosom. Med.*, 13: 242, 1951.

19. Shagass, C. The sedation threshold: A method for estimating tension in psychiatric patients. *Electroencephalog. & Clin. Neurophysiol.*, 6: 221, 1954.

20. Shagass, C. Differentiation between anxiety and depression by the photically activated electroencephalogram. *Am. J. Psychiat.*, 112: 41, 1955.

21. Shagass, C. Anxiety, depression, and the photically driven electroencephalogram. *A.M.A. Arch. Neurol. & Psychiat.*, 74: 3, 1955.

22. Shagass, C., and Naiman, J. The sedation threshold as an objective index of manifest anxiety in psychoneurosis. *J. Psychosom. Res.*, 1: 49, 1956.

23. Shagass, C., and Naiman, J. The sedation threshold, manifest anxiety, and some aspects of ego function. *A.M.A. Arch. Neurol. & Psychiat.*, 74: 397, 1955.

24. Sheldon, W. H., and Stevens, S. S. *The Varieties of Temperament*, New York, Harper, 1945.

25. Weinstein, E. A., *et al.* The diagnostic use of amobarbital sodium ("Amytal Sodium") in brain disease. *Am. J. Psychiat.*, 109: 889, 1953.

21

THEORY AND TREATMENT OF STUTTERING AS AN APPROACH-AVOIDANCE CONFLICT

JOSEPH G. SHEEHAN

Department of Psychology, University of California

A. The Problem

Seldom is the rôle of conflict, so important in every problem of adjustment, so clearly portrayed as in the disorder of stuttering. Stuttering behavior is essentially a hesitancy, an interruption in the forward flow of speech, a holding back in a situation which calls for going ahead. In the author's view, this hesitant or avoidant aspect of stuttering reflects the fundamental nature of the disorder:

> Stuttering is a result of approach-avoidance conflict, of opposed urges to speak and to hold back from speaking. The "holding back" may be due either to learned avoidances or to unconscious motives; the approach-avoidance formulation fits both (45).

This is, briefly stated, the theory to be presented in this paper. It seeks to <u>integrate advances in speech pathology, psychopathology, and learning theory into a systematic theory of stuttering</u>.

In recent years Miller (40) and Dollard and Miller (10) have formulated in systematic terms the nature of conflicts, especially those involving simultaneous approach and avoidance tendencies. Lewin (36) analyzed conflicts between driving and restraining forces in relation to positive and negative valences. Travis (53, 54), Glauber (24), and Fenichel (16) have developed psychoanalytic theories of stuttering based in part on conflict between conscious and unconscious wishes. Johnson (17, 30), Bryngelson (8), Van Riper (60, 61), and speech pathologists of the Iowa tradition have evolved, under different theoretical banners, systems of treatment which stressed non-avoidance and reduction of fears.

Aspects of conflict in stuttering have been noted by a number of investigators. More than 80 years ago the German writer Wyneken called the stutterer a *Sprachzweifler*, a "speech-doubter," comparing his plight to that of one seized with uncertainty at the moment of attempting a leap (63). In 1936 Johnson and Knott (32) defined stuttering as the manifestation of a conflict between the communicative drive or impulse and the impulse to inhibit expected stuttering. Knott and Johnson noted ". . . an experimental conflict . . . marked by the attempt of the stutterer to perform two mutually opposed tasks simultaneously; one to talk, the other not to stutter (34).

As part of his analytically oriented theory, Travis held stuttering to be "a compromise between 'letting out' and 'holding in' (54) . . . The stutterer wishes to express himself, and at the same time fears doing so" (53). Fenichel stated: "The symptom of stuttering reveals a conflict between antagonistic tendencies; the patient shows us that he wishes to say something and yet does not wish to" (16, p. 311). Closely related observations of conflict in stuttering may be found in Blanton and Blanton (3), Bluemel (5, 6), Dunlap (11), Fletcher (18, pp. 231–232), Froeschels (22, 23), Glauber (24), Hill (26), Johnson (29, 30, 32), Solomon (51, 52), Van Riper (57, 60, pp. 269, 277, 287, 321–322, 61, pp. 19–20), Wischner (62, p. 330), and Wyneken (63).

Wide divergence has appeared among various writers as to the nature of the conflict and its relation to the stuttering. For some it has been a conflict over gratification of instincts, for others a conscious interference with an automatic process, for still others a rivalry between cortical hemispheres. Many apparently competing theories attack the problem at different levels and do not necessarily contradict one another. In like manner, the approach-avoidance conflict theory presented here involves only its own level of analysis and is sufficiently broad to be compatible with many other interpretations of stuttering.

B. Two Essential Questions

If we reduce stuttering behavior to the simplest possible terms, we find that it is a *momentary blocking*. Almost mysteriously the stutterer is stuck on a word, and then, for reasons just as baffling, he is able to continue. An explanation of stuttering must account for these twin features of the stutterer's behavior.

Most theories of stuttering have focused on the hesitancy, on what produces the blocking. But from the standpoint of systematic theory as well as therapy, it is just as important to explain termination of the block as the block itself. This problem has been considered in an earlier study: "What seems to determine the moment of release, the moment at which the stutterer can finally say the word?" (44, p. 69).

Two questions then become essential in the explanation of the stutterer's behavior: (1) What makes him stop? (2) What enables him to continue? To answer them fully, with support for the answers, requires the complete spelling out of the theory portion of this paper.

The two central hypotheses, however, may be stated quite briefly:

(1) *The Conflict Hypothesis.* The stutterer stops whenever conflicting approach and avoidance tendencies reach an equilibrium.

(2) *The Fear-Reduction Hypothesis.* The occurrence of stuttering reduces the fear which elicited it, so that *during* the block there is sufficient reduction in fear-motivated avoidance to resolve the conflict, permitting release of the blocked word.

The discussion that follows will take up each of these in turn.

C. THE CONFLICT HYPOTHESIS

1. STATEMENT

If stuttering occurs whenever approach and avoidance tendencies reach an equilibrium, we should be able to analyze the process in terms of relative strengths of gradients of each. Miller (40, 41) and Dollard and Miller (10) have provided us with an excellent theoretical model for such an analysis (Figure 1).

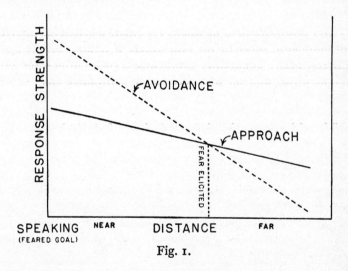

Fig. 1.

For the stutterer, the speaking of a difficult word involves a goal, that of communication, but also a fear, that of inability to communicate. The stutterer thus has a "feared goal" in Miller's sense. Conflicting tendencies in the stutterer to approach and to avoid are represented by solid and broken lines respectively. From the fact that the fear-motivated avoidance gradient is steeper than the reward-motivated approach gradient, it can be seen that an organism put in an approach-avoidance conflict situation will *go part-way and then stop*, or oscillate helplessly in the zone where the gradients cross. This is exactly the be-

havior the stutterer shows in attempting a feared word, or upon entering a feared situation. He says "K-K-K-Katy" or blocks silently after
having begun the word. He freezes at the instant of picking up the
phone, or halts on the threshold of a strange office.

If this formulation is essentially correct, we are in a position to
answer the first question. The stutterer stops after advancing part-way
because he is in a conflict situation, and the moment of his stopping is
determined by the relative strengths of approach and avoidance
gradients. Stuttering behavior itself has a hesitant character because
it is the result of a conflict. Such an interpretation of stuttering accords
well with Freud's classic view of the nature of neurotic conflict:

> ". . . neurotic symptoms . . . are the result of a conflict. The two
> powers which have entered into opposition meet together again in the symp-
> tom and become reconciled by means of the *compromise* contained in the
> symptom-formation" (19, p. 313).

In the compromise, i.e., the symptom of stuttering, the conflict is neatly
externalized.

Many of the secondary symptoms of stuttering, as analyzed by Van
Riper (57), may be interpreted as compensatory efforts to overcome
avoidance, to go forward in the face of fear. Others, as he has pointed
out, are just reactions to fear, directly expressed avoidance. Among the
compensatory measures to overcome avoidance are the devices of starting, antiexpectancy, and release. These are, in effect, attempts to reach
the goal by a roundabout route, a characteristic of conflict behavior
noted by Lewin (37, p. 263). Devices of avoidance and postponement,
on the other hand, are essentially reactions to fear, direct expressions
of the approach-avoidance conflict.

The primary symptoms of stuttering can equally be attributed to
approach-avoidance conflict. Repetition and prolongation may represent
oscillating and stopping, respectively, near the point where the gradients
cross, at the point of equilibrium in the conflict. Both Johnson and Van
Riper have pointed out that syllable repetition and other forms of non-
fluency in children characteristically appear in the midst of many conflicting speech pressures, e.g., vocabulary acquisition, phrase choices,
and sentence building. Adults similarly tend to speak hesitantly in
pressure situations.

Speech is a sequence of movements, and stuttering is a breakdown
in the sequence. Whatever the involvements of the disorder, the point
at which the breakdown occurs must bear a relation to these involvements. The breakdown occurs early in the sequence, but seldom prevents initiation of the sequence. Stuttering is, in other words, chiefly a
disorder of *release*, of going partway and then stopping. Froeschels (22)

has called repetition and prolongation ("clonus and tonus") the only symptoms common to all stutterers, an observation supported by the author's findings (44, p. 62). The stopping and oscillation which these symptoms may express are the features common to approach-avoidance behavior.

For clarity in presentation, this discussion has centered on stuttering as simple approach-avoidance conflict. Speaking has been the approach response; not speaking the avoidance response. But at times there are approach and avoidance tendencies to the act of speaking itself as well as to the act of not speaking. This involves some additional assumptions and a further analysis, in terms of Miller's double approach avoidance conflict (Figures 2 and 3), which may account better for certain occurrences of stuttering.

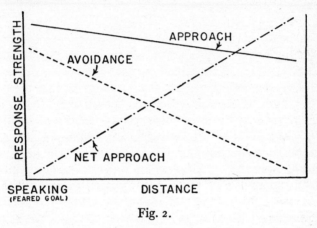

Fig. 2.

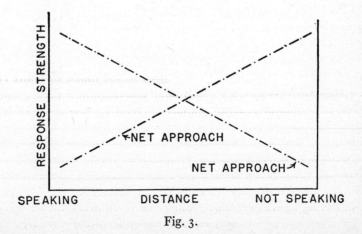

Fig. 3.

The conflict on speaking is as follows: There is an approach tendency for speaking, since it is socially demanded. But since speaking entails the danger of stuttering, there is an avoidance tendency based on the fear elicited by this danger. This is the type of conflict which Johnson and Knott (32) held responsible for stuttering.

The conflict on not speaking is as follows: There is an approach tendency for not speaking, because silence becomes an attractive alternative to the danger situation of speaking. But this alternative also is to be feared.

In a situation which calls for speech, not speaking or not being able to speak in itself involves a threat. Many stutterers show a *fear of silence*, and any dead stop in their communication spurs panicky efforts to release the block. Many of the irrelevant and apparently unintelligent symptoms of the stutterer can be understood as a filibustering, a measure taken against the fear of silence.

Consequently, there is an avoidance tendency for not speaking as well as an approach tendency for not speaking. Movement toward either feared goal elicits more fear, so that the net approach tendency will be greater toward the more distant goal. As this is approached, e.g., as the stutterer gets closer to the speech attempt or as he gets further away from it, the alternative goal becomes more distant, hence less dangerous and more attractive. The stutterer will then turn and approach the other goal until it becomes too feared. Dollard and Miller's prediction for this type of situation is "one of stable equilibrium like that of the pendulum" (10, pp. 366–367). Such behavior toward feared words and situations is characteristic of the stutterer.

The paradoxical increase in "fear elicited" as lowered avoidance permits a closer approach to the feared goal is equally true of simple approach-avoidance conflict (1).

2. EVIDENCE

What predictions flow from conflict theory, and what evidence can be brought to bear on these predictions? If stuttering is a form of conflict, a resultant of competing urges to approach and avoid, then it should vary systematically as follows: Stuttering should be increased by (a) a heightening of the avoidance drive through an increase in the penalty upon which fear and avoidance are based; (b) by a lowering of the approach drive. Stuttering should be decreased by (a) reduction in the avoidance drive (fear, penalty); (b) by an increase in the approach drive.

What are the findings? The effect of penalty upon stuttering was shown in an important early study by Van Riper (58), who found that frequency of stuttering is increased by expectation of electric shock to be administered according to the number of blocks. Trial shocks only were administered, so that Van Riper's procedure was essentially a shock threat situation, a neat experimental paradigm for the relationship between stuttering and fear. Recently these results have been repeated by Frick as part of a comprehensive investigation of the relationship between punishment and stuttering. In other portions of his experiment, Frick administered shock for each stuttered word, in one condition at the end of the passage and in another immediately after the block. In each case the added penalty resulted in greater frequency of stuttering (21). Porter found that the frequency of stuttering is increased by greater social penalty, as measured by the number of persons in the audience (43). On the other hand, the frequency of stuttering is decreased by a reduction in penalty as measured by the meaningfulness of the material (Eisenson and Horowitz, 13), and by degree of communicative responsibility (Eisenson and Wells, 14). Bloodstein (4, p. 296) has suggested that the adaptation effect, the reduction in frequency of stuttering with repeated readings of the same passage, may be explained on the basis of a reduction in propositionality. As in the Eisenson studies, this involves a reduction in penalty. These findings accord well with the predictions of the approach-avoidance theory.

So much for penalty, and increases or decreases in the avoidance drive. What about the approach drive? The evidence on this is sparse. That which we do have, mostly clinical observation, supports our formulation. Stutterers, like people generally, show markedly more hesitancy when dealing with material they are reluctant to reveal. Literature is full of descriptions of small boys stammering their excuses and of the hesitant speech of marriage proposals. Stuttering has been known to start from a parental demand of an oral confession of guilt. The reduction of communicatory drive in such a situation is fairly obvious. On the other hand, increases in the approach drive brought about through hypnosis, suggestion (4) or speaking under strong or unusual stimulation (4) brings increased fluency. Stutterers sometimes surprise themselves and their associates by speaking normally in a crisis situation. Anger or sudden stress may produce a spectacular fluency. Such events point to the effect of a temporary increase in the approach drive.

A recently completed study bears directly on the strengthening of approach behavior in stutterers. Twenty adult stutterers read two 200-word passages five consecutive times under different conditions. The control condition was a standard adaptation situation, in which the subject simply read the passage each time as naturally as possible. Under the experimental condition, the subject repeated each stuttered word until he had attacked it once successfully. This technique led to more normal speech and less stuttering (P = .02). Under the assumptions stated in the study, the approach response of speaking was thereby strengthened while the avoidant response of stuttering was moved further away from the point of reinforcement and correspondingly weakened (46).

3. LEVELS OF CONFLICT

In order to present the conflict hypothesis directly and simply, more thorough analysis of the different levels at which conflict may occur in stuttering has been reserved for separate presentation. Five distinct levels emerge: word-level; situation-level; emotional content level; relationship level, and ego-protective level.

At the *word level* the conflict is between the urge to speak the word and the urge not to speak the word. For example, the stutterer wants to say "hello," i.e., he approaches this word, but fear holds him back, because "h" sounds have through past experience acquired cue value.

At the *situation level* there is a parallel conflict between entering and not entering a feared situation. The stutterer's behavior toward using the telephone, reciting in classes, or introducing himself to strangers illustrates this conflict. Many situations which demand speech hold enough threat to produce a competing drive to hold back.

These two levels are based upon Van Riper's distinction between specific expectancy, or word-fear, as contrasted with general expectancy or situation-fear (57, 60). Such fears are usually based on past speech experiences and involve directly learned avoidance. How conflict based on word fear and situation fear can lead to blocking has been illustrated briefly by our diagram, Figure 1, and analyzed in detail elsewhere (46).

Conflict due to the *emotional content* of words, apart from their phonetic properties, such as has been described by Travis (53, p. 202), involved unconscious motivation for avoidance. This is illustrated by the stutterer whose speech grows worse in describing a traumatic experience, or upon giving information he is reluctant to divulge. It is the emotional and verbal content that is involved, not the situation or the words in themselves. Dunlap (11) said of the stutterer: "Sometimes he is in constant fear lest he inadvertently reveal something he would rather his elders did not hear." The inhibition of emotional content, especially hostile feeling, is a common denominator in many instances of stuttering (1).

At a closely related level of conflict, the occurrence of stuttering is in part a function of the *relationship* between the stutterer and his listener. Some stutterers experience no fear when they play a dominant rôle. One may give a fluent public address but stutter to individuals in the audience before and afterward. A child may block severely before one parent but speak easily to the other. An army enlisted man could never say "sergeant" until he became one. The fact that many stutterers can act in plays seems to show the effect of changed rôle. Several of the conditions listed by Bloodstein (4) as involving the behavior of the listener may equally be interpreted in terms of relationship. Pointing out that the stutterer can usually talk well when alone, Adler concludes, ". . . I can only interpret his stammer as the expression of his attitude toward others" (2, p. 63). Fletcher (18), Travis (53), Fenichel (16, pp. 311–314), Abbott (1), and many others have stated in one way or another the importance of the relationship between the stutterer and his listener.

Since stuttering may be termed a compromise between speech and silence, we should consider the symbolic significance of all three in analyzing what is expressed toward the listener. Depending upon our initial reference points, we may get widely differing results: (a) stuttering may be considered an act of aggression against the listener; fluency then would be nonaggressive or friendly behavior; (b) speech may be considered an aggressive, competitive, phallic (in psychoanalytic terms) act; silence here is presumably neutral; (c) silence in itself may be viewed as hostile. Noting that in dreams to be mute is a symbol of death, Fenichel (16, pp. 311–313) likened stuttering to a partial mutism resulting from a turning inward against the stutterer's own ego of hostile urges originally directed against the listener. From his discussion it is possible to infer all three of the above meanings. Perhaps it should be concluded simply that either stuttering or speech or silence can be used to express hostility or more positive feelings at various times, but that no constant or universal meaning can be offered. Whatever the behavior through which the feeling is expressed, the occurrence of stuttering will in part be determined by degree of conflict at the relationship level.

At the *ego-protective level,* stuttering serves as a lifelong defense mechanism keeping its possessor out of dangerous competition. Through the stuttering, certain aspirations may be abandoned which might involve threat of failure, or threat of success.

Although our formulation of the ego-protective level stresses life aspirations and goals, the concept is sufficiently broad to include any defensive function of stuttering. Travis' excellent formulation more nearly represents the classic Freudian view of symptoms as defenses against forbidden impulses:

". . . stuttering is a defense created with extraordinary skill and designed to prevent anxiety from developing when certain impulses of which the stutterer dares not become aware, threaten to expose themselves" (53, p. 193).

That stutterers do tend significantly to avoid threat of failure is shown by their behavior in an experimental level of aspiration situation. Compared to normal controls, stutterers set less exacting (though more realistic) goals for themselves, predicted more modest performances, and showed in general a lower level of aspiration (49).

Any particular moment of stuttering may be understood in terms of the interplay of conflicting forces at these levels. Whatever the level of conflict, the overt conflict is experienced at the word-level. Conflict at the ego-protective level, for example, might explain a stutterer's resistance in therapy. It would not explain his blocking on a word, except through the mediation of word-fear. In like manner, the pressure of the situation, emotionality of the utterance, or nature of the interpersonal relation must ultimately be expressed at the word-level. It is in this fundamental sense that stuttering is a conflict between speaking and not speaking.

D. THE FEAR REDUCTION HYPOTHESIS

I. STATEMENT

If stuttering results from a conflict, how is the conflict resolved? According to the conflict hypothesis, the stutterer stops when approach and avoidance tendencies reach an equilibrium. Why then doesn't the stutterer remain permanently in a conflict situation? How is he able to obtain release from the block?

At the beginning of a block the stutterer is stuck. He cannot get the word out. By the end of the block some change has taken place, so that he can now utter the word. What has happened between these points? If the stutterer cannot say the word for a time, why is he able to say it at all? To account for this, the hypothesis is advanced that the occurrence of stuttering brings about a reduction of the fear which elicited it.

During the moment of stuttering, there must be sufficient reduction of fear, avoidance tendency and conflict to "release" the blocked word. Were it not for this fact, once the stutterer became stuck on a word, he would remain stuck indefinitely.

How can the occurrence of stuttering reduce the fear that elicits it? Why should the stutterer be in any better position to speak the word at the end of a block than at the beginning? After all, the symptoms of stuttering frequently bear little relevance to the actual speaking of the word (57, 44).

The occurrence of stuttering may effect a reduction of fear in several ways:

First, since the stutterer's fear is tied up with his avoidance and is an effort to hide the disapproved symptoms, once the stuttering begins to occur it can no longer be hidden. The stuttering block itself forces the stutterer to "face" his stuttering to a certain extent. This reduces the conflict. The thing the stutterer feared has now occurred. He can no longer avoid it completely, and this partially reduces the fear. On the other hand, successful avoidance builds up tension.

Second, once the stuttering block begins to occur it is a known entity. As the stutterer begins to approach a block, he has a vague dread, a generalized expectancy. As he nears the actual moment of stuttering, he recognizes more familiar landmarks (initial sound, length of word, cf. Brown, 7) and is even able to predict the duration of the block with some precision (study by Milisen and Van Riper, 39). Hence, he gets some feeling of control, the fear is now more specific and there is less fear of the unknown, and there is a reduction of the element of fear from a sense of helplessness (study by Mowrer and Viek, 42).

Third, to the extent that stuttering can be interpreted as an aggressive act directed against the listener (Fenichel, 16) the stuttering relieves the aggression (frustration-aggression hypothesis), hence reduces the inhibition to aggression, hence reduces the approach-avoidance conflict of the stuttering.

To test these corollary hypotheses is obviously beyond the scope of this paper. They are stated here for the completeness of the theory and as problems for future research.

2. EVIDENCE

Among studies which may be interpreted as revealing the effect of stuttering on fear are the following:

1. The study by Meissner (38) in which voluntary non-fluency reduced stuttering.

2. The studies of Johnson and Knott (33), Johnson and Inness (31), Shulman (50), and other studies showing the adaptation effect. From the fear-reduction hypothesis, we may infer that the occurrence of stuttering in the first reading dissipates sufficient anxiety so that there is less stuttering in the second reading, etc. Such an interpretation of adaptation is in agreement with and in large part contained in Johnson's current published view:

> The adaptation effect would appear to be a particularly clean-cut example of the effect of improved adjustment to the reading situation, lowered anxiety about stuttering resulting from "doing the thing feared" and discovering on the spot that the dreaded consequences turn out to be less dreadful than expected (30, p. 210).

3. The study by Brown (7) showing that stutterers tend to stutter more on the first word in a sentence. According to our hypothesis, the

stuttering which occurs on the first word will, through generalization, make subsequent words in that sentence easier.

4. The effectiveness of the technique of negative practice as reported by Dunlap (11, 12), Case (9), and Fishman (17). Duplicating the stuttered performance voluntarily should "satisfy" the fear, lower the avoidance drive, and diminish the conflict causing the stuttering.

5. Van Riper's study of thoracic breathing (56) in which stutterers show a rehearsal of the block during an expectancy period. The rehearsal behavior is here interpreted as an effort to reduce the fear by stuttering subvocally first.

6. As a specific test of the fear-reduction hypothesis presented here, the author and Robert Voas of U.C.L.A. carried out a study of physiological tension patterns of 12 stutterers during the moment of stuttering (47, 48). Masseter muscle action currents and other measures showed a rise in amplitude (tension) from the beginning of the block to the moment of release. Since lowering the avoidance gradient in approach-avoidance conflict produces an initial increase in manifest tension as the individual moves closer to the feared goal, this finding on tension patterns in stuttering is in accordance with approach-avoidance conflict theory. Upon the speaking of the word — the reaching of the goal — the resolving of the conflict — a marked reduction in tension occurred as the muscle group returned to the resting state. It should be pointed out that this type of tension reduction occurs normally with the speaking of a word whether stuttered or not. The theoretically important feature is that sufficient fear reduction occurs *during* the stuttering block to permit release of the blocked word.

7. Two other findings may be cited in support of the fear-reduction hypothesis. First, in applying a non-reinforcement procedure to a group of stutterers, it was possible to obtain a normal speaking of the word simply by asking the subject to repeat the word, i.e., to stutter on it until all fear present was "satisfied." That the subjects were able to do this, that they could speak the word more easily the second, third, and fourth attempt, is in itself strong evidence for a mechanism of fear reduction resulting from stuttering (46). In another study (44, p. 25), a tendency was noted toward stuttering with succeedingly larger portions of the word, e.g., "th-thir-thirty." From our hypothesis, the stuttering which occurred on the first attempt reduced fear and avoidance sufficiently so that succeeding points of stoppage occurred closer to the goal, i.e., nearer the speaking of the word.

3. IMPLICATIONS

These results have interesting ramifications. Van Riper states that successful avoidance increases the stutterer's fear and causes more trouble in the long run (60, pp. 284–285). The concept of stuttering as a fear-reducer clarifies this relationship. When the stutterer is able to avoid stuttering he does not dissipate the anxiety, the tension builds up and even though he may continue to be fluent, he is building up future trouble through the avoidance. On the other hand, when he stutters or pretends to stutter, he is reducing his fears and building toward greater fluency later on. Hence we have a paradoxical relation — the stuttering produces the fluency and the fluency produces the stuttering. This paradoxical relation provides a possible explanation of something frequently observed, namely, that stuttering tends to occur in waves.

We could thus view stuttering as having a function similar to that of tics, asthma, and many neurotic symptoms, that it "binds" the anxiety and has the property of reducing it. We would have a parallel here to compulsive acts. When the person cannot stutter or success-fully does not, the fear builds up. Stuttering may be thus viewed as an expression of accumulated anxiety. When the behavior occurs, the anxiety erupts and is let out. This concept may go a long way toward explaining the apparently paradoxical fact that we can build up a stutterer's tension by asking him to be fluent and we can reduce his fear by encouraging him to engage freely in the expression of the symptom.

On the concept of anxiety binding Freud gives as one view, ". . . all symptom formation would be brought about solely to avoid anxiety. The symptoms bind the psychic energy which would otherwise be dis-charged as anxiety . . . if a compulsion neurotic is prevented from washing his hands after touching something, he becomes a prey to al-most insupportable anxiety" (20, p. 85).

In the same context, the concepts of the stuttering symptom as a defense against anxiety has long been stressed by Travis (53, 54, p. 35).

It is as though each stutterer carries around with him a "stutter potential," a *reservoir of fear* which is tapped from time to time by the occurrence of stuttering. Such a concept, while more figurative than real, may help us understand the seemingly neurotic stutterer who suffers agonies in anticipation of stuttering that never quite happens. It is precisely because the individual never stutters that he never ob-tains relief. His need for stuttering, as Travis aptly put it, becomes acute. In a psychological sense he is much worse off than the indi-vidual who can express his conflict, and reduce his fear, through out-ward stuttering behavior. Such a concept has interesting possibilities: not only does it provide theoretical support for procedures used by Johnson and Vin Riper with stutterers, but it suggests potentialities for *symptom expression* as a psychotherapeutic technique with any problem based on fear.

4. THEORETICAL RELATIONSHIPS

A paradoxical effect of fear-reduction during the block may be inferred from the nature of the conflict. By the lowering of the avoidance gradient, the stutterer is brought closer to the feared goal and hence may experience a paradoxical increase in "fear elicited." Thus a reduction in fear shifts the equilibrium of the forces in conflict and brings the stutterer closer to the speaking of the word, but simultaneously he is experiencing more fear as he nears the goal.

From the basic diagram of approach-avoidance conflict (our Figure 1), Dollard and Miller state their assumption that *fear elicited* is fixed by the height of the intersection of the two gradients, and proceed with the following analysis:

. . . When the avoidance is strong relative to the approach, the two gradients intersect far from the goal. . . . At this distance the approach tendency is so weak that the subject is not strongly tempted to do frightening things. . . . Extinguishing the fear of the goal or making it seem less dangerous . . . will lower the entire gradient of avoidance . . . this will produce a paradoxical effect . . . as the apparent danger is reduced the subject will be more strongly tempted to do things which frighten him. Stronger fear and conflict will therefore be elicited (10).

At this point the situation must sound discouraging, but Dollard and Miller further point out:

This deduction holds only for the range within which the gradients of approach and avoidance intersect. If the gradient of avoidance is weakened so much that it no longer intersects the gradient of approach, the subject will advance to the goal and further decreases in the gradient of avoidance will decrease the amount of fear and conflict (10).

This discussion may help us distinguish between the fear reduction *during* the block which permits release and that which results from the release, because the goal of speaking the word is reached. The fear-reduction which determines the release may be obscured somewhat by a simultaneous increase in fear, conflict, and avoidance strength with the nearing of the feared goal.

Two shifts are occurring at once. For a given amount of fear and avoidance tendency, the point at which the stutterer initially stops is determined in part by the strength of the approach drive, which is in turn a function of his need to communicate and ability to tolerate anxiety. When he reaches the point of stoppage the stuttering begins to occur, reducing the fear which elicited it and lowering the avoidance gradient so that he moves closer to the goal. Thus the amount of fear subjectively experienced may remain relatively constant throughout the block. If the stutterer does not complete the block, but leaves the field or engages in some instrumental escape response, or if by using a device or trick he successfully reaches the goal in a roundabout manner, he does not "satisfy the fear" present and may continue to experience tension after the block. The unsatisfied fear may transfer over to a subsequent word and be dissipated on that word. When the opposite happens and there is rehearsal or sub-vocal satisfying of the fear first, there may be a stuttering on the word preceding the word originally feared, an observation made by Hill (26). Since fear-reduction reinforces the instrumental acts which bring it about, and reinforced responses tend to move up in the response sequence (25, pp. 212–215), the stuttering tends to become anticipatory. Van Riper has shown that the actual form of the block may be rehearsed in breathing patterns prior to speech attempt (39). Through secondary reinforcement such rehearsal behavior will be fear-reducing, which indeed appears to be its function. Proprioceptive feedback from this rehearsal behavior enables the stutterer to anticipate his blocks, even to predicting their duration with some accuracy.

Thus there are indications of fear-reduction occurring during at least the first two of the three stages of the stuttering process as analyzed by Johnson: pre-spasm, spasm, and post-spasm (28). From a fear-reduction occurring before and during the block and at the moment of release, the symptom is reinforced and maintained, the anxiety is "bound" within it, and a vicious circle is perpetuated.

E. TREATMENT

If stuttering is basically an approach-avoidance conflict, then the fundamental goal of treatment becomes the elimination of all tendency to avoidance, whatever the source. Since the avoidance is based on fear, stuttering is to be treated as a fear problem. Successful treatment then requires gaining a mastery over fear and finding expression of whatever needs, feelings, and tendencies have been locked up in the symptom. In terms of therapeutic approach, two specific values of the approach-avoidance formulation should be mentioned: (a) Approach-avoidance theory relates fear, avoidance and conflict to stuttering, and theory to treatment in a systematic way. The paramount importance of reducing fears and avoidances becomes clearly apparent from the theory itself. (b) The analysis of levels of conflict and the distinction between learned avoidances and unconscious motives for avoidance provides for an integration of psychotherapy and speech therapy not always apparent in the writings of psychologists and speech pathologists.

The relative utilization of speech therapy and psychotherapy in present-day clinical work offers many contrasts. On one hand a few stragglers still use a purely symptomatic treatment which tries to ignore fears, prevent blocks, and build fluency directly through "confidence" measures. These people neglect all psychotherapy and, in a modern sense, speech therapy as well. At the opposite pole are many able clinicians, often psychoanalytically oriented, who insist that we must "ignore the symptom" and work toward the original cause, presumably something in the stutterer's past. For these people the speech pathologist could offer the stutterer nothing except in terms of whatever general psychotherapeutic abilities he might possess.

However, when stuttering is treated as a form of conflict, speech therapy and psychotherapy are not in competition, but have a common goal: the reduction of all tendencies to avoidance and of the fears which motivate them.

Although the stutterer's need for psychotherapy is now widely accepted, many of those who see this need most clearly continue to ask, "Why work on the speech at all?" To answer this question, and to defend the rôle that speech pathologists have come to assume in helping stutterers, we list the following points:

First, if we are really justified in viewing stuttering as an externalized conflict, should we not avail ourselves of this ready avenue to other levels? Conflict at the relationship level, for example, is mediated through situation and word-fear; why then not begin where the stuttering occurs and work back to the stutterer's relationships? The stutterer's blocks and his reactions to them mirror his self-concepts, attitudes toward others, mechanisms for handling conflicts, and many other aspects of his personality. Each time the stutterer has a block he is reliving in a small way one of the most significant experiences of his life.

Second, if we accept the hypotheses that stuttering reduces to some degree the fear that elicits it, possibilities suggest themselves for planned use of stuttering behavior as a tension reducer or outlet for fear. The "negative practice" techniques employed by Dunlap (12) probably owed some of their efficacy to this effect, though he advocated their use on different grounds. Such Iowa School methods as a voluntary repetition of "bounce," smooth prolongation or "slide," and duplication of the true pattern have been used successfully for years to reduce the stutterer's anxiety. Some of the best successes have been obtained with cases who had little outward stuttering to begin with and who underwent no discernible speech changes. But through such speech therapy, with very little conventional psychotherapy, they have been freed from the taxing strain of anticipation.

Third, profound personality changes can result from successful speech therapy. Teaching a stutterer how to handle his fears and his blocks, helping him develop healthier attitudes toward his problem, toward himself, and toward others — these things are not mere symptom treatment. Encouraging the stutterer to attack feared and difficult situations may support him strongly in something he really has wanted to do. Many stutterers relate that they get tired of running away; it is a deeply moving experience to master situations from which they have always retreated.

Fourth, a certain amount of direct speech therapy is necessary to deal with the maintaining causes of stuttering. Van Riper states, "Stuttering is peculiarly able to maintain itself once it gets started (60, p. 276) . . . in the secondary stage . . . the disorder has become 'chronic' or self-perpetuating . . . a vicious circle" (60, p. 239). Johnson observes: "Stuttering is something like our fear of thunder — there is no inherent or rational necessity for it, but once started it tends to be maintained, generation after generation" (30, p. 194). Both these authorities, as well as Dunlap (11, p. 199), Case (9), Wischner (62, pp. 330–331), and others, have pointed out how stuttering may perpetuate itself on a learned behavior or habit level. Wischner considers stuttering as learned behavior which seems to resemble responses set up by instrumental avoidance training (62, p. 327), hence difficult to extinguish (62, p. 332).

An experiment by the author has shown that when reinforcement of the stuttering can be prevented, modified or decreased, stuttering is reduced. In this way the vicious circle may be broken (46, pp. 61–62). Van Riper's method of "cancellation," as well as a host of other techniques of the Iowa School, are directed toward the same result (60, pp. 348–371). With such techniques available, it is unnecessary to let the stutterer struggle helplessly with his blocks for an indefinite period while searching for buried complexes. And in long-range terms, if the therapist disdains all direct work on speech, he offers the stutterer only a purely verbal system for coping with long-reinforced habitual responses that are permitted to remain intact.

Treatment may begin at the topmost level of conflict and work downward. Conflicts due to immediate word fear and situation fear are dealt with through that specialized portion of the therapeutic process known as speech therapy. Conflicts at deeper levels are straight problems in psychotherapy, which may be handled concurrently. To the extent that such conflicts express themselves through outward stuttering behavior, they may be reached via the speech therapy. The stutterer's reaction to speech therapy frequently reveals the nature and extent of his resistances.

At the beginning the stutterer is caught in a vicious circle. He doesn't have the tools with which to work. Increasing his motivation at that point only increases the penalty on stuttering, therefore fear, conflict, and number of blocks. Speech therapy of the non-avoidance type can serve two important functions: first, for those whose stuttering has become self-maintaining or functionally autonomous, reducing drives toward avoidance may be sufficient to break up the "vicious circle" and free the stutterer; second, speech therapy gives the stutterer tools for dealing with word and situation fears he had not formerly possessed. When a stutterer rejects this opportunity he provides a focal point for the analysis and understanding of his own resistances. Such analysis is considered an essential first step in therapy by Fenichel (15, p. 46), who recommends that analysis of resistance precede analysis of content. This leads to the problem of dealing with unconscious sources of avoidance and conflict, i.e., psychotherapy for the stutterer.

Since the emotionality of the utterance is so frequently a source of conflict in the stutterer, an important goal in psychotherapy is *release of feeling*. Pent-up feelings or repressed emotional material responsible for producing blockings in speech require free expression and adequate outlet. Such goals are common in psychotherapy, and numerous techniques to achieve them are familiar terms in its literature: release of feeling, clarification of feeling, catharsis, abreaction, working through, play therapy, psychodrama, and others. It is interesting that one of the few modern therapists reporting fair success with stutterers is David Levy (35, pp. 77–79), whose "release therapy" is aimed primarily at the expression of feeling.

Many of the speech therapy techniques of the "Iowa School" may be interpreted as exercises in the expression of aggression. The stutterer who changes his mind about "faking" to a clerk because, "He seemed so nice, I couldn't do it to him," may illustrate a common underlying attitude. A "spluttering" or choking up of speech, behavior which at least superficially resembles stuttering, is a cultural caricature for inexpressible aggression. If stuttering may be viewed this way, in accord with Fenichel, then such techniques as negative practice and "bouncing" not only provide a means of abreaction but reduce the need to be aggressive. Such needs on the stutterer's part may be reduced in two ways: through the use of stuttering behavior itself, and through release of feelings behind it.

All maladjustments are in a sense due to a lack of satisfactory *relationships* in early life. People are neurotic to the extent that they lack good interpersonal relations. Psychotherapy, as the undoing process of maladjustment, must be directed toward establishing that which has been lacking — warm and satisfying relationships. In the beginning phases the therapist himself supplies the relationship. Later on, as treatment begins to be effective, the individual's improved adjustment is reflected in more congenial relations outside therapy.

Stuttering not only expresses the nature of the stutterer's relationships but is in part determined by them. When there is considerable conflict at this level, the working through of certain crucial relationships becomes essential to success. Fletcher showed awareness of this in regarding stuttering as a "social morbidity" (18, pp. 222–240), symptomatic of the victim's attitude toward all society. Recognition of the stutterer's need for better relationships has undoubtedly stimulated the development of group therapy methods with stutterers.

Dollard and Miller's analysis of the nature of approach-avoidance conflict may serve as a warning against bringing the stutterer too quickly into new and dangerous rôles. They point out that because of the paradoxical effect of a lowering of avoidance tendencies in eliciting greater fear, it is necessary to "dose anxiety" or to pace the individual so that he will not experience too much conflict at once and drop out of therapy (10, pp. 400–403). A further danger of reducing avoidance too quickly, and in all attempts at sudden cures, emerges from the ego-protective level of conflict.

At some point in the treatment of a stutterer it is necessary to consider the effect of the handicap, and possible recovery from it, upon goals and aspirations, upon what the individual has planned to do with his life. Specially constructed sentence completion test items, or open-ended questions, may elicit revealing projective material in this area. Examples: "What kind of a person would you be if you didn't stutter?" or "If your stuttering suddenly disappeared, what difference would it make in your life?" or "If I could get over stuttering, I would. . . ."

Frequently such questions make the stutterer anxious. Because the defeat may have become a peg upon which to hang all his shortcomings, or perhaps because of the capacity of the human organism to adapt itself to disturbance, the stutterer is likely to feel a little strange without his symptom. The individual may have lived with his stuttering so long that functioning without it involves a radical change in self-concept which must be gradual. To put it in another way, fluency may have become ego-alien. In the later stages of treatment the stutterer must learn to accept his new rôle with its fluency, just as in the early stages he needed to accept his old rôle with its stuttering.

As changes during treatment begin to occur, there should be a certain amount of *preparation for recovery*. Such preparation should include a careful psychotherapeutic exploration of the adaptiveness of the stutterer's goals, and the relation of these to the disorder. If the stutterer has enslaved himself to a striving toward unattainables, the therapist should help him find freedom. If the stutterer's level of aspiration is lower than his capabilities warrant, the therapist may help him realize the new possibilities opening up before him. All these have the effect of reducing avoidance and conflict due to ego-protective functions of the symptom.

From the foregoing, it may be seen that therapy is carried out at all five of the levels at which conflict occurs in stuttering — word and situation, feeling, relationship, and ego-protective. Psychotherapy and speech therapy are twin avenues to the common goal of reducing fear and avoidance. In the course of treatment, as well as in theory, the problem of stuttering may be handled and understood in terms of approach-avoidance conflict.

F. Summary

1. Stuttering is a resultant of approach-avoidance conflict, of opposed urges to speak and to hold back from speaking.

2. The "holding back" may be due either to learned avoidances or to unconscious motives.

3. Principal hypotheses concerning stuttering behavior spring from two fundamental questions: (a) What produces blocking? (b) What determines release?

4. The Conflict Hypothesis: The stutterer blocks or stops whenever conflicting approach and avoidance tendencies reach an equilibrium.

5. The Fear-Reduction Hypothesis: The occurrence of stuttering reduces the fear which elicits it sufficiently to permit release of the blocked word, resolving the conflict momentarily and enabling the stutterer to continue.

6. In this way the symptom is reinforced and maintained, the anxiety is "bound" within it, and a vicious circle is perpetuated.

7. Conflict is directly expressed in primary symptoms of repetition and prolongation, which reflect a breakdown in the sequence of movements necessary to speech.

8. Secondary symptoms involve learned behavior representing compensatory efforts to overcome avoidance or to reach the goal by a roundabout route.

9. Conflict may occur at several levels — word, situation, emotional content, relationship, and ego-protective levels; any particular moment of stuttering is determined by interplay of forces at these levels.

10. Approach-avoidance theory relates fear, avoidance, and conflict to stuttering in a systematic way, so that goals of treatment become apparent from the theory itself.

11. Treatment proceeds through an integrated psychotherapy and speech therapy, aimed at attacking feared words and situations, releasing feelings, improving relationships, and freeing the individual from unadaptive goals, thereby achieving a total reduction of the fear and avoidance tendency responsible for the stutterer's conflict.

References

1. Abbott, J. A. Repressed hostility as a factor in adult stuttering. *J. Speech Disor.*, 1947, 12: 428–430.
2. Adler, A. *Problems of Neurosis*, London: Kegan Paul, Trench, Trubner, 1929.
3. Blanton, M. G., & Blanton, S. *Speech Training for Children*, New York: Century, 1924.
4. Bloodstein, O. N. Conditions under which stuttering is reduced or absent: A review of literature. *J. Speech Disor.*, 1949, 14: 295–302.
5. Bluemel, C. S. *Stammering and Allied Disorders*, New York: Macmillan, 1935.
6. ——— Stammering and inhibition. *J. Speech Disor.*, 1940, 5: 305–308.
7. Brown, S. F. The loci of stutterings in the speech sequence. *J. Speech Disor.*, 1945, 10: 182–192.
8. Bryngelson, B., Chapman, M. E., & Hansen, O. K. *Know Yourself: A Workbook for Those Who Stutter*, Minneapolis: Burgess, 1950.
9. Case, H. M. Stuttering and speech blocking: A comparative study of maladjustment. Ph.D. dissertation, University of California at Los Angeles, 1940. Pp. 78.
10. Dollard, J., & Miller, N. E. *Personality and Psychotherapy*, New York: McGraw-Hill, 1950.
11. Dunlap, K. *Habits: Their Making and Unmaking*, New York: Liveright, 1932.
12. ——— Stammering: Its nature, etiology and therapy. *J. Comp. Psychol.*, 1944, 37: 187–202.
13. Eisenson, J., & Horowitz, E. The influence of propositionality on stuttering. *J. Speech Disor.*, 1945, 10: 193–197.
14. Eisenson, J., & Wells, C. A study of the influence of communicative responsibility in a choral speech situation for stutterers. *J. Speech Disor.*, 1942, 7: 259–262.
15. Fenichel, O. *Problems of Psychoanalytic Technique*, Albany: Psychoanalytic Quarterly, 1939.
16. Fenichel, O. *The Psychoanalytic Theory of Neurosis*, New York: Norton, 1945.
17. Fishman, H. C. A study of the efficacy of negative practice as a corrective for stammering. *J. Speech Disor.*, 1937, 2: 67–72.
18. Fletcher, J. M. *The Problem of Stuttering*, New York: Longmans, Green, 1928.
19. Freud, S. *A General Introduction to Psychoanalysis*, New York: Garden City Publ., 1943.
20. ——— *The Problem of Anxiety*, New York: Norton, 1936.
21. Frick, J. V. An exploratory study of the effect of punishment (electric shock)

upon stuttering behavior. Ph.D. dissertation, State University of Iowa, Feb., 1951.

22. Froeschels, E. Stuttering and nystagmus. *Monatschr. f. Ohrenh.*, 1915, 49: 161–167.

23. ——— Uber des Wesen des Stotterns. *Wien, Med. Wchnschr.*, 1914, 64: 1067–1076.

24. Glauber, I. P. Psychoanalytic concepts of the stutterer. *Nerv. Child*, 1943, 2: 172–180.

25. Hilgard, E. R., & Marquis, D. G. *Conditioning and Learning*, New York: Appleton-Century, 1940.

26. Hill, H. An interbehavioral analysis of several aspects of stuttering. *J. Gen. Psychol.*, 1945, 32: 289–316.

27. Johnson, W. *People in Quandaries*, New York: Harper, 1946.

28. ——— An interpretation of stuttering. *Q. J. Speech*, 1933, 19: 70–76.

29. Johnson, W. (and others) A study of the onset and development of stuttering. *J. Speech Disor.*, 1942, 7: 251–257.

30. Johnson, W., Brown, S. F., Curtis, J. F., Edney, C. W., & Keaster, J. *Speech Handicapped School Children*, New York: Harper, 1948.

31. Johnson, W., & Inness, M. Studies in the psychology of stuttering: XIII. A statistical analysis of the adaptation and consistency effects in relation to stuttering. *J. Speech Disor.*, 1939, 4: 79–86.

32. Johnson, W., & Knott, J. R. The moment of stuttering. *J. Genet. Psychol.*, 1936, 48: 475–480.

33. ——— Studies in the psychology of stuttering: I. The distribution of moments of stuttering in successive readings of same material. *J. Speech Disor.*, 1937, 2: 17–19.

34. Knott, J. R., & Johnson, W. An interpretive demonstration of ten observable facts about stuttering. In *Proceedings of the American Speech Correction Association*. Madison: College Typing Company, 1936, 6: 150–154.

35. Levy, D. Release therapy. In Tomkins, S. S. (Ed.), *Contemporary Psychopathology*, Cambridge: Harvard Univ., 1947.

36. Lewin, K. *Dynamic Theory of Personality*, New York: McGraw-Hill, 1935.

37. ——— *Field Theory in Social Science*, New York: Harper, 1951.

38. Meissner, J. H. The relationship between voluntary non-fluency and stuttering. *J. Speech Disor.*, 1946, 11: 13–23.

39. Milisen, R., & Van Riper, C. A study of the predicted duration of the stutterer's blocks as related to their actual duration. *J. Speech Disor.*, 1939, 4: 339–345.

40. Miller, N. E. Experimental studies of conflict. In Hunt, J. McV. (Ed.), *Personality and the Behavior Disorders*, New York: Ronald Press, 1944. (Vol I, pp. 431–465.)

41. Miller, N. E. Comments on theoretical models illustrated by the development of a theory of conflict. *J. Personal.*, 1951, 20: 82–100.

42. Mowrer, O. H., & Viek, P. An experimental analogue of fear from a sense of helplessness. *J. Abn. & Soc. Psychol.*, 1948, 43: 193–200.

43. Porter, H. v. K. Studies in the psychology of stuttering: XIV, Stuttering phenomena in relation to size and personnel of audience. *J. Speech Disor.*, 1939, 4: 323–333.

44. Sheehan, J. G. A study of the phenomena of stuttering. M.A. thesis, University of Michigan, 1946.

45. ——— A theory of stuttering as approach-avoidance conflict. *Amer. Psychol.*, 1950, 5: 469.

46. —— The modification of stuttering through non-reinforcement. *J. Abn. & Soc. Psychol.*, 1951, 46: 51–63.

47. —— Fear-reduction during stuttering in relation to conflict, "anxiety-binding" and reinforcement. *Amer. Psychol.*, 1952, 7: 530 (Abstract).

48. Sheehan, J. G., & Voas, R. Tension patterns during stuttering in relation to conflict, fear-reduction, and reinforcement. *Speech Monog.*, (in press).

49. Sheehan, J. G., & Zelen, S. A level of aspiration study of stutterers. *Amer. Psychol.*, 1951, 6: 500 (Abstract).

50. Shulman, E. A study of certain factors influencing the variability of stuttering. Ph.D. dissertation, State University of Iowa, 1944.

51. Solomon, M. Stuttering as an emotional disorder. *Proc. Amer. Speech Correct. Assoc.*, 1932, 2: 118–121.

52. Solomon, M. Stuttering as an emotional and personality disorder. *J. Speech Disor.*, 1939, 4: 347–357.

53. Travis, L. E. The need for stuttering. *J. Speech Disor.*, 1940, 5: 193–202.

54. —— My present views on stuttering. *Western Speech*, 1946, 10: 3–5.

55. Travis, L. E., Tuttle, W. W., & Cowan, D. W. A study of the heart rate during stuttering. *J. Speech Disor.*, 1936, 1: 21–26.

56. Van Riper, C. A study of the thoracic breathing of stutterers during expectancy and occurrence of stuttering spasm. *J. Speech Disor.*, 1936, 1: 61–72.

57. —— Effect of devices for minimizing stuttering on the creation of symptoms. *J. Abn. & Soc. Psychol.*, 1937, 32: 185–192.

58. —— The effect of penalty upon frequency of stuttering. *J. Genet. Psychol.*, 1937, 50: 193–195.

59. —— The relation of tremors to perpetuation and release from the stuttering spasm. Unpublished paper read at 1939 meeting of the American Speech Correction Association, Chicago, Ill. See A.S.C.A. Program, *J. Speech Disor.*, 1939, 336.

60. —— *Speech Correction; Principles and Methods*, (2nd ed.) New York: Prentice-Hall, 1947.

61. —— *Stuttering*, Chicago: National Society for Crippled Children and Adults, 1949.

62. Wischner, G. J. Stuttering behavior and learning: A preliminary theoretical formulation. *J. Speech & Hear. Disor.*, 1950, 15: 324–335.

63. Wyneken, C. Ueber das Stottern und dessen Heilung. (Concerning stuttering and its cure.) *Zeitschrift für Rationelle Medicin.* 1868. 31: 1–20.

Part III

SCHIZOPHRENIC PSYCHOSES

22

RESPONSIVENESS IN CHRONIC SCHIZOPHRENIA

ROBERT B. MALMO, CHARLES SHAGASS, AND A. ARTHUR SMITH

Allan Memorial Institute of Psychiatry, McGill University, Montreal, Canada

Experimental studies of schizophrenia [1] have produced a considerable amount of objective evidence that schizophrenics differ from normal controls in various ways (4, 14). There are, however, no integrating principles which can account for all these deviations.

Angyal, Freeman and Hoskins (3) have called attention to the pervasiveness of "withdrawal" in schizophrenia, and they have sought an explanation for this symptom in terms of low physiological reactivity. The companion symptom of "affective dulling" has also been related to the physiological findings of hyporeactivity (3, 22), and some authors have concluded that the results of the physiological experiments show how capacity for emotional response has been generally reduced in schizophrenia. In its simplest form, this theory holds that all (or nearly all) effector mechanisms are "damped" or "braked" so that changes which are normally effective in eliciting responses are no longer effective in the schizophrenic.[2]

It is a matter of great importance to examine the evidence bearing on the question of whether cardinal symptoms of schizophrenia can possibly be explained in terms of this simple physiological principle of hyporeactivity. The available evidence include the following observations: diminished response to agents such as thyroid extract (6), dinitrophenol (9), adrenalin (10), and adrenocorticotrophic hormone (ACTH) (25); abnormally low response to inhalation of heated air (11); diminished post-rotational sway (12); and pupillary hypofunction in response to pain, light, and muscular reaction (22). Several additional examples of hyporeactivity are cited by Hoskins in his review (14).

However, the experimental evidence does not uniformly support

From *Journal of Personality*, 19: 359, 1951.

[1] We employ the unitary term "schizophrenia" for the sake of brevity. The designation "schizophrenic disorders" would probably be more appropriate.

[2] Actually, the extreme form of this theory would make the term "withdrawal" something of a misnomer. "Withdrawal" implies active (voluntary or "purposeful") reaction *away* from something, whereas, according to the theory, absence of positive action can be explained simply in terms of generalized reduction in effector action.

the contention that diminished reactivity characterizes schizophrenia. Data indicating normal or even greater than normal reactivity have been reported. Altschule and Sulzbach (2) found evidence of normal vasodilation and increased vasoconstriction in a study of the effect of carbon dioxide on acrocyanosis in schizophrenia. Their main conclusions were supported by the work of Freeman (8) and Cameron (5) on temperature regulation. Cohen and Patterson (7) observed abnormally prolonged elevation of pulse in response to painful stimulation in their schizophrenic subjects. Adrenocortical function in response to insulin shock, electroshock and adrenalin injections has been found essentially normal in schizophrenics (23). From recent work, Altschule and his co-workers (1) concluded that reaction of the adrenal cortex to certain physical stresses and to the injection of ACTH in their schizophrenic subjects was not diminished, as compared with the changes observed in nonpsychotic subjects. Further instances of normal physiological reaction to stimulation in chronic schizophrenia have been cited in Hunt and Cofer's (15) review of emotional behavior in schizophrenia.

The stage of the disease presents one source of variation in physiological responsiveness of schizophrenics. Available data are fairly uniform in revealing increased reactivity in *early* schizophrenia (associated with the frequent presence of high levels of anxiety at this stage). Malmo and Shagass (17) found that early schizophrenics were as hyperreactive physiologically as a group of psychoneurotics with severe anxiety. Pfister (24) found increased cardiovascular responsiveness in the early stages of schizophrenia; however, he concluded that as the disease progressed, reactivity diminished, until it was less than normal.

The evidence makes it clear that the "hyporeactitvy theory" in its simplest form is untenable. Yet there is no doubt that schizophrenics' reactions deviate from normals' in terms of what may be tentatively considered as continua of responsiveness. In order to provide the further data needed for the development of a more valid concept of responsiveness in schizophrenia, attention to certain features of experimental design seems desirable. As Sands and Rodnick (28) have argued, more attention should be paid to the specific nature of the stimulus and to the particular aspects of response. Experimental design should provide several stimulating conditions for concurrent observation of several physiological and behavioral indicators.

The purpose of the present report is to present certain data which were taken with these requirements in mind. These data were obtained during the course of a survey investigation of behavioral and physiological reactions of psychiatric patients under stress. The experimental design included the following features: (1) comparison of chronic schizophrenics with psychoneurotics, acute psychotics and nonpatient controls; (2) study of relative responsiveness in the same chronic schizophrenic group under three different conditions of stress; and (3) continuous and simultaneous recording of several physiological and behavioral indicators.

METHODS

Subjects. Our 17 chronic schizophrenic subjects were all cases of relatively long commitment to a mental hospital. They were all males, with ages ranging from 19 to 37 years, with a mean of 28.5 years. Duration of hospitalization ranged from 1.5 to 6 years, averaging 3 years. Duration of illness ranged from 2 to 9 years, with a mean duration of 4.5 years. A clear remission since onset of illness had occurred in only one patient who, however, had required continuous commitment for one year before participating in the present experiments. All cases manifested either delusions, hallucinations or both. Classification as to type of schizophrenia was: paranoid, 10 cases; simple, 4; catatonic, 2; undetermined, 1.

In one respect these cases constituted a selected group, in so far as all were candidates for lobotomy, since insulin and electroconvulsive therapy had been found unsuccessful and they presented problems of management.

For comparative purposes we employed data from 58 unselected patients from the psychiatric wards of a general hospital, which does not accept patients on a commitment basis, and from 21 nonpatient control subjects. For purposes of data analysis the 58 unselected patients were further subdivided into two groups, composed of 44 psychoneurotics and 14 acute psychotics.

Procedure. EMG's from the neck and right arm, heart rate, blood pressure and pneumograph tracings of respiration were all recorded continuously as part of a battery of physiological measurements, taken simultaneously under three standard conditions of stress: Pain-Stress, Rapid Discrimination, and Mirror Drawing. In the Pain-Stress Test the subject received 12 thermal stimulations on his forehead. These stimuli were of painful intensity, and were spaced at intervals of $1\frac{1}{2}$ minutes. The subject's finger rested on a button on which he was instructed to press "when he felt that the stimulus was about to become painful." Five different intensities were employed in fixed order (in watts: 500, 270, 340, 400, 270, 340, 400, 270, 340, 400, 500, 500). All stimuli were 3 seconds in duration except the last which was 1 second.

The Rapid Discrimination Test was an apparatus-paced size discrimination test. The subject, seated in a darkened room, viewed a screen on which were projected 6 numbered circles which varied slightly in size. His task was to choose the largest circle and to call out the appropriate number. The subject was instructed further to press down on the button each time he called out a number. There were 20 sets of circles which always appeared in the same order. This series was run off three times for each subject, allowing first 5 seconds for each discrimination in the series, then 3 seconds, and finally 2 seconds.

There were two Mirror Drawing Tests: drawing of a diagonal line from one point to another (MDT–1), and tracing a circle inside and outside (MDT–2) while viewing the paper in a mirror.

Further details concerning these tests have been presented elsewhere (21).

Results

Muscular tension. The results from EMG measurements in the Pain-Stress Test are plotted in Figures 1 and 2. In Figure 1, mean arm tension for each group is plotted separately for each of the following 10-second periods: before stimulus, during and immediately fol-

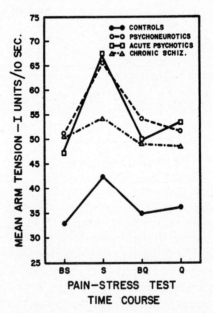

Fig. 1. Mean arm tension during different phases of the Pain-Stress Test in the four subject groups. BS, before stimulus; S, during stimulus; BQ, before questions; Q, during questions.

lowing stimulation, before questioning, and during questioning. Since there were 12 stimulations, tension values (for each subject) were based on 12 separate measurements. I units (or integrator units) refer to an arbitrary scale which was found expedient in connection with the use of electronic integrators. Validation experiments showed that this scale faithfully represented degree of muscular tension (21). Figure 1 shows that with respect to background level of tension (points BS and BQ) chronic schizophrenics resembled the other patients in

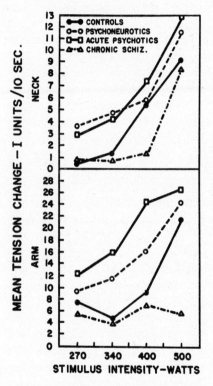

Fig. 2. Mean change in arm and neck tension plotted against intensity of thermal stimulation. Only stimuli of 3 seconds' duration are plotted; stimulus 12 (500 watts for 1 second) is omitted.

showing considerably more tension than controls. Analysis of variance showed that this difference was very significant (P less than .01). The nonsignificant interaction variance, together with the nonsignificant BS-BQ variance indicates that for points BS and BQ, difference in level was the only significant difference between the two groups. Further, there was no significant change from BS to BQ for either group. On the other hand, the schizophrenics' *change* in tension upon stimulation (S) was smaller than that shown by any other group, including normals. The difference, in amount of change, between chronic schizophrenics and the other two patient-groups combined, was a reliable one (P less than .02). There was no significant difference, in change, between chronic schizophrenics and controls.

Rise in arm tension during the stimulation period (S) was associated with the act of pressing on the button to signal pain. The correlation between muscle potential change and frequency of button pressure was 0.57 (based on data from the psychoneurotics and acute psychotics). Consistent with this was the finding that mean frequency of button pressures in the chronic schizophrenic group was significantly lower than that for controls (and other patients).

Figure 2 also shows this lowered responsiveness [3] to the actual pain stimulus in the chronic schizophrenics. Here the ordinates are scaled in terms of amount of *change* in muscle tension during the stimulation period. The lower graphs show arm change for each of the different intensities of stimulation. Note that all curves, except the one for the chronic schizophrenics, show a correlation of amplitude of response with intensity of stimulation. The schizophrenic curve is flat. This flat curve reflects low responsiveness of the chronic schizophrenic group to the actual thermal stimulations, throughout the range of stimulus intensities employed.

The most striking finding in the schizophrenic group was that despite high level of arm tension, the *act* of pressing on the button (to signal pain) was relatively infrequent in this group. Lower responsiveness to the pain stimulus in the chronic schizophrenics is further shown in the graphs for neck tension (see upper graphs, Figure 2). There were fewer instances of head withdrawal in the group of chronic schizophrenics than in any other group (including controls). There were no significant intergroup differences in *level* of neck tension.

Figure 3 presents the muscle potential data from the Rapid Discrimination Test. The figure shows that mean arm tension in the chronic schizophrenic group exceeded the control value in each of the five 30-second periods of measurement (before the test, during each of the three performance priods, and after the test). The largest and most reliable difference between chronic schizophrenics and controls was the one for the 30-second period immediately following instructions

---

[3] There is an important distinction here: between the *specific* response, as measured by change in tension during the 3-second thermal stimulation, and a more general kind of "responsiveness," reflected in the level of tension. This latter may be a response to broad features of the experimental situation. It may, equally, be related to the subject's own thought processes, and hence to a large degree may be independent of any easily denotable aspects of the situation.

and just before test performance commenced ("Before" in Figure 3).

Reliable differences were also found between the tension values of these two groups for the first performance series, and for the period following performance ("I" and "After" in Figure 3). The differences between chronic schizophrenics and controls for the latter two-thirds of performance (II and III in the figure) did not meet the criterion for statistical reliability (5 per cent confidence level).

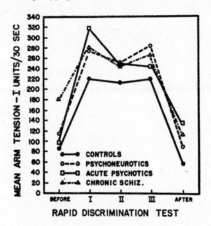

Fig. 3. Mean arm tension during Rapid Discrimination Test. I. First presentation, 5-second rate. II. Second presentation, 3-second rate. III. Third presentation, 2-second rate.

In the Mirror Drawing Tests muscular tension in the chronic schizophrenic group was higher than that of controls, during the "rest" period before instructions, during instruction, and during performance.

Respiration. Respiration was scored in two ways: (a) *Respiratory deviation percentage*: This was obtained by counting the number of respirations which deviated (in either rate or amplitude beyond certain limits arbitrarily set) from the subject's own pre-stimulation averages. For the rate a 30 per cent deviation was set as the limit, and for the amplitude a 50 per cent deviation. Five separate percentage values were computed for each group (see Table I). A percentage was computed by dividing the number of deviating respirations by the total expected from the mean rate. (b) A *respiratory irregularity* rating was made in order to score the effect of thermal stimulation on the contour of the respiration curve at the time of stimulation. Examples of respiration rated plus and minus have been published (17, see Figure 3, p. 13). Respiration was recorded only in the Pain-Stress Test.

The results from these respiratory measurements are presented in Table I. In comparison with the other groups, the chronic schizophrenics were relatively unresponsive in terms of the measure of *respiratory irregularity*. This was particularly evident at the higher intensities (400 and 500 watts) where the chi-square test showed reliable differences between the chronic schizophrenics and the other two groups.

In terms of *total respiratory deviation percentage*, however, there were no significant differences between groups. In contrast to the meas-

TABLE I. GROUP DIFFERENCES IN RESPIRATORY SCORES
PAIN-STRESS TEST

Stimulus Intensity (watts)	Mean Per Cent Respiratory Irregularity				
	500 (1 sec)	270	340	400	500
Controls................	9.52	24.76	30.95	59.05	83.33
Psychon. and Acute Psychot.	24.56	43.62	49.31	69.65	85.86
Chron. Schiz..............	18.75	20.63	28.75	34.38	62.50

	Median Per Cent Respiratory Deviations				
	Amplitude		Rate		Total
	Increase	Decrease	Increase	Decrease	Deviation*
Controls................	7.87	3.23	4.72	3.04	19.33
Psychon. and Acute Psychot.	6.89	3.43	4.14	2.86	23.45
Chron. Schiz..............	4.95	6.62	3.28	3.04	22.45

* Use of medians precludes summation of rows to equal total.

ure of *respiratory irregularity* which reflects abrupt and brief changes in the respiratory curve in response to pain stimulation, this "respiratory" deviation measure reflects unsteadiness of respiration over a longer period of time. Examination of Table I reveals that deviations in the direction of decreased amplitude were more frequent in the chronic schizophrenic group. Differences between this group and the other two groups were statistically reliable (chi-square test). This finding indicates that there was more shallow breathing in our chronic schizophrenic group.

Heart rate. Mean heart rate for chronic schizophrenics during the Pain-Stress Test was reliably higher than that of normal controls (3 per cent level of confidence).

Figure 4 presents heart rate data from the Rapid Discrimination Test. The ordinate is scaled in T-scores which take both age and sex into account, and thus permit direct comparison of heart rates (18).

Note the rise in the curve for chronic schizophrenics, from before performance to during performance, in contrast to the relatively flat curve for normal controls. During performance the mean heart rate of the schizophrenic group reached levels approximating mean heart rates for the psychoneurotic and acute psychotic groups. The schizophrenic group was the only one which showed a statistically reliable increase in heart rate during this test.

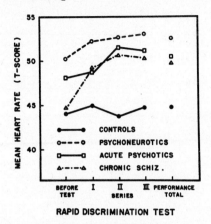

Fig. 4. Mean heart rate during Rapid Discrimination Test. Note rise in heart rate of chronic schizophrenics.

Figure 5 presents heart rate data from the Mirror Drawing Tests. The same trend — toward higher heart rate for chronic schizophrenics than for controls — is again present. The differences, however, are not statistically reliable.

Blood pressure. The systolic blood pressure reactions of the chronic schizophrenics in all tests were very similar to those of the normal controls (lower than the values for psychoneurotics and acute psychotics). Diastolic blood pressure, which was recorded only in connection with the Pain-Stress Test, was significantly higher for chronic schizophrenics than for any other group. Statistical analysis showed the mean pulse pressure for the chronic schizophrenic group to be reliably lower than the corresponding values for any of the other three groups. This finding was consistent for auscultatory measurements, and for machine values both before and during the Pain-Stress Test. These blood pressure data have been presented in greater detail elsewhere (19).

Behavioral indices, performance tests. Twelve chronic schizophrenics co-operated to the extent of attempting the discriminations. This group of 12 cases made significantly fewer correct responses than the controls (and also significantly fewer than the psychoneurotics and acute psychotics). Omissions rather than erroneous responses were responsible for the lower mean score in the chronic schizophrenic group. Detailed analysis of the scores on this test have been presented elsewhere (20).

Thirteen chronic schizophrenics completed the first Mirror Drawing Test and nine completed the second task. In terms of time taken to complete the task, the chronic schizophrenics were inferior to the

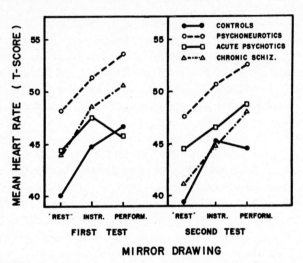

Fig. 5. Mean heart rate during Mirror Drawing Tests. Discussion on page 332.

normal controls in the two Mirror Drawing Tests. Mean scores for these two groups in the first test were 28.00 seconds and 11.67 seconds; and, in the second test, 99.00 and 43.81. Both differences were statistically significant.

DISCUSSION

Present findings are consistent with the conclusion reached from a brief survey of the literature in the introductory section of this paper. Our data do not support the contention that the chronic schizophrenic is generally characterized by low physiological responsiveness. In this discussion we shall first consider our individual findings in relation to previous published data. Secondly, we shall discuss the data within the framework of an analysis of the concept of responsiveness in schizophrenia. Finally, a tentative hypothesis concerning the neural mechanisms underlying deviant responsiveness in schizophrenia will be presented.

Our finding of consistently high heart rates in the chronic schizophrenic group is in agreement with the finding of Cohen and Patterson

(7). Present data on blood pressure are in agreement with Rheingold's finding of lower pulse pressure in schizophrenics (26). High diastolic blood pressure and increase of diastolic pressure under stress appears similar to Freeman and Carmichael's findings in schizophrenics given injections of epinephrine (10). Further, the high diastolic blood pressure observed in our chronic schizophrenic patients may be associated with the frequent finding of acrocyanosis in schizophrenia. Altschule and Sulzbach (2) have shown that this acrocyanosis is due to prolonged vasoconstriction and that it is reversible, even after many years, by the use of carbon dioxide. Since peripheral vasoconstriction is one of the more important factors causing elevation of diastolic blood pressure, it appears likely that the high diastolic blood pressure which we noted in the present schizophrenic patients depended upon this mechanism of vasoconstriction.

One clear instance of low responsiveness in the chronic schizophrenic group was noted in the Pain-Stress Test. The schizophrenics did not press the button to signal pain as often as did the normal controls. Here it is tempting to conclude that pain stimulation was less stressful for the schizophrenics. But this explanation fails to account for the higher *level* of muscular tension in the right arm, the higher heart rate and higher diastolic blood pressure which the schizophrenics showed in comparison with the normal controls.

In order to understand this finding we must distinguish between those aspects of responsiveness which involve background physiological activities (such as heart rate, blood pressure and level of muscular tension), and those aspects which involve "purposive" acts (such as pressing the button to indicate pain, performing size discriminations, and mirror drawings). The first class of activities are diffuse in character, largely involuntary, and frequently associated with emotional arousal. "Purposive" acts are selective rather than diffuse in character, largely voluntary, and less regularly associated with emotional arousal.

Employing this distinction, we find that the schizophrenic group gave evidence of normal or greater than normal background physiological activity in all three stress situations. On the other hand, the "purposive" acts required by the stress tests were less frequently or less well executed by the schizophrenics. In the Pain-Stress Test the act of pressing the button to signal pain was relatively infrequent, even though the level of tension in the signaling arm was high. In the Rapid Discrimination Test, the schizophrenics made no more errors in size judgment than any other group, but they did *omit* significantly more responses. At the same time they showed more heart rate reaction and more evidence of diffuse motor activity (20) than

any other group. In the Mirror Drawing Test, the drawing performance of the schizophrenic group was definitely inferior, whereas background physiological activity was relatively high.

Our data thus indicate that in schizophrenia those aspects of responsiveness which are associated with emotional arousal may remain
intact, while the mechanisms underlying overt, "purposive" acts may
be defective or inoperative. This conclusion is counter to the traditional view that "affect is flat" in chronic schizophrenia. Typically,
the run-of-the-mine *chronic* schizophrenic *appears* emotionally unresponsive to the observer (e.g., in a psychiatric interview).

But this observation may be due more to lack of "purposive"
response to the questions of the examiner than to any general decrease in affectivity. Our chronic schizophrenic group, it should be
emphasized, would similarly have been judged as unresponsive, had
only measures of response to the specific painful stimuli been available. However, measures reflecting general level of activity suggested the opposite — that the chronic schizophrenic was quite "responsive." It is also important to consider that in some cases this
responsiveness may have had determinants which were largely independent of any easily denotable aspects of the situation.

The thought processes of the patients could be one such determinant. This suggestion is strengthened by the subjective reports
given by chronic schizophrenics during a post-test interview, following the Pain-Stress Test. Thus, Subject No. 58: "I was raising some
feelings in myself in relation to the woman psychologist — from the
time I was asked to take the test I was mostly thinking about women
I would see and talk to." Subject No. 67 thought "about going home,"
and was "a little scared." Subject No. 92 was thinking "about their
finding a cancer, or seeing if I was all there."

Similarly, the introspective data from Jonathan Lang [4] support
the view that the actual loss of affective strength in schizophrenia is
considerably less than it has seemed:

From my own experience, I am inclined to the view — taken by some
psychiatrists . . . — that the actual loss of affective strength is considerably
less than it seems. For me, external stimuli still retain a considerable degree
of affective potential even after nine and one half years of the psychosis.
Foods, particularly sweets, still arouse in me pleasant feelings which maintain
a good appetite. My attitude towards my relatives contains a higher affective
content at the present time than it did previous to the psychosis. I go to

[4] In 1939 "Jonathan Lang" (pseudonym) was 32 years old, had attended college three
years and was widely read in psychology. He developed schizophrenic psychosis with
paranoid and catatonic trends in 1929; in 1939 he was still psychotic and was in a sani-
tarium.

shows about once each week and enjoy going to them. My interest in what goes on around me is very little, if any, less than it was before the development of the diseased condition. . . . While the capacity for affective discharge has continued with little abatement, there has been an increasing tendency for affective discharges to be centered around ideation (16, p. 195).

This account supports the hypothesis that mechanisms of emotional arousal may be relatively intact in chronic schizophrenia. Lang's suggestion that affective discharges in schizophrenia come to be centered around ideation is of particular interest and it is in line with the indications from our present physiological data. It may be that the major functional pathology in schizophrenia is to be sought in the mechanisms which underlie "purposive" motor activity.

As the basis for a tentative hypothesis concerning the nature of disturbed "purposive" activity in schizophrenia, we may point out that there is much evidence of a generally higher degree of spontaneous central nervous system activity in schizophrenics than in nonpsychotic persons (by "spontaneous" is meant activity not determined by immediate environmental stimulation). The evidence for this assertion is both clinical and experimental. Hallucinations and delusions are the product of spontaneous central nervous activity. Ideational preoccupation may be interpreted in this way. Rodnick and Shakow's (27) evidence for defective preparatory set in schizophrenia is probably indicative of spontaneous activity interfering with instructions to respond in their reaction time experiments.

If we accept the premise that schizophrenia is characterized by an unusually high amount of spontaneously occurring central nervous activity, we may proceed to examine the finding of disrupted "purposive" activity in the light of the theory of neural action proposed by Hebb (13). In terms of Hebb's phase sequences, stimulation from environmental changes will influence behavior if the neural effects (environmentally initiated phase sequences) happen to "mesh" with the ongoing autonomous central processes (spontaneously occurring phase sequences). In schizophrenia the spontaneous phase sequences appear to dominate neural action to such a large extent that phase sequences set up by environmental stimulation would have less chance of "meshing" and resulting in unitary, effective "purposive" action (action which an observer would consider appropriate in terms of the environmental context).

Furthermore, as Hebb has pointed out, when sensory and central facilitations conflict they produce phase sequences which are mutually incompatible, and emotional disturbance may result. The diffuse aspects of emotional reaction which according to Hebb's theory are caused by such conflicts could appear in the absence of the mechanisms of "purposive" action. However, some of the usual components of emotional reaction such as facial expression and verbal communication may be absent because of interference with their mechanisms by other, spontaneously active mechanisms. This may be the physiological basis of the "split" in schizophrenia.

Since our group of chronic schizophrenics was, to some extent, a selected one and of relatively small size, we must be cautious about generalizing too far from present data. On the other hand, the data clearly showed the need for carefully analyzing the concept of responsiveness. We did obtain evidence which might have been interpreted as supporting the "hyporeactivity" theory had not the simultaneous presence of contradictory data forced a more detailed analysis and a different interpretation.

REFERENCES

1. Altschule, M. D., Promisel, E., Parkhurst, B. H., and Grunebaum, H. Effects of ACTH in patients with mental disease. *Arch. Neurol. Psychiat.*, Chicago, 1950, 64: 641–649.

2. Altschule, M. D. and Sulzbach, W. M. Effect of carbon dioxide on acrocyanosis in schizophrenia. *Arch. Neurol. Psychiat.*, Chicago, 1949, 61: 44–55.

3. Angyal, A., Freeman, H., and Hoskins, R. G. Physiologic aspects of schizophrenic withdrawal. *Arch. Neurol. Psychiat.*, Chicago, 1940, 44: 621–626.

4. Bellak, L. *Dementia praecox*, New York: Grune and Stratton, 1948.

5. Cameron, D. E. Heat production and heat control in the schizophrenic reaction. *Arch. Neurol. Psychiat.*, Chicago, 1934, 32: 704–711.

6. Cohen, L. H., and Fierman, J. H. Metabolic, cardiovascular, and biochemical changes associated with experimentally induced hyperthyroidism in schizophrenia. *Endocrinology*, 1938, 22: 548–558.

7. Cohen, L. H., and Patterson, M. Effect of pain on the heart rate of normal and schizophrenic individuals. *J. gen. Psychol.*, 1937, 17: 273–289.

8. Freeman, H. Skin and body temperatures of schizophrenic and normal subjects under varying environmental conditions. *Arch. Neurol. Psychiat.*, Chicago, 1939, 42: 724–734.

9. Freeman, H. Heat-regulatory mechanisms in normal and in schizophrenic subjects: under basal conditions and after the administration of dinitrophenol. *Arch. Neurol. Psychiat.*, Chicago, 1940, 43: 456–462.

10. Freeman, H., and Carmichael, H. T. A pharmacodynamic investigation of the autonomic nervous system in schizophrenia: I. Effect of intravenous injections of epinephrine on the blood pressure and pulse rate. *Arch. Neurol. Psychiat.*, Chicago, 1935, 33: 342–352.

11. Freeman, H., and Rodnick, E. H. Autonomic and respiratory responses of schizophrenic and normal subjects to changes of intra-pulmonary atmosphere. *Psychosom. Med.*, 1940, 2: 101–109.

12. Freeman, H., and Rodnick, E. H. Effect of rotation on postural steadiness in normal and in schizophrenic subjects. *Arch. Neurol. Psychiat.*, Chicago, 1942, 48: 47–53.

13. Hebb, D. O. *The organization of behavior,* New York: Wiley, 1949.

14. Hoskins, Roy G. *The biology of schizophrenia,* New York: Norton, 1946.

15. Hunt, J. McV., and Cofer, C. N. Psychological deficit. In J. McV. Hunt (ed.), *Personality and the behavior disorders,* New York: Ronald, 1944, II, 971–1032.

16. Lang, J. The other side of the affective aspects of schizophrenia. *Psychiatry,* 1939, 2: 195–202.

17. Malmo, R. B., and Shagass, C. Physiologic studies of reaction to stress in anxiety and early schizophrenia. *Psychosom. Med.,* 1949, 11: 9–24.

18. Malmo, R. B., and Shagass, C. Variability of heart rate in relation to age, sex and stress. *J. appl. Physiol.,* 1949, 2: 181–184.

19. Malmo, R. B., and Shagass, C. Studies of blood pressure in psychiatric patients under stress. *Psychosom. Med.* (in press).

20. Malmo, R. B., Shagass, C., Bélanger, D. J., and Smith, A. A. Motor control in psychiatric patients under stress. *J. abnorm. soc. Psychol.* (in press).

21. Malmo, R. B., Shagass, C., and Davis, J. F. Electromyographic studies of muscular tension in psychiatric patients under stress. *J. clin. exp. Psychopath.,* 1951, 12: 45–66.

22. May, P. R. A. Pupillary abnormalities in schizophrenia and during muscular effort. *J. ment. Sci.,* 1948, 94: 89–98.

23. Parsons, E. H., Gildea, E. F., Ronzoni, E., and Hulbert, S. Z. Comparative lymphocytic and biochemical responses of patients with schizophrenia and affective disorders to electroshock, insulin shock, and epinephrine. *Amer. J. Psychiat.,* 1949, 105: 573–580.

24. Pfister, H. O. Disturbances of the autonomic nervous system in schizophrenia and their relations to the insulin, cardiazol and sleep treatments. *Amer. J. Psychiat. Suppl.,* 1938, 109: 94–118.

25. Pincus, G., Hoagland, H., Freeman, H., Elamadjian, F., and Romanoff, L. P. A study of pituitary-adrenocortical function in normal and psychotic men. *Psychosom. Med.,* 1949, 11: 74–101.

26. Rheingold, J. C. Autonomic integration in schizophrenia. *Psychosom. Med.,* 1939, 1: 397–413.

27. Rodnick, E. H., and Shakow, D. Set in the schizophrenic as measured by a composite reaction time index. *Amer. J. Psychiat.,* 1940, 97: 214–225.

28. Sands, S. L., and Rodnick, E. H. Concept and experimental design in the study of stress and personality. *Amer. J. Psychiat.,* 1950, 106: 673–679.

23

A STUDY OF FAIRBAIRN'S THEORY OF SCHIZOID REACTIONS

H. GUNTRIP

Department of Psychiatry, Leeds University, England

I. The Schizoid Condition

The psychotherapist must be greatly concerned with those states of mind in which patients become inaccessible emotionally, when the patient seems to be bodily present but mentally absent. A patient, *A*, recently said 'I don't seem to come here' as if she came in body but did not bring herself with her. She found herself in the same state of mind when she asked the young man next door to go for a walk with her. He did and she became tired, dull, unable to talk; she commented: 'It was the same as when I come here: I don't seem to be present.' Her reactions to food were similar. She would long for a nice meal and sit down to it and find her appetite gone, as if she had nothing to do with eating. One patient, *B*, dreamed: 'My husband and I came to see you and he explained that I wasn't here because I'd gone to hospital.' Complaints of feeling cut off, shut off, out of touch, feeling apart or strange, of things being out of focus or unreal, of not feeling one with people, or of the point having gone out of life, interest flagging, things seeming futile and meaningless, all describe in various ways this state of mind. Patients often call it 'depression,' but it lacks the heavy, black, inner sense of brooding, of anger and of guilt, which are not difficult to discover in depression. Depression is really a more extraverted state of mind, in which the patient is struggling not to break out into angry and aggressive behaviour. The states described above are rather the 'schizoid states'. They are definitely introverted.

External relationships seem to have been emptied by a massive withdrawal of the real libidinal self. Effective mental activity has disappeared into a hidden inner world; the patient's conscious ego is emptied of vital feeling and action, and seems to have become unreal. You may catch glimpses of intense activity going on in the inner world through dreams and phantasies, but the patient's conscious ego merely reports these as if it were a neutral observer not personally

From *British Journal of Medical Psychology*, 25: 86, 1952, published by Cambridge University Press.

involved in the inner drama of which it is a detached spectator. The attitude to the outer world is the same; *non-involvement and observation at a distance without any feeling*, like that of a press reporter describing a social gathering of which he is not a part, in which he has no personal interest, and by which he is bored. When a schizoid state supervenes, the conscious ego appears to be in a state of suspended animation in between two worlds, internal and external and having no real relationships with either of them. It has decreed an emotional and impulsive standstill, on the basis of keeping out of affective range and being unmoved.

These schizoid states may alternate with depression, and at times seem to be rather confusingly mixed with it so that both schizoid and depressive signs appear. They are of all degrees of intensity ranging from transient moods that come and go during a session, to states that persist over a long period, when they show very clearly and distinctly the specific schizoid traits.

An example of a patient, *C*, describing herself as depressed when she is really schizoid may be useful at this point. She opened the session by saying: 'I'm very depressed. I've been just sitting and couldn't get out of the chair. There seemed no purpose anywhere, the future blank. I'm very bored and want a big change. I feel hopeless, resigned, no way out, stuck. I'm wondering how I can manage somehow just to get around and put up with it.' (Analyst: 'Your solution is to damp everything down, don't feel anything, give up all real relationship to people on an emotional level, and just "do things" in a mechanical way, be a robot.') Her reaction brought out clearly the schizoid trait: 'Yes, I felt I didn't care, didn't register anything. Then I felt alarmed, felt this was dangerous. If I hadn't made myself do something I'd have just sat, not bothered, not interested.' (Analyst: 'That's your reaction in analysis to me: don't be influenced, don't be moved, don't be lured into reacting to me.') Her reply was: 'If I were moved at all; I'd feel very annoyed with you. I hate and detest you for making me feel like this. The more I'm inclined to be drawn towards you, the more I feel a fool, undermined.'

The mere fact of the analyst's presence as another human being with whom she needed to be emotionally real, i.e. express what she was actually feeling, created an emotional crisis in her with which she could only deal by abolishing the relationship. So her major defence against her anxieties is to keep herself emotionally out of reach, inaccessible, and keep everyone at arm's length. She once said: 'I'd rather hate you than love you,' but this goes even further. She will neither love nor hate, she won't feel anything at all, and outwardly in sessions often appears lazy, bored at coming, and with a 'laissez faire' attitude.

This then is the problem we seek to understand. What is really happening to these patients and why?

II. Fairbairn's Theory of Schizoid Reactions

The purpose of this paper is to state Fairbairn's theory of schizoid reactions and to illustrate it by clinical material. His revolutionary rethinking of psycho-analytical theory was first presented as a recasting of the classic libido theory and as a revised psychopathology of the psychoses and psycho-neuroses. Only two points in his theory need be mentioned here.

(1). First he laid it down that the goal of the individual's libido is not pleasure, or merely subjective gratification, but the object itself. He says: 'Pleasure is the sign-post to the object' (1941, p. 255). The fundamental fact about human nature is our libidinal drive towards good object-relationships. The key biological formula is the adaptation of the organism to the environment. The key psychological formula is the relationship of the person to the human environment. The significance of human living lies in object-relationships, and only in such terms can our life be said to have a meaning.

Quite specially in this region lie the schizoid's problems. He is driven by anxiety to cut off all object-relations. Our needs, fears, frustrations, resentments and anxieties in our inevitable quest for good objects are the real problem in psychopathology, because they are the real problem in life itself. When difficulties in achieving and maintaining good object-relations are too pronounced, and human relations are attended with too great anxiety and conflict, desperate efforts are often made to deny and eliminate this basic need. People go into their shell, bury themselves in work of an impersonal nature, abolish relations with actual people so far they can and devote themselves to abstractions, ideals, theories, organizations,[1] and so on. In the nature of the case these manoeuvres cannot succeed and always end disastrously, since they are an attempt to deny our very nature itself. Clearly we cannot do that and remain healthy.

The more people cut themselves off from human relations in the outer world, the more they are driven back on object-relations in their inner mental world, till the psychotic lives only in his inner world. But it is still a world of object-relations. We are constitutionally incapable of living as isolated units. The real loss of all objects would be equivalent to psychic death. Karen Horney (1946) says: 'Neuroses are generated by disturbances in human relationships.' But Horney thinks

---

[1] This does not imply that such activities are necessarily always schizoid. That depends on how much personal feeling enters into the activity.

only in terms of relations to external objects at the conscious level. The real heart of the matter is a far less obvious danger, a repressed world of internalized psychic objects, bad objects, and 'bad-object situations.' What is new in all this is the theory of internal objects as developed in more elaborate form by Melanie Klein and Fairbairn, and the fact that Fairbairn makes object-relations, not instinctual impulses, the prior and important thing. It is the object that is the real goal of the libidinal drive. We seek persons not pleasures. Impulses are not psychic entities but reactions of an ego to objects.

What is meant by a world of internal objects may be expressed as follows: in some sense we retain all our experience in life and 'carry things in our minds'. If we did not, we would lose all continuity with our past, would only be able to live from moment to moment like butterflies alighting and flitting away, and no relationships or experiences could have any permanent values for us. Thus in some sense everything is mentally internalized, retained and inwardly possessed; that is our only defence against complete discontinuity in living, a distressing example of which we see in the man who loses his memory, and is consciously uprooted.

But things are mentally internalized and retained in two different ways which we call respectively *memory* and *internal objects*. Good objects are, in the first place, mentally internalized and retained only as memories. They are enjoyed at the time, the experience is satisfying and leaves no problems, and can later on be looked back to and reflected on with pleasure. In the case of a continuing good-object relationship of major importance as with a parent or marriage partner, we have a combination of memories of the happy past and confidence in the continuing possession of the good object in an externally real sense in the present and future. There is no reason here for setting up internalized objects. Outer experience suffices to meet our needs. On this point Fairbairn differs from Melanie Klein.

Objects are only internalized in a more radical way when the relationship turns into a bad-object situation through, say, the object changing or dying. When someone we need and love ceases to love us, or behaves in such a way that we interpret it as cessation of love, that person becomes, in an emotional, libidinal sense, a bad object. This happens to a child when his mother refuses the breast, weans the baby, or is cross, impatient and punitive, or is absent temporarily or for a longer period through illness, or permanently through death: it also happens when the person we need is emotionally detached and aloof and unresponsive. All that is experienced as frustration of the most important of all needs, as rejection and desertion or else as persecution and attack. Then the lost object, now become a bad object, is mentally internalized in a much more vital and fundamental sense than memory. Bereaved people dream vividly of the lost loved one, even years afterwards, as still actually alive. A patient, beset by a life-long fear of dying, was found under analysis, to be persistently dreaming of dead men in coffins. In one dream, the coffined figure was behind a curtain and his mind was on it all the time while he was busy in the dream with cheerful social activities. A fatal inner attraction to, and attachment to, the dead man threatened him and set up an actual fear of dying. The dead man was his father as he had seen him actually in his coffin. Another patient had a nightmare of his mother violently losing her temper with him, after she had been dead twelve years. _An inner psychic world_ (see Riviere, 1952) _has been set up duplicating the original situation, but it is an unhappy world in which one is tied to bad objects and feeling therefore always frustrated, hungry, angry, and guilty, and profoundly anxious._

It is bad objects which are internalized, because we cannot accept their badness and yet cannot give them up, cannot leave them alone, cannot master and control them in outer reality and so keep on struggling to possess them, alter them and compel them to change into good objects, in our inner psychic world. They never do change. In our inner unconscious world where we repress and lock away very early in life our original bad objects, they remain always rejecting, indifferent or hostile to us according to our actual outer experience. It must be emphasized that these internalized objects are not just phantasies. The child is emotionally identified with his objects, and when he mentally incorporates them he remains identified with them and they become part and parcel of the very psychic structure of his personality. The phantasies in which internal objects reveal their existence to consciousness are activities of the structures which constitute the internal objects. Objects are only internalized later in life in this radical way by fusion with already existing internal-object structures. In adult life situations in outer reality are unconsciously interpreted in the light of these situations persisting in unconscious, inner, and purely psychic reality. We live in the outer world with the emotions generated in the inner one. The fundamental psychopathological problem is: how do people deal with their internalized bad objects, to what extent do they feel identified with them, and how do they complicate relations with external objects. It is the object all the time that matters, whether external or internal, not pleasure.

(2) From this point of view Fairbairn constructed a revised theory of the psychoses and psychoneuroses, the second point relevant for our purpose. In the orthodox Freud-Abraham view, these illnesses were due to arrests of libidinal development at fixation points in the first five

years: schizophrenia at the oral sucking stage, manic-depression at the oral biting stage, paranoia at the early anal; obsessions at the late anal; and hysteria at the phallic or early genital stages. Fairbairn proposed a totally different view, based not on the fate of libidinal impulses, but on the nature of relationships with internal bad objects. For him, *the schizoid and depressive states are the two fundamental types of reaction in bad-object relationships, the two basic or ultimate dangers to be escaped from.* They originate in the difficulties experienced in object-relationships in the oral stage of absolute infantile dependence and he treats of paranoia, obsessions, hysteria and phobias as four different defensive techniques for dealing with internal bad objects so as to master them and ward off a relapse into the depressed or schizoid states of mind. This makes intelligible the fact that patients ring the changes actually on paranoid, obsessional, hysteric and phobic reactions even if any particular patient predominantly favours one technique most of the time. The psychoneuroses are, basically, defences against internal bad-object situations which would otherwise set up depressive or schizoid states; though these situations are usually re-activated by a bad external situation.

Thus what has to be done in deep treatment is to help the patient to drop these unsatisfactory techniques which never solve the problem, and find courage to become conscious of what lies behind these symptom-producing struggles with internal bad objects; in other words, to risk going back into the basic bad-object situations in which they feel they are succumbing to one or other of the two ultimate psychic dangers, depression or schizoid loss of affect. Naturally depressive and schizoid reactions constantly break through into consciousness, in varying degrees of severity, in spite of defences.

(3) The nature of the two ultimately dangerous situations may be simply described. When you want love from a person who will not give ① it and so becomes a bad object to you, you can react in either or both of two ways. You may become angry and enraged at the frustration and want to make an aggressive attack on the bad object to force it to become good and stop frustrating you: like a small child who cannot get what it wants from the mother and who flies into a temper-tantrum and hammers on her with his little fists. This is the problem of hate or love made angry. It is an attack on a hostile, rejecting, actively refusing bad-object. It leads to *depression* for it rouses the fear that one's hate will destroy the very person one needs and loves.

But there is an earlier and more basic reaction. When you cannot get ② what you want from the person you need, instead of getting angry you may simply go on getting more and more hungry, and full of a sense of painful craving, and a longing to get total and complete possession of your love-object so that you cannot be left to starve. _Love made hungry is the schizoid_ problem and it rouses the terrible fear than one's love has become so devouring and incorporative that love itself has become destructive. Depression is the fear of loving lest one's hate should destroy. Schizoid aloofness is the fear of loving lest one's love should destroy, which is far worse.

This difference of the two attitudes goes along with a difference in appearance, so to speak, of the object. The schizoid sees the object as a desirable deserter, or as Fairbairn calls it, an exciting _needed object_ [2] whom he must go after hungrily but then draw back from lest he should devour and destroy it in his desperately intense need to get total possession of it. The depressive sees the object as a hateful denier, or in Fairbairn's term a _rejecting object_ to be destroyed out of the way to make room for a good-object. Thus one patient constantly dreams of wanting a woman who goes away and leaves him, while another dreams of furious, murderous anger against a sinister person who robs him or gets between him and what he wants. The schizoid is hungry for a desirable deserter, the depressive is murderous against a hateful robber.

Thus the two fundamental forms of internal bad objects are, in Fairbairn's terminology, the needed object and the rejecting object. In the course of years many externally real figures of both sexes may be absorbed, by layering and fusion, into these two internal bad objects, but at bottom they remain always two aspects of the breast-mother. They are always there, and parts of the ego (split off, disowned, secondary or subsidiary 'selves') are always having disturbing relationships with them, so that the depressive is always being goaded to anger, and the schizoid always being tantalized and made hungry.

The depressive position is later and more developed than the schizoid, for it is ambivalent. The hateful robber is really an aspect of the same person who is needed and desired, as if the mother excites the child's longing for her, gives him just enough to tantalize and inflame his appetite, and then robs him by taking herself away. This was neatly expressed in patient _C_'s dream. 'I was enjoying my favourite meal and saved the nicest bit to the end, and then mother snatched it (the breast, herself) away under my nose. I was furious but when I protested she said "Don't be a baby".' There is the guilt reaction, agreeing with the denier against oneself and giving up one's own needs. Fairbairn holds that depression has occupied too exclusively the centre of the picture of psychopathological states as a result of Freud's concentration on obsessions with their ambivalence, guilt and super-ego problems. He believes the schizoid condition is the fundamental problem and is pre-ambivalent.

[2] Fairbairn now prefers simply the term 'Exciting Object' (E.O.).

Melanie Klein (1932, 1948) stressed how ambivalence rises to its maximum over the weaning crisis at a time when the infant has learned to bite and can react sadistically. Love and hate block each other. The infant attacks and also feels identified with, the object of his aggression, and so feels guilty and involves himself in the fate, factual or phantasied, of the object. Hate of the object involves hate of oneself, you suffer with the object you attack because you cannot give up the object and feel one with it. Hence the familiar guilt and depression after a bereavement: you feel guilty as if you have killed the lost person and depressed as if you were dying with him or her. Three patients who all suffered marked guilt and depression recovered repressed and internalized death-bed scenes of a parent.

What is the meaning of hate? It is not the absolute opposite of love; that would be indifference, having no interest in a person, not wanting a relationship and so having no reason for either loving or hating, feeling nothing. Hate is love grown angry because of rejection. We can only really hate a person if we want their love. Hate is an expression of frustrated love needs, an attempt to destroy the bad rejecting side of a person in the hope of leaving their good responsive side available, a struggle to alter them. The anxiety is over the danger of hate destroying both sides, and the easiest way out is to find two objects and love one and hate the other.

But as we have seen, the individual can adopt an earlier simpler reaction. Instead of reacting with anger, he can react with an enormously exaggerated sense of need. Desire becomes hunger and hunger becomes greed which is hunger grown frightened of losing what it wants. He feels so uncertain about possessing his love-object that he feels a desperate craving to make sure of it by getting it inside him, swallowing it and incorporating it. This is illustrated by patient B, who phantasied standing with a vacuum cleaner (herself, empty and hungry), and everyone who came near she sucked them into it. At a more normal and ordinarily conscious level this is expressed by patient C thus: 'I'm afraid I couldn't make moderate demands on people, so I don't make any demands at all.' Many people show openly this devouring possessiveness towards those they love. Many more repress it and keep out of real relations.

This dream brings out the schizoid situation. So much fear is felt of devouring everyone and so losing everyone in the process, that a general withdrawal from all external relationships is embarked on. Retreat into indifference, the true opposite of the love which is felt to be too dangerous to express. Want no one, make no demands, abolish all external relationships, and be aloof, cold, without any feeling, do not be moved by anything. The withdrawn libido is turned inwards, introverted. The

patient goes into his shell and is busy only with internal objects, towards
whom he feels the same devouring attitude. Outwardly everything seems
futile and meaningless. Fairbairn considers that a sense of 'futility' is
the specific schizoid affect. Just as the depressive is identified with the
one he attacks and so hurts himself, so the schizoid is identified with
the object he devours and loses, and so loses himself; e.g. the snake
eating its own tail. The depressive fears loss of his object. The schizoid,
in addition, fears loss of his ego, of himself.

III. The Schizoid's Relation to Objects (Need and Fear of
     Object-Relations)

A. ACTIVE. FEAR OF LOSS OF THE OBJECT

(1) *The object as a desired deserter or 'needed object'*

Theory only lives when it is seen as describing the actual reactions
of real people, though the material revealing the schizoid position only
becomes undisguisedly accessible at deep levels of analysis, and is often
not reached when defences are reasonably effective. In the very unstable schizoid it breaks through with disconcerting ease, a bad sign.

A headmaster, *D*, described himself as depressed, and went on to
say, 'I don't feel so worried about the school or hopeless about the
future.' He had said the same things the week before and regarded it
as a sign of improvement, but the real meaning emerged when he remarked 'Perhaps my interest in school has flagged' and it appeared
that his loss of the sense of hopelessness about the future was due
simply to his not thinking about the future. He had cut it off. He then
reported a dream of visiting a camp school. 'The resident head walked
away when I arrived and left me to fend for myself and there was no
meal ready for me.' He remarked: 'I'm preoccupied with what I'm
going to eat and when, yet I don't eat a lot. Also I want to get away
from people and am more comfortable when eating alone. I'm concerned at my loss of interest in school. I don't feel comfortable with
father and prefer to be in another room. I'm very introverted; I feel
totally cut off.'

Here is a gradually emerging description, not of depression but of a
schizoid state, loss of interest in present and future, loss of appetite
for food, getting away from people, introverted, totally cut off. The
situation that calls out the reaction is that of being faced with a desired
but deserting object, the head in the dream who prepares no meal for
him, and leaves him to fend for himself when he is hungry. The head is
the father, of whom he complains that he can never get near him: also
the analyst to whom he says: 'you remain the analyst, you won't indulge
me in a warm personal relationship, you won't be my friend. I want

something more personal than analysis.' The schizoid is very sensitive and quickly feels unwanted, because he is always being deserted in his inner world.

Faced with these desired deserters he first feels exaggeratedly hungry, and then denies his hunger, eats little and turns away from people till he feels introverted and totally cut off. He has withdrawn his libido from the objects he cannot possess, and feels loss of interest and loss of appetite. There is little evidence of anger and guilt as there would be in depression; his attitude is more that of fear and retreat.

(2) *The object as being devoured*

This entire problem is frequently worked out over food. The above patient is hungry but rejects both food and people. He can only eat alone. The patient *C* says that whenever her husband comes in she at once feels hungry and must eat. Really she is hungry for him but dare not show it. The same turning away from what one feels too greedily and devouringly hungry for is shown very clearly by this same patient in other ways. Visiting friends she was handed a glass of sherry, took a quick sip and put it down and did not touch it again. She had felt she wanted to swallow it at one gulp. Her general attitude to food was one of rejection. Appetite would disappear at the sight of food, she would nibble at a dish and push it away, or force it down and feel sick. But what lay behind this rejecting attitude was expressed in a dream in which she was eating an enormous meal and just went on and on and on endlessly. She is getting as much as she can inside her before it is taken away as in the dream where her mother whipped it away under her nose. Her attitude is incorporative, to get it inside where she cannot be robbed of it, because she has no confidence about being given enough. The breast one is sure of can be sucked at contentedly and let go when one feels satisfied: one knows it will be available when needed again. The breast that does not come when wanted, is not satisfying when one has it because it might be snatched away before need is met. It rouses a desperate hungry urge to make sure of it, not by merely sucking at it but by swallowing it, getting it inside one altogether. The impulse changes from 'taking in from the breast' into an omnivorous urge to 'take in the whole breast itself.' The object is incorporated. The contented baby sucks, the angry and potentially depressive baby bites, the hungry and potentially schizoid baby wants to swallow, as in the case of the vacuum cleaner phantasy. A patient who at first made sucking noises in sessions, then changed to compulsive gulping and swallowing and nausea.

Fairbairn (1941, p. 252) writes: "The paranoid, obsessional, and hysterical states — to which may be added the phobic state — essentially represent, not products of fixations at specific libidinal phases, but simply a variety of techniques employed to defend the ego against the effects of conflicts of oral origin.'

Now, as Fairbairn says: 'You can't eat your cake and have it.' This hungry, greedy, devouring, swallowing up, incorporating attitude leads to deep fears lest the real external object be lost. This anxiety about destroying and losing the love-object through being so devouringly hungry is terribly real. Thus the patient C, who has become more conscious of her love-hunger with the result that on the one hand her appetite for food has increased enormously, and on the other her anxious attitude to her husband has become more acute, says: 'When he comes in I feel ravenously hungry, and eat, but towards him I'm afraid I'm a nuisance. If I make advances to him I keep saying "I'm not a nuisance am I, you don't 'not want me' do you?" I'm terribly anxious about it all, it's an appalling situation, I'm scared stiff, it's all so violent. I've an urge to get hold of him and hold him so tight that he can't breathe, shut him off from everything but me.' She has the same transference reaction to the analyst. She dreamed that 'I came for treatment and you were going off to America with a lot of people. Someone dropped out so I went and you weren't pleased.' Her comment was 'you didn't want me but I wasn't going to be thrown off. I was thinking to-day of your getting ill, suppose you died. Then I got in a furious temper. I'd like to strangle you, kill you.' That is, get a strangle-hold on the analyst so that he could not leave her, but then he might be killed. The schizoid person is afraid of wearing out, of draining, or exhausting and ultimately losing love-objects. As Fairbairn says, the terrible dilemma of the schizoid is that love itself is destructive, and he dare not love. Hence he withdraws into detachment and aloofness. All intimate relationships are felt in terms of eating, swallowing up, and are too dangerous to be risked. The above patient says: 'I lay half awake looking at my husband and thinking, "What a pity he's going to die." It seemed fixed. Then I felt lonely, no point of relationship with all I could see. I love him so much but I seem to have no choice about destroying him. I want something badly and then daren't move a finger to get it. I'm paralysed.'

(3) *Schizoid reactions to food and eating*

From the foregoing we may summarize the schizoid's reactions to food and eating, for since his basic problems in relation to objects derive from his reactions to the breast, food and eating naturally play a large part in his struggles to solve these problems. His reactions to people and to food are basically the same. Thus patient C says: 'Two men friends make me excited but it's not even a taste, only a smell of a good meal. I'm always feeling I want to be with one or the other of them, but I can't do it or I'll lose them both. One of them kissed me and I gave him a hug and a kiss and enjoyed it and wanted more. Ought I? I've sought desperately for so long and now I feel I must run away from it. I don't want to eat these days. I couldn't sleep. I felt I'd lost him: what if he or I had an accident and got killed. It's ridiculous but I'm in a constant furore of anxiety, I must see him: nothing else matters. I knew I'd be like this if I didn't see him but I didn't go. It's funny, I don't think I'm in love with him, yet I need him desperately. I can't engage in any other activity. I felt the same with a fellow ten years ago. He went away for a day and I was in an agony of fear; what if he were killed, an awful dread. It feels it must happen. I don't even like mentioning it in case this present friend gets killed, and I feel I'll have an accident, too. I get desperately tired, and feel empty inside and have to buy sweet biscuits and gobble them up.'

Thus she has the kind of relation with this man (and with all objects) that compromises her stable existence as a separate person when she is not with him: she goes to bits. She wants to eat him up as it were, and feels swallowed up in her relation to him, and feels the destruction of both is inevitable whether she is with him or apart from him.

The patient *B*, before she started analysis, was having visual hallucinations of leopards leaping across in front of her with their mouths wide open. At an advanced stage of treatment these faded into phantasies and she had a phantasy of two leopards trying to swallow each other's head. She would enjoy a hearty meal and then promptly be sick and reject it. *There is a constant oscillation between hungry eating and refusal to eat, longing for people and rejecting them.*

(4) *The transference situation*

The necessary and inevitable frustration of a patient's libidinal needs in the analytical situation is peculiarly well adapted to bring out schizoid reactions, as we have already noted. The patient longs for the analyst's love, may recognize intellectually that a steady, consistent, genuine, concern for the patient's well-being is a true form of love, yet, because it is not love in a full libidinal sense (Fairbairn reminds us that it is *agape*, not *eros*), the patient does not 'feel' it as love. He feels rather that the analyst is cold, indifferent, bored, not interested, not listening, busy with something else while the patient talks, rejective. Patients will react to the analyst's silence by stopping talking to make him say something. The analyst excites by his presence but does not libidinally satisfy, and so constantly arouses a hungry craving.

The patient will then begin to feel he is bad for the analyst, that he is wasting his time, depressing him by pouring out a long story of troubles. He will want, and fear, to make requests lest he is imposing on the analyst and making illegitimate demands. He may say 'How on earth can you stand this constant strain of listening to this sort of thing day after day?' and in general feels he is draining and exhausting, i.e. devouring, the analyst.

He will oscillate between expressing his need and feeling guilty about it. The patient *A* says: 'I felt I must get possession of something of yours. I thought I'd come early and enjoy your arm chair and read your books in the waiting room.' But then she switches over to: 'You can't possibly want to let me take up your time week after week.' Guilt and anxiety then dictate a reversal of the original relationship. The patient must now be passive and begins to see the analyst as the active devourer. He drains the patient of recources by charging fees, he wants to dominate and subjugate the patient, he will rob him of his personality. A patient, after a long silence, says: 'I'm thinking I must be careful, you're going to get something out of me.' The analyst will absorb or rob the patient.

This terrible oscillation may make a patient feel confused and not know where he is. Thus a patient, *E*, says: 'I've been thinking I might lose your help, you'll make an excuse to get rid of me. I want more analysis but you don't bother with me. Analysis is only a very small part of a week. You don't understand me. There's a part of me I don't bring into analysis. I might be swallowed up in your personality and lose my individuality, so I adopt a condescending attitude to you. What you say isn't important, you're only a bourgeois therapist and don't understand the conditions of my life, your focus of analytical capacity is tiny, you're cabined within bourgeois ideas. But if I said what I felt, I'd make you depressed and lose your support. You ought to be able to give me specific advice to help me when I feel helpless and imprisoned. I feel much the same with my girl. In analysis I feel I should get out, and away from it I feel I should be in. This week I feel in a "no man's land." '

Here the whole dilemma of 'craving for' yet 'not being able to accept' the needed person, comes out in transference on the analyst. The swing over in transference to the opposite, from 'devouring' to 'being devoured,' leads to the specific consideration of the passive aspect of the schizoid's relation to objects.

B. PASSIVE. FEAR OF THE LOSS OF INDEPENDENCE

(1) *The object as devouring the ego*

The patients' fears of a devouring sense of need towards objects is paralleled by the fear that others have the same 'swallowing up" attitude to them. Thus patient *C* says: 'I can't stand crowds, they swallow me up. With you I feel if I accept your help I'll be subjugated, lose my personality, be smothered. Now I feel withdrawn like a snail, but now you can't swallow me up. I get a "shutting myself off" attitude which lessens my anxiety.'

The patient *B*, a very schizoid married woman of 30, has for a long time been talking out devouring phantasies of all kinds, and slowly emerging from her schizoid condition. She was thin, white, cold, aloof, frigid: often it was some time before she could start talking in session, and would arrive terrified but hiding it under an automatic laugh or bored expression. When she did start talking she would begin to look tense, and tears would roll silently down and she would say she felt frightened. Gradually she has begun to talk more freely and put on weight and colour and be capable of sexual relationships with her husband. Her phantasies included those of his penis eating her and of her vagina biting off his penis. On one occasion she said: 'Last night I felt excited at coming here to-day, and then terrified and confused. I couldn't sleep for thinking of you. I felt drawn towards you and then shot back. Then I felt I was one big mouth all over and just wanting to get you inside. But sometimes I feel you'll eat me.'

A male patient, *F*, of 40, living in a hostel reported that he had begun to get friendly with another very decent type of man there, and commented: 'I've begun to get frightened. I don't know why but I feel it's dangerous and I just cut myself off. When I see him coming I shoot off up to my bedroom.' Then he reported a nightmare from which he had awakened in great fear. A monster was coming after him and its huge mouth closed over him like a trap and he was engulfed. Then he burst out of its head and killed it. So the schizoid not only fears devouring and losing the love-object, but also that the other person will devour him. Then he becomes claustrophobic, and expresses this in such familiar ways as feeling restricted, tied, imprisoned, trapped, smothered, and must break away to be free and recover and safeguard his independence: so he retreats from object-relations. With people, he feels either bursting (if he is getting them into himself) or smothered (if he feels he is being absorbed and losing his personality in them) These anxieties are often expressed by starting up in the night feeling choking, and is one reason for fear of going to sleep.

(2) Relationships as a mutual devouring

We are now in a position to appreciate the terrible dilemma in which
the schizoid person is caught in object-relationships. Owing to his intensely hungry and unsatisfied need for love, and his consequent incorporating and monopolizing attitude towards those he needs, he cannot help seeing his objects in the light of his own desires towards them.
The result is that any relationship into which some genuine feeling
goes, immediately comes to be felt deep down, and unconsciously
experienced, as a mutual devouring. Such intense anxiety results that
there seems to be no alternative but to withdraw from relationships altogether, to prevent the loss of his independence. Relationships are felt
to be too dangerous to enter into.

IV. THE SCHIZOID RETREAT FROM OBJECTS

(1) The 'in and out' programme

The chronic dilemma in which the schizoid individual is placed,
namely that he can neither be in a relationship with another person nor
out of it, without in various ways risking the loss of both his object and
himself, is due to the fact that he has not yet outgrown the particular
kind of dependence on love-objects that is characteristic of infancy:
namely identification in an emotional sense, and the wish to incorporate
in a conative, active sense. He and those he loves feel to be part and
parcel of one another, so that when separated he feels utterly insecure
and lost, but when reunited he feels swallowed, absorbed, and loses his
separate individuality by regression to infantile dependence. Thus he
must always be rushing into a relationship for security and at once
breaking out again for freedom and independence: an alternation between regression to the womb and the struggle to be born, between the
merging of his ego in, and the differentiation of it from, the person he
loves. The schizoid cannot stand alone, yet is always fighting desperately to defend his independence: like those film stars who spend
their best years rushing into and out of one marriage after another.

This 'in and out' programme, always breaking away from what one
is at the same time holding on to, is perhaps the most characteristic
behavioural expression of the schizoid conflict. Thus a young man engaged to be married says: 'When I'm with Dorothy I'm quiet, I think
"I can't afford to let myself go and let her see that I want her. I must
let her see I can get on without her." So I keep away from her and
appear indifferent.' He experienced the same conflict about jobs. He
phantasied getting a job in South America or China, but in fact turned
down every job that would take him away from home. A girl in the

twenties says: 'When I'm at home I want to get away and when I'm away I want to get back home.' Patient A, who is a nurse residing in a hostel, says: 'The other night I decided I wanted to stay in the hostel and not go home, then I felt the hostel was a prison and I went home. As soon as I got there I wanted to go out again. Yesterday I rang mother to say I was coming home, and then immediately I felt exhausted and rang her again to say I was too tired to come. I'm always switching about, as soon as I'm with the person I want I feel they restrict me. I have wondered if I did get one of my two men friends would I then want to be free again.' The patient F, a bachelor of 40 who is engaged, says: 'If I kiss Mary my heart isn't in it. I hold my breath and count. I can only hug and kiss a dog because it doesn't want anything from me, there are no strings attached. I've always been like that, so I've got lots of acquaintances but no real close friends. I feel I want to stay in and go out, to read and not to read, to go to Church and not to go. I've actually gone into a Church and immediately come out again and then wanted to return in.'

So people find their lives slipping away changing houses, clothes, jobs, hobbies, friends, engagements and marriages, and unable to commit themselves to any one relationship in a stable and permanent way: always needing love yet always dreading being tied. This same conflict accounts for the tendency of engaged or married couples to phantasy about or feel attracted to someone else: as if they must preserve freedom of attachment at least in imagination. One patient remarked: "I want to be loved but I mustn't be possessed.'

(2) Giving up emotional relations to external objects

The oscillation of 'in and out,' 'rushing to and from,' 'holding on and breaking away' is naturally profoundly disturbing and disruptive of all continuity in living, and at some point the anxiety aroused becomes so great that it cannot be sustained. It is then that a complete retreat from object-relations is embarked on, and the person becomes overtly schizoid, emotionally inaccessible, cut off.

This state of emotional apathy, of not suffering any feeling, excitement or enthusiasm, not experiencing either affection or anger, can be very successfully masked. If feeling is repressed, it is often possible to build up a kind of mechanized, robot personality. The ego that operates consciously becomes more a system than a person, a trained and disciplined instrument for 'doing the right and necessary thing' without any real feeling entering in. Fairbairn makes the highly important distinction between 'helping people without feeling' and 'loving.' Duty rather than affection becomes the key word. Patient A sought temporary relief from her disruptive conflict over her man friend by putting it away and making a list of all the things she ought to do, and systematically going through them one by one, routinizing her whole life — and that had been a life-long tendency. She had always had to 'do things in order'; even as a child she made a note-book list of games and had to play them in order.

The patient F, a man with strongly, in fact exclusively, religious interests, showed markedly this characteristic of helping people without really feeling for them. He said: 'I've no real emotional relations with people. I can't reciprocate tenderness. I can cry and suffer with people. I can help people, but when they stop suffering I'm finished. I can't enter into folks' joys and laughter. I can do things for people but shrink from them if they start thanking me.' His suffering with people was in fact his identifying himself as a suffering person with anyone else who suffered. Apart from that he allowed no emotional relationship to arise.

It is even possible to mask more effectively the real nature of the compulsive, unfeeling zeal in good works, by simulating a feeling of concern for others. Some shallow affect is helped out by behaviour expressive of deep care and consideration for other people; nevertheless, genuine feeling for other people is not really there. Such behaviour is not, of course, consciously insincere. It is a genuine effort to do the best that one can do in the absence of a capacity to release true feeling. What looks deceptively like genuine feeling for another person may break into consciousness, when in fact it is based on identification with the other person and is mainly a feeling of anxiety and pity for oneself.

Many practically useful types of personality are basically schizoid. Hard workers, compulsively unselfish folk, efficient organizers, highly intellectual people, may all accomplish valuable results, but it is often possible to detect an unfeeling callousness behind their good works, and a lack of sensitiveness to other people's feelings, in the way they will over-ride individuals in their devotion to causes.

The schizoid repression of feeling, and retreat from emotional relationships, may however go much further and produce a serious breakdown of constructive effort. Then the unhappy sufferer from incapacitating conflicts will succumb to real futility: nothing seems worth doing, interest dies, the world seems unreal, the ego feels depersonalized. Suicide may be attempted in a cold, calculated way to the accompaniment of such thoughts as 'I am useless, bad for everybody, I'll be best out of the way.' The patient F had never reached that point, but he said: 'I feel I love people in an impersonal way; it seems a false position; hypocritical. Perhaps I don't do any loving. I'm terrified when I see young people go off and being successful and I'm at a dead bottom, absolute dereliction, excommunicate.'

V. The Fundamental Problem: Identification

(1) *Identification and infantile dependence*

It has already been mentioned that schizoid problems arise out of identification, which Fairbairn holds to be the original infantile form of relation to, and dependence on, objects. The criticism is sometimes made that psycho-analysis invents a strange terminology that the layman cannot apply to real life. We may therefore illustrate the state of identification with the love-object in the words of Ngaio Marsh (1935), a successful writer of detective fiction. In *Enter a Murderer* she creates the character of Surbonadier, a bad actor who expresses his immaturity by being a drug addict and blackmailer. Stephanie Vaughan, the leading lady, says: 'He was passionately in love with me. That doesn't begin to express it. He was completely and utterly absorbed as though apart from me he had no reality.' In other words, the man was swallowed up in his love-object, had no true individuality of his own, and could not exist in a state of separation from her. He had never become born out of his mother's psyche and differentiated as a separate and real person in his own right, and identification with another person remained at bottom the basis of all his personal relationships.

The patient *E* said: 'If I go away from home I feel I've lost something, but when I'm there I feel imprisoned. I feel my destiny is bound up with theirs and I can't get away, yet I feel they imprison me and ruin my life.' The patient *A* dreamed of being 'grafted on to another person.' The patient *F* said: 'Why should I be on bad terms with my sister? After all I am my sister,' and then started in some surprise at what he had heard himself say. The patient *B*, struggling to master a blind compulsive longing for a male relative she played with as a child, said: 'I've always felt he's me and I'm him. I felt a terrible need to fuss around him and do everything for him. I want him to be touching me all the time. I feel there is no difference between him and me.' Fairbairn holds that identification is the cause of the compulsiveness of such feelings as infatuation. Identification is betrayed in a variety of curious ways, such as the fear of being buried alive, i.e. absorbed into another person, a return to the womb; also expressed in the suicidal urge to put one's head in a gas oven: or again in dressing in the clothes of another person. Patient *C*, feeling in a state of panic one night when her husband was away, felt safe when she slept in his pyjamas.

(2) *Dissolving identification: separation-anxiety, and psychic birth*

The regressive urge to remain identified for the sake of comfort and security conflicts with the developmental need to dissolve iden-

tification and differentiate oneself as a separate personality. This conflict, as it sways back and forth, sets up the 'in and out' programme.
Identification, naturally, varies in degree, but the markedly schizoid
person, in whom it plays such a fundamental part, begins to lose all
true independence of feeling, thought and action as soon as a relationship with another person attains any degree of emotional reality. A
single illuminating example will suffice.

The patient C says: 'I feel I lack the capacity to go out. I can never
leave the people I love. If I go out I'm emptied, I lose myself. I can't
get beyond that. If I become dependent on you, I'd enjoy my dependence on you too much and want to prolong babyhood. Being shut in
means being warm, safe, and not confronted with unforeseen events.'
But this kind of security is also a prison, so the patient goes on to say:
'I feel I'm walking up and down inside an enclosed space. I dreamed
of a baby being born out of a gas oven (i.e. reversal of the suicide
idea). I was struck with the danger of coming out, it was a long drop
from the oven to the floor. I feel I'm disintegrating if I go out. The
only feeling of being real comes with getting back in and being with
someone. I don't feel alone inside even if there's no-one there. Sometimes I feel like someone falling out of an aeroplane, or falling through
water and expecting to hit the bottom and there isn't one. I have strong
impulses to throw myself out of the window.' This 'birth symbolism'
shows that suicidal impulses may have opposite meanings. The gas
oven means a return to the womb, a surrender to identification with
mother. Falling out of the window means a struggle to separate and
be born (and also casting out the person with whom one is identified). The struggle to dissolve identification is long and severe, and
in analysis it recapitulates the whole process of growing up to the
normal mixture of voluntary dependence and independence characteristic of the mature adult person. One of the major causes of anxiety
is that separation is felt to involve, not natural growth and development, but a violent, angry, destructive break-away, as if a baby, in
being born, were bound to leave a dying mother behind.

VI. Schizoid Characteristics

There are various characteristics which specifically mark the schizoid
personality, and the most general and all-embracing is:

(1) *Introversion.* By the very meaning of the term, the schizoid
is described as cut off from the world of outer reality in an emotional
sense. All his libidinal desire and striving is directed inwards towards
internal objects and he lives an intense inner life, often revealed in
an astonishing wealth and richness of phantasy and imaginative life

whenever that becomes accessible to observation; though mostly this varied phantasy life is carried on in secret, hidden away often even from the schizoid's own conscious self. His ego is split. But the barrier between the conscious and the unconscious self may be very thin in a deeply schizoid person and the world of internal objects and relationships may flood into and dominate consciousness very easily.

(2) _Narcissism_ is a schizoid characteristic that arises out of the predominantly interior life he lives. His love-objects are all inside him, and moreover he is greatly identified with them, so that his libidinal attachments appear to be to himself. This subtly deceptive situation was not recognized by Freud when he propounded his theory of auto-eroticism and narcissism, and ego-libido as distinct from object-libido. The schizoid's physically incorporative feeling towards his love-objects is the bodily counterpart, or rather foundation, of the mentally incorporative attitude which leads to mental internalization of objects and the setting up of a world of internal psychic objects. But these mentally internalized objects, especially when the patient feels strongly identified with them, can be discovered, contacted and enjoyed, or even attacked, in his own body, when the external object is not there. One patient, who cannot be directly angry with another person, always goes away alone when her temper is roused and punches herself. She is identified with the object of her aggression which leads to a depressive state, though, of course, it is a libidinal attachment at bottom. The normally so-called autoerotic and narcissistic phenomena of thumb-sucking, masturbation, hugging oneself and so on are based on identification. Autoerotic phenomena are only secondarily autoerotic; autoerotism is a relationship with an external object who is identified with oneself, the baby's thumb deputizes for the mother's breast. Narcissism is a disguised object-relation. Thus the patient B felt depressed while bathing and cried silently, and then felt a strong urge to snuggle her head down on to her own shoulder, i.e. mother's shoulder in herself, and at once she felt better. Again sitting with her husband one evening reading, she became aware that she was thinking of an intimate relation with him and found she had slipped her hand inside her frock and was caressing her own breast. These phenomena lead to a third schizoid characteristic:

(3) _Self-sufficiency._ The above patient was actually taking no notice of her husband as an external person: her relation with him was all going on inside herself and she felt contented. This introverted, narcissistic self-sufficiency which does without real external relationships while all emotional relations are carried on in the inner world, is a safeguard against anxiety breaking out in dealings with actual people. Self-sufficiency, or the attempt to get on without external

relationships, comes out clearly in the case of patient *C*. She had been talking of wanting a baby, and then dreamed that she had a baby by her mother. It was suggested that having a baby meant getting something of her husband inside her, and deep down that felt to be getting something of mother inside her. But since she had often shown that she identified herself very much with babies, it would also represent being the baby inside the mother. She was wanting to set up a self-sufficiency situation in which she was both the mother and the baby. She replied: 'Yes, I always think of it as a girl. It gives me a feeling of security. I've got it all here under control, there's no uncertainty.' In such a position she could do without her husband and be all-sufficient within herself.

(4) *A sense of superiority* naturally goes with self-sufficiency. One has no need of other people, they can be dispensed with. This overcompensates the deep-seated dependence on people which leads to feelings of inferiority, smallness and weakness. But there often goes with it a feeling of being different from other people. Thus a very obsessional patient reveals the schizoid background of her symptoms when she says: 'I'm always dissatisfied. As a child I would cry with boredom at the silly games the children played. It got worse in my teens, terrible boredom, futility, lack of interest. I would look at people and see them interested in things I thought silly. I felt I was different and had more brains. I was thinking deeply about the purpose of life.' She could think about life in the abstract but couldn't live it in real relationships with other people.

(5) *Loss of affect* in external situations is an inevitable part of the total picture. A man in the late forties says: 'I find it difficult to be with mother. I ought to be more sympathetic to her than I can be. I always feel I'm not paying attention to what she says. I don't feel terribly drawn to anyone. I can feel cold about all the people who are near and dear to me. When my wife and I were having sexual relations she would say: "Do you love me?" I would answer: "Of course I do, but sex isn't love, it's only an experience." I could never see why that upset her.' Feeling was excluded even from sexual activity which was reduced to what one patient called 'an intermittent biological urge which seemed to have little connexion with "me."'

(6) *Loneliness* is an inescapable result of schizoid introversion and abolition of external relationships. It reveals itself in the intense longing for friendships and love which repeatedly break through. Loneliness in the midst of a crowd is the experience of the schizoid cut off from affective rapport.

(7) *Depersonalization,* loss of the sense of identity and individuality, loss of oneself, brings out clearly the serious dangers of the schizoid

state. Derealization of the outer world is involved as well. Thus the patient C maintains that the worst fright she ever had was a petrifying experience at the age of two years. 'I couldn't get hold of the idea that I was me. I lost the sense for a little while of being a separate entity. I was afraid to look at anything; and afraid to touch anything as if I didn't register touch. I couldn't believe I was doing things except mechanically. I saw everything in an unrealistic way. Everything seemed highly dangerous. I was terrified while it lasted. All my life since I've been saying to myself at intervals "I am me." '

VII. FAIRBAIRN AND FREUD

When one surveys the material here set out, it becomes apparent that Fairbairn's theory of the schizoid problem represents a radical revision in psycho-analytical thinking. Freud rested his theory of development and of the psychoneuroses on the centrality of the Oedipus situation in the last phase of infancy. Failure to solve the Oedipus conflict of incestuous love and jealous hate of the parent of the same sex led to regression to pregenital levels of sexual and emotional life and a lasting burden of guilt. This now looks rather like a pioneer's rough sketch-map of uncharted territory by comparison with Fairbairn's detailed ordnance survey map of infantile development which is based on, but goes a long way beyond, Melanie Klein's discoveries about internal objects and the depressive position. The Oedipus problem as Freud saw it was, in fact, no more than the gateway opening into the area of the psychopathology of infancy. Yet Fairbairn's position is essentially simple. Once stated it should be apparent that man's need of a love-relationship is the fundamental thing in his life, and that the love-hunger and anger set up by frustration of this basic need must constitute the two primary problems of personality on the emotional level. Freud's 'guilt over the incestuous tie to the mother' now resolves itself into the primary necessity of overcoming infantile dependence on the parents, and on the mother in particular, in order to grow up to mature adulthood. The Oedipus conflict theory in a purely biological and sexual sense is seen to have misrepresented and distorted the real problem, and sidetracked inquiry. The fundamental emotional attitude of the child to both parents is the same and is determined, not by the sex of the parent but by the child's need for libidinal satisfaction and protective love, and a stable environment, and by the fact that all its relationships start off on the basis of identification. In its quest for a libidinally good object the child will turn from the mother to the father, and go back and forth between them many times. The less satisfactory the object-relationships with his parents prove to be in the course of development, the more the child remains embedded in relationships by identification, and the more it creates, and remains tied to, an inner world of bad internal objects who will thereafter dwell in its unconscious as an abiding fifth column of secret persecutors, at once exciting desire and denying satisfaction. A deep-seated ever unsatisfied hunger will be the foundation of the personality, creating the fundamental danger of the schizoid state.

VIII. Cultural Expressions of Schizoid Fears

Academic psychologists are fond of accusing psycho-analysts of dealing with abnormal minds and drawing from them unjustified conclusions about normal minds. In fact psycho-analysis shows conclusively that this is an entirely misleading distinction. It would be easy to demonstrate every psychopathological process from the study of so-called normal minds alone. Nowadays many people seek analysis not for specific neurotic breakdowns but for character and personality problems, and many of them are people who continue to hold effectively positions of responsibility and who are judged by the world at large to be 'normal' people. Thus psychopathology should be capable of throwing an important light on many aspects of ordinary social and cultural life. This is far too large a theme to be more than touched on here. A few hints must suffice.

(1) *Common mild schizoid traits.* One has only to collect up some of the common phrases that describe an introvert reaction in human relationships to realize how common the 'schizoid type' of personality is. One constantly hears in the social intercourse of daily life, such comments as 'he's gone into his shell', 'he only half listens to what you say', 'he's always preoccupied', or 'absent-minded', 'he lives in a world of ideas', 'he's an unpractical type', he's difficult to get to know', 'he couldn't enthuse about anything', 'he's a cold fish', 'he's very efficient but rather inhuman', and one could multiply the list. All these comments may well describe people whose general stability in any reasonable environment is quite adequate, but who clearly lack the capacity for simple, spontaneous, warm and friendly responsiveness to their humankind. Not infrequently they are more emotionally expressive towards animals than towards the human beings with whom they live or work. They are undemonstrative: it is not merely that they are the opposite of emotionally effervescent, but rather that their relationships with people are actually emotionally shallow. It is as well to recognize, from these schizoid types, that psychopathological phenomena cannot be set apart from the so-called 'normal'.

(2) *Politics.* All through the ages politics has rung the changes,

with monotonous regularity, on the themes of 'freedom' and 'authority'. Men have fought passionately for liberty and independence; freedom from foreign domination, freedom from state paternalism and bureaucratic control, freedom from social and economic class oppression, freedom from the shackles of an imposed religious orthodoxy. Yet at other times men have proved to be just as willing, and indeed eager, to be embraced in, and supported and directed by, some totalitarian organization of state or church. No doubt urgent practical necessity often drives men one way or the other at different periods of history and in different phases of social change. But if we seek the ultimate motivations of human action, it is impossible not to link up this social and political oscillation of aim, with the 'in and out' programme of the schizoid person. Man's deepest needs make him dependent on others, but there is nothing more productive of the feeling of being tied or restricted than being overdependent through basic emotional immaturity. Certainly human beings in the mass are far less emotionally mature than they suppose themselves to be, and this accounts for much of the aggressiveness, the oppositionism, and the compulsive assertion of a false, forced, independence that are such obvious social behaviour trends. The schizoid person frequently 'has a bee in his bonnet' about freedom. The love of liberty has been for so long the keynote of British national life that what Erich Fromm (1942) calls 'the fear of freedom' found in totalitarianism, and in political as well as religious authoritarianism seems to us a strange aberration. It is well to realize that both motives are deeply rooted in the psychic structure of human personality.

(3) *Ideology.* Much has been said of 'depressed eras' in history, but when one considers the cold, calculating, mechanical, ruthless, and unfeeling nature of the planned cruelty of political intellectuals and ideologists, we may well think this to be a 'schizoid era'. The cold and inscrutable Himmler showed all the marks of a deeply schizoid personality and his suicide was consistent. The schizoid intellectual wielding unlimited political power is perhaps the most dangerous type of leader. He is a devourer of the human rights of all whom he can rule. The way some of the most ruthless Nazis could turn to the study of theology was significant of a schizoid splitting of personality. But if we turn to the purely intellectual and cultural sphere it is not difficult to recognize the impersonal atmosphere of schizoid thinking in Hegelianism. Its dialect of thesis breeding antithesis seems an intellectual version of the schizoid need for unity which in turn breeds the need for separation. Still more apparent is the schizoid sense of futility, disillusionment, and underlying anxiety in Existentialism. These thinkers, from Kierkegaard to Heidegger and Sartre, find human existence

to be rooted in anxiety and insecurity, a fundamental dread that ultimately we have no certainties and the only thing we can affirm is 'noth-
ingness', 'unreality', a final sense of triviality and meaninglessness. This
surely is schizoid despair and loss of contact with the verities of emotional reality, rationalized into a philosophy; yet Existentialist thinkers,
unlike the Logical Positivists, are calling us to face and deal with
these real problems of our human situation. It is a sign of the mental
state of our age.

SUMMARY

We may finally summarize the emotional dilemma of the schizoid
thus: he feels a deep dread of entering into a real personal relationship, i.e. one into which genuine feeling enters, because, though his
need for a love-object is so great, yet he can only sustain a relationship
at a deep emotional level, on the basis of infantile and absolute dependence. To the love-hungry schizoid faced internally with an exciting
but deserting object all relationships are felt to be 'swallowing-up
things' which trap and imprison and destroy. If your hate is destructive you are still free to love because you can find someone else to
hate. But if you feel your love is destructive the situation is terrifying.
You are always *impelled into* a relationship by your needs and at once
driven out again by the fear either of exhausting your love-object by
the demands you want to make or else losing your own individuality
by over-dependence and identification. This 'in and out' oscillation
is *the typical schizoid behaviour*, and to escape from it into detachment and loss of feeling is *the typical schizoid state.*
The schizoid feels faced with utter loss, and the destruction of both
ego and object, whether in a relationship or out of it. In a relationship,
identification involves loss of the ego, and incorporation involves a
hungry devouring and losing of the object. In breaking away to independence, the object is destroyed as you fight a way out to freedom,
or lost by separation, and the ego is destroyed or emptied by the loss
of the object with whom it is identified. The only real solution is the
dissolving of identification and the maturing of the personality: the
differentiation of ego and object and the growth of a capacity for co-
operative independence and mutuality.

REFERENCES

Fairbairn, W. R. D. (1941). A revised psychopathology of the psychoses and
psychoneuroses. *Int. J. Psycho-Anal.*, 22, p. 250.
Fairbairn, W. R. D. (1944). Endopsychic structure considered in the light of
object-relationships. *Int. J. Psycho-Anal.*, 25, p. 70.

Fromm, E. (1942). *The Fear of Freedom*, London: Kegan Paul.

Horney, K. (1946). *Our Inner Conflicts*, London: Kegan Paul.

Klein, M. (1932). *The Psychoanalysis of Children*, London: Hogarth Press.

Klein, M. (1948). *Contributions to Psychoanalysis*, London: Hogarth Press.

Marsh, N. (1935). *Enter a Murderer*, London: Penguin Books.

Riviere, J. (1952). The unconscious phantasy of an inner world. *Int. J. Psycho-Anal.*, 33, p. 160.

24

A STUDY OF THE FREUDIAN THEORY OF PARANOIA BY MEANS OF THE RORSCHACH TEST

MARVIN L. ARONSON, Ph.D.

Postgraduate Center for Psychotherapy, New York

A. Introduction

During the latter half of the nineteenth century, psychiatric thought on paranoia was focused largely on the diagnostic aspects of the disease and few systematic attempts were made to explain its underlying dynamics. During this period, conceptions of paranoia were, for the most part, dominated by the symptomatological descriptions of Kraepelin in Germany, Krafft-Ebbing in Austria, and Magnan in France. (London, 1931.)

In 1895, Freud and Breuer suggested that sexual disturbances might play a significant role in the etiology of paranoid delusions. One year later, Freud (1896) postulated that projection was the primary defence mechanism in paranoia. In 1911, Freud presented a detailed analysis of the case of Dr. Jur. Daniel Paul Schreber, a prominent German judge who had developed a remarkably elaborate system of paranoid delusions. On the basis of his analysis of the Schreber case, Freud postulated that unconscious homosexual conflicts lie at the root of most cases of paranoia. According to Freud's theory, all of the major types of paranoid delusions can be represented as contradictions of the basic unconscious feeling that *"I (a man) love him (a man)."* In his theoretical discussion of the Schreber case, Freud (1911) outlined the specific processes by which each of the major types of paranoid delusions is utilized to cope with homosexual threats, as follows:

1. *Delusions of Persecution.* The proposition *"I (a man) love him (a man)"* is contradicted by the formulation "I do not *love* him — I *hate him.*" The paranoid cannot accept this formulation consciously, and consequently, he transforms it, by the mechanism of projection, into another one: "He *hates* (persecutes) *me* which will justify me in hating him." As a result of this projection, "the unconscious feeling, which is, in fact, the motive force, makes its appearance as though

From the *Journal of Projective Techniques*, 16: No. 4, 1952.

it were the consequence of an external perception: 'I do not *love* him — I *hate* him because *he persecutes me.*' " Freud (1922) contended that the chief persecutor in paranoia is invariably a previously loved one of the same sex.

2. *Erotomania.* The unconscious proposition "I do not love *him* — I love *her*" is transformed by projection into 'I notice that *she* loves me." The final formulation then becomes "I do not love *him* — I love *her* because *she loves me.*"

3. *Delusions of Jealousy.* Here, the unconscious homosexuality is contradicted by the formulation "It is not *I* who loves the man — *she* loves him." In women, the final formulation becomes "It is not *I* who loves the women, *he* loves them."

4. *Megalomania.* The homosexual threat is warded off by asserting "I do not love at all — I do not love anyone." This is psychologically equivalent, according to Freud, to the proposition "I love only myself," and it constitutes, essentially, a "sexualized overestimation of the ego."

Within a few years after Freud's presentation of the Schreber case, a number of other analysts reported the results of their therapeutic experience with paranoid patients. In 1914, Payne, who had reviewed the psychoanalytic literature on paranoia, found that homosexuality was described as the core conflict in every case of paranoia which had been presented up until that time. In the same year, Shockley (1914) concluded that Freud's theory of paranoia could be "regarded as proven since it has been observed by so many writers." More recent summaries of the analytic literature on paranoia may be found in publications by Fenichel (1945), Gardner (1931), Klein and Horwitz (1949) and Miller (1941).

Only one psychoanalyst, Gardner (1931), has investigated the Freudian theory of paranoia in a research study involving a large number of cases. Gardner studied the incidence of repressed homosexuality in forty unselected cases of paranoid schizophrenia and eighty cases of paranoid condition. His criteria for repressed homosexuality were: (1) homosexual acts; (2) statements by the patients that they had been attacked homosexually; and (3) symbolic expressions of homosexuality. Using these relatively gross criteria, Gardner found evidence for repressed homosexuality in 45% of his total sample. Among the paranoid schizophrenic patients, the incidence of repressed homosexuality was 55%, while among the paranoid condition patients, the incidence was 40%.

Miller (1941), a non-analyst, found that the Freudian theory of paranoia was applicable in only twelve out of the 400 cases of paranoia which he had studied. On the basis of his research, Miller concluded that paranoid mechanisms may be caused by a large variety of etiological factors. According to Miller, all of the following factors can lead to paranoia: (1) incomplete psychosexual development; (2) physical inferiorities; (3) impotence; (4) deafness; (5) blindness; (6) failing faculties; (7) organic brain disease and (8) life situations giving rise to feelings of frustration, inadequacy, anxiety, etc.

Recently, Klein and Horwitz (1949), also using a case study approach, investigated various psychosexual characteristics of a group of forty male and forty female paranoids. They found that the Freudian theory of paranoia was applicable in some of their cases but by no means in all. Only about one fifth of their patients showed preoccupations with homosexuality, even at the height of their illness when their defences were presumably weakened. In many of these cases the patients' fears of becoming homosexual appeared to be related to consistent failures to reach life goals, blows to the ego, a generalized distrust of people's acceptance, and other fears which the authors felt were not specifically related to unconscious homosexuality in the Freudian sense.

B. STATEMENT OF PROBLEM

As revealed in the above summary of the literature, the Freudian theory of paranoia has, thus far, been subjected to only a limited amount of investigation. The analysts, as a group, accepted the theory almost immediately after its initial presentation in 1911, and since that time, the chief evidence which they have offered in support of the theory is the fact that homosexual conflicts have been clinically detected in most analyzed cases of paranoia.

To the non-analytically oriented worker, this kind of evidence does not provide an adequate test of the theory's validity. Thus, for example, one can argue that criteria for evaluating the kind of material obtained in psychoanalytic interviews are so subjective, that it is not surprising that investigators who accept the basic postulates of the Freudian system can find evidence for homosexual conflicts in most cases of paranoia. Another criticism that might be made is that the mere detection of homosexual conflicts in individual cases of paranoia, without control studies of its incidence in nonparanoid individuals, does not constitute proof of the theory, since as Freud (1911) himself contended, some degree of homosexual conflict is present in everybody.

These and other criticisms point up the need for an independent evaluation of the theory. The present study constitutes an attempt at such an evaluation. It seeks to determine whether or not certain predictions of the Freudian theory of paranoia have demonstrable validity on an instrument which psychologists frequently employ for investigating psychosexual disturbances — the Rorschach Test.

C. PROCEDURE

I. A group of individuals were categorized into each of the following three groups on the basis of the extent to which they utilized paranoid mechanisms in their adjustment [1]:

A. _Paranoid Group_ (Pa) — thirty psychotic patients in whom paranoid delusions were the most prominent symptoms.

B. _Psychotic Group_ (Ps) — thirty psychotic patients, relatively less delusional than the patients in the paranoid group but similar to them on matched criteria. This group was included in the study in order to help determine whether differences obtained between the paranoids and the normals (See Group C below) were related to psychosis, in general, or to paranoid delusions, specifically.

C. _Normal Group_ (N) — thirty non-hospitalized individuals, presumably less delusional than the patients in either the paranoid or the psychotic groups, but similar to them with respect to same matched criteria, described below.

II. The thirty subjects in each of the three groups were then tested individually by means of the Rorschach Test.

The assumption was made, in the present study, that the Rorschach Test is an adequate measure of homosexual conflict. If this assumption is warranted, one would expect, on the basis of the Freudian theory of paranoia, that a group of individuals whose major mechanisms of adjustment are of a primarily paranoid nature, would show greater evidence of homosexual conflict on the Rorschach than would groups of individuals who utilize primarily non-paranoid mechanisms. Accordingly, the _major hypothesis of this study was that the subjects in the paranoid group would show a greater amount of homosexual conflict (or more broadly, psychosexual disturbances) on the Rorschach, than would the subjects in either of the control groups._ No differences were predicted between the psychotics and the normals with regard to homosexual conflict because it was felt that psychoanalytic theory is not clear on this point.

D. THE RORSCHACH AS A MEASURE OF HOMOSEXUAL CONFLICT

Although the Rorschach is probably used more frequently for the detection of both latent and overt homosexuality than any other psychological instrument, only a handful of research studies have specifi-

[1] See Section E below for a more detailed description of how the three groups were selected.

cally dealt with the relationship between Rorschach responses and the dynamics of homosexuality. In all of these studies, the emphasis has been almost entirely on the content of Rorschach responses rather than on the "structural" aspects of personality as revealed by the Rorschach psychogram.

In the first of these studies, Bergman (1945) analyzed the content of the Rorschach records of twenty acknowledged male homosexual soldiers and reported five kinds of "typical" responses which he had found in these records. Due and Wright, also in 1945, studied the Rorschach protocols of forty-two males who were either overt homosexuals or who were going through situational maladjustment due to homosexual conflicts. These authors listed seven kinds of responses, with examples of each, as typical of their homosexual subjects. Lindner (1946) listed forty-three separate Rorschach responses, which he had found, empirically, to be related to various types of psychiatric syndromes. Six of these responses were presented as indicative of homosexual preoccupations.

Wheeler (1949) criticized all of these earlier studies on the grounds that they did not follow uniform testing procedures, allowed subjective elements to enter into the treatment of their data, used inadequate statistical techniques, and failed to provide the necessary control groups. Wheeler selected some of the responses suggested by these earlier studies and by other Rorschach workers and constructed a check list of twenty "signs" of homosexuality. He then conducted an investigation to determine the extent to which these twenty signs were internally consistent with each other and externally consistent with therapists' ratings of homosexuality. In Wheeler's study, the Rorschach was administered to 100 patients who had received eight or more therapeutic interviews at an outpatient mental hygiene clinic, and a distribution was obtained of the number of homosexual signs occurring in each record. The obtained distribution was then dichotomized between two and three signs. All those records in which three or more signs occurred were considered "indicative of homosexual trends." The therapeutic staff at the clinic was asked to categorize each of the 100 patients into one of the following four classifications with respect to degree of homosexuality: (1) "repressed," (2) "suppressed," (3) "overt" and (4) "absent." Since the number of cases classified as either "overt" or "suppressed" was very small, Wheeler combined all of the subjects in his sample into the following two contrasting groups (1) "repressed, suppressed, overt," and (2) "absent." The degree of correspondence between the two measures of homosexuality — Rorschach content indices and therapists' ratings — was then computed by means of Yule's Coefficient of Association (Q).

It was found that the twenty individual homosexual signs had a wide range of consistency both with the total number of signs and with the therapists' judgments. Althought most of the individual signs were not very discriminative, a fairly high positive relationship (.42) was obtained at this particular clinic between the *total* number of homosexual signs and the ratings of the entire therapeutic staff. The relationship between the two criteria was much higher for psychiatrists (.90) than for psychologists (.28), while the ratings of social workers at the clinic showed no relationship to the total number of homosexual signs (.01).

Reitzell (1949) tabulated the frequency with which Wheeler's twenty signs of homosexuality, plus two signs which she added to Wheeler's list, occurred in the Rorschach protocols of a group of homosexuals, a group of hysterics, and a group of alcoholics. Although her results were somewhat inconclusive statistically, Reitzell's data indicated a trend for the homosexual signs to occur more frequently in the records of the homosexual subjects than in those of either the hysteric or the alcoholic subjects.

In summary, previous studies have suggested that the Rorschach Test can yield valuable information concerning the dynamics of homosexuality. The validation of Rorschach content indices of homosexuality is still far from complete. However, there does seem to be sufficient evidence accumulated to warrant their usefulness as measures of homosexuality in the present study.

E. Selection of the Groups

The main criterion for placing subjects into one of the three groups described above was the extent to which paranoid delusions predominated in their clinical picture. Since negative results on the Rorschach Test could be attributed to an initially inadequate separation of the groups, considerable care was taken to ensure that the groups were clearly differentiated on the criterion of delusions.

All of the subjects in the normal group were selected from the following organizations in Ann Arbor, Michigan: (1) The American Legion Post, (2) The Veterans of Foreign Wars Post, and (3) The Ann Arbor Branch of the Michigan Unemployment Commission. All of the normal subjects had to meet the following requirements: (1) white, (2) veterans of World War II, (3) not over forty years of age, (4) not more than twelve grades of education, (5) no previous psychiatric treatment, and (7) no medical discharge from the armed services.

Although some of the normal subjects might possibly have shown some tendency toward paranoid behavior, the assumption was made that the normal control group, as a whole, was minimally delusional compared to the paranoid group. There was no way of ascertaining the incidence of overt homosexuality in the normal group, but the fact that 26 out of the 30 normal subjects were married suggests that in these cases, at least, there was probably little or no overt homosexual behavior.

All of the sixty psychotic patients were selected from the patient population of the Veterans Hospital at Fort Custer, Michigan. This is a large mental hospital caring for veterans of World Wars I and II. The majority of the patients in this hospital are psychotic; relatively few are diagnosed as neurotic.

The task of differentiating the two psychotic groups (paranoid and non-paranoid) on the criterion of delusions presented considerable difficulties because of the fact that delusions are not specific to patients diagnosed as Paranoid Schizophrenia, but rather, may occur in a large variety of psychotic reactions.

One way to separate the two psychotic groups would have been on the basis of diagnosis — that is, to compose the paranoid group of patients who had been psychiatrically diagnosed as Paranoid Schizophrenia and the non-paranoid psychotic group of patients who had been given some other diagnosis. This approach was discarded for the following reasons:

1. Psychiatrists differ widely in the criteria which they utilize for diagnosing patients as either paranoid or non-paranoid.

2. Some patients who are not diagnosed paranoid, may, nevertheless, exhibit many paranoid delusions.

3. Diagnostic classifications do not ordinarily indicate the *extent* to which paranoid delusions are present or absent.

Instead of relying exclusively on diagnostic labels for differentiating the patients into either of the two psychotic groups, it was decided to make use of *all* clinical material which was available at the Fort Custer Veterans Hospital. Most of the available clinical data on patients in this hospital may be found in their case folders. Following is a list of the different kinds of records which are typically available in these folders: (1) routine admission interviews, (2) psychiatric interview notes, (3) nurses' ward notes, (4) records of physical or shock therapy, (5) commitment papers and other legal documents, (6) records of social service contacts with the patients' relatives, (7) correspondence with other institutions, and (8) observations of behavior during psychological testing (protocols and test interpretations were not read in order to avoid contamination).

The author read through about 75 case folders, and on the basis of the above kinds of data, selected the twenty cases which seemed to be most extreme with regard to the presence or absence of paranoid delusions. The remainder of the cases were discarded. The twenty extreme cases were then presented for rating to two graduate students from the University of Michigan.

The raters were instructed to read through the clinical folders of each of these twenty patients and to rate them for each of the four kinds of paranoid delusions which Freud (1911) had specifically linked with homosexual conflict: (1) delusions of persecution, (2) erotomania, (3) delusions of jealousy, and (4) megalomania. The author rated the same cases independently. Following is the rating scale on which the patients were rated for *each* of the four kinds of paranoid delusions:

0 — minimally delusional
1 — very slightly delusional
2 — slightly delusional
3 — fairly delusional
4 — markedly delusional
5 — extremely delusional
6 — maximally delusional

The raters were instructed to give high ratings to those patients whose entire symptomatology was dominated by one or more of the four kinds of paranoid delusions, and to give low ratings to those patients who exhibited primarily other types of symptoms (e.g. catatonic withdrawal). The entire psychotic population of the hospital was used as the reference group for all of these ratings. It will be noted that these ratings were not necessarily ratings of the *strength* of the delusions, but rather, of the *extent* to which the delusions pervaded the patient's symptomatology.

Since the Freudian theory of paranoia maintains that all of the four kinds of paranoid delusions are related to homosexual conflicts, it was decided to take the highest rating obtained by each patient on *any* of the four kinds of delusions as the basis for selecting him for either the paranoid or the psychotic groups. Using the *highest* rating obtained by each patient on any of the four kinds of paranoid delusions as the basis for comparison, agreement between all three raters was then computed by means of the Pearson product — moment correlation formula. The results of this analysis showed a high agreement between the three raters in their evaluations of the twenty cases. The author's ratings correlated .956 with those of one of the raters and .916 with those of the other. The ratings of the other two raters correlated .883. In 85% of the twenty cases, all three raters agreed unanimously in placing given patients into either the "high delusional group" (ratings of 4–6) or the "low delusional group" (ratings of 0–3). The agreement between the raters on these twenty cases was considered high enough to warrant the author's selection of the entire sixty cases for both of the psychotic groups, by himself.

The author read through approximately 500 case folders in selecting the thirty patients for each of the two psychotic groups. All patients who were selected for the paranoid group received ratings of "4" or more on delusions of persecution, while all patients in the non-paranoid psychotic group received ratings of "2" or less on delusions of persecution. The mean rating on delusions of persecution in the paranoid group was 4.90. The mean rating for the psychotic group was .63.

After all of the ratings on delusions had been made, it was noted that delusions of persecution were rated as occurring far more frequently than were any of the other three types of paranoid delusions. Only ten of the paranoid patients received ratings of "4" or more on megalomania, while none of the paranoid patients received ratings of "4" or more on either erotomania or delusions of jealousy. In the psychotic group, none of the patients received ratings of more than "2" on *any* of the four kinds of delusions.

There seem to be several possible explanations for the preponderance of delusions of persecution in the paranoid group. One explanation may be that delusions of persecution actually occur more frequently among paranoids than do any of the other kinds of delusions. Another reason might be that psychiatrists tend to place more emphasis on delusions of persecution than on any of the other kinds of delusions, in their diagnostic evaluations. This is particularly true in the case of erotomania and delusions of jealousy, both of which are rarely emphasized in present-day diagnoses.

Actually, since Freud (1911) maintained in the Schreber case that regardless of their outward content, *all* of the major types of paranoid delusions can be regarded as attempts to ward off homosexual threats, it should make no difference, theoretically, which of the four kinds of paranoid delusions was used as the criterion for selecting patients for the paranoid group. To test this hypothesis, comparisons were made on the Rorschach indices of homosexuality between the ten paranoids who showed both delusions of persecution and megalomania and the remaining twenty paranoids who showed only delusions of persecution. No significant differences were found. In addition, both of these paranoid groups were compared with the normals and with the psychotics on the Rorschach Test. It was found that the paranoid subjects with both kinds of delusions did not differ more markedly from either of the control groups than the paranoids with only delusions of persecution did.

Following are comparisons of the groups with respect to diagnosis, age, intellectual level, education, occupation, religious affiliations, and in the case of the two psychotic groups, length of hospitalization at the time of testing.[2]

1. *Diagnosis.* All but two of the cases selected for the paranoid group had been given a diagnosis of Paranoid Schizophrenia by the hospital psychiatrists, while none of the patients in the psychotic group was diagnosed Paranoid Schizophrenia. Eighteen of the patients in the psychotic group were diagnosed as Schizophrenia, Unclassified, five were diagnosed as Schizophrenia, Mixed, three as Simple Schizophrenia, two as Catatonic Schizophrenia, one as Hebephrenic Schizophrenia, and one as Schizophrenic Reaction. The very small overlap in the diagnoses of the two psychotic groups reflects the fact that only patients who were *extreme* with respect to the presence or absence of paranoid delusions were selected for either group.

2. *Age.* The mean age of the paranoids was 30.80 years, that of the psychotics 28.97 and that of the normals 26.93. The standard deviations for the three groups respectively were 4.58, 4.49, and 3.50. It was found that the paranoids were significantly older than the normals at the .01 level of statistical confidence. However, it is doubtful if the few years' difference in age between the paranoids and the normals was of much psychological significance, particularly in view of the fact that Freudian theory of paranoia does not stipulate age as an important variable. To check this hypothesis, a correlation was computed between age and homosexual responses on the Rorschach; no significant correlation was obtained. It will be noted that all of the subjects in this study were relatively young; none of the subjects in any of the groups was over forty years of age. This age limit was purposely set in order to eliminate individuals with involutional, organic, and senile conditions, some of whom show delusions which are not related to homosexual conflict, according to the Freudian theory of paranoia.

3. *Intellectual Level.* The intellectual level of the subjects was estimated from the mean weighted score obtained on the Vocabulary Subtest of the Wechsler-Bellevue Scale (Wechsler, 1944). The mean weighted scores for the paranoids, psychotics, and normals respectively were 11.27, 10.97, and 11.57. The standard deviations of the three groups respectively were 2.24, 1.94, and 1.63. Since no significant differences were found between the groups, it would appear that there were no gross differences between the three groups in their general level of intellectual functioning.

---

[2] Unless otherwise stated, all statistical comparisons of the three groups in this study were made by means of Fisher's (1936) small sample t test.

4. *Education.* Educational level was measured by the number of grades of schooling. The mean number of grades spent in school by the paranoids, psychotics, and normals respectively, were 10.90, 11.13, and 10.93. The standard deviations for the three groups were 3.10, 2.26, and 1.53, respectively. There were no significant differences between any of the three groups on this measure.

5. *Occupation.* The majority of the subjects in all three groups were engaged either as unskilled or as semi-skilled laborers. There was only one professional worker in the entire sample (he was in the paranoid group). There were no owners of businesses at all.

6. *Religious Affiliations.* In the paranoid group, there were 17 Protestants, 11 Catholics, and 2 Jews. There were 22 Protestants, 8 Catholics, and no Jews in the psychotic group. In the normal group, there were 24 Protestants, 6 Catholics, and no Jews. These data were based on the religious affiliations as listed by the patients and normal subjects. No data on actual church attendance were available for these groups. The distribution of religious affiliations for the entire sample seems to be fairly representative of the national distribution.

7. *Length of Hospitalization.* Both psychotic groups had been in the hospital a relatively short period at the time of testing. The paranoids had been in the hospital an average of 5.57 months (σ 5.07 months), and the psychotics had been in the hospital 4.97 months (σ 3.62 months) at the time of testing. There were no significant differences between the groups.

In summary, most of the subjects from this sample came from the lower and lower-middle classes of the United States. They were roughly of average intelligence, had a somewhat above average amount of education, were engaged primarily as unskilled or semi-skilled laborers before institutionalization, and reflected the national distribution in their religious affiliations. On most of these peripheral variables, these subjects differed from Schreber (Freud, 1911) and probably from the majority of the psychoanalytically treated patients, most of whom tend to be drawn from the upper-middle and upper classes. However, since the Freudian theory of paranoia does not stipulate that any of these variables is important, but rather, implies that the relationship between homosexuality and paranoia is a universal one, it appeared that these subjects could legitimately be used for testing the validity of the theory.

F. RORSCHACH TEST RESULTS

Each of the sixty psychotic patients was tested individually at the Veterans Hospital, Fort Custer, Michigan, by graduate students of the

University of Michigan. Approximately one-quarter of the psychotic patients were tested by the author. All thirty of the normal subjects were tested by the author in one session each.

The Rorschach protocols of all ninety subjects in the total sample were then carefully scrutinized and a tabulation was made of the number of Wheeler's (1949) twenty signs of homosexuality, plus one additional homosexuality sign suggested by Reitzell (1949).[3]

In the course of this tabulation, it was noted that there were very marked differences between the paranoid group and each of the other groups on total number of responses (R) on the Rorschach. The mean number of responses given by the paranoids was 33.93, while the psychotics gave only 22.23 responses, and the normals gave 22.00 responses. The standard deviations for the paranoids, psychotics, and normals, respectively, were 19.92, 9.20, and 5.08. The differences between the paranoids and each of the control groups were significant at the .01 level of statistical confidence. The fact that the paranoids gave significantly more Rorschach responses than either of the other groups has no specific bearing on the Freudian theory of paranoia; it simply indicates that the paranoids were more productive than either of the control groups. Since the three groups were initially matched for intelligence on the Wechsler-Bellevue weighted Vocabulary Subtest scores, these differences between the paranoids and both of the other groups on Rorschach R were probably more a function of personality variables than of intellectual ones.

As might be expected, it was found that there was a definite positive correlation between number of homosexual signs and Rorschach R for each of the three groups separately, and also, for the entire combined sample. The correlation between homosexual signs and Rorschach R for the paranoid group was .646, for the psychotic group .537, for the normal group .303, and for the combined ninety subjects .675. The implication of these findings for this study was that the larger the Rorschach R, the greater the number of homosexual signs that were likely to be obtained. Therefore, if the three groups were compared solely on mean *absolute* number of homosexual signs, and the paranoids exceeded both of the other groups on that measure, one could have argued that the obtained differences were due, at least partially, to the fact that the paranoids gave many more responses than either of the other groups.

In view of these considerations, it was decided to supplement comparisons of the groups on mean number of homosexual signs (Table

---

[3] Reitzell added two signs to Wheeler's list of twenty: "household furnishings," and "eyes." Only "household furnshings" was used in this study, since "eyes" is commonly considered a "paranoid sign" on the Rorschach.

I, Comparison A) with the following three alternative kinds of analyses:

1. The ratio of homosexual signs to Rorschach R was computed for each individual and the groups were compared on the mean per cent of homosexual signs to Rorschach R (Table I, Comparison B). In these comparisons, the ratio of homosexual signs to Rorschach R for each subject was converted into a per cent and treated as a score. The three groups were then compared by means of Fisher's (1936) t test.

2. A tabulation was made of the number of homosexual signs obtained on the first, second, third, fourth, and fifth or more responses to each Rorschach card. The groups were then compared on the mean number of homosexual signs obtained on the first response to each card (Table I, Comparison C). This analysis, in effect, constituted a means of controlling for Rorschach R since the same number of responses was analyzed for each of the three groups (10 responses x 30 subjects equals 300 responses for each group).

3. The total distribution of per cent scores of homosexual signs to Rorschach R was divided into the highest, middle, and lowest thirds. A tabulation was then made of the number of individuals from each group who fell into each third of the distribution. The hypothesis was tested, by means of the chi-square technique, that there were no significant differences between the groups (Table I, Comparison D).

Comparison A in Table I reveals that the paranoids obtain a significantly large number of homosexual signs than either of the other groups does. It also shows that the psychotics tend to get more signs than the normals, but that this difference does not achieve statistical significance. However, as pointed out previously, both of these findings are ambiguous because the paranoids give significantly more Rorschach responses than either of the other groups does.

Comparison B in Table I reveals that the paranoids obtain a significantly higher mean per cent of homosexual signs to Rorschach R than either of the other groups does. The psychotics get a significantly higher mean per cent than the normals do, but they do not differ as significantly from the normals as the paranoids do from both of the other groups. The relative position of the three groups is exactly the same as it was in the comparison of the groups on absolute number of homosexual signs (Comparison A).

Comparison C in Table I shows that the paranoids obtain a significantly larger number of homosexual signs on the first responses to each Rorschach card than does either control group. The psychotics and the normals do not differ significantly in this respect. It will be noted that each of the three groups obtains approximately half of its

TABLE I. COMPARISONS OF PARANOID, PSYCHOTIC AND NORMAL GROUPS
ON RORSCHACH HOMOSEXUAL RESPONSES

Group	Comparison A. Absolute Number of Homosexual Signs				
	Mean	σ	Comparison	t	p
Paranoids	7.10	4.21	Pa vs N	7.43	.001
Psychotics	1.90	1.96	Pa vs Ps	6.04	.001
Normals	1.10	1.10	Ps vs N	1.92	.05–.10

Group	Comparison B. Per Cent of Homosexual Signs to Rorschach R				
	Mean	σ	Comparison	t	p
Paranoids	22.9	12.3	Pa vs N	7.21	.001
Psychotics	8.5	7.5	Pa vs Ps	5.37	.001
Normals	4.9	5.4	Ps vs N	2.10	.02–.05

Group	Comparison C. Homosexual Signs on First Response to Each Card				
	Mean	σ	Comparison	t	p
Paranoids	3.47	2.05	Pa vs N	7.09	.001
Psychotics	.87	.88	Pa vs Ps	6.32	.001
Normals	.57	.92	Ps vs N	1.27	.20–.30

Comparison D. Subjects from Each Group in Highest, Middle, and Lowest
Thirds of Distribution of Ratio Scores

Third	Paranoids	Psychotics	Normals	Total
Highest	22	6	2	30
Middle	7	14	9	30
Lowest	1	10	19	30

Comparison	Chi-Square	P
Pa vs N	33.12	.001
Pa vs Ps	18.84	.001
Ps vs N	5.88	.05–.10

total number of homosexual signs on the first response to each card. Again, the relative positions of the three groups with respect to homosexual signs is the same as in Table I, Comparison A: paranoids, psychotics, and normals. It was not feasible to conduct this type of analysis beyond the first response per card because there was no assurance that all individuals had given the same number of Rorschach responses.

Comparison D in Table I shows clearly that the paranoids obtain higher ratio scores of homosexual signs to Rorschach R than either of the other groups does. The psychotics tend to get higher ratio scores than the normals do, but this difference does not achieve statistical significance. The relative position of the three groups is exactly the same as it was in Comparisons A, B, and C in Table I.

In summary, Comparisons B–D in Table I have all shown that even when differences in R are taken into account, the paranoids still show much more of a homosexual pattern on the Rorschach than does either of the other groups.

Table II shows the frequency with which each of Wheeler's (1949) twenty homosexual signs, plus one sign suggested by Reitzell

(1949) (Sign 21 in Table II), was selected by subjects in each of the three groups. It also shows the number of subjects in each of the

TABLE II. FREQUENCY OF OCCURRENCE OF HOMOSEXUAL SIGNS AND NUMBER OF SUBJECTS RESPONDING ONE OR MORE TIMES TO EACH SIGN

Sign No.	Pa F	Pa n	Ps F	Ps n	N F	N n	Totals F	Totals n
1	4	4	5	5	3	3	12	12
2	10	10	0	0	1	1	11	11
3	5	5	1	1	1	1	7	7
4	6	6	2	2	1	1	9	9
5	4	4	1	1	2	2	7	7
6	12	12	6	6	5	5	23	23
7	11	11	2	2	4	4	17	17
8	4	4	1	1	0	0	5	5
9	0	0	1	1	1	1	2	2
10	14	14	1	1	0	0	15	15
11	6	6	0	0	0	0	6	6
12	7	7	0	0	1	1	8	8
13	7	7	0	0	1	1	8	8
14	1	1	1	1	0	0	2	2
15	12	10	3	3	2	1	17	14
16	10	6	1	1	0	0	11	7
17	6	5	0	0	4	4	10	9
18	17	12	3	3	1	1	21	16
19	57	18	25	10	3	2	85	30
20	12	10	2	2	0	0	14	12
*21	8	5	2	1	3	3	13	9

Key: F = frequency of each sign; n = number of subjects responding one or more times to each sign; * = Reitzell's Sign.

three groups who responded one or more times to each sign. It will be noted that for Signs 1–14, the frequency of selection of each sign exactly equals the number of subjects responding one or more times to the sign. This is due to the fact that Signs 1–14 can be scored only once in each record, since they refer to specific areas of the Rorschach cards. Signs 15–21 are scored each time they occur anywhere in the record.

It can be seen from Table II that the paranoids exceed both of the other groups in frequency of response to all of the homosexual signs except Signs 1, 9, and 14. None of the individual signs occurs with great frequency except Sign 19 ("Male or female genitalia") which is given frequently by subjects in both of the psychotic groups. Both psychotic groups obtain a significantly higher mean per cent of Sign 19 to total number of homosexual signs than the normals do (significant in each case at the .01 level). The larger number of Sign 19 responses reported by the psychotic groups probably reflects a general lessening of sexual inhibitions on their part. However, even when Sign

19 is dropped out, the paranoids still obtain a significantly higher mean per cent of homosexual signs to Rorschach R than either of the other groups does (significant at the .001 level). The psychotics, however, do not differ significantly from the normals when Sign 19 is dropped out.

In Comparison B, Table I, it was revealed that the psychotics obtain a significantly higher per cent of *total* homosexual signs to Rorschach R than the normals do. It would appear, on the basis of the present analysis, that this difference was primarily due to the fact that the psychotics were less inhibited than the normals in expressing their sexual preoccupations (Sign 19).

Table III lists all those homosexual signs which were responded to by ten or more paranoid subjects. It also lists the "tentative rationale" which Wheeler (1949) suggested for each sign.

G. Conclusions

The results of this study have shown that paranoid subjects report an overwhelmingly greater number of homosexual signs on the Rorschach Test than do either non-paranoid psychotics or normals. In view of Wheeler's (1949) empirical demonstration that these homosexual signs are both internally consistent with each other and externally consistent with therapists' judgments of homosexual conflict, the obtained results appear to be strongly supportive of the Freudian theory of paranoia. These results do not, of course, prove that homosexual conflicts have a direct causative effect in the etiology of paranoid delusions, as Freud's theory maintains. They do, however, suggest that there is a definite relationship between these two variables, at least in terms of the Rorschach.

Unfortunately, it is not possible to make unequivocal statements about the dynamics of the paranoid subjects on the basis of their responses to the particular Rorschach signs of homosexuality used in the present study because the precise rational significance of these signs is still unknown. The rationales suggested for these signs by Wheeler (1949) seem to have some face validity, but they must be considered only as tentative explanations until further investigations yield more information on their specific relationship to the dynamics of homosexuality.

An interesting finding of this study was the fact that the psychotic patients reported significantly more responses dealing with male or female genitalia (Wheeler's Sign 19) than the normal subjects did. This finding suggests that *all* psychotic patients, regardless of whether or not they have paranoid delusions, are disturbed in the sexual area.

TABLE III. HOMOSEXUAL SIGNS RESPONDED TO BY TEN OR MORE
PARANOID SUBJECTS

Sign	Card	Location	Content	Wheeler's Rationale
2	I	Lower Center D	Male or muscular female torso	Confusion in "body-picture," confused male-female anatomy.
6	III	W or W	Animals or animal-like (dehumanized)	People seen as "less than human." Consequent avoidance of sex.
7	IV	W or W	Human or animal; contorted, threatening	Feminine (passive) identification with male figure seen as threatening, etc.
10	VII	W or W or Top D	Human: female with derogatory specification	Derogatory attitude toward women; hostile feminine identification.
15			Human or animal oral detail	Preoccupation with oral (pregenital) areas — perhaps as sexualized.
18			Human object or architecture; with religious specification	(Paranoid) preoccupation with religious (guilt laden?) objects or acts.
19			Male or female genitalia	Preoccupation with sex. Perhaps indicative of lack or satisfaction.
20			Feminine clothing	Feminine identification; perhaps related to transvestism.

This table is based on a table by Wheeler (1949, pp. 104–106).

It remains for future research to determine the specific *kinds* of sexual disturbance which distinguish paranoids from non-paranoid psychotics. Needless to say, such research must await more precisely defined homosexual indices than are currently available.

Finally, the results obtained on the Rorschach test suggest that Wheeler's signs of homosexuality may prove to be useful aides in diagnosing paranoia clinically. It would appear from these data that the presence of a large number of homosexual signs on the Rorschach, particularly in a psychotic record, is suggestive of some paranoid involvement. Further research is indicated in this area.

REFERENCES

Bergmann, M. 1945. Homosexuality on the Rorschach test. *Bull. Menninger Clinic*, 9: 78–84.

Due, F. & Wright, M. 1945. The use of content analysis in Rorschach interpretations: differential characteristics of male homosexuals. *Rorschach Res. Exch.*, 9: 169–177.

Fenichel, O. 1945. *The Psychoanalytic Theory of Neurosis*, New York: Norton & Co.

Fisher, R. 1936. *Statistical Methods for Research Workers*, Edinburgh: Oliver & Boyd.

Freud, S. & Breuer, J. 1895. *Studienueber Hysterie*, Leipzig und Wien: F. Deuticke.

Freud, S. 1896. Further remarks on the defense neuro-psychoses. In *Collected Papers. Vol. I*, 1924. London: Hogarth.

Freud, S. 1911. Psychoanalytic notes upon an autobiographical account of a case of paranoia. In *Collected Papers. Vol. III*, 1924 London: Hogarth.

Freud, S. 1922. Certain neurotic mechanisms in jealousy, paranoia and homosexuality. In *Collected Papers, Vol. II*, 1924. London: Hogarth.

Gardner. G. 1931. Evidences of homosexuality in one hundred and twenty unanalyzed cases with paranoid content. *Psychoanal. Rev.*, 18: 57–61.

Klein, H. & Horwitz, W. 1949. Psychosexual factors in the paranoid phenomenon. *Amer. J. Psychiat.*, 105: 697–701.

Lindner, R. 1946. Content analysis in Rorschach work. *Rorschach Res. Exch.*, 10: 121–130.

London, L. 1931. Mechanisms in paranoia with report of a case. *Psychoanal. Rev.*, 18: 391–412.

Miller, C. 1941. The paranoid syndrome. *Arch. Neurol. Psychiat.*, 45: 953–963.

Payne, C. 1914. Freudian contributions to the paranoia problem. *Psychoanal. Rev.*, 1: 76–187, 308, 445.

Reitzell, J. M. 1949. A comparative study of hysterics, homosexuals and alcoholics using content analysis of Rorschach responses. *J. Proj. Tech. and Rorschach Res. Exch.*, 13: 127–141.

Shockley, F. 1914. The role of homosexuality in the genesis of paranoid conditions. *Psychoanal. Rev.*, 1: 431–438.

Wechsler, D. 1944. *Measurement of Adult Intelligence*, Baltimore: Williams and Wilkins.

Wheeler, W. 1949. An analysis of Rorschach indices of male homosexuality. *J. Proj. Tech. and Rorschach Res. Exch.*, 13: 97–126.

25

PSEUDOHOMOSEXUALITY, THE PARANOID MECHANISM, AND PARANOIA

An Adaptational Revision of a Classical Freudian Theory

LIONEL OVESEY

The classical psychoanalytic theory of paranoia in the male was first proposed by Freud in his celebrated paper on the Schreber case.[1] This theory is formulated within an instinctual frame of reference and is based on the concept of constitutional bisexuality. It holds that the paranoid delusion in its various forms is a defense against repressed homosexual impulses. Many subsequent papers have been written by the adherents of Freud in support of this theory, and it has remained essentially unaltered with the passage of time. It has been extended to include nondelusional paranoid responses in the neurotic, and it has also been applied to paranoia in women, but with somewhat less conviction than in the case of men. The theory has found widespread acceptance in psychiatric circles, and most psychiatrists today would probably subscribe quite uncritically to the Freudian proposition that there is an exclusive etiological relationship between paranoia and homosexuality.

Such unanimity is particularly remarkable in view of the repeated observation that cases of paranoia not infrequently fail to show evidence of a homosexual motivation, either in their conscious or their unconscious productions. In such cases, Freud's theory is nevertheless invoked with the implication that the homosexual impulses are really present, but are so deeply repressed that they cannot be uncovered. This discrepancy has been noted by many clinicians, but subjected to formal investigation by only a few. Of special significance is a study by Klein and Horwitz,[2] who searched for homosexual content in the case records of a large number of hospitalized paranoid patients of

Reprinted by special permission of the William Alanson White Psychiatric Foundation, Inc. from *Psychiatry*, 18: 163–173, 1955.

[1] Sigmund Freud, "Psychoanalytic Notes upon an Autobiographical Account of a Case of Paranoia (Dementia Paranoides)," in *Collected Papers* 3: 387–470; London, Hogarth Press, 1948.

[2] H. R. Klein and W. A. Horwitz, "Psychosexual Factors in the Paranoid Phenomena," *Amer. J. Psychiatry* (1949) 105: 697–701.

both sexes who had undergone psychotherapy. The investigators classified as homosexual content not only erotic homosexual needs, feelings, and conflicts, but also fears of being considered homosexual, fears of being or becoming homosexual, and fears of homosexual attack. Their findings are extremely revealing. To begin with, such content was found in only one-fifth of the total group; furthermore, within this fraction, even at the height of the illness, most of the patients neither showed any behavior of a homosexual nature nor expressed during treatment any erotic homosexual feelings, in spite of the fact that many of these patients were so disorganized that effective defense would seem impossible. The authors draw the following conclusion, which is pertinent to the adaptational orientation of this paper: "In many patients the fear of being or becoming homosexual was an expression of failure, blow to pride, or general distrust of acceptance. These fears did not of necessity represent homosexual strivings." [3] This conclusion is completely in accord with the concept of pseudohomosexuality as I have developed it in two previous papers.[4]

The term *pseudohomosexual* was devised to facilitate the understanding of anxieties about homosexuality. The instinctual frame of reference used by Freud offers, without discrimination, a single explanation for all such anxieties — an explanation conceived in terms of a sexual instinct in search of gratification. I have attempted to show, however, that adaptationally these anxieties can be broken down into three distinctly separate motivational components: the sexual component, the dependency component, and the power component. The sexual component is the only one of these three that seeks sexual gratification as its motivational goal. The anxiety generated in this search is, therefore, a true homosexual anxiety, and should be so labeled. The dependency and power components, however, as denoted by their names, seek completely different, nonsexual goals, although they make use of the genital organs to achieve them. In consequence, the goals appear to be sexual, but in reality are not. For this reason, I have designated these two components, dependency and power, the pseudohomosexual components; and the anxiety incident to the operation of these components constitutes the pseudohomosexual anxiety — that is, an anxiety about dependency and power strivings that is misinterpreted by the patient as a true homosexual anxiety.

This paper will present an adaptational revision of the Freudian

[3] Reference footnote 2; p. 701.
[4] See Lionel Ovesey, "The Homosexual Conflict: An Adaptational Analysis," Psychiatry (1954) 17: 243–250; and "The Pseudohomosexual Anxiety," Psychiatry (1955) 18: 17–25. The present paper, in proposing an adaptational revision of the Freudian theory of paranoia, carries through to a logical conclusion one of the lines of thought begun in these two earlier papers, and preferably should be read in sequence.

theory of paranoia through the application of the concept of pseudo-homosexuality, and will include those extensions of the original theory that deal with nondelusional manifestations of the paranoid mechanism. I shall demonstrate that the paranoid phenomena can stem from nonsexual adaptations to societal stimuli, and motivationally need have nothing to do with homosexuality whatsoever.

THE FREUDIAN THEORY OF PARANOIA

Before presenting my own revision, I should like to review Freud's essential formulations on the mechanism of paranoia as they are proposed in his discussion of the Schreber case. The basic premise is stated by Freud in the following quotation: "We consider, then, that what lies at the core of the conflict in cases of paranoia among males is a homosexual wish-phantasy of *loving a man*." He goes on to show that the principal forms of paranoia can all be represented as contradictions of the single proposition, "I (a man) *love him* (a man)":[5]

(1) *The delusion of persecution* contradicts the *verb*: "I do not *love* him — I *hate* him." The latter idea is transformed by projection into another one: "He *hates* (persecutes) *me*, which will justify me in hating him." Thus, the final formula is: "I do not *love* him — I *hate* him, because HE PERSECUTES ME." Freud concludes: "Observation leaves room for no doubt that the persecutor is some-one who was once loved."

(2) *Erotomania* contradicts the *object*: "I do not love *him* — I love *her*." Projection transforms this formulation into: "I do not love *him* — I love *her*, because SHE LOVES ME."

(3) *The delusion of jealousy* contradicts the *subject*: "It is not *I* who *love* the man — *she* loves him." Freud completes this formulation with the explanation: ". . . and he suspects the woman in relation to all the men whom he himself is tempted to love." Delusions of jealousy in women, he feels, are exactly analogous.

(4) *Megalomania* contradicts the proposition as a whole: "*I do not love at all — I do not love anyone*." Freud concludes: "And since, after all, one's libido must go somewhere, this proposition seems to be the psychological equivalent of the proposition: 'I love only myself.' So that this kind of contradiction would give us megalomania, which we may regard as a *sexual over-estimation of the ego* and may thus set beside the overestimation of the love-object with which we are already familiar."

Thus Freud's theory of paranoia begins with a repressed homosexual wish expressed in the formula, "I (a man) *love him* (a man)," and

[5] Reference footnote 1; pp. 448–451.

then goes on to describe the various ways in which this wish can be denied and projected. Freud, of course, was not unaware that the most prominent clinical feature in paranoia was the patient's complaint of social humiliation. He even commented on this:

Paranoia is a disorder in which a sexual aetiology is by no means obvious; on the contrary, the strikingly prominent features in the causation of paranoia, especially among males, are social humiliations and slights. But if we go into the matter only a little more deeply, we shall be able to see that the really operative factor in these social injuries lies in the part played in them by the homosexual components of affective life. So long as the individual is functioning normally and it is consequently impossible to see into the depths of his mental life, there is justification for doubting whether his emotional relations to his neighbours in society have anything to do with sexuality, either actually or genetically. But the development of delusions never fails to unmask these relations and to trace back the social feelings to their roots in a purely sensual erotic wish.[6]

This is a good example of the reasoning made necessary by an inflexible frame of reference incapable of encompassing the empirical facts; rather, the facts must be molded to fit the frame of reference. As I shall attempt to show, social humiliation is the end result of a failure in social adaptation and can be explained in purely adaptational terms without recourse to a sexual instinct.

The Adaptational Psychodynamics of the Pseudohomosexual Conflict

The pseudohomosexual conflict can develop only in those men who fail to meet successfully the societal standards for masculine performance. There are two ways to account for such failures: either the man never learned how to meet these standards; or he learned how, but it does him little good because he suffers from an inhibition of assertion and cannot put his knowledge to effective use. Since I am concerned here only with the latter possibility, it is important to establish from the outset where inhibitions of assertion come from: they originate in childhood from power struggles between the growing child and either his parents or his siblings. These struggles are inevitably perceived unconsciously in symbolic terms of murderous violence in which each of the adversaries seeks to kill the other. Since the forces arrayed against the child are so great that he dare not risk an aggressive move for fear of lethal retaliation, an inhibition of aggression is the logical outcome of such a power struggle. Once an inhibition of aggression is laid down, it is not long before the child symbolically extends his violent conception

[6] Reference footnote 1: p. 445.

of aggression to encompass nonhostile assertion as well. The end result in the adult is an inhibition of assertion in all its forms, with or without hostile intent.[7]

The nonassertive male may unconsciously react to his failures in terms of a symbolic equation that sets in motion the pseudohomosexual anxiety. This equation is the following: I am a failure = I am not a man = I am castrated = I am a woman = I am a homosexual. In essence, therefore, the pseudohomosexual conflict represents a failure in 'masculine' assertion, and each idea in this equation reflects a social value judgment. It follows, then, that this failure in assertion does not exist in social isolation, but is perceived as a competitive defeat by other men. The defeat, in turn, is placed in a dominance-submission context in which the weaker male is castrated by the stronger male and forced to submit to him as a woman. The weaker male attempts to avoid this fate, and to avoid the pseudohomosexuality anxiety that goes with it, by resort to one or both of two defensive measures, neither of which is successful.

Motivationally, these measures have to do with strivings for power and dependency. Paradoxically, they serve only to perpetuate the very anxiety they were designed to alleviate. The power-driven male tries to dissipate his weakness in a compensatory fashion through a show of strength, and to this end he is continuously engaged in competition with other men. There is no discrimination about this competition; it is about anything and everything. Unfortunately, his conviction of inadequacy is so strong that he concedes defeat in advance. The result is a chronic pseudohomosexual anxiety. Resort to dependency fares no better. The dependent pseudohomosexual male seeks the magical protection of an omnipotent father-substitute via the equation, penis = breast. He aspires to repair his castration through a magical reparative fantasy of oral or anal incorporation of the stronger man's penis, thus making the donor's strength available to him. This maneuver is doomed not only because it is magical, and hence cannot succeed in any case, but also because the fantasied act of incorporation is misinterpreted as truly homosexual in its motivation. Thus, as in the case of power, the dependency fantasy intensifies the pseudohomosexual anxiety.

The Power Motive. — All these facets of the pseudohomosexual conflict can be easily demonstrated in clinical material. The following sequence of two dreams is an example of the power motive. The patient, the second of three brothers, found himself involved in a competitive transference in which he reproduced his sibling rivalry. The immediate

[7] For a discussion of the distinction between assertion and aggression, see "The Pseudohomosexual Anxiety," reference footnote 4.

stimulus for the first dream was the patient's hostile preoccupation with the therapist's greater income in contrast to his own:

I was fighting with my older brother. He was much bigger and stronger than me. He threw me on my back and pinned my arms to the ground with his knees. Then he pried open my mouth and forced his penis into it and made me suck it.

The patient found the dream extremely unpleasant and was reluctant to report it. He remembered that as a boy his older brother on several occasions had pinned him to the ground, pried open open his mouth, and spat into it, but there had never been anything sexual between them. The patient had experienced no erotic homosexual feelings in the dream, nor, for that matter, at any other time in his life; yet the dream created a concern that he might be a homosexual. Motivationally, however, the dream has nothing to do with sex, but makes use of a homosexual act to symbolize his competitive defeat at the hands of the therapist, represented in the dream as his older brother. The dream, therefore, is a paranoid expression of his competitive hostility couched in terms of oral rape. The patient left the interview in which he reported this dream considerably relieved to find that he was not a homosexual, but he was hardly delighted with the implication of competitive inferiority to the therapist.

That night he had another dream, an exact replica in its action of the first, but this time he did to his younger brother what previously his older brother had done to him. In this dream the therapist was represented by the younger brother, and the patient's hostile impulse came through without projection. Now the score was even; the patient had made a woman out of the therapist, and in so doing had retrieved his lost masculinity.

The hierarchal integration of this patient's relationships with other males is typical of the pseudohomosexual conflict. The integration is on the basis of an old army principle. Simply stated, the principle is the following: There's always a bigger bastard.

In the next example, another patient, a doctor, made use of the same principle, but introduced the added feature of castration. This dream was prompted by a competition with the therapist about professional status:

There were two dogs — that is, either people or dogs. One was big and one was little. The big one was a giant; the little one was a child, a puppy. Both dogs were males. The big dog walked the little dog to the sofa, bent him over and had anal intercourse with him. Then the big dog bent down and bit off the little dog's genitals, clean off, everything.

Here, the dog-eat-dog philosophy inherent in the power struggle was expressed somewhat more literally than in the previous example. The patient awakened with feelings of repulsion and disgust and an anxiety about homosexuality, but without erotic motivation. In his report of the dream, it became clear that the sofa was the analyst's couch, defining the locale of the dream. The patient identified the big dog as the therapist, the puppy as himself. The tremendous disparity in size between the two dogs made him think of father and son. His subsequent associations made it clear that the transference component of the dream derived from his infantile relationship with his father.

One more example will suffice to illustrate the pseudohomosexual elaborations of the power struggle. An illustrator who had had a series of drawings rejected by a desirable magazine, reported the following dream:

The magazine printed one of my drawings, but under another artist's name, and they made the drawing so small you could hardly see it. Then a bull was attacking me. He had me impaled on his horns and was biting my thumb and running around and around with me on his head. I yelled for my cousin to act like a cow so the bull would get interested in him and let me go.

The bull that castrated and anally raped the patient represented his competitors, who had been more successful than he in getting their work published. His cousin, whom he exhorted to act like a cow, was an unskilled laborer, and in comparison with the patient, a complete vocational failure. Thus, vocational success was symbolically equated with masculine strength; vocational failure with feminine weakness. The penalty for failure was not only social humiliation, but also castration, rape, and subjugation as a woman by the victorious male competitors. The patient, of course, did not like such treatment in the least, and so he protested defensively that his cousin, a real failure, was more suited to the feminine role than he was. This dream, therefore, contained all the elements of the symbolic equation previously cited: a vocational failure led to social humiliation and then via the paranoid mechanism was simultaneously expressed in terms of homosexuality, castration, and femininity. The patient produced no homosexual motivation, nor in such a dream would any be expected. The motivation was solely that of power, and the associated anxiety was solely a pseudohomosexual anxiety.

The Dependency Motive. — The resort to dependency represents the seeking of magical solutions to the failures in assertion which I have already described. Consider, for example, the following case of a dependent male with a marked inhibition of assertion.[8] He found it

---

[8] I am indebted for this example to Dr. Julian Barish.

next to impossible to make an independent decision in any activity whatsoever. Instead, he became paralyzed by endless procrastination, and usually ended up by doing nothing. He came to treatment presumably to achieve self-sufficiency, but his unconscious productions pointed to a diametrically opposite motivation. In reality, he sought an omnipotent parent-figure, who would magically take over and run his life for him. This was his sixth attempt at therapy; he had tried five previous psychiatrists, with whom he remained in treatment for varying periods from a few months to as long as two years. In each instance the patient broke off with the complaint that nothing was being done for him. Nevertheless, he had not yet given up hope. This he indicated in this opening dream at the end of the second week in his current therapy. The dream not only revealed his magical expectations, but demonstrated also an underlying pseudohomosexual response to his failure in "masculine" assertion:

I was watching a television program of Eisenhower leading a round table discussion. It seemed foreboding. I was scared. A little girl was reprimanded for making too much noise.

The action in the dream was symbolic of the therapeutic procedure. He represented himself as a little girl, the therapist as Eisenhower. The derogatory self-image was a measure of his helplessness in two dimensions: _infantilism and femininity;_ likewise, the identification of the therapist with the President was a measure of the omnipotence with which he had once endowed his father and which he now wished to recapture in the therapist. The patient's sexual adaptation was entirely heterosexual, with no evidence of homosexual desire. However, dependency through the protective love of a man is inevitably misinterpreted as homosexuality. It is, therefore, safe to predict that as the therapy continues a pseudohomosexual anxiety will be found attached to the dependency wish and to the deflated image that accompanies it. In the dream he took a rather dim view of the present therapist's ability to render magical aid, and he anticipated only a rebuke for his infantile demands. Needless to say, such an approach to the therapy augured ill for the prognosis, and there was little reason to hope that the sixth psychiatrist would fare any better than the preceding five.

The desire for dependency through the paternal love of a father-substitute is the most superficial form of the dependency fantasy. The same fantasy on a deeper unconscious level is integrated in a more primitive fashion through the equation, breast = penis. The patient who resorts to this equation attempts to gratify his dependency needs through the oral or anal incorporation of the stronger man's penis. Clinically, the oral route seems to be the more common. A typical example occurred in a patient with an interesting elaboration of a severe inhibition of aggression.[9] He was afraid to learn how to drive, even though he was under constant pressure from his wife to do so. Finally, one day, she lost her temper and tauntingly scoffed that he was not a man. That same night he dreamed that he went to a butcher shop and ate several hunks of meat. He identified the butcher as the therapist. After waking, he felt the meat had been tainted, and he had a bad taste in his mouth. At the same time he experienced feelings of wrong-doing, revulsion, and guilt. In his next therapeutic hour, he remarked that the bad taste made him fear a homosexual implication in the dream. Then he spontaneously associated "penis" to the meat, and suggested that it was up to the therapist to provide what he lacked. Thus the dream had satisfied this demand through a fellatio fantasy in which he orally incorporated the therapist's penis. Equipped in this way, he felt that he could magically go ahead, resolve his inhibition of aggression, learn to drive a car, and so stand up as a man to his wife. The penalty for this fantasy, however, was a pseudohomosexual anxiety — the result of his misinterpretation of the magical device as homosexual, rather than dependent, in its motivational intent. In patients with a more malignant pathology, the fellatio fantasy not infrequently is acted out. Such patients, at times of great anxiety, may seek out men upon whom they perform fellatio, but with no sexual sensation on their own part.

Anal incorporation can be illustrated by the masturbation fantasy of a patient who developed an ambidextrous technique for simultaneous genital and anal masturbation. He manipulated his penis with one hand while he pumped a thermometer in and out of his anus with the other. In the fantasy that accompanied this act, he imagined himself sandwiched between his mother and father as they were having intercourse. The father's penis entered the patient's anus, emerged as the patient's penis, and then penetrated the mother's vagina. The incorporative fantasy here had a mixed heterosexual, homosexual, and pseudohomosexual motivation. The patient not only secured sexual gratification of both varieties, but he also incorporated the father's penis and magically made use of its strength to repair his own weakness, not just in sexual situations, but in nonsexual situations as well. The homosexual motivation was completely latent, for he had never had any homosexual experiences and engaged exclusively in heterosexual relationships. As one would suspect, however, he had an anxiety about being homosexual; but from the motivational breakdown of his fantasy, it is clear that only a part of this anxiety was a true homo-

[9] I am indebted for this example to Dr. Herbert Hendin.

sexual anxiety; the rest was a pseudohomosexual anxiety. The sexual motivations were primary during masturbation, but on other occasions the pseudohomosexual motivation of dependency took precedence. Nonsexual situations that called for assertion but generated severe anxiety were thus handled by the patient in a characteristic fashion. He would retire to the nearest lavatory, give his anus a few quick strokes with a thermometer, and then go out and try to assert himself. He always carried a spare thermometer with him for just such a contingency. While the use of the thermometer on such occasions might arouse erotic sensation, it was not primarily a sexual act; rather it was a magical attempt to achieve strength through dependency on the father. Here is a case, therefore, where the magical reparative fantasy of anal incorporation of the penis, when symbolically acted out, was at least temporarily successful, but the cost was an accentuation of both the homosexual and pseudohomosexual components of the patient's anxiety. This case is a good example of the motivational complexities of thoughts, feelings, and acts concerned with actual or symbolic homosexuality.

THE PSYCHOTIC INTEGRATION OF THE PSEUDOHOMOSEXUAL CONFLICT

The various aspects of the pseudohomosexual conflict described above have been nondelusional in their manifestations. Not one of the patients cited suffered from paranoia, although several made use of the paranoid mechanism. At this point one must distinguish between content and form in psychopathological disturbances. The former is concerned with what the conflict is about; the latter is concerned with how the conflict is handled. Content reflects the impact of social institutions upon the patient; form reflects the psychological integration of that content by the patient. It follows, then, that the same conflict can be integrated psychologically by different patients in different ways. Thus, the pseudohomosexual conflict can occur in either a psychotic or a neurotic setting, and, therefore, can have a delusional, as well as a nondelusional, expression. The psychotic integration of this conflict is characteristically found in paranoia with or without the concomitant presence of true latent homosexuality. Such an integration is demonstrated in the clinical vignette that follows. It will come as no surprise, if one keeps in mind the distinction between content and form, to find that the essential features of the pseudohomosexual conflict, as they have been described, are in no way altered.

The patient, who was 34 years old, married and with two children, was suffering from incipient paranoid schizophrenia. He was a talented, enormously ambitious, and highly successful young executive who had advanced with phenomenal rapidity to a top position as sales manager of a large business organization. His presenting symptomatology was organized around a growing conviction that he was changing into a woman; he came to the psychiatrist through the intervention of an endocrinologist to whom he had applied for injections of male hormone in the hope that they would halt the supposed transformation.

The patient had always had the fear that he was "effeminate," even though objectively he was completely masculine in his physical appearance and in his behavior. However, this fear had never seriously interfered with his capacity to function until the past year, when it had begun to assume delusional proportions.

Strangely enough, the intensification of his anxiety coincided in time with his promotion to sales manager. At first glance, this might seem a paradox; it would be more reasonable for such a success to enhance his masculinity, rather than to undermine it. However, in this case, the unexpected occurred, but not without a hidden logic that will soon be made apparent. The patient was now, by the time he came to treatment, practically convinced that a bodily alteration was in process — that his voice was higher, that his hips were larger, and that he was beginning to walk with a flounce. None of this, of course, was true; but nevertheless, it was what he believed. He was convinced that at the rate things were going it wouldn't be long before his genitals were affected, and then the alteration would be complete. He was terrified at this prospect and repeatedly examined his genitals for signs of shrinkage. As yet, he admitted to no change, but he was convinced the outlook was bleak. He offered a neat explanation for these difficulties: they were all due to excessive masturbation in childhood. As he put it, there were only so many shots in the magazine, and once you used them up, transformation into a woman was inevitable.

The preoccupation with femininity gave rise to a series of related symptoms characteristic of paranoia. Foremost among these were ideas of reference in which he repeatedly misinterpreted the remarks and actions of people around him. He believed they referred to him as effeminate and as a homosexual. To make matters worse, these ideas, almost imperceptibly but quite definitely, were beginning to shade off into delusions of persecution. His potency had always been and remained normal, but there had been a marked lessening of sexual activity since the onset of his illness. This was due not so much to an absence of sexual desire, but rather to his reluctance to engage in intercourse even when the desire was present. This reluctance had its source in his ideas about masturbation — intercourse would further deplete his supply of semen and, hence, it was best avoided. But although abstinence might suit the patient's needs, his wife was starting to complain, and he feared momentarily that she might look for other men. He was gradually becoming more and more suspicious, although he still conceded that her behavior was above reproach. Doubts of this kind, however, are the early precursors of delusions of jealousy.

The patient also confessed to repetitive fantasies in which he performed fellatio, always on the same man — his uncle, a business tycoon of considerable prominence, whom the patient greatly admired and whom he would like to emulate. These were typical pseudohomosexual oral incorporative fantasies. They were unaccompanied by erotic sensation, but the patient misinterpreted them as truly homosexual and offered them as further evidence of his progress toward femininity. In reality, he had never experienced any homosexual desire, nor had he ever engaged in any homosexual activity.

The early history of the patient included the following data:

The patient was a fraternal twin; he and his twin brother were the youngest of twelve siblings, six males and six females. The father had died before the patient was 6 months old. The mother was a decent sort who did her best; but with twelve children, the competition for her attention was fierce. The patient was born into a family of giants. Each of his brothers, including his twin, was over six feet tall, and each of his sisters was five feet eight or taller. Unhappily, the patient himself was only five feet six. The psychological problem this created for him resulted in his embarking on an endless but unsuccessful competitive effort designed to disprove his conviction of inferiority. This effort was doomed to failure from the start, for the simple reason that he could never surmount the disparity in size, no matter how hard he tried, nor how successful were his accomplishments.

Finally the patient had come to attribute his failure to masturbation — a superficial rationalization which served mainly to hide from him where the real problem lay. The heart of the matter was the sibling struggle, first for dependency and then for power, and it was the psychological derivatives of this struggle that were the prime movers in his paranoid breakdown.

The basic psychodynamic pattern climactically emerged at the end of six months of psychotherapy. First, there was a brief period of relative quiescence, manifestly a transference improvement; then, as the unconscious conflict began to approach the surface, the patient's anxiety became more and more intense. There was talk of quitting his job, and with it, of course, the therapy, and retiring in obscurity to a small country town where he would see out his days free from competitive strain running a gasoline station. As it turned out, this was no idle threat. Abruptly one day he resigned from his job, and came to take his leave from the therapy. Fortunately, for the purpose of understanding the pseudohomosexual conflict, he brought with him a dream that laid bare the underlying psychodynamics and explained the precipitate haste with which he made his final decision.

Mother gave me a pint of food, a salad, on a plate. A half a dozen young boys with spears were chasing me. They wanted to take the salad away from me. They wanted it for themselves. I tripped over a rock and the plate dropped into a small pond. The salad stayed on top of the water, but the plate sank. I put my hand into the water to get the plate, but then I couldn't pull my arm out. It was held tight by a lot of worms. The gang of boys cornered me and they started to prod me from behind like savages with their spears. I don't know whether I got out of there alive or not.

This was an obvious sibling rivalry dream in which the patient made use of primitive symbols to express the lethal nature of the original competition for the mother, both as a dependency and as a sexual object. This competition in childhood had first been conceived in the usual terms of murderous violence and then, later, subjected to pseudohomosexual elaboration. Consequently, as an adult, the patient anticipated as retaliation for any competitive effort not only death, but also the retaliatory measures that are a part of the pseudo-homosexual conflict: castration and oral/anal rape. The dream brings to light an intermediate step in this man's illness. This step is commonly referred to as a *success phobia* and defines the patient's inability to tolerate the successful achievement of ambitious goals because he foresaw the retaliation from his competitors as inevitable. It is this conflict that ultimately found expression through the paranoid mechanism; and rather than face it, the patient ran away from both his job and the therapy. In retrospect, it is a moot question whether the better choice would have been to stay and meet the problem head-on. In view of the malignancy of the patient's pathology, a good case can certainly be made out for the course he took, but that is another matter which is beyond the scope of this paper.

The success phobia clarifies an issue that was left hanging; it explains the paradoxical observation that the patient broke down at the peak of his vocational success. This was the moment of greatest danger, and to the patient it represented a delusional materialization of the expected retaliation. At this instant the delusion of femininity was established and the overt paranoid psychosis was set in motion.

AN ADAPTATIONAL THEORY OF PARANOIA

I am now in a position to attempt an adaptational revision of the Freudian theory of paranoia in the male. This revision is based on the concept of pseudohomosexuality and is equally applicable to nondelusional manifestations of the paranoid mechanism. The material for such a revision has been organized in Table I under five sequential headings, as follows:

True Motivation. — This is teleologically determined — that is, in terms of the ultimate adaptational goal.

Symbolic Distortion. — This describes how the meaning of the true motivation is altered in the unconscious mind.

Apparent (False) Motivation. — This is the motivation as it is perceived by the patient after the true motivation has undergone symbolic distortion.

Projected Idea. — This is the paranoid defense against the apparent motivation.

Anxiety. — This defines the related anxiety. The table makes clear the distinction between the homosexual anxiety and the pseudohomosexual anxiety: the former stems from a true homosexual motivation; the latter stems from an apparent (false) homosexual motivation symbolically derived from the unconscious distortion of the true motivations of power and dependency.

TABLE I

True Motivation	Symbolic Distortion	Apparent (False) Motivation	Projected Idea	Anxiety
Homosexual: I want homosexual gratification from him.	*None.*	*None.*	He wants homosexual gratification from me.	Homosexual
Power (Aggression): I want to subject him to competitive defeat.	I want to kill him.	Power (Aggression = Murder): I want to kill him.	He wants to kill me.	Survival
	I want to castrate him and make a woman (homosexual) of him.	Power (Aggression = Castration): I want to castrate him and make a woman (homosexual) of him.	He wants to castrate me and make a woman (homosexual) of me.	Castration and Pseudohomosexual
	I want to subjugate him as a woman (homosexual) = I want to subject him to oral/anal rape.	Homosexual: I want oral/anal homosexual gratification from him.	He wants oral/anal homosexual gratification from me = He wants to subject me to oral/anal rape.	Pseudohomosexual
Dependency: I want to be dependent on him = I want him to love me (nonsexually).	I want him to love me (sexually).	Homosexual: I want homosexual gratification from him.	He wants homosexual gratification from me.	Pseudohomosexual
	I want to incorporate his penis orally/anally.	Homosexual: I want oral/anal homosexual gratification from him.	He wants oral/anal homosexual gratification from me = He wants to subject me to oral/anal rape.	Pseudohomosexual
Dependency + Frustration → Aggression = I hate him because he won't let me be dependent on him.	I want to kill him.	Aggression = Murder: I want to kill him.	He wants to kill me.	Survival

In demonstrating by means of this table the various motivations that can give rise to the paranoid mechanism, I have not totally discarded the original Freudian conclusion that true homosexuality is always the base of paranoia, but have modified and incorporated it in the revision. The table explains the clinical discrepancy in the Freudian theory previously noted that paranoid patients have repeatedly been studied who showed no evidence of true homosexuality. The table makes clear that the homosexual motivation is in no way exclusive; in fact, I would go so far as to suggest that it is the pure power (aggression) motivation without any pseudohomosexual elaboration that is the constant feature in paranoid phenomena, and that the essential related anxiety is, therefore, a survival anxiety. In contrast, the pseudohomosexual components of both the power and the dependency motivations, the true homosexual motivation, and the survival component of the dependency motivation are all variables which can be present or absent, as the case may be. Furthermore, in my clinical experience, the pseudohomosexual motivations occur with far greater frequency than does the homosexual one. This is especially true in nondelusional manifestations of the paranoid mechanism, where true homosexuality appears to be relatively rare. The table also shows that the hatred that stems from dependency-frustration can ultimately be experienced as a projected attack by the dependency-object. The most simple delusional representation of this attack is murder. A more complicated form, the delusion of being poisoned, is integrated through the equation: penis = breast = food. Dependency-gratification is equated with good food; dependency-frustration with bad food. Poison then symbolically derives from the latter. Here, the patient's reasoning is either black or white. If the dependency-object isn't for him, then he's against him; if he doesn't intend to feed him, then he intends to poison him. The nature of paranoia does not permit of a neutral position. In those cases where the dependency-object is a woman, the equation is reduced to its nucleus: breast = food. There are many other interesting elaborations of this equation, but their description is not in the main stream of this paper, and, therefore, must be omitted.

Alternative pseudohomosexual explanations for each of the four principal forms of paranoia cited by Freud now become self-evident.

(1) *The delusion of persecution* is amply explained in the table.

(2) *Erotomania* is a compensatory attempt to repair a pseudohomosexual failure in "masculine" assertion by resort to the sexual conquest of women.

(3) *The delusion of jealousy* expresses the conviction of the pseudohomosexual male that he cannot hold a woman against the competition of stronger men. He may then have pseudohomosexual fantasies

involving his more powerful rivals, and these fantasies will be misinterpreted by him as truly homosexual.

(4) *Megalomania* is a compensatory attempt at ego-inflation where the self-esteem is woefully weak. Pseudohomosexuality plays a role in megalomania to whatever extent it contributes to such low-esteem. The same, for that matter, can also be said of homosexuality, and, adaptationally, that is the only connection between homosexuality and megalomania. Restating this adaptational premise in libidinal terms, in my opinion, adds nothing to one's understanding of it. For this reason, the energetic explanation of megalomania offered by Freud seems to me purely a flight of fancy made necessary by his adherence to the libido theory.

The adaptational theory of the paranoid mechanism and paranoia described in this paper, unlike the classical Freudian theory, agrees completely with the observable clinical facts. The revision was made possible by altering the frame of reference within which the paranoid phenomena were examined. The adaptational formulation that has emerged is not merely of academic interest, but can have great practical significance for dynamic psychotherapy. Such a therapy cannot succeed unless it is based on an accurate motivational breakdown of the patient's behavior. The proposed theory provides this breakdown for the male patient with paranoid manifestations.

26

PSYCHOTHERAPY OF SCHIZOPHRENIA

FRIEDA FROMM-REICHMANN, M.D.

When I received the invitation to talk to you about psychotherapy of schizophrenia, I gave a good deal of thought to the question of how you might like me to approach the topic. Finally, I felt it might be most appropriate to report the development in the understanding and the technique of our clinical work since 1948 when I had the privilege to talk to you about it at the schizophrenia symposium during the annual meeting in Washington.

The goal of psychotherapy with schizophrenics was seen then, as it is now, as helping them by a consistent dynamically oriented psychotherapeutic exchange to gain awareness of the unconscious motivations for and curative insight into the genetics and dynamics of their disorder.

As a result of the continued research which is inherent in dynamic psychotherapy, I have gained some further insight into the dynamics of schizophrenic symptomatology from which have evolved some variations in the details of the treatment. Briefly, they are:

1. The old hypothesis according to which the schizophrenic's early experiences of warp and rejection were of over-all significance for the interpretive understanding and treatment has been somewhat revised.

2. The conflict-provoking dependent needs of schizophrenic patients have been seen more clearly.

3. The devastating influence of schizophrenic hostility on the patients themselves has been understood more clearly in connection with their states of autism and partial regression (weak ego — autistic self-depreciation).

4. This has led to a therapeutically helpful reformulation of the anxiety of schizophrenic patients as an outcome of the universal human conflict between dependency and hostility which is overwhelmingly magnified in schizophrenia.

5. The multiple meaning of some schizophrenic communications and

From *The American Journal of Psychiatry*, December 1954.

its influence on the psychiatrist's interpretive endeavors has been clarified.

Before I begin to elaborate these topics, I have to ask you to forgive me for lack of reference to publications of other workers in the
field. There is unfortunately not time enough to comment on the published work of our colleagues, to indicate what I owe to them, and also
to develop my own conceptions. So, I felt I ought to decide to do the
latter.

I would like to begin by stating that my discussion will comprise
the treatment of hospitalized disturbed psychotics as well as that of
manifestly less disturbed ambulatory patients whom we treat in the
same way through all phases and all manifestations of their illness.
This position is not new, but it has recently become more controversial
due to opposite techniques which other authors have propagated.

From a social and behavioral standpoint and from the viewpoint
of the special care which manifestly psychotic patients may need
in order to be protected from harming themselves and others, the difference between these two types of patients may seem tremendous. Psychodynamically speaking, I see no difference between the symptomatology of actively psychotic and more conformative schizophrenics.

All schizophrenic patients live in a state of partial regression to
early phases of their personal development, the disturbed ones more
severely regressed than the conformative ones. All of them are also
living simultaneously on the level of their present chronological age,
the conformative ones more obviously so than the severely disturbed
ones. Irrespective of the degree of regression and disturbance, we try
to reach the regressed portion of their personalities by addressing the
adult portion, rudimentary as this may appear in some severely disturbed patients. Also, the general psychodynamic conception that
anxiety plays a central role in all mental illnesses and that mental
symptoms in general may be understood simultaneously as an expression of and as a defense against anxiety and its underlying conflicts
holds regardless of the severity of the picture of illness, and regardless of its more or less dramatic character. Hence we make the explora-
ation of the dynamic roots of the schizophrenic's anxieties our potential goal through all phases of illness.

Lack of immediate communicative responses to treatment in acutely
disturbed patients is no measuring rod for their actual awareness of
and for their inner response to our psychotherapeutic approach. This
old experience has been further corroborated in more recent dealings
with several recovered patients. They did refer to various aspects of
our psychotherapeutic contacts, after their emergence, while we were
working through the dynamics of their problems, or later while we

were reviewing treatment and illness during the recovery period.

While symptomatic psychotherapy of acute psychotic manifestations may be necessary with some patients, for situational reasons, many of us consider it not too important to be overconcerned with the duration of the acutely disturbed states of patients while they are under psychotherapy.

My experience during the last 20 years has been mainly with schizophrenic patients who came to our hospital in a state of severe psychotic disturbance, from which the majority emerged sooner or later under intensive dynamic psychotherapy. After their emergence, they continued treatment with the same psychiatrist through the years of their outwardly more quiet state of illness, with the aim of ultimate recovery with insight. During both phases the patients were seen for 4 to 6 regularly scheduled weekly interviews lasting one hour or longer. Sometimes relapses occurred. Such relapses were due to failure in therapeutic skill and evaluation of the extent of the patient's endurance for psychotherapy, to unrecognized difficulties in the doctor-patient relationship, or to responses to intercurrent events beyond the psychiatrist's control. As a rule, these relapses could be handled successfully if the psychiatrist himself did not become too frightened, too discouraged, or too narcissistically hurt by their occurrence.

From the experience with these patients we learned about one more reason for advocating the same type of psychotherapeutic approach through all phases of the illness: part of the work which a patient has to accomplish during treatment and at the time of his recovery is, in my judgment, to learn to accept and to integrate the fact that he has gone through a psychotic illness, and that there is a "continuity," as one patient called it, between the person as he manifested himself in the psychosis and the one he is after his recovery. The discussion of the history of the patients' illness and treatment after their recovery serves of course the same purpose. This is in contrast to the therapeutic attitude of some psychiatrists who hold that recovering patients should learn to detest and eject their psychotic symptomatology, like a foreign body, from their memory.

The difficult task of integrating the psychotic past, which we advocate, will be greatly facilitated if it can be done on the basis of patient's memory of a psychiatrist who has maintained the same type of psychotherapeutic relationship with them through the whole course of treatment. Changes in the doctor's therapeutic approach may easily become a mirror of the lack of continuity in the patient's personality, and, incidentally, may become an inducement for patients to dwell in one or the other phase of their illness, depending upon their preference for this or the other type of therapeutic relationship.

The following experience with a patient illustrates the difficulties of integrating the experience of a past psychosis.

This patient emerged from a severe schizophrenic disturbance of many years duration, for which she was finally hospitalized for 2 years at Chestnut Lodge and then treated as an ambulatory patient for another 2 years. Eventually she became free of her psychotic symptomatology except for the maintenance of one manifest symptom: she would hold on to the habit of pulling the skin off her heels to the point of habitually producing open wounds. No attempt at understanding the dynamics of this residual symptom clicked, until the patient developed one day an acute anxiety state in one of our psychotherapeutic interviews in response to my commenting on favorable "changes" that had taken place in her. After that, the main dynamic significance of the skin-pulling became suddenly clear to her and to me. "I am still surprised and sometimes a little anxious about the change which I have undergone," she said, "and about finding and maintaining the continuity and the identity between the girl who used to be so frightfully mixed up that she had to stay locked up on the disturbed ward of Chestnut Lodge, and the popular and academically successful college-girl of today." The skin-pulling as a symptom similar to another self-mutilating act of burning herself, which she repeatedly committed while acutely ill, helped her to maintain her continuity. It made it possible to be ill and well at the same time, because it was only she who knew about the symptom which could be hidden from everybody else with whom she came in contact as a healthy person. After this discovery, the symptom eventually disappeared.

Incidentally, important as the understanding of this one dynamic aspect of the patient's symptom was for therapeutic reasons, this does not mean that it constituted its only significance.

It was stated that mental symptoms in general can be understood as a means of expressing and of warding off anxiety and the central conflicts which are at the root of this anxiety, and that the exploration of this anxiety is most important in psychotherapy with schizophrenics. If this is true, we have to ask for a specific psychodynamic formulation of the causal interrelatedness between schizophrenic symptomatology and the conflicts underlying the anxiety in schizophrenic patients. A correct workable conception of the psychodynamic correlation between anxiety and schizophrenic symptom-formation is a prerequisite for the development of a valid method of dynamic psychotherapy with schizophrenic patients.

We know the historically determined deadly fear of schizophrenics of being neglected, rejected, or abandoned, and their inability to ask for the acceptance and attention they want. Consequently, most psychiatrists who did psychotherapy with schizophrenics in the early days suggested treating them with utter caution, as I did, or with unending maternal love, permissiveness, and understanding as did Schwing and more recently Sechehaye. While doing so, psychiatrists faced another dynamically significant problem of the schizophrenic, the unconscious struggle between his intense dependent needs and his recoil from them. These we learned to understand genetically as the correlate to the patients' experience of neglect by the "bad mother" at a time when her attention was indispensable for the infant's and the child's survival.

We also know about the resentment, anger, hostility, fury, or violence, with which the infant and child, the "bad me" as Sullivan called it, and later the schizophrenic patient, responds to the early damaging influences of the "bad mother," as he experienced her.

In order to understand the devastating significance of his hostility for schizophrenic patients, we have to realize the following developmental facts of their lives. As we first learned from Freud and Bleuler, schizophrenics are people who responded to the early misery of their interpersonal contacts not only with anger and hostility, but also with a partial regression into an early state of ego-development and of autistic self-concern and self-preoccupation. This early traumatization and the partial regression make for a weak organization of the schizophrenic's ego. Consequently, he feels more threatened than other people by all strong emotional experiences, and above all, by the realization of his own hostile impulses.

Another reason for the specific hardship which schizophrenic hostility creates for the patients is that their autistic self-preoccupation makes for their being painfully concerned with their own "bad me," with their own hostility and fury, or their fantasies of violence and destruction against themselves and others.

Besides, their grandiose concept of power in these states of regression to an early state of interpersonal development makes for their preoccupation with themselves as more or less dangerous people.

Where other types of patients are mainly concerned with the fear of disapproval, of the withdrawal of love which they may elicit in other people by their hostile impulses or other emanations of their "bad me," schizophrenic patients are more concerned with their own status as dangerously hostile people with the damage which may be done to others who associate with them, and with their impulses of punitive self-mutilation.

Yet, neither the fearful and grandiose self-preoccupation with his dangerous hostility, nor the threat of the primary abandonment by mother, nor the resulting dependent needs from which the patient simultaneously recoils, nor the secondary rejection he may have elicited in the mother and other significant persons in his environment because of his "badness" are in themselves potent enough to elicit schizophrenic anxiety.

Schizophrenics suffer, as all people in our culture do even though to a much lesser degree, from the tension between dependent needs and longing for freedom, between tendencies of clinging dependence and of hostility. For the above-mentioned reasons the degree of the schizophrenic's need for dependency, the extent to which he simultaneously recoils from it, and the color and degree of his hostile tendencies and fantasies toward himself and others are much more intense than in other people. As a result, the general tension engendered by the clash of each of these single powerful emotional elements becomes completely overwhelming. In other words, the quantitative difference between the schizophrenic's anxiety and similarly motivated tensions in people who have not been emotionally traumatized as early in life as the schizophrenic, and who could therefore develop a stronger ego organization, is so great that it acquires a totally different quality. It is this tremendous volume of the schizophrenic's anxiety which makes it unbearable in the long run. It then has to be discharged by symptom-formation; *i.e.*, schizophrenic symptomatology is seen as the expression of and defense against schizophrenic anxiety, engendered by the tremendous tension between his great dependent needs, his fear to give them up, his recoil from them, his hostility, his thoughts and fantasies of destructiveness against himself and others.

In delineating the dynamic interrelatedness between schizophrenic anxiety and symptomatology, I do not claim, of course, to solve the total problem of schizophrenic symptomatology. I am referring only to such portions of the dynamics as seems necessary for the clarification of my therapeutic conceptions. Our treatment of many schizophrenic manifestations has been corrected or markedly improved in the light of the hypothesis offered.

Take for example the meaning of the schizophrenic's "fear of closeness," a formulation which, incidentally, has been much abused. In the early years of psychotherapy with schizophrenics we used to understand this fear of intimacy as an expression of anxiety that all closeness, much as it was simultaneously desired, might be followed by subsequent rejection; then we learned that this fear of closeness seemed also strongly determined by the fear which the partially regressed schizophrenic with his weak ego-organization felt, that closeness might endanger his identity, might destroy the boundaries between his own ego and that of the other person.

In the meantime, I learned from my work with quite a number of further patients, that their fear of closeness is tied up with their anxiety regarding the discovery of their secret hostility or violence against persons for whom they feel also attachment and dependence. They give a mitigated, non-dangerous expression to this hostility, and try simultaneously to hide it as a secret by staying away from people.

Let me mention, in this context, an experience which I had repeatedly with patients whom I saw in an office connected with my home: they became tense and anxious when we met after my secretary and maid had left the house. The patients commented on the lack of protection against their hostile impulses.

One young paranoid patient formulated this outrightly, by asking, "Do you realize that I can knock you down in no time?" Unfortunately, I became preoccupied with my role of demonstrating the lack of fear which at the time was luckily mine. Thus, I failed to notice how frightened the patient felt by the realization of his potential violence against a woman doctor, with whom he had established at the same time a dependent relationship. Later on I realized that he was warning me against and asking for protection from future acts of violence, by which he felt we were both threatened. Subsequently, such threats against me or other doctors whom he accidentally saw in my house, against the house itself, and against the attendants who came to take care of him, were the unfortunate result. All these assaultive acts were accompanied by marked signs of anxiety.

I continued seeing the patient in a wet pack, until he agreed to abstain from all violent actions and to express his hostile feelings verbally. This he did for some time, alternately with verbal expressions of his dependent attachment and with nonverbal signs of anxiety, until he developed a marked manifest psychotic symptomatology. Since then, it became more difficult to have the patient face his dependent needs and his hostility or the anxiety engendered by both. Had I caught on immediately to the patient's anxiety regarding his own hostility, he might have been spared the necessity of transforming it into overt psychotic symptomatology.

Let us now take a look at states of catatonic stupor in the light of our hypothesis. I believe it is of interest to state that many clinicians have been accustomed to describe stuporous states as a result of the schizophrenic's withdrawal of interest from outward reality. Hence the oversimplification of interpreting them only as a response to catatonic fear of rejection becomes quite understandable.

Actually, a patient in stupor has not withdrawn his interest from the environment. As we know from reports about the experiences while in stupor, which these patients furnish after their emergence, they are, more frequently than not, keen observers of what is going on in their environment. Withdrawal of the ability for interpersonal communication is what characterizes the condition of the patient in stupor, not withdrawal of interest in the environment *per se*. As we know now, this comes about not only in response to the threat of rejection by others, but much more for fear of the patient's own hostility or violence in response to actual or assumed acts of rejection from other people.

I remember in this connection the catatonic patient previously reported who became stuporous when she did not receive my message that I had to postpone a scheduled interview. Upon discovering this unfortunate omission, I painstakingly explained the situation to the patient. When she heard and understood me, she emerged from the stuporous state and psychotherapeutic contact could be resumed.

Incidentally, while telling you about my therapeutic approach to this or other patients, I have to fight off a temptation to dramatize; this in spite of the fact that dramatization does certainly not go with what I would consider good taste in delivering a scientific paper. Upon asking myself about the reason for this temptation, I discovered that actually it is not as illegitimate as it appears to be. It is promoted by the fact that I feel inclined to duplicate tone and inflections of the patient's and my voice, the concomitant gestures, changes in facial expression, etc. This comes about because the doctor's nonverbal concomitants of the psychotherapeutic exchange with schizophrenic patients, in and outside of manifestly psychotic episodes, are equally if not at times more important than the verbal contents of our therapeutic communication.

The particular emotional stimulus to which a stuporous schizophrenic will respond, which instigated this digression, must be much stronger than one that can be produced by the content *per se* of what is said. An academic type of delivery to the patient will not do the trick.

Of course, to a certain extent nonverbal elements play a great role in all interpersonal communications, but the degree of expressive skill with which the patient himself uses means of nonverbal communication, and his specific sensitivity to the meaning of its use by the psychotherapist is such that for all practical purposes the difference in quantity, here again, turns actually into one of quality.

This great perceptive sensitivity of schizophrenic patients was one of the reasons for my overcautious approach to them in bygone times. We used to look at the sensitiveness of these patients in a merely descriptive way and labelled it as one of their admirable characteristics. If we investigate it psychodynamically we realize that it develops actually in response to their anxiety as a means of orientation in a dangerous world, and we can use it as a signpost on our road toward the psychodynamic investigation of schizophrenic anxiety. Also we should not overlook the possibility that many of the initially correct results of the schizophrenic's perceptive sensitivity may be subsequently subject to distorted psychotic interpretation and misevaluation.

To return to our discussion of the psychodynamics of states of catatonic stupor, I too used to interpret them as a sign only of the patients' having withdrawn because of the lack of consideration or rejection of them. I believe now that this is neither the primary nor the only cause, and that withdrawal into stupor is more strongly motivated by the anxiety of patients who realize the danger of their own hostile responses to such neglect by people on whom they depend and to whom they are attached. Several patients corroborated the validity of this hypothesis by spontaneous comments after their recovery.

The symptoms that patients in stupor show concomitant with their withdrawal of interest from communication furnish another proof. Stuporous patients regress to a period of life when they used food-intake and elimination as an expression of their hostility against and of their wish to exert control over their environment.

The hostile meaning of disturbances in elimination can also be demonstrated outside of stuporous states. I had impressive proof of it in my dealings with a schizophrenic woman patient, who is also mentioned in the Stanton and Schwartz paper, "A Social Psychological Study of Incontinence."

One day, this patient urinated, before I came to see her, on the seat of the chair on which I was supposed to be seated during our interview. I did not see that the chair was wet. The patient did not warn me and I sat down. I became aware of the situation only after the dampness had penetrated my clothing. I thereupon expressed my disgust in no uncertain terms. Then I stated that I had to go home. The patient asked anxiously about my coming back, which I refused with the explanation that the time allotted to our interview would be over by the time I would have taken a bath and attended to my soiled clothes.

Obviously, the patient's wetting my chair was an expression of hostile aspects in her dependent relationship with me. However, I did not say so in so many words, because I felt that the verbalization of this insight should come from the patient. In subsequent discussions of the event, she responded first with symptom-formation and nonverbal communication, wavering back and forth from expressions of hostility against me to expressions of attachment and dependence, until she was finally able to reveal that this had been a planned expression of resentment against me. The patient wished to punish me for what she had experienced as excessive therapeutic pressure during an interview preceding the chair-wetting.

Certain symptoms of several hebephrenic patients of our observation could also be psychodynamically understood and therapeutically approached as an expression of the anxiety connected with their hostility toward people on whom they likewise felt extremely dependent. These patients withdrew their interest from their interpersonal environment except for a kind of tolerant and peaceful, if incomprehensible, give-and-take with some of their fellow patients, until it all was suddenly interrupted by an outburst of hostility against these patients or against the personnel. As far as their dealings with me went, they did what hebephrenic patients will do at times, as we all know: a kind of mischievous smile or laughter accompanied or interrupted their scarce communications or was in itself the only sign of their being in some kind of contact with me. Two patients stated, after they were ready to resume verbal contacts with me, that their laughter was a correlate of hostile derogatory ideas against and fantasies about me. As they at last established a close relationship of utter dependence upon me, this was accompanied by a marked increase in intensity and duration of these spells of derogatory, tense laughter. The anxiety connected with the establishment of a dependent relationship expressed itself and was warded off by the increased derogatory laughter. The laughter subsided eventually, in response to the psychotherapeutic investigation and the working through of the various aspects of the patients' relationship with me.

With regard to paranoid patients, one of their dynamisms is, as we know, that they project onto others the blame for what they consider blameworthy in themselves. Upon investigation of the contents of their blameworthy experiences we always discover that they are extremely hostile in nature. The suspiciousness of these people points in the same direction.

Again, their suspicion and hostility increase parallel with the realization of their friendly dependent relationship with the psychiatrist. This showed quite impressively in the above-mentioned violent man patient. The fact that the office where we initially met was part of my home became to him, to use Mme. Sechehaye's expression, a "symbolic realization" of his wish to be my friend and houseguest. As he fantasied that I shared his wishes and hallucinated that he heard me say so, he became more and more hostile and anxious.

If our hypothesis about the interrelatedness between craving for and recoiling from dependency, dangerous hostility and violence against themselves and others, overwhelming anxiety and schizophrenic symptomatology is correct, we must ask how the therapeutic approaches of consistent love and permissive care, as they used to be given to schizophrenic patients by some therapists, including myself, could be helpful. We used to think that they were successful (1) because they gave a patient the love and interest he had missed since childhood and throughout life; (2) because his hostility could subside in the absence of the warp which had originated it; and (3) because the patient was helped to re-evaluate his distorted patterns of interpersonal attitudes toward the reality of other people.

We now realize that what we have long known to be true for neurotic

patients also holds true for schizophrenics. The suffering from lack of
love in early life cannot be made up for by giving the adult what the
infant has missed. It will not have the same validity now that it would
have had earlier in life. Patients have to learn to integrate the early
loss and to understand their own part in their interpersonal difficulties
with the significant people of their childhood.

I also know now, and can corroborate this with spontaneous statements of recovered patients, that the love and consideration given to
them is therapeutically more significant because they interpret it as
proof that they are not as bad, as hostile in the eyes of the therapist,
as they feel themselves to be.

The few fragments of therapeutic exchange with patients quoted
so far may serve as examples of the change in our psychotherapeutic
attitude, part of which I already elaborated in my contribution to the
1950 Yale Symposium on Psychotherapy with Schizophrenics.

Of course, we give our schizophrenic patients all the signs of empathic consideration that they need because they suffer. If possible,
we prefer to do so by implication or in nonverbalized innuendoes. Too
marked sympathetic statements may enhance fear of intimacy and
they may unnecessarily increase patients' dependence on the therapist,
putting into motion the psychopathological chain of dependent attachment, resentment, anxiety, symptom-formation.

However, we no longer treat the patients with the utter caution
of by-gone days. They are sensitive but not frail. If we approach them
too cautiously, or if we do not expect them to be potentially able to
discriminate between right and wrong, we do not render them a therapeutically valid service. We contribute to their low self-evaluation,
instead of helping them to develop a healthier attitude toward themselves and others.

Also, if there was lack of parental interest in infancy, this entails
lack of guidance in childhood. This fact deserves more therapeutic
consideration than it has been given so far. There are therapeutically
valid variations of the guidance needed and missed in early childhood,
which can be usefully included in psychotherapy with schizophrenics
in adulthood.

One exuberant young patient, the daughter of indiscriminately "encouraging" parents, was warned against expecting life to become a garden of roses
after her recovery. Treatment, she was told, should make her capable of
handling the vicissitudes of life which were bound to occur, as well as to enjoy
the gardens of roses which life would offer her at other times. When we reviewed her treatment history after her recovery, she volunteered that this
statement had helped her a great deal, "not because I believed for a moment
that you were right, doctor, but because it was such a great sign of your con-

fidence in me and your respect for me, that you thought you could say such a serious thing to me and that I would be able to take it."

In line with our attempts at raising patients' low opinion of themselves, we replace offers of interpretations by the therapist, if possible, by attempts at encouraging patients to find and formulate their interpretations themselves, as demonstrated in my exchange with the patient who wet the chair.

So far we have discussed the psychodynamics of schizophrenics symptom-formation in general as a response to their anxiety. Let us now consider the double and multiple meaning that is inherent in many of the schizophrenic's cryptic and distorted manifestations. Many of them elude the psychiatrist's understanding, but they may yield indirectly to therapeutic endeavors in other areas. Insight into their dynamics may thus be gained in subsequent discussions.

Others, such as hallucinations and delusions, I found frequently accessible to a direct psychotherapeutic approach. They would be successfully examined with the patient as they occurred in his experience and in terms of his own formulations. I stated, however, explicitly to the patient that I did not share his hallucinatory or delusional experience.

There is one more access to understanding schizophrenic communications which has not been mentioned as yet. Schizophrenics are able to refer in their productions simultaneously to experiences from the area of their early childhood, from their present living in general, and, if they are under treatment, from their relationship with the therapist, like dreamers do in their dreams. Sometimes we are able to understand the meaning of and their reference to various chronological levels of the patients' experience, sometimes not.

At any rate, it is most important for the psychiatrist to realize this multiple meaning of many schizophrenic symptoms and communications. This realization should make us replace the old therapeutic attitude that therapists ought to be able to find and offer to the patient the only correct meaning of a symptom or communication by the suggestion that they should train themselves to become able to feel which of several meanings of a schizophrenic symptom or communication (if they catch on to several of them) is the therapeutically most significant one at a given time. This ability of the psychiatrist to select sensitively when and what to present to the patient is most desirable, because of the narrowed ways of the schizophrenic's thinking and his short span of attention which limits his capacity to listen.

The insights into the possibilities and the limitations of understanding schizophrenic communications should do away with the endless discussion that used to go on between various members of groups of psychotherapists as to whether a patient's communication in word or action meant only what Dr. A. heard or exclusively what Dr. B. heard. Depending upon the scope of personal and clinical experience and the personality of the therapist and on his ability to understand patient's communications via identification, each among several psychotherapists may catch on to one of the different meanings of a patient's communication.

The insight into the manifold meanings of patients' symptoms or other manifestations may also do away with the continuing discussions in our literature of the question whether or not schizophrenic patients understand their own communications. I believe it should be stated that they sometimes do and sometimes do not. Sometimes they may, above all, be aware of the descriptive content of their communication, but not of its dynamic significance. While this whole question holds great theoretical interest, I believe now that for therapeutic purposes its solution is not too important. This holds true all the more since the main trends in treatment no longer go in terms of translating the descriptive meaning of the content of any single symptom.

There are two facts that have led us more and more away from working with patients in terms of interpreting their various symptoms and other cryptic communications. One is negative and is determined by the fact that most isolated interpretations of the content of a single symptom or other communication will not cover all its meanings in a therapeutically significant way. The other is an important positive one: it follows from the knowledge of the psychodynamic fact that schizophrenic patients, like any other mental patients under treatment, repeat with the therapist the interpersonal experiences which they have undergone during a lifetime.

Hence we have moved increasingly in the direction which I have already elaborated in previous papers: we make the therapeutic exploration and clarification of schizophrenic anxiety and symptomatology, as they manifest themselves in the patient-doctor relationship, as integral a part of psychotherapy with schizophrenics as it is with neurotic patients. Some modifications are, of course, required in view of the difference between schizophrenic and neurotic modes of relatedness with the psychiatrist and with other people. But in both cases, our therapeutic attention is focused on the dynamic investigation and clarification of the conscious and the unconscious aspects of the patient-doctor relationship in its own right and in its transference aspects. Special attention is paid to the exploration of the anxiety aroused by the therapist's probing into the patients' problems, and to his security operations against it.

Here is an example from the treatment history of the patient who pulled the skin off her heels, which illustrates both the multiple meaning of schizophrenic symptoms on various experiential levels and our approach to its basic dynamic significance in terms of investigating its manifestations in the patient-doctor relationship:

We are already familiar with the dynamic validity of the skin-pulling as a way for the patient to establish her "continuity." As we learned in the course of its further investigation, the localization of this symptom was determined by mischievously ridiculing memories of her mother's coming home from outings to prepare a meal for the family, going into the kitchen, removing shoes and stockings but not coat and hat, and walking around the kitchen on bare feet.

The self-mutilating character of the symptom proved to be elicited by the patient's resentment against me. In her judgment, I misevaluated the other act of self-mutilation from which she suffered during her psychotic episodes, the compulsion of burning her skin. The patient thought of them as a means of relieving unbearable tension, whereas she felt that I thought of them only as a serious expression of tension. In maintaining the skin-pulling, while otherwise nearly recovered, she meant to demonstrate to me that skin injuring was not a severe sign of illness.

During the treatment period after the dismissal from the hospital, the patient tried for quite a while to avoid the recognition of her hostility against me and the realization of her dependent attachment to me which she resented, by trying to cut me out of her every-day life. She did so, repeating an old pattern of living in two worlds, the world which she shared with me during our therapeutic interviews, and life outside the interviews, during which she excluded me completely from her thinking. Previously, the patient had established this pattern with her parents by living for 11 years in an imaginary kingdom which she populated by people of her own making and by the spiritual representations of others whom she actually knew. They all shared a language, literature, and religion of her own creation. Therapeutic investigation taught us that the patient erected this private world as a means of excluding her prying parents from an integral part of her life. It was her way of fighting her dependence on them and of demonstrating how different she was from them in all areas where she disliked and resented them.

The patient recognized the significance of the dichotomy in her dealings with me as a means of escape from her resentment against and dependence on me, only after going twice through a sudden outburst of hostility and anxiety which led to brief periods of re-admission to the hospital where she regressed to her old symptom of burning herself.

After a few stormy therapeutic interviews, she understood the dynamic significance of her need for readmission; she felt so dependent on me and so hostile against me that she had to come back to live in the hospital and to burn her skin.

During the ambulatory treatment periods which followed, the patient learned eventually to recognize that her excluding me from one part of her life was a repetition of the exclusion of her parents from her private kingdom.

After that, she saw too that her resentment against me was also a revival of an old gripe against her parents; they had a marked tendency to make her out to be dumb, as I tried to do, in her judgment, by putting over her my misevaluation of the skin burning. They kept her for many years in a state of overdependence, as I had done too, by virtue of our therapeutic relationship.

All these transference facets of the patient's relationship with me, as well as the problems of the doctor-patient relationship in their own right had to be worked through several times before the patient could ultimately become free from her interpersonal difficulties with me, with her parents and other people, and from the anxiety which they engendered.

While we consider the suggestions about psychotherapy with schizophrenics, which we have offered, to be psychodynamically valid and helpful rules, we believe, on the other hand, that the ways and means to go about using them will be inevitably subject to many variations, depending on the specific assets and liabilities of the personality of the therapist, and, hence, on the specific coloring of his interaction with his patient.

Psychotherapy with schizophrenics is hard and exacting work for both patients and therapists. Every psychiatrist must find his own style in his psychotherapeutic approach to schizophrenic patients. About technical details such as seeing patients only in the office, walking around with them, seeing them for nonscheduled interviews I used to have strong feelings and meanings. Now I consider them unimportant, as long as the psychotherapist is aware of and alert to the dynamic significance of what he and the patient are doing, and what is going on between them. What matters is that he conducts treatment on the basis of his correct appraisal and exploration of the psychodynamics of the patient's psychopathology and its manifestations in the doctor-patient relationship. Successful histories of treatment with the principles suggested, but conducted in various and sundry interpersonal and environmental settings, are a living proof of the validity of my present corrected attitude.

Since the work with schizophrenics makes great and specific demands on the psychiatrist's skill and endurance, no discussion of psychotherapy with schizophrenics is satisfactory as long as the consideration of the specific personal problems of the therapist is omitted. In view of the extensive previous discussions of this topic by others and by myself, I shall only briefly enumerate the specific problems and requirements which ought to be met and solved by psychiatrists who wish to work with schizophrenics: they should be able to realize and constructively handle unexpected emotional responses, such as fears or anxieties, at times inevitably aroused in each of them by anxious, violent, overdependent, or lonely schizophrenic patients.

There is one special point I might add. Psychotherapists who share the fear of loneliness, which is the fate of men in our time, must watch out specifically lest their need to counteract their own loneliness makes them incapable of enduring the inevitable loneliness and separation that their schizophrenic patients may bring home to them in their isolating cryptic communications. An undesirable urge to translate cryptic schizophrenic communications prematurely may interfere in such therapists with the more sound tendency to patiently wait and listen to the patients' own explanations of their communications.

SUMMARY

1. The goal of dynamic psychotherapy with schizophrenics is the same as that of intensive psychotherapy with other mental disturbances, i.e. to help both ambulatory and hospitalized patients gain awareness of and curative insight into the history and unknown dynamic causes which are responsible for their disorder.

2. The same type of psychotherapeutic approach to schizophrenic patients during all phases and manifestations of the disorder and discussions of illness and treatment after their recovery are recommended for the purpose of helping such patients to integrate their recovery with their psychotic past.

3. An attempt is made to understand schizophrenic symptomatology and to approach it therapeutically as an expression of and as a defense against anxiety. The hypothesis is offered that the universal human experience of tension between dependency, fear of relinquishing it, recoil from it, and interpersonal hostility becomes, in the case of schizophrenic persons, so highly magnified and so overwhelming that it leads to unbearable degrees of anxiety and then to discharge in symptom-formation.

4. The multiple meaning of many schizophrenic symptoms, communications, and other manifestations has been discussed. The need for understanding and translating them descriptively for therapeutic reasons has been questioned, and the significance of nonverbal communications with schizophrenic patients has been stressed.

5. Psychodynamic investigation and clarification of schizophrenic anxiety and symptomatology in its conscious and unconscious manifestations in the patient-psychiatrist relationship is presented to be equally crucial for psychotherapy with schizophrenics as for other mental patients.

27

THE TREATMENT OF SCHIZOPHRENIC PSYCHOSIS BY DIRECT ANALYTIC THERAPY

With Discussion

JOHN NATHANIEL ROSEN, M.D.

This paper is an attempt to describe — with an illustrative case history — the method the writer has employed in the apparently successful treatment of 37 cases of so-called deteriorated schizophrenia. This group included the three chief categories that are used diagnostically, hebephrenic, catatonic and paranoid. I wish frankly to admit that it is not at all clear in my mind what the fundamentals in this method are; but I have every reason to believe that the foundations upon which this therapy is based, although still obscure, are nonetheless sound.

An absolute essential in the equipment of the therapist is the deepest possible knowledge of the unconscious. It will soon be seen — when I describe what actually goes on between the patient and myself — that I was called upon to converse with the patient in the language of the unconscious and to be in a position to interpret the unconscious to him at every single available opportunity.

Each symptom, each remark, every symbol must be untwisted, clear down to its earliest ontogenetic and even philogenetic roots in the unconscious. Only when the symptom is so clearly unmasked to the patient that it will no longer serve its purpose, will he be able to relinquish it for a more sensible way of handling his instinctual drives. The task is not completed with the resolution of the psychosis and can only be considered concluded when the transference is as completely worked out as we aim to do in ordinary analytic procedures.

Those who have read my paper on "A Method of Resolving Acute Catatonic Excitement" [1] will note that an empirical procedure resulted in an enormous diminution of the psychotic anxiety. It was this simple discovery of talking directly to the unconscious, which was incidentally the only mental activity operating in those patients, that gave me the hope that some kind of elaboration of this formula might

From *The Psychiatric Quarterly*, 21:3, 1947. © 1947 by *The Psychiatric Quarterly*.
[1] *Psychiat. Quart.*, 20:2, 183, April 1946.

succeed in more chronic cases where the "scar tissue" and other evidences of pathological repair were in greater abundance.

Early years of training in pathology prompted me to describe the deteriorated schizophrenic in these organic terms, although at no point along the line have I ever been persuaded that there exists in these patients an organic or even constitutional factor that could begin to fulfill the criteria of Koch's postulates. In each case, in accordance with well-known authors, I also found environmental factors of such distressing intensity that, if they could be duplicated, I believe they would produce the same type of psychosis in many other individuals which was produced in the unfortunate victims.

Before giving excerpts from the treatment of an apparently deteriorated schizophrenic of the paranoid type, it must be said that the method must be modified to meet the needs of each individual case. For instance, one of my patients in a catatonic state never uttered a word to me for over a period of nine months, whereas a hebephrenic of many years duration hardly ever gave me an opportunity to get a word in edgewise. I believe, however, that something in the therapy is common to all.

In the case of the hebephrenic, the words "gotten in edgewise" finally had effect. In that of the catatonic, the words cast into an apparent vacuum proved to have taken effect. The patient, a married woman in her late twenties, spoke at last. The physician had tended her, fed her, treated her like a baby for nine months. For two of them, he had been with her for 10 hours a day, for the next seven, for four. When she started to improve, her progress was rapid. Today she has been well for a year, making an adjustment far above her prepsychotic level. She is mature in relations with her children, against whom she formerly had much unconscious hostility, and is active in child study association work. She has taken charge of her own family affairs and has forbidden her mother to shop for her, as the older woman formerly did. She has asserted her independence to her husband who, as a result, thinks more of her than ever. Her pre-psychotic sexual relations were in obedience to her husband's demands and performed with very little feeling; she now has intercourse frequently and on a mature level and with normal enjoyment of both fore-play and intercourse itself. Formerly shy and schizoid, she now has many friends and leads an active social life in which she generally dominates.[2]

In 36 of these cases the psychosis was resolved. The thirty-seventh

SUMMARY OF 37 CASES TREATED BY DIRECT ANALYTIC THERAPY *

Patient	Sex	Marital status	Age	Diagnosis	Symptomatology	Duration of psychosis	Total hospitalization time	"SHOCK" TREATMENTS Type	Number	Duration	Results	Type and duration of other treatments	Time between "shock" treatment and direct psychoanalysis	Average daily hours of direct psychoanalysis	Duration of direct psychoanalysis	Present length of remission
1	F	M	34	Schizophrenia	Depressed, anxious self-centered, retarded	7 mos.	9 mos.	ECT Insulin	9 conv. 49 comas	3 wks. 11 wks.	Unimproved Unimproved	Ambul. Insulin 1 mo.	None	2	4 mos.	21 mos.
2†	F	M	27	Schizophrenia	Confused, visual and auditory hallucinations, excited, temperature rose shortly after admission	6 yrs.	5 mos.	Unknown				Sedation		8	3 days	36 mos.
3	F	M	31	Schizophrenia	Contact superficial, sentences disconnected and illogical, blocking, depressed, fearful, crying, visual and auditory hallucinations, feelings of unreality and depersonalization	2 yrs.	6 mos.	ECT Insulin	22 conv. 40 comas	2 mos. 3 mos.	Improved but relapsed	None	7 mos.	2	2 mos.	2 wks.
4	F	M	41	Schizophrenia	Profound depression, bizarre and illogical ideas, archaic thinking	11 mos.	11 mos.	ECT Insulin	9 conv. 50 comas	3 wks. 2 mos.	Unimproved Unimproved	Ambul. Insulin 2 mos.	3 mos.	2	3 mos.	34 mos.

No.	Sex		Age	Diagnosis	Symptoms			Previous treatment		Result						
5	F	S	34	Schizophrenia	Depression, obsessions, auditory hallucinations, periods of excitement	5 yrs.	5 yrs.	ECT ECT with Insulin	20 conv. 20 conv. 33 comas	Unimproved Unimproved	Ambul. Insulin 1½ mos.	3 mos.	1–3	11 mos.	16 mos.
6	F	M	43	Schizophrenia	Claustrophobia, confusion, fear of homicidal intent, delusions, agoraphobia	16 yrs.	None	None			None		1	2 wks.	4 wks.
7	F	S	31	Schizophrenia	Vague anxiety, headaches, insomnia, depression, inability to work	6 mos.	5 mos.	None			None		1	5 mos.	25 mos.
8	F	S	22	Schizophrenia	Excitement, overactivity, assaultiveness, hallucinations, screaming, tearing clothes and bed clothes	7 mos.	5 mos.	ECT	30 conv.	Unimproved	Ambul. Insulin 4 mos.	4 mos.	1–3	2 mos.	31 mos.
9	M	M	36	Schizophrenia	Suicidal attempt, reticent, said someone was creeping under his skin, destructive, abusive, assaultive, irrelevant remarks, auditory hallucinations, depressed, resistive, insight and judgment impaired, self-absorbed, blocking	21 yrs.	7½ yrs.	None			None		1½–2	1 mo.	18 mos.

* Statistics as of January 15, 1947.

† Treatment of this patient was terminated at Brooklyn State Hospital against the therapist's advice after the psychosis was resolved but before the treatment was completed. The writer does not know the present whereabouts of this patient, but his latest information was that she was well.

Summary of 37 Cases Treated by Direct Analytic Therapy

Patient	Sex	Marital status	Age	Diagnosis	Symptomatology	Duration of psychosis	Total hospitalization time	"SHOCK" TREATMENTS				Type and duration of other treatments	Time between "shock" treatment and direct psychoanalysis	Average daily hours of direct psychoanalysis	Duration of direct psychoanalysis	Present length of remission
								Type	Number	Duration	Results					
10	F	M	24	Schizophrenia	People following her, auditory hallucinations, especially a whistling sound which represented a code, fear that she was an orphan, depressed, suicidal ideas, suicidal attempt	7 yrs.	OPD 6 mos.	None				Sedation		4–5 2	1 mo. 1 mo.	19 mos.
11*	F	S	32	Schizophrenia	Extremely poor contact, inferior conscious control over thought processes, inability to prolong voluntary attention, uncontrolled and delusional thinking, all responses irrational	11 yrs.	11 yrs.	ECT Insulin Metrazol with Insulin	75 conv. 120 comas 20 conv.	Unknown	Unimproved Unimproved Unimproved	None	5 yrs.	2–3	7 wks.	2½ mos.
12	F	M	23	Schizophrenia	Mutism, stupor, excitement, aggression, viciousness, assaultiveness	5 yrs.	5 yrs.	ECT Insulin Metrazol	8 conv. 53 comas 8 conv.	3 wks. 3 mos. 3 wks.	Unimproved Unimproved Unimproved	None	None	1–3	4 mos.	19 mos.

No.	Sex	M.S.	Age	Diagnosis	Symptoms	Duration	Prev. treatment	Type	Type 2	No.	Result
13	M	S	27	Schizophrenia	Delusions, hallucinations, terror	2 yrs.	None	None	None	1	10 mos. 39 mos.
14	F	M	33	Schizophrenia	Acute anxiety, panic, palpitations, feelings of unreality, insomnia, anorexia, vomiting, weakness, depression	3 yrs.	4 mos.	None	None	2	4 mos. 24 mos.
15†	M	S	22	Schizophrenia	Complained that his mind was separating from his body, became excited, placed in restraint, loss of weight, sharp elevation of temperature, talked continually, paid no attention to questions	7 mos.	2 mos.	None	Sedation	10 / 3	3 days 38 mos. / 1 mo., 12 days
16	M	S	22	Schizophrenia	Delusions, periods of excitement, stupor	3 yrs.	None	None	Yr. Psychoanalysis	1	8 mos. 19 mos.
17	M	S	26	Schizophrenia	Delusions, visual hallucinations, women's faces float in air upside down	9 yrs.	None	None	Sedation	1	4 mos. 16 mos.
18	M	M	43	Schizophrenia	Withdrawn, depersonalization	2 yrs.	None	None	None	1	3 mos. 7 mos.
19	F	M	52	Schizophrenia	Visual hallucinations, suicidal drive	11 yrs.	None	None	Psychotherapy	2	1 mo. 16 mos.

* Patient (11) showed marked impairment of intellectual functioning, resembling organic deterioration.
† Treatment of this patient was terminated at Brooklyn State Hospital against the therapist's advice after the psychosis was resolved but before the treatment was completed. The writer does not know the present whereabouts of this patient, but his latest information was that he was well.

Summary of 37 Cases Treated by Direct Analytic Therapy

Patient	Sex	Marital status	Age	Diagnosis	Symptomatology	Duration of psychosis	Total hospitalization time	"SHOCK" TREATMENTS				Type and duration of other treatments	Time between "shock" treatment and direct psychoanalysis	Average daily hours of direct psychoanalysis	Duration of direct psychoanalysis	Present length of remission
								Type	Number	Duration	Results					
20	M	S	17	Schizophrenia	Hears voices ordering him to kill his father, jump off the roof and jump under a subway train, depressed, anxious, cries constantly	2 yrs.	2½ mos.	None				None		3–4	2½ mos.	37 mos.
21	F	W	33	Schizophrenia	Depression, crying, tremendous anxiety, constant exhaustion, delusions	7 yrs.	9 mos.	None				Psychotherapy		2	6 mos.	30 mos.
22	F	S	18	Schizophrenia	Mutism, cerea flexibilitas, wetting, soiling	Unknown	5 mos.	Insulin	35 comas and fever	3 mos.	Unimproved	None	None	1–3	1 mo., 20 days	27 mos.
23	F	M	33	Schizophrenia	Overactivity, grandiose ideas, incoherent, shifting of mood, bizarre postures, facial grimacing, echolalia, overtalkative, irrelevant, scattered, discordant activity	6 yrs.	3 mos.	None				Psychoanalysis 5 yrs.		1–2	5 wks.	3 wks.
24	F	S	18	Schizophrenia	Active auditory hallucinations, excitement	9 mos.	9 mos.	ECT	20 conv.	1½ mos.	Little improvement	None	4 mos.	1	1 mo.	28 mos.

No.	Sex		Age	Diagnosis	Symptoms			Treatment			Result					
25	F	S	21	Schizophrenia	Delusions, hallucinations, blocking, untidiness, suicide attempt by cutting wrists	3 yrs.	None	ECT	20 conv.	2 mos.	Unimproved	Psychoanalysis 6 mos.	1 yr.	1	6 mos.	13 mos.
26	F	S	35	Schizophrenia	Anxiety symptoms, fear of fainting, fear of crowds, anxiety attacks	2½ yrs.	6 mos.	None				None		2	2 mos.	26 mos.
27	F	M	33	Schizophrenia	Feelings of incompetence and inferiority, little drive or initiative, insomnia, irritability, crying spells, agitated, depressed, suicidal attempt, hazy, confused, paranoid delusions	3 yrs.	6 mos.	None				Psychotherapy		1	6 mos.	28 mos.
28	F	M	30	Schizophrenia	Paranoid delusions, incoherent, intense psychomotor activity, mutism, negativism, resistiveness	9 mos.	1 mo.	ECT	8 conv.	2 wks.	Unimproved	None	3 wks.	10 / 4	2 mos. / 7 mos.	12 mos.
29*	M	S	15	Schizophrenia	Moody, retarded, mute, anti-social, felt everything was disintegrating about him, thought he was "dying and evaporating," auditory hallucinations, went into catatonic stupor with negativism, mutism and moderate cerea flexibilitas	12 mos.	17 mos.	Insulin / Metrazol	42 comas / 3 conv.	1½ mos.	Some improvement / Worse	Thyroid 3 mos.	1 wk.	12	3 days	36 mos.

* Treatment of this patient was terminated at Brooklyn State Hospital against the therapist's advice after only three days. Nevertheless, the boy's psychosis was resolved, and he was released from the hospital. He remained out of the hospital for approximately three years, was returned on December 12, 1946, and is still a patient.

Summary of 37 Cases Treated by Direct Analytic Therapy

Patient	Sex	Marital status	Age	Diagnosis	Symptomatology	Duration of psychosis	Total hospitalization time	"SHOCK" TREATMENTS				Type and duration of other treatments	Time between "shock" treatment and direct psychoanalysis	Average daily hours of direct psychoanalysis	Duration of direct psychoanalysis	Present length of remission
								Type	Number	Duration	Results					
30	F	S	19	Schizophrenia	Frightened, confused, feelings of unreality, rich fantasy life, daydreams in color	6 yrs.	OPD	None						1	3 mos.	21 mos.
31	M	S	30	Schizophrenia	Paranoid trends, hypomania, delusions of grandeur, obscene language, aggressive, assaultive	9 yrs.	15 mos. (Approx.)	ECT	20 conv.	1 mo.	Unimproved	Hydro. Sedation Vitamins Psychotherapy 5 mos.	1 yr.	1	4 mos.	14 mos.
32	M	M	39	Schizophrenia	Over talkative, religious, discovered philosophy of life, begs for forgiveness, voices talking about him, put his hands in boiling water to boil them	1 mo.	3 wks.	None				None		2	3 wks.	38 mos.
33	F	S	26	Schizophrenia	Delusions, hallucinations, suicide attempt with 60 luminal tablets	3 yrs.	2 wks.	None				Psychotherapy		3	3 mos.	21 mos.

No.	Sex	M.S.	Age	Diagnosis	Symptoms	Duration	Previous psychotherapy	Previous treatment	Conv./Comas	Duration	Result	Adjunctive therapy	No.	Duration	Follow-up
34	M	S	21	Schizophrenia	Depression, sudden religious fervor, felt he had a personal God, withdrawn, obsessions and compulsions	3 yrs.	None	None				Psychotherapy	1	5 mos.	22 mos.
35*	F	M	37	Schizophrenia	Silly, childish, dilapidated, deteriorated, active auditory hallucinations, bizarre delusions, excitement, incoherence, primitive, archaic expressions	2 yrs.	11 mos.	ECT Insulin	28 conv. 50 comas	1½ mos. 2½ mos.	Unimproved Unimproved	None	5	5 mos.	27 mos.
36	M	S	21	Schizophrenia	Acute excitement, felt he was somebody else who burned to death in airplane, feared he was going insane, felt his insides were soft and offered no resistance to thoughts penetrating his body	1 mo.	2 days	None				Sedation	3	1 mo.	6 wks.
37	M	S	49	Schizophrenia	Auditory hallucinations, "seizures," persecutory delusions	27 yrs.	4 yrs.	ECT Insulin	20 conv. 60 comas	1 mo. 5 mos.	Unimproved		2	8 mos.	7 mos.

* This is the patient referred to in the introduction who had a relapse following a suicide attempt by her sister. The relapse lasted only a few weeks and she is now back at home and free from psychotic symptoms, showing evidence of having gained insight as a result of this pseudo-psychotic experience.

patient, still psychotic,[3] has been with me for eight weeks. Some patients have been discharged as "recovered" and others are still in analysis. One of the patients, after a two-year lapse of time, and while still being analyzed, again manifested psychotic behavior. The immediate cause was a suicidal attempt by her sister, who was very dear to this patient. The patient is now being studied to determine to what extent her insight altered the present picture. The impression I get from her at this time is dilemma and confusion rather than the deteriorated psychosis she originally had.[4]

Regarding recovered patients: Let me define "recovery." As I use this term, it does not mean merely that the patient is able to live comfortably outside an institution, but rather that such a degree of integrity is achieved that the emotional stability of the patient and his personality and character-structures are so well organized as to withstand at least as much environmental assault as is expected of a normal person, that is, of a person who never experienced a psychotic episode.

The findings to date are empirical ones. They are expressions of some natural law of human behavior, just as surely as thunder and lightning are expressions of a natural law. At the present time I cannot come up with the right answers, but there is no doubt that they exist. Freud, Federn and others have indicated the existence of general psychodynamic laws in their theoretical concepts of the ego, the super-ego and the id. When the gaps in this knowledge are filled, the secret of the etiology of schizophrenia will be revealed.

The diagnoses of schizophrenia were in all cases made by physicians other than the present writer, in most cases concurred in by more than one physician. Because the question of diagnosis is certain to be raised by a presentation of this sort, the writer has purposely excluded from this report four other cases — also diagnosed schizophrenia by other psychiatrists — but in which he feels the symptomatology was mainly manic-depressive. It has been the aim, in investigating the possibilities of this therapy, to treat initially only patients who were severely schizophrenic beyond the possibility of a doubt. It should be said that the four where the writer found manic-depressive features have made apparently complete recoveries also.

Honi Soit Qui Mal y Pense

This paper is in large part a clinical report dealing with the treatment of a single patient. Unavoidably, it reports the patient's lan-

---

[3] The psychosis of this patient has been resolved since this was written.

[4] The relapse lasted only a few weeks and the patient is now back at home and free from psychotic symptoms. She shows evidence of having gained insight as a result of this pseudo-psychotic experience.

guage — his exact language. The language of schizophrenia is often offensive. Although the psychotherapist must learn neither to take nor to feel offense, it is only fair to say that there is much reported here which even the professional reader will find startling and revolting. But to disguise it with the euphemisms of scientific terms would be to distort the whole picture inexcusably, to present it with an air of unreality, to rob it of affect. It would be a complete misrepresentation to say that having had a spoon put in R. Z.'s mouth reminded him of fellatio; it did not; it reminded him of "cock-sucking." And it would be even more of an absurdity to say that the patient told the physician to have intercourse with himself, to avoid the belligerent, affect-laden command, "Fuck yourself!" The writer feels, nevertheless, that there is so much of this material that he owes even the psychiatrist reader this note of warning and apology.

CASE HISTORY

R. Z. (No. 37 in the table), aged 49, is a single, white man, born in New York City. He attended grammar school and is a Protestant. He is a tall man, well-built; and physical examination reveals no abnormalities. His anamnesis is sketchy, because his talk was scattered and his orientation was poor. He came to me because he heard voices and he could not work. The voices started in 1922 and were still with him. In 1922, the voices told him to join the Masons, to get an apron and then to hell with it. He accounted for the voices on the basis of some form of electrical telepathy. During the previous four years, on and off, he had been at a mental hospital, where he had had a series of electric shock treatments and then a series of insulin. What was most disturbing to him were attacks of pain throughout his body which he called "those terrific seizures."

There were two voices particularly familiar to him. The principal voice was a woman's. Whatever he did had a special meaning, but just what that meaning was, he didn't know. He was vague about his past life and his family. His parents, Austrian-born, and emigrants to this country, were both dead. He had a very hazy recollection of them and of when they died, but thought they were kind-hearted persons. He has two siblings, the older, a brother, whom he hasn't seen in he "doesn't know how many" years, and an older sister, who is married and lives in Texas. The first session was disappointing indeed. During an hour's time, he spoke only once: "Suck my ass.[5] Kiss my ass. I am not afraid of anything."

On the following day he seemed somewhat more relaxed and was

[5] Arse.

able to sit still in the chair. He said: "Open your mouth." (*The analyst* [6]): *Who told you this?* "I can't be sure. A voice." *What does it mean?* "To suck a cock." *Do you?* "No, I never did." *Did anyone do it to you?* "No. I remember before I went to school, I was very young, some one took me into the cellar and gave me a bag of candy. I have never felt ashamed of it. I lived through plenty of misery and pain for it. When I was 11, some kids were playing 'dog' with their 'pricks' out, lapping each other. They asked me to play. I did. One of the kids did it for me and I gave him presents and then money. I liked the sensation. It started me off with masturbation. Some years later at a bar I met the boy. After I had a few beers, I offered him 50 cents. He said if I didn't leave him alone he'd tell his mother. I forgot all about those things until 1940."

Bearing in mind what Freud teaches us about the homosexual aspects of paranoia, it was simple enough to interpret, "Open your mouth." Although the patient had at first denied his homosexual tendencies, he apparently poured forth considerable material indicating them.

The physician assumed a permissive rôle and acted as if he didn't understand why the patient was worried. The analyst said that many persons had homosexual experiences, especially children, and he added that he recalled stories of "things like that" where he was brought up. The patient made a point of denying any interest in this type of sexual activity, but indicated that he was constantly suspicious of persons who went into subway toilets. For many years, he was a motorman on a subway train, and he remembered tales told by guards of how they made a lot of money by letting fellows "do that" to them. If he had wanted to, he could have made plenty of money "that way." The patient left the interview apparently greatly reassured; and the writer learned something that he didn't ascertain from the history, namely, that the patient had been working as a motorman.

At the next interview, R. Z. stated: "Open wide. Hold your breath. Don't be afraid to tell him it. The voice said: 'Piss on your mother's grave. Kiss my ass. Don't say that.' " What he ascribes to the voice here is his own Oedipal fantasy, and it was not surprising that his associations had to do with intercourse. "I had intercourse twice in 11 year. I often tried to go with women, but the voice and my fears prevented it. A long time ago, when I was living home with my mother and suffering with this illness, my sister came home. I heard her say: 'Get undressed. Wash your dick. How do you fuck a whore? I am a whore. I will show you how. I will suck you off.' She was kneeling near the radio and I walked over to her to be sucked off because I'd do

---

[6] Analyst's remarks italicized throughout case history.

anything to get well. She stood up and walked away. I couldn't understand it. When I see a woman, the voice says to her: 'Look out, he is a cop.' And then she turns away." He was asked, *Why a cop?* in the hope that somehow it might be explained to him about the hidden wish which has to do with getting women (mother) to turn away from father, i.e., the "cop." He seemed unimpressed and continued: "Hold your breath. Ah! You're a cheap fuck. Why are you smiling now? Swallow! Oh. What a dope. Tell him what you know. Liar! How shall I look? Down. Why don't you do it? Do it." *Do what?* "Jerk off. I have been thinking about it a lot. I also told it to that psychologist. He advised me to try it. I can't see it. I want to go out and get a woman. In my thought it comes to me that I can free myself by jerking off. In 1936, I was very sick and had to stay off the job for five months. In those days I went to the whorehouse. It came to me to jerk off, and I fought it. One day I did. The people on the street stopped speaking and laughed as I passed them by. They said out loud, 'He jerked himself off.' I didn't do it since, honest. I had a number of erections." Since he told the physician here what a good boy he was, the physician made much of what a good boy he was. Apparently some transference reaction was taking place in which the physician became identified with his father because the patient continued: "The girls make advances to me. In the park, in my house and at other places. I just walk away from them. I don't bother with them." The implication here being: "I won't disturb your women, father, if you will continue to love me and take care of me."

At about the tenth visit, the physician began to test the consistency of the patient's defenses. Regarding the problem of the voices and the names people called him, the question of validity was raised. R. Z. held steadfast to the concept of this as "thought transference." He mentioned, however, that it was incredible that he should be such a center of attraction. In the last few days he had begun to wonder if his sister was really a whore. He told of an occasion when, acting in his official capacity as a Mason, he was expected to go to a funeral service. As he circled the dead man, he became very hot. When he threw the leaves on the coffin, his hand suddenly became stiff. He heard the nephew of the dead man call public attention to his act. The physician had him associate to this experience as to dream material. "Hot" was "passion" and a "stiff arm," a "stiff prick." Since his associations were so clearly sexual, the meaning of the disguised wish was disclosed to him and the emphasis was placed on the way forbidden sexual wishes come out under pressure in a disguised form. Some indication of how the unconscious is a reservoir of hidden sexual drives was pointed out to him. The last bit of analysis gave a new kind of superego relationship to the ego and resulted in a rush of homosexual memories.

The next time that the patient said: "Hold your breath," the physician told him there was no reason to hold back and that he could tell him his secrets. As if in direct response to this request from the patient's unconscious, the man began: "Do you mean about that woman? It was around 1926. We were on strike. One of the men took me home. These people were friendly with the trainman, who was a fag. We went to a masquerade fairy ball. I was introduced to a woman and we had a box. We looked down at the fairies dancing. I didn't dance with them. After this experience, my sickness got very much worse. Wherever I went in the street, people looked at me and said: 'That is a woman.' No matter where I went, even in other cities, it was the same thing. I never went even to another fairy ball." Once at a doctor's office, he had a rectal examination for hemorrhoids. The rubber finger-cot broke, and he was seized with a pain that went from his rectum over his entire body. (Probably an orgasm.) At another time, while he was in "some kind of a hospital," he received an enema which resulted in the same kind of terrible pain. After this, he found that he couldn't see things. He thought that his eyes were out of focus. Again, he went to a hospital, and they found that his vision was normal.

He went home and found his brother sleeping on the couch. "My brother seemed to say, 'On account of you I got fucked in the ass.' My mother seemed to say, 'Shut up. Don't say these things to him.' A terrible odor suddenly came out of my body. I thought it must come from my armpits. I went to many doctors. They put their noses to my body and they couldn't get that smell. They gave me medicine for it, but it didn't help." PAUSE. "You stink." *Who?* "Me, I guess." *If you tell a fellow he stinks, what does it mean?* "He smells bad or he is a bad guy." *If it happens to be that he is a bad guy, can you smell it?* "No." This was interpreted to him as the voice of his punishing conscience in relation to the material he had just described. It called him a stinker. *Now how in the hell could those doctors smell a stinking character?*

The clarity with which the psychotic recognizes symbols is pointed out as follows: "I go to the restaurant and ask for a piece of cake. They walk away from me. A 'piece' is a 'hump' and 'cake' is eat it. Cock-sucking or cunt-lapping. All food has different meanings. 'They' told it to me. A cruller is a 'prick.' A doughnut is a 'cunt.' Rye bread is an 'ass-hole.' Mustard is 'shit.' When I went past a church or a synagogue, I spit. I did it for a long time, then it came to me, and I stopped." *What came to you?* "It was my father. A lot of these things are due to a form." *What do you mean by a form?* "Form of insanity." The obvious reason for repressing "insanity" was discussed.

R. Z. blithely continued that many things were due to a form and that he always feared that perhaps he was "insane," but, he continued, he would battle a voice if it told him to do something like, "Wreck the train." Just before he had quit work as a motorman, he had gotten up to go to work and "was told" to take a shower. While in the shower, he was told that "this day" he would wreck the train. He began to twist in the tub and suddenly tumbled out, falling in such a way as to fracture his wrists. He went to "report sick;" and when his story was heard, he was discharged. He was unable to understand this, and decided to communicate his difficulties to the F. B. I. He wrote many letters to the F. B. I., but every time he went to mail one, the "seizures" were so terrible that he was unable to do so. He got the idea that he was a psychiatrist and a hypnotist. This thought continued for some weeks during which time he felt he controlled people. When it was determined that this was a reaction-formation against his passivity, i. e., against being controlled, he gave up the delusion.

The patient now perceived a marked increase in his positive feelings toward the physician. He observed that he was getting better and could do anything but telephone. He could write, draw, read a paper and go out into the street in relative comfort. He missed the analyst over the week-end. In the midst of the session, he suddenly became angry and stated he was going to Yonkers. "You are a son of a bitch. Cock-sucker. Your father put his cock in your mother's mouth, and that is how you were born. I had a feeling stronger than ever to throw myself under an elevated train." (*Analyst*): *Father will fuck you in the ass. The train is a big, powerful penis and you wish to lay under it.* The patient stated that everything had a meaning. "I could never understand it." It seemed that he was beginning to understand something about his homosexual wishes in relation to the physician; but, as yet, no transference interpretation on this score was made. He developed two psychosomatic symptoms as a defense against his mounting anal-attitudes toward the physician: diarrhea and headache. *This diarrhea is a way of shitting on somebody, isn't it?* "You know, when I was five years old, I used to sleep with my mother. I would be awakened by my father calling out to her to come into his room. She would go, and I would cry. After a while I would run in to get my mother. I just thought of this." *No wonder you hate your father. No wonder you hate your mother.* "But my father was nice to me." *Then the way to get close to father is to be a woman like mother?* "When I was very, very young, I guess I must have been a baby, one night I had a condition and I couldn't get my breath. My father carried me in his arms from room to room and they called the doctor. The doctor put a spoon in my mouth that cured me. The whole story reminds me of cock-sucking. The spoon is a penis." *I don't see why you call all these things cock-sucking. You're not a homosexual. It seems to me that this is clearly a case in which your life was saved because your father loved you; and the doctor, a man, loved you and saved you. You show a great need to be loved by a man.* "I guess that's a father and son relationship."

The patient was impressed, by the physician, with the importance of these screen-memories for the purpose of stimulating such memories further. The patient's anger toward the physician mounted in subsequent visits. Each session was: "Fuck yourself. Kiss my ass," and so forth and so forth. He seemed constantly to refer to father taking mother from his bed. His fantasy-life was preoccupied with all kinds of thoughts of intercourse with his sister. During the next few days, he described himself as being hypnotized, and he was compelled to walk on his toes and shake from side to side. He was asked to demonstrate this walk for the physician. It was characteristic of theatrical demonstrations of a "pansy." He felt that crowds of people were following him, jeering at him. *The interpretation of this may be painful to you, but what it means is that you want to be a woman and you want to attract a man.* "I used to walk for years with my eyes almost shut. When I opened them again, the light actually hurt my eyes. I did it so that I should not see men." *Did men tempt you?* "I don't know." *What about the voice that told you to take men's "pricks" in your mouth?* "That came from me. I don't hear that anymore." *If your eyes were shut you couldn't see yourself either.* "I was ashamed. Tell him you want to suck his cock." *Who?* "You. A funny thing happened to me in 1928. The hair fell off my chest and it never came back." The physician examined the patient to verify this psychosomatic compliance. Although his body had more than the usual amount of hair — well distributed — his chest was smooth.

R. Z. began to bring in material which showed more and more his fear and hatred of women. He hated nuns, nurses, and the Christian Science Church, where the parental figure is a woman — Mary Baker Eddy. "When I was 29 and going to whorehouses, I couldn't get an erection. I went to a doctor, and he gave me medicine for it. When the whore got undressed, I began to shake inside. It was a frightening, unpleasant feeling." *Why do you feel this way about women?* He could not understand, but the question reminded him of an experience he had once had with a Spanish whore. She undressed, and he failed with her. He asked her to sit on his lap and try it that way. She did and he got an immediate erection. She jumped up and said, "No, not that." "She thought I wanted to put it in her ass-hole." *Perhaps you did. Why do you think you were able to have an erection?* He replied promptly, "It's like fucking a man in the ass." *Sure you didn't see the feared organ of the female?* This interpretation excited him considerably and pleased him. He felt that he understood so much now.

He recalled a sudden interest in the school for the deaf. After seeing a motion picture of lip reading, he practised it all the way home on the subway. *Why does this interest you?* "Cock-sucking." *Exactly, again using your mouth.* The patient was overjoyed with this new trick of understanding. "Last night it came to me that I had to go to Jersey to shop. I had such conflicts I couldn't buy anything. I went in and out of the store many times. I felt the salesmen were angry with me. Finally I went to a place to eat. I saw a cop and thoughts came to me: crook, pickpocket." (During this recitation, he was visibly agitated.) *Did you attempt to analyze all this?* "Sure, cock-sucking." *How do you arrive at that?* After some hesitation the patient said, "I don't know." *Everything isn't cock-sucking.* "Well I used to think of female clothes. I had that thought when I discovered silk or rayon in things I bought. I always wanted to return things, but no store will take things back after you wore them." *What would you rather be, a crook or a "fag"?* [7] "Neither." *If you had to make a choice?* "A crook." *The cop was your punishing and tempting father. He gave you a feeling of guilt and you hid from yourself the source of the guilt-feeling and accepted a lesser charge. That is why the thought, crook, etc., comes to you about yourself, instead of "fag." Why didn't you call me on the telephone when this disturbance was going on?* "To tell the truth, it wasn't so bad. I didn't have the severe sensations of pain this time."

The followng day, the patient proudly announced he had bought a pair of shoes and a shirt. To him, this was an exciting adventure. It was the first clothing he had been able to buy in years. "And you know, the shoes fit. I used to have to buy shoes many sizes too small. I used to go through torture to break in these small shoes. Then I had to get narrow shoes that were open at the toe and heel." *What does that mean?* "A cunt." *You remember how you walked on your toes with your heels lifted. How does that fit in with all this?* "I was being a woman and wearing women's shoes." The material continued to pour out in the same vein, his wish to be a homosexual and his symptomatic action-defenses. When the going got too tough, he invariably experienced a "seizure" and this was being interpreted in terms of super-ego chastisement. He described the "seizure" as a sudden stiffening of the body in various attitudes. The pain he described as pain in the groin, but he pointed to his stomach. He knew where the groin was but for-

[7] "Faggot" — male homosexual.

got when questioned. He suddenly got the thought that he was being punished "for fucking that man's wife." *Who's wife?* "Dr. C——'s—— that is the way it comes to me." The fear of punishment for intercourse was further introduced to the patient as a more plausible reason for his avoiding intercourse all these years. He was reminded of how he had explained this as not knowing where to find a woman and that if he did, she thought he was a cop, and so forth. As an additional thought, it was suggested: *I wonder if you ever thought of fucking your mother when you used to sleep with her? What would father have done to you if you had?* His great struggle now was with his temptation to run away from the analysis. He would have liked to visit his sister in Texas. He went to the Grand Central Terminal every day before his visit to my office, with the intention of buying a ticket to "almost any place" and taking a trip. He had his first dream since he became sick.

Dream: "I was in the kitchen of the house we used to live in. I sat sideways on a chair in front of the window. The shade was drawn. Suddenly I was blind. All was pitch blackness. I struggled fiercely to see. I pulled at my eyes, and suddenly I got my left eye open, and I saw light. I opened the shade to look out and it was cloudy and murky outside. My right eye seemed to stick tight, and the skin on that side of my face got wrinkled tight. Just then my mother and sister came in. I opened the door for them. My mother said, 'Look at what is wrong with your face.' My sister remarked casually, 'Things will be all right again.' "

Associations. "It must be our old apartment." He was unable to talk about the dream. A thought came to him: "I am man and woman. I was able to telephone to you twice over the week-end but it was very difficult. I visited a friend up-town and the family remarked on how I didn't seem to be 'nervous' any more."

Interpretation. It was pointed out, mostly from the manifest content, that since the analysis, R. Z. saw some light, versus the utter darkness of the not-understanding when he first became sick; his fierce struggle to see was to get the light, to see meanings, and to understand his illness. He fulfilled a wish also to be back with mother and sister.

The following day, the patient arrived in a state of intense excitement. His face was very pale, and perspiration covered his forehead. Instead of sitting down or lying on the couch, he assumed a menacing attitude in front of where the physician was seated. He took a knife from his pocket, released a spring and the blade sprung open. He said that for hours he had been sitting in Grand Central Station planning to run away; but it came to him that he had to go home to get the knife and cut the physician's throat. The physician was not unmindful of the precariousness of his position — but, although prepared to defend himself in the event of any further movement on the part of the patient, continued a steady barrage of interpretation of a strictly transference nature. *You want to kill me because I tempt you. Baby wants to suck my cock. He is hungry. He is frightened. He wants mother. He wants to destroy father who takes mother away from him. All you want is love and protection. I will love and protect you. Put the knife on the desk. Sit down. Lie down. No one will hurt you.* The physician got up and insisted that the patient hand him the knife, which he did with obvious relief. For some time the patient was dizzy, and he began to cry. The physician consoled him, and at the termination of the interview, he was informed that the knife would be returned to him tomorrow.

On the following day, when the patient returned, he was again agitated, but this time his manner seemed to be pleading. The knife was placed on the desk and permission was given to take it if he wished to. He picked it up and sheepishly put it in his back pocket. He mumbled something about: "Oh, that, I wouldn't use it. I just brought it here to show you." On the couch, he again repeated the thought: "You must go kill him," meaning the doctor. He added something about money. The Masons took his money and Dr. C—— took his money, and "at the Masons," they took his money and never explained the ritual. *How about wanting to kill me because I took your money?* "I don't mean that at all. You gave me protection, power, strength. You explain things to me." He was able to be aggressive toward the physician because he found that he could trust him. An interpretation of the knife-thrust as a gratification of an unconscious sexual wish was made to the patient. The following day the patient said that he was happy about the way he felt and that he was optimistic that better days were coming, in fact, better days were here.

All along in this case, I was expecting some kind of a blow-up, which seemed indicated, with the defenses constantly being undermined through the therapy. With all psychotic patients, positive and negative transferences are always more intense than with psychoneurotics. Failing to gratify the infantile wishes with the analyst, sooner or later the honeymoon-period terminates, and dramatic consequences usually follow. Just as the ego prevented R. Z. from wrecking the train, so this same ego prevented him from wrecking the analyst. For this reason, I felt that the risk was not too great in continuing to treat him outside an institution. With each day, the patient showed more and more evidence that he was accepting and adjusting to a world of reality; and the intensity of the symptoms continued to diminish.

The patient asked the physician to go with him to purchase a suit. In the past, he had tried on outlandish clothes that didn't fit; and,

even though salesmen argued with him against making such purchases, he nevertheless made them. He was fearful that he might repeat this. He now longed to have friends and to go back to work. The
part of him that wanted "to suck a cock" was still there, but got
weaker. He said that after he left my office "yesterday," and was
walking along the street, he suddenly got very dizzy and very nauseated.
He said that he just got that feeling again as he was about to come to
my office "today." He talked at great length about what a tough
neighborhood he was brought up in and how he always had to fight
for himself. If he went to his father for help, his father would not
help him, but would force him to fight. "I am not a coward. I am not
afraid of a beating." *I believe the reaction you had yesterday and again
today was due to my agreeing to help you buy a suit. This is like your
father helping you to fight, which would be an expression of love. This
intensified your wish to, and fear of, sucking my cock; and the symptomatic response from your stomach stated: I will not accept eating
from your penis. I will reject that by vomiting it out. Don't try to
make a sissy out of me. I came from a tough neighborhood.*

The patient admitted that he was excited and happy at the thought
that I would go with him to buy a suit, but somehow it all became
incorporated in psychotic thought, and he then got the idea that I
was only fooling. "Yesterday I went up to the job to ask my friends
where I could get a 'hump.' The trouble with me is that I couldn't tell
people what I wanted to. Now I can. I am going to make friends.
Maybe I can talk on the phone and get a job. I went to C———'s
office today and talked to his secretary. I asked him to send you the
report on my case, and I paid him $5.00 that I owed him." It was
agreed that we would go "tomorrow" to purchase the suit.

All the next morning, he was nervous, but the actual purchasing
of the suit occurred in a perfectly normal manner. As we left the store,
he seemed greatly relieved and called it quite an experience. He was
annoyed at his landlady neglecting his room. He went down and complained to her in a "nice way." She explained it as "maid-trouble." He
didn't want to fight with her because when he was so very sick, she
tried to be nice to him. He had gone to a show yesterday, and had
gotten cramps "like he wanted to move his bowels." Since this had
happened many times before and proved to be a mental feeling only,
he had decided to ignore it. On the way home, he had to go so badly,
he just barely made his house. He lost the voice and the talking in
his head, but expected it to return momentarily. He found it difficult
to believe that normal experiences were real.

"It came to my thought within the past few days that when I was
about two years old, my brother put his cock in my mouth. My family

caught him and from then on, after school he had to go to the home of relatives until my father came home from work. I can't be sure if this is a true experience or not, but I think I can find out. It may be like the thoughts I had about my sister being a whore. My brother had part of his leg shot away in the last war. He wears a high shoe and gets along with hardly a limp. He is not quite all right. If I talk to him about this, he will begin to cry."

On the following day he stated: "I feel so like a normal person again today. I took a bath without trouble. It's such a beautiful day. I sat in the park. What I miss most is a human companion. Could we go out for a walk?" (The physician agreed.) Outside, R. Z. felt that the world and people were normal. He continued to feel "real" during the entire period we were out. He mentioned that he had had "hot nuts" last night. This thought reminded him of a fellow he knew who had syphilis. The association was used to point out to him his fear of a heterosexual relationship because of its castrative threat. He wore his new suit. In many ways, he indicated his great love for his physician, and when this was interpreted to him he said: "In a pig's ass, I love you." This denial was not accepted; but, instead, the concrete evidences of his devotion to the analyst were pointed out to him. He then declared he feared to love any man. If he did (and here he gave an example of a friend who was a stamp collector), he would be inextricably bound to that man — fused, as it were — and it would last forever. This thought was interpreted as homosexual, however well sublimated. As a matter of fact, there was a profound incestuous sexual need in him. A wish again to be fused with mother, in mother's womb, or to be one with mother at mother's breast. This is the basic ultimate goal in any homosexual relationship.

Following this, the patient again began to have thoughts that he was attracting the attention of men. In connection with this, he had thought of the wonderful food his mother fed him — the quantity of it, the quality of it, etc. Because of the sexual nature of the intimacy he craved with his mother, he returned to the homosexual pattern, but this time, not without insight.

Smoking, eating, sleeping, etc., all his thoughts, had a strong sexual significance accompanied by intercourse hallucinations. When asked why, he was unable to explain, although he admitted being aware that all his thoughts led to sex. This hallucinatory experience was pointed out to him as a consequence of his homosexual wishes, which were intolerable, and of his incestuous wishes, which were intolerable, and of his normal genital drives which continued to go ungratified. *It is essential to the satisfactory conclusion of the case that you permit yourself to seek and obtain a normal sexual outlet.*

R. Z. is now seeking employment and is registered with the United States Employment Service. He has also interviewed a man about a position in his store as a clerk. He called up an old girl-friend to make a date, but discovered that she no longer "lived there." He went to the home of a friend — the stamp collector — who arranged with his girl-friend to get another girl so that the four could go out. This was the plan for the week-end. The physician informed R. Z. of the date of his own vacation and the patient's voice began to quiver, as if he might cry. He said he didn't understand it, but that it gave him a "queer feeling." He went out with his "date" and complained that she was a homely woman. He tried very hard to be sociable, and it gave him a "dull ache." He did some "necking" and the party was out until 6:00 a. m.

R. Z. says that the hair has grown back on his chest during the past three months and it started ever since he got "hot nuts." During the vacation period, he had a good time going to the beaches, to movies, going out on dates, and visiting with friends. He is making some money with a friend in the cigarette business. Only once did he get upset, and this occurred when he made up his mind to go to Lake George to visit the physician. He took the day-liner to Albany; and in Albany he became confused, found himself in a conflict and finally "decided to Hell with it," and took a train and went back to New York City. At the present time, the analysis continues. R. Z. now has no psychotic symptoms and his adjustment is on an increasingly mature level.

Conclusion [8]

R. Z. was presented in person so that the doctors attending the seminar where this paper was read in part could evaluate his present mental health. It was unanimously agreed that he was no longer psychotic. As far as possible, when the patients in the foregoing series appeared to be free from psychosis, I had my findings checked by my colleagues. In this way, my opinions regarding the resolution of the psychosis were confirmed.

This leads to the next inevitable question: Will these results withstand the test of time? That question cannot be answered at present; time alone will tell. In the meantime, however, 37 persons, who according to prognoses might face lives of institutionalization, have lived comfortably with society if only for a time. Even if it should be necessary for these patients to return to mental hospitals tomorrow, at least they have been able to enjoy their periods of happiness. Should

---

[8] The "Conclusion" was not part of the original paper, but has been added for publication (in The Psychiatric Quarterly).

this prove to be the only gain of my experiment, I would still consider my efforts justified. I hope to report the details of treatment in all of these cases, and others as research expands, and also to publish accounts of the progress of the patients listed in the foregoing in the years to come.

The method of treatment is rather sharply divided into two parts. The first part, the direct psychoanalysis, resolves the psychosis by dealing mostly with that level of mentation which occurs in the preverbal period of life and shortly thereafter. The second part is a more orthodox form of psychoanalysis, where the aim is to construct a stable personality and a mature character. The faults in earlier development which are revealed during the study of the psychosis are longitudinally structuralized into later years and, because the patient remembers so much of the psychosis and its meaning, abundant material is obtained that can be utilized subsequently. It is not my intention in this paper to dwell on theoretical concepts; but there is one point on the counter-transference that I believe to be so valid that I shall state it now for the benefit of those who plan to use this method.

The counter-transference is like the attitude of the parent to the child, as distinguished from the transference, which is like the attitude of the child to the parent. The child's ability to disturb the peace of mind of his parent is the earliest known means by which he obtains gratification and protection. When the child is not at rest, it results in the parent feeling unhappily disturbed, and he resents this feeling. Almost in self-defense he attempts to re-establish the former equilibrium. This is constantly recurring in the daily relationship between the parent and the child. The parent is expected to give up his peace of mind again and again to establish peace of mind in the baby. The extent of parental narcissism will determine how much love he can spare from himself for the needs of the child. The immature parent, i. e., the intensely narcissistic one, can withstand only minor assaults and, beyond this, he attacks the annoying little aggressor, thereby establishing an increasingly vicious cycle of attack and counter-attack. Perhaps this is the earliest source of parental death wishes[9] against children. I believe that these unconscious wishes on the part of the parent are perceived by the unconscious of the child and constitute to him an "unholy peril" with all the accompanying terrifying anxiety thereby provoked. The extent, therefore, of parental narcissism and lack of love for the child as an object must be an important determinant in the degree to which one is susceptible to schizophrenic reactions. Such a parent is in great need of love and protection himself and is doubly assaulted by the child who can love only himself.

[9] Be dead — that is quiet or still — in that way I will be let alone.

In the case of direct psychoanalysis the counter-transference must be of the nature of the feelings a good parent would have for a highly disturbed child. The therapist, like the good parent, must identify with the unhappy child and be so disturbed by the unhappiness of the child, that he himself cannot rest until the child is again at peace. Then the parent can again be at peace. If this feeling is present, the patient will *invariably* perceive it unconsciously. This does not mean that the therapist may not react automatically to physical attack, but if the basic unconscious relationship is as described, any conscious reaction on the part of the therapist will not be misunderstood by the patient as an alteration of the basically sound interplay of feeling. Schizophrenia, as is well known, is characterized by the most intense narcissism. The schizophrenic, at the very first interview, makes it plain that he has no love to spare for his physician, i.e., for the parental figure. The physician may not understand this helpless behavior in the patient and may very well respond like an irate, annoyed parent and proceed to treat the patient with institutionalization, shock therapy and other "riddance" mechanisms. This is not necessarily a reflection of the extent to which the physician is narcissistic. If the patient were really an infant, the physician might quite easily respond with loving care, but what he sees at this interview, is a physically mature adult who only feels and behaves like an infant. In the beginning then, the physician can expect no more love from a patient than a parent gets from a baby. What he gets instead is the patient's total dependency on him.

In order to treat the schizophrenic, the physician must have such a degree of inner security that he is able to function independently, whether he is loved by the patient or not. Or perhaps it would be better to state that the physician must be able to manage with the least possible amount of love from the patient. He must make up for the tremendous deficit of love experienced in the patient's life. Some people have this capacity for loving as a divine gift. But it is possible to acquire this the hard way — by psychoanalysis. It is the *sina qua non* for the application of this method in the treatment of schizophrenia.

It may be well to mention another fact concerning the present adjustments of the writers' recovered patients. The opinion has already been expressed that they have achieved such a degree of integrity and emotional stability and that their character and personality-structures are so well organized that they can withstand at least as much environmental assaults as is expected of a normal person. But it should be stressed that in addition to this, they are superior in respect to their amazing understanding of the existence and meaning of the unconscious. I am constantly plagiarizing from their unusual insights in order to understand better some of the bizarre symptomatic actions and symbolic representations of patients I am currently treating. The following examples will explain what is meant.

A patient of mine is the mother of a two-year-old girl. For a period of a week, the child awoke in the middle of the night tearful and frightened. When the mother went to the child, the child told her to, "Go away, Mommie. I want Daddy." She made this request of her Daddy on each occasion, "Give me my crayon. I want to draw with my crayon." The patient explained to me, "Of course she would have to get it from Daddy. What she really wants is the penis that she feels only Daddy, like God, has the power to give her. After all, who provides things for the various members of the family, except Daddy? My husband thought the child was just being perverse and naughty, but I understood immediately that she was aware of the fact that she didn't have a penis; and what she was attempting to do was to remedy this deprivation."

One might think that the patient had read Freud, but what she was doing in reality was to utilize the same source of information that Freud did — the knowledge of the unconscious.

Another example is the paranoid schizophrenic, whom I invited in the latter stages of his treatment to assist me in understanding the peculiar behavior of a catatonic patient. What was puzzling to me was the fact that when the catatonic patient was seated he showed hardly any anxiety. On arising, however, he presented a picture of increasing panic. He seemed to be searching for something. He gazed around the room, looked in his pockets, pulled out his handkerchief, put it back again — all to the tune of increasing distress. I had made many interpretations to the effect that he thought he was castrated and was looking for his penis that had been sacrificed — and so on. None of these proved effective.

It took my paranoid patient to add the ingredient that solved the riddle. He told me:

"He is not worried whether he has a penis or not while he is sitting down because when he is sitting down, he is a girl and that is the way girls do it. [Meaning urination.] When he stands up, he is doing it like a boy, but he is not sure that he is a boy and what he is searching for is the answer to this question."

I felt that if this understanding were valid, my problem was to convince the patient that he was a man, that is, that he had a penis. I tackled it directly at the very next visit. When the patient stood up, I told him to put his hand on his penis and assisted him in this maneuver. As soon as he felt his penis, he was immediately reassured and the diminution in anxiety was at once apparent. He ceased searching and followed me out of the waiting room with an evident lack of concern. This symptom did not recur.

It seems reasonable to conclude from these experiences that everybody's unconscious perfectly understands everybody else's unconscious; and, whereas, most of us cannot command this fund of knowledge in our daily life, it is available to the schizophrenic because of the intimacy in which he lived with it. I hope these remarks will not be construed as an advertisement for schizophrenia because the ringside seats that they have had to the pyrotechnics of the unconscious is hardly compensation for the suffering schizophrenics have experienced.

Many of the writer's patients were treated within the confines of the institutions in which they resided. It was my good fortune to have treated two trained nurses who were schizophrenic patients at the New York State Psychiatric Institute. Because these two former patients now work with me in the treatment of other schizophrenic patients (their insight and understanding of schizophrenia is something amazing to behold and far surpasses mine), I am able to place patients in a controlled environment outside an institution with complete safety. They, with me, assume full responsibility for the protection of the patients and of persons who come in contact with the patients for 24 hours a day, seven days a week. I find that the resolution of the psychosis takes place much more rapidly outside an institution because the amount and character of distractions can be completely controlled.

There are many problems still to be solved: Two are reduction of the enormous amount of time required for this treatment and reduction of its relatively high cost. And one must consider that results, however good, must still be called tentative; and it must be emphasized that no claim of anything whatever is made in this series beyond the evidences supplied by this report.

DISCUSSION [10]

Paul Federn, M.D.

I am grateful to Dr. Rosen for having shown me his paper and to Dr. Eisenstein for having asked me to discuss it. Although Rosen has been working out his method of psychoanalyzing psychotics for four years, he still gives only preliminary papers. He began his work without knowing about this discussant's experiences, published in three papers in the 1943 *Psychiatric Quarterly*. Later, he read the papers, and, since then, we had some discussions about his method. The method is a promising and important original contribution. Like every pioneer

[10] By participants in the seminar.

he carried on his work against a good deal of resistance. However, the Psychiatric Institute gave him the opportunity to continue his way, which seems to be the right one.

I do not know whether it is Rosen's opinion that his cases are cured in the sense of having been freed of the unknown pathological entity, causing schizophrenic or paranoiac psychosis. I myself do not think so. His method consists in attacking by direct psychoanalytical understanding traumatic events of infancy and childhood, and coping with them as being still there, because there is regression to the ego-states of infancy and childhood. Our optimistic viewpoint assumes that this method removes so much of the cause that a satisfactory maturation of the ego catches up with previous failures of development and with gaps in integration. Rosen's good results can be explained — without advancing any new theory — by attributing a great traumatic effect to early sex experiences. Freud assumed such a sexual etiology once in regard to hysteria; later he modified his etiological theory in regard to the part played by such traumata, yet never abandoned this etiology. Rosen's findings revive this etiological factor in psychotic cases. However, his cases are freed or relieved of their psychotic states, characterized by a false reality of the psychotic's own making and consequently by badly distorted conceptions of the outside world.

It is common experience that many psychotic cases, by themselves, come back to healthier states, some even to states of health, and some even more quickly under the influence of different organic treatments. We do not yet know the cause and nature of spontaneous improvement.

In contradistinction to spontaneous restoration with the psychoanalytic treatment by Dr. Rosen, or the analogous but less direct techniques of this discussant, or of Fromm-Reichmann, we know exactly the helping agency that relieves the patients in their regressive states, of fear, of guilt, and of aggression.

The agency is not one but at least two agents — the one is common to all psychotherapy, to all therapy even — it is the *positive transference. The other is the participation of the psychiatrist in the psychotic reality of the patient*, when objective reality became unbearable to the patient left alone with his conflicts — which were unconscious during the pre-psychotic period but gained consciousness during the psychotic state.

Rosen uses the positive transference to participate in the patient's psychotic mental life. He not only participates insofar that he accepts their psychotic reality — with all that appears, absurd, "nuts," crazy, inconsistent, disintegrated and moronic to the normal mind. He goes deeper.

His participation is a psychoanalytical one. By means of psycho-analytical understanding, the psychotic reality ceases to be absurd, "nuts," crazy, inconsistent, disintegrated and moronic for the *normal* mind of the therapist. Through psychoanalytic translation, all the psychotic, *senseless* realities have sense and meaning — not the common-sense-meaning of the adult, but the specific sense-meaning of the child-hood-state, to which the patient's ego has regressed.

Sometimes Rosen translates a hallucination into its deeper instinctual meaning. In most cases, he uses psychoanalysis directly to recognize what the patient experiences factually. Always, Rosen sincerely accepts the emotional reaction of the patient as adequate to his regressive feelings and helps him directly by explaining to him the feelings which are adequate to the regressive ego-state, in which he has already been living a long period of years. Thus, his technique exactly, and differently, deals with the patient's typical perceptions, conceptions and emotional cathexes; such participation is no easy job.

Rosen's method is in full accordance with this discussant's own assertions in regard to psychoanalysis of psychoses. No free association is used to provoke more unconscious material; the psychotic symptoms and productions are enough material for psychoanalysis. Rosen deals with conflicts and mental pains of the patient and sides with him in his conflicts; he sides with him also in the residues of normal life, when he helps him in shopping and on other occasions.

He deals with the different ego-states with full understanding of the specific conflicts in every *single state*.

It is astonishing that, as far as my knowledge goes, nobody has ever used before the method of *direct psychoanalytic* [11] approach to the psychotic unconscious products. Even while Jung was convinced that morbid complexes themselves are the toxic agents which create the schizophrenic state, he did not proceed to try to fight the complexes directly.

Sometimes Rosen's method is like a neo-catharsis, when the patient frees himself of his accumulated emotional cathexis by crying, by swearing, by coprolaliac and obscene talking, and even by menacing with death the object of his transference, whose understanding friendship does not give more than that. To a great extent, Rosen is giving belated, but most necessary, sex-education and sex-information to his patients, who are still living in an invisible mental nursery.

It is clear to me that this technique and its good results can only be used by psychiatrists who are as fully convinced of Freud's inter-

---

[11] EDITOR'S NOTE: — Dr. Rosen wishes at this point to express his gratitude and appreciation to Dr. Federn for having coined the phrase "direct psychoanalysis" to describe Dr. Rosen's method of treatment.

pretation of the Unconscious as Rosen is. Rosen's findings are also another proof of the truth of Freud's tenets. It may be allowable to compare Federn's (mine) and Rosen's techniques. Federn interprets the psychosis in the sense of Freud, for one's own better understanding, and then uses one's understanding to make the patient slowly understand himself better and face his own problems with the healthy part of his ego, then slowly to restore more and more health to the ego. Furthermore, Federn's method is focussed on re-repression.

Rosen's method is a direct fighting of the unconscious that became conscious, without caring much about its re-repression. To use this method is possible when the patient's ego is still, to a great part, healthy and able to cooperate with the psychoanalyst. It appears, however, that many more cases can be approached by his direct psychoanalysis than we may assume.

We should not forget that psychotics come to the psychiatrist in a state made worse by the necessity of defending their psychotic reality against a host of normal persons, who do not believe the patient's reality. And the normal part of the patient's ego cannot side either with the psychotic part or with the normal persons. Therefore, the healthy part usually soon loses all strength and reacts with all kinds of complicating neurotic behavior, especially with anxiety states and obsessions. The security of being understood by the psychiatrist, by the nurse, and by other people, allows the normal part of the ego to regain its strength.

To understand the psychotic, one must fully understand the Unconscious. I pay my tribute to Dr. Rosen that, as a psychiatrist, he has incorporated Freud's work into his own mind, with great clarity combined with pioneer enthusiasm; I also pay tribute to the therapeutic methodological progress. Most cases will need further watch and social help. Records will be checked by other workers. Such checking presupposes the same understanding of the Unconscious which Rosen attained by reading Freud.

For this reason, I venture a word of caution concerning too wide experimentation with this treatment. It was devised as a last resort to save the life of a boy dying of exhaustion in a state of acute catatonic excitement — a situation where any effort whatever would have been warranted. Justification of this treatment in other cases has so far been mostly empiric. It may have dangers which have not yet been recognized. Since danger to life would require recognition by the physician; and, since the therapy as a whole is based on psychoanalysis, I suggest that for the present it might be well to confine experimentation with it to trained psychiatrists who are also fully qualified psychoanalysts. It may be safe for the psychiatrist who has not been analyzed to attempt use of this method; but it would be well to make certain of this before extending its scope.

Paul Hoch, M.D.

I think that Dr. Rosen's paper and his previous paper which was published in *The Psychiatric Quarterly* brings up a number of questions which we will have to discuss. First are some of the points which he raises as to the therapy of schizophrenia in general.

The textbooks which deal with schizophrenia usually start out with the statement that the treatment of schizophrenia is impossible because a schizophrenic patient is unable to form any sort of transference relation with the physician; therefore, any form of psychoanalytic therapy with a patient is not feasible. A great number of psychiatrists before Rosen voiced the opinion that this idea was wrong. The case which he presented this evening also demonstrates that the patient is able to form a transference relationship with the therapist. However, this transference is a very weak one, a very precarious one. If you go back to the childhood relationship of the schizophrenic patient, you will find one thing which is maintained practically all his life, namely, a sole — I would say restricted or monopolistic — emotional relationship to one or another member of the family which later on is probably transferred to one person who pays attention to him. This relationship, however, has a very narrow base. The patient is unable to broaden the base and branch out to form other emotional attachments. Nevertheless he has developed a firm attachment with one or the other parent and this attachment can be used to some extent for therapy.

Another point in the transference situation, Dr. Rosen indicated in his paper quite clearly, especially when the patient started to threaten him, that this transference relationship with the therapist is a very precarious one, a very ambivalent one. The analytic relationship which characterizes the schizophrenic rather than the neurotic patient is based on a simultaneous love-hate relationship. The patient suddenly can break up the transference or turn around and threaten, or even kill, the therapist. Ferenczi and others, who used a method very similar to Dr. Rosen's, were on several occasions threatened by their patients, and there were some who even paid the penalty for not taking into consideration the ambivalent transference relationship of the patient. But all this shows that it really is possible to form a transference relationship with the patient, even though this transference relationship is only maintained for a while.

Until now, it has been impossible to cure the majority of schizophrenics with any method, organic or psychoanalytic. A great many therapies which have been used in the treatment of schizophrenia have not lasted more than five years. No therapy for the treatment of schizophrenia has survived this five-year followup. I hope that Dr. Rosen's will survive this time span.

I should like to take up another issue which is constantly confused: the concept of deterioration. This term is very loosely used and many patients are judged deteriorated who are not. Symptoms of regression are usually interpreted as signs of deterioration, and no therapy is given. I emphasize that a great many patients who appear to be deteriorated are not deteriorated. Schizophrenic regression is different from deterioration. In regression, the patient's ability to make contact remains, although he is unable to use it. The patient can bounce back again to some degree from any type of regression. Nevertheless, if we are dealing with a patient who is truly deteriorated, it is clear that the therapy will be very difficult. I cannot accept the case presented by Dr. Rosen as deteriorated because a fully deteriorated patient would not have established transference in 10 sessions as well as this patient did and verbalize his difficulties as well as this patient did. I am sure that this patient showed only signs of regression, but was actually not deteriorated and that, therefore, contact was possible.

Dr. Rosen mentioned in his paper, as is also mentioned in the literature of psychoanalysis, that the treatment of the schizophrenic should actually be a treatment of his ego. This concept assumes that in schizophrenia a very strong ego regression is present and, if we are able to support the ego, we might be able to life the patient out of the psychosis. The therapy aims at strengthening the ego which is weak. It is obvious today that schizophrenia is not alone an impairment of the ego, but is an impairment of all three layers of the psyche (Freudian interpretation of the psychic organization). The patient not only shows a weak ego, but a weak super-ego which goes down very fast during the psychosis. The id is also impaired and the interrelation of the three layers is badly coordinated. Because all three layers are affected, the treatment of such patients is very difficult and in many cases unsuccessful.

Schizophrenia can be treated with many methods, and all these methods until now have demonstrated one thing: that if you employ a continuous drip method containing affection and protection, the patient is able to lift out from the psychotic state to some extent and is able to function. But very few patients, if you follow up their cases for a number of years, are capable of maintaining this form of recovery against everyday stress when the treatment is discontinued. Here my skepticism comes in, because, until several years have elapsed, after the termination of treatment, I am not prepared to accept this patient as cured. These patients are functioning better, are lifted out of psychotic states, but the underlying structure on which the psychosis grows is maintained.

No therapy known today will alter the basic structure. All therapies have until now accomplished just one thing: They have reduced the emotional pitch which is behind the symptoms of the patient and reduced the marked anxiety which is present in many patients. I had the privilege several years ago of discussing the paper of Dr. Schilder, who originally expressed the opinion that if we are able to limit this great panic, this great anxiety in the schizophrenic patient, which, he surmised, is probably based on catastrophic infantile experiences, we would be able to cure the patient. He experimented with psychotherapeutic methods; and he even treated some with group therapy. This lasted a few years, and then he said: "The improvements are mostly only temporary. Today I am more inclined to believe schizophrenia is an organic psychosis." In other words, his ability to make permanent cures was very meager. These "cured" patients, under some stress from an unexpected quarter, very suddenly relapsed. One of the interesting things to watch in schizophrenia is how a supposedly cured patient under stress of some sort suddenly blossoms out full-fledged with the previous symptoms. How is it possible that in a few days the patient is again back in the same state when we believed him cured?

Another point: In a large number of schizophrenic patients, acute and chronic, the disorder is oscillating and cyclical. If this is not taken into consideration, therapeutic results can be obtained which are bound to the cycle of the patient, but not actually to the therapy. Psychotherapy, psychoanalysis, homeopathic methods, "shock" treatments — I could name 15 other methods, all of which effect temporary cures.

We have to be cautious in appraising Dr. Rosen's method, but I am glad he has the optimism to experiment with this kind of treatment. We shall have to approach his method with the necessary caution and with the necessary criticism. The treatment of schizophrenia is full of claims of cure, with claims of recovery, and if we look into these claims, we see a temporary reduction of anxiety, a temporary meeting of stress situations; but the individual's immunity to stress and to emotional upheavals is very low and it usually remains, even after treatment, rather brittle.

Jule Eisenbud, M.D.

I have no prepared discussion; nevertheless, I should like to comment on the paper and on one or two of the points raised by Dr. Hoch.

We have witnessed a rather remarkable case presentation this evening and we ought to evaluate it very carefully and be very careful not to lump it in with other statistics which have been referred to. I don't want to quibble on the question of whether or not this patient began therapy in a deteriorated state or whether his cure, if it is a cure, will last five years. (Why we set a date of five years in any case, we don't know. It is a rather arbitrary figure. It is questionable whether life can guarantee five years of stability to any person.) What we have seen, however, whether or not this patient was deteriorated when he began, whether or not his cure will last, is that he made the beginnings of a remarkable recovery under purely psychological auspices. I don't feel quite right in comparing this method to homeopathic methods or frontal lobotomy or "shock." This is a purely psychological method.

If we try to dissect what we have heard and assay the therapeutic factor from the welter of material, it is apparent that we are going to run into difficulty; and it was apparent to no one more quickly than to Dr. Rosen, who began by stating that many factors are still obscure. At the outset, however, I don't think that we have the right even to consider the question of spontaneous remission in this case. The man had been ill for 27 years; if he started to become well at the time the physician began to handle him, I am prepared to agree that there is a connection, regardless of what may be said about a schizophrenic cycle.

Now, what does Dr. Rosen do? Speak directly to the unconscious? It is questionable whether anyone can speak directly to the unconscious, but we know what he means. I am prepared to hazard that Dr. Rosen speaks to a person, not to an unconscious — a person who has an unconscious, perhaps, but whose unconscious is, nevertheless, bounded by some sort of an ego, however rudimentary. When Rosen says he speaks directly to the unconscious, we know what he means. He gets right in with direct interpretation. He recognizes undoubtedly that he is dealing with a disturbed ego. He treats the patient as if the early traumata, the early ghosts, were still present and on the scene. Time has no meaning. He feels that, as Dr. Federn said, this patient is still in an invisible nursery. There are a number of interpretations which he has read you which one could quibble about. It looks very easy, just as it looks easy when Tilden plays tennis! Everything goes in the right place. We can't question whether the interpretations were absolutely correct; we don't know. There's one thing, however, which has impressed me about the work of Dr. Rosen during the time that I have been privileged to observe it, and that is the fact that, so far as I can observe, Dr. Rosen has absolutely no hostility toward the patient, toward the psychotic patient. This, I think, is a very important factor.

If we read the papers of Frieda Fromm-Reichmann, for instance, we get the impression that the transference, in the case of the psychotic, is a very exquisite, delicately balanced affair, for the slightest misstep on the part of the physician will result in catastrophe in the therapy. I believe that this is the case, not only because of the ambivalence of the patient, but because of the ambivalence of the physician, where a physician has to be watching at every moment to see that — because of the unfortunate effects — he doesn't slam the door in the patient's face or interrupt the patient to answer a phone call. Such a treatment will be dangerous at every moment.

I have observed Dr. Rosen with several of his patients, and at first I was astounded to notice the casual way in which he just threw overboard the exquisite instruction of Frieda Fromm-Reichmann. I watched, and I watched, and I said to myself, that *I* could never treat a patient with such a casual attitude. But I noticed one thing, that as far as I could observe, Rosen is not afraid to do this because he has no hostility toward the patient whatsoever. The average physician prefers not to treat psychotics to start with. If he does, he feels safe in having his own ego between him and the psychotic process, and safe if he has a good hunk of the patient's ego between the two participating parties.

Rosen isn't afraid of mixing right up with the patient, isn't afraid of being engulfed by the process. He is not afraid of the seductive lure of the world of fantasy to which psychotic individuals cling, nor is he afraid, apparently, of the extreme dependency of the psychotic which at times can be vicious and which most of us regard as an unwanted burden. I think it is these factors which are, as much as anything I can observe, responsible for the excellent results which Dr. Rosen gets.

I think many of us could make interpretations almost as good as Dr. Rosen has given, if we really believed in the unconscious. (Many of us don't.) But I don't believe that there are many people who could approach the psychotic with the complete absence of fear, the complete absence of hostility, the identification without the need to shuttle back and forth frequently to a safety zone, that characterizes Dr. Rosen's approach. And for these reasons, I wonder whether Dr. Rosen's method will ultimately turn out to be generally applicable. However, we have lots of time before us.

Other people will try this method, and Rosen himself will unquestionably see the five-year mark and give us statistics. Whether or not the transference can be resolved so that the strength that he is able to infuse into these people will take as a permanent graft, and whether he will be able firmly to cement the building blocks of reality into these regressive egos, we don't know. But we shall see.

Melitta Schmideberg, M.D.

I agree with Dr. Eisenbud's remarks, in particular those concerning the counter-transference. This is important in every treatment, but especially so with patients beyond the pale of ordinary society, such as psychotics and criminals.

I have achieved full cure with two patients, a boy of 16 suffering from paranoid dementia and a schizophrenic man of 23, both of whom were followed up for a period of nine years. Both fell in love, married happily and were able to handle difficult situations. I followed up the improvement in a schizophrenic defective woman patient of 28 for 14 years. She manages her life successfully and without relapse, though she probably still had some delusions. I achieved an I.Q. of 100 in a schizophrenic defective child of three and one-half who could not talk nor do anything when she came to me. On the other hand, I had two cases which did not show improvement. I have treated 25 schizophrenic, schizophrenic-defective or dementia paranoid cases, and one of true paranoia, achieving varying degrees of improvement. One patient with dementia paranoides showed improvement after eight interviews, and I followed him up for two years. I achieved a good improvement in a schizophrenic woman of 60 who had been in institutions a number of times. I treated only those patients who were not too disturbed to be seen at my office. One had been certified; several were certifiable, and some had had "shock" treatment without results.

Dr. Rosen is to be admired for achieving results in 37 out of 38 cases, a record better than my own. It is possible that it is easier to bring about improvement in the worst cases because they do not have the normal defenses. My technique differs slightly from Dr. Rosen's — I do not wait for the patient's free associations, but interpret whatever material I get. I analyze delusions, hearing of voices, etc., just as I do a neurotic symptom. I try above all to analyze the aggression and anxiety, and constantly watch the transference. It is very unstable and likely to change from moment to moment because of intense anxiety and ambivalence, but if the patient receives relief and sympathy, he becomes more attached than any other patient. He clings to the analyst as a protection against his overwhelming anxiety, regarding the analyst as his last contact with reality.

Joseph Meiers, M.D.

I have taken the liberty to insert myself into this discussion, in spite of the little time left, only because I think I may be able to contribute a bit from the point of view that is of interest today, in the public eye, more than anything else — mainly the potential gain from Dr.

Rosen's procedure, to a better possibility of coping with the more chronic manifestations of mental illness (psychoses) as we have them in an overwhelming majority in the state and other large public mental hospitals — a fact which is, as you all know, of such paramount concern both from a purely psychiatric viewpoint and, at the same time, also from the vantage point of national health. And it so happens that, after all, Dr. Rosen *did* obtain his primary incentive and idea for his present endeavor while working in a large state hospital. . . .

Thus he will agree with me, I think, if I say that he could be easily supplied with a couple of hundred, or even thousands of carefully selected — what he would call "deteriorated" — cases of various types of schizophrenia in order to try his method, as described here today, on them with all possible controls and variations. Right now, I recall a case of a young girl who had been in the hospital (one where I worked) from age 11 to 16 and one-half. I started to try the method of "direct approach" and actional-interpretive dialogue with her, with a modicum of success. I had not then read of Rosen's procedure, and was departing from somewhat different bases, largely those of the psychodramatic method . . . I cannot now go into the details of that case and its tentative management. I have mentioned it *merely* to underscore that the case of this young girl had become, after a short series of electric shock treatments, completely "inactivated" as to treatment. She was moderately catatonic, grabbed her own and other patients' food, was most of the time in a camisole, inert, indifferent apparently. In short, she was what not only Dr. Rosen here tonight, but most colleagues might consider as "typically deteriorated." You will forgive me, if I want to make it *a point* that we must (for very important reasons, *differentiate* between a really "deteriorated" and a merely "inveterated" case.

True mental deterioration is, of course, as all of you know, not hard to establish when we see it in senility, certain forms of alcoholism, etc. On the other hand, one often is induced to assume "deterioration" falsely — mostly in certain forms of catatonics, and mixed catatonic-paranoids, where a thorough testing is near-to-impossible because of the patient's inaccessibility.[12] To refer to the case of my unfortunate child patient once more — while she seemed to nurses and others for all practical purposes, somewhat of a living "mummy," a few shots well aimed at her ego, revealed that she not only was able to write (after five years of well-nigh complete inactivity!) but that she also recalled memories of her puberty and before. Thus, I hope to have your agreement, to some extent, at least, when I say that it is crucial — just from

---

[12] Roe, A., and Shakow, D. *Intelligence in Mental Illness.* New York Academy of Sciences, New York, 1940.

the viewpoint of selecting cases for the "Rosen method" — to avoid carefully the real "mentally deteriorated," inasmuch as they would unnecessarily tip the scales of the results.

However, it is essential to stress the features of "inveteration," i. e., of sheer *long duration* of a psychosis (and even neurosis) on the psyche of the patient as such — a point that is not too often brought to our attention. There seems to me — if you permit a very sketchy hint — to be these *two* principal sides in inveteration:

1. The patient, whether hospitalized or extramural, is more and more put on his defensive and thus develops an ever-thickening maze of both intra-psychic and inter-personal defenses. 2. All the sum total of his thoughts, convictions (and errors!) about his environment and himself, his illness, etc., becomes almost impermeable. *None* of us, whether psychotic, neurotic or "normal," wants to be *"all wrong"* in his judgments, recollections and conclusions. Thus, we observe so often a persistence of "delusional" material from the past, where there is no actual delusional thinking at present. These two features, interlocked, tend to form (in the "inveterated" case much more than the fresh one) the almost cretacaous *"crust of inveteration"* which is superadded to the original "core" of the psychotic trauma and its constitutional matrix. It is this which we are up against in dealing with inveteration — even without factual "deterioration."

In regard to this problem, I think three discussional approaches we heard here tonight were most remarkable. As for Dr. Paul Federn's contribution — to which I largely agree in its evaluation of Dr. Rosen's work — I am sure had he been here in person, he might have participated in the discussions of the "deterioration" ("inveteration") problem, too. As it is, I think we all are deeply grateful for what he has given in his message to the discussion.

On the other hand, I feel that Dr. Hoch's cautious approach is fully warranted. Even so, he did *not* seem to deny, even from the official viewpoint — as it were — of the New York Psychiatric Institute, of which we may consider him factually, if not formally representative, that Dr. Rosen's method of "direct (and as I would add, 'interactional'!) approach" is worth being tried out further, final judgment being reserved for a duration of a few years of maintained cures.

Now, as to that "time limit" of *five* years — arbitrary as it may seem, some line of duration has to be chosen! How happy would all of us be, including Dr. Hoch and all the state authorities, if the curative results in Dr. Rosen's cases prove to last even slightly less than five years. May I point out, by the way, that these *five* years have an important practical significance, as the law stands, from the point of view of the "established" duration of the "incurable mental illness"

case, as it comes up in marriage annulment, etc., law suits. The consequences that would ensue from cures of "inveterated" psychoses *after*
they had been declared "incurable" — well, we need not go into that
here and now.

The important question — and one which will have to be scrutinized
carefully in subsequent investigations — is the following: How much
of the curative result in Rosen's cases is due entirely to the "purely"
and typically psychoanalytic-interpretive approach, no matter how
much widened and extended beyond the customary boundaries of the
classic method? How much, on the other hand, is due to that inter-
actional, "dramatic" element, of the 'living together,' as it were, of
therapist and patient through mutual experiences, as described tonight
by Rosen and earlier in his article in *The Psychiatric Quarterly* of April
1946? On the basis of my own experiences I am greatly inclined to
attribute a lion's share to the inter-actional, "dramic" nature of the
approach.[13] An authority in orthodox analysis, like Kubie, warns
against the "direct interpretation" or confrontation of the patient with
results of free association *not* understood by the patient himself — in
typical psychoanalysis; as this often leads to embarrassing results, if
not worse.[14] Nothing like that can be observed in true psychodramatic,
inter-actional work with the patient — for the simple reason, as it
appears, that it is the patient, and only he who does the interpretation
that affects him and that he "acts out" the emotions connected with
or brought up by that "interpretation."

Hyman Spotniz, M.D.

About seven years ago I became interested in treating a series of
post-psychotic patients who had previously been hospitalized for their
psychoses. After I had treated them for a while, I became impressed
with the same factors and had the same type of feeling that Dr. Rosen
has summarized tonight with the words, "talking directly to the unconscious." About three years ago, I stopped most of my work in this
field. However, I am glad to be able to confirm that this experience
actually did exist for me, too. It is possible to feel as if one is talking
to the unconscious of the patient. Patients sense the feeling of com-
munion with them and immediately begin to respond; and the material,
which is readily interpreted, leads to a rapid amelioration of symptoms
over a period of weeks or months.

My last work of this type was done at a local hospital with a case
of ulcerative colitis. The patient was referred to me for psychoanalytic

[13] Meiers, Joseph L. *Origins and Development of Group Psychotherapy.* Beacon House,
New York, 1946.
[14] Kubie, Lawrence S. The Nature of Psychotherapy. *Bull. N. Y. Acad. Med.*, 1943.

therapy, because a gastro-enterologist considered that he was on his deathbed and would have to have an operation immediately or die within a few days. The psychiatric service wanted to demonstrate what could be done with psychotherapy. I "spoke directly to his unconscious," that is, whatever he said was immediately interpreted with what appeared to me to be its symbolic meaning. This patient walked out of the hospital within three weeks with a dramatic improvement. I had at that time known and predicted that he would relapse. The feeling I had was that his improvement was due to the pain he was experiencing and his desire to escape from rapid-fire interpretations. He later did have a partial relapse and was treated subsequently along more standard analytical lines. He has now been symptom-free for a year and a half.

I want to compliment Dr. Rosen on his courage and on his deep insight in this field. I feel it requires a great deal of courage, devotion and sincerity to do this type of work.

EDITORIAL COMMENT (The Psychiatric Quarterly)

HONI SOIT QUI MAL Y PENSE

> Oh perish the use of the four-letter words
> Whose meanings are never obscure;
> The Angles and Saxons, those bawdy old birds,
> Were vulgar, obscene and impure.
> But cherish the use of the weaseling phrase
> That never says quite what you mean.
> You had better be known for your hypocrite ways
> Than vulgar, impure and obscene.[15]

The "vulgar, impure and obscene" words which English has inherited from the Angles and the Saxons loom large in the vocabularies of psychotic patients. But when an investigator and earnest student attempts to rescue a deteriorated patient sunk in the morass of catatonic stupor by interpreting his delusions and hallucinations and speaking to him in the same infantile words flung at him by accusing voices — thus to draw out his mental content, to be understood, and to gain a response — he must watch his step or he will be misunderstood by the uninformed and suspected of evil-mindedness. The editor has asked patients at discharge conferences (staff meetings) to repeat the exact words heard by them, words which the patients had just described as unreal or imaginary "voices." Rarely can a patient be induced to do so. Often he excuses himself by saying he "cannot re-

[15] From "Ode to the Four-Letter Word." Anonymous?

member"; but sometimes by frankly saying: "Oh no! There are ladies present."

The unconscious, when coming to verbal expression, does not choose the "weaseling phrase" but the hearty Anglo-Saxon words which mean just what they say. Every experienced psychiatrist has heard from the lips of patients known to come from homes of culture and refinement, torrents of vulgarity and obscenity when in a maniacal rage. One is prompted to exclaim: "Where *could* she have learned such words!" And the deteriorated hebephrenic or catatonic — without the spur of rage or excitement, without any appearance of shame — uses words and phrases that so shock the prudish that interns and nurses have asked to be excused from service on certain wards.

The editor and his associates feel that a keen sense of clinical duty makes it imperative upon them to quote — when quotations are essential to an unbiased presentation of clinical material — patients' and therapists' remarks exactly as they are made. An attempt to "purify" the clinical record by substituting parlor or scientific phraseology of the twentieth century for four-letter words known to everyone would be a species of prudish hypocrisy unworthy of a medical publication. The members of the editorial staff are not addicted to the employment of scatology in their own conversation. They regret that prudes may find on the pages of *The Quarterly* words employed — when essential to the context — that may give offense to the Miss Nancies of both sexes; but the regret is wholly for the state of mind of such prudes; and there is no intention whatever of modifying the editorial policy of truthfulness to details in quotations.

We submit here and now that psychiatry is a profession for adults and that it is time for psychiatrists in general to act adult. It is not a profession for the sort of lady, male or female, who shudders at four-letter words and the mental images they invoke.

These remarks are occasioned by the fact that in this issue of *The Psychiatric Quarterly* we are publishing the second report on the successful treatment of psychotics by a method which is purely psychotherapeutic. This report summarizes the results of treatment in 37 successfully-treated cases; but it is for the most part a clinical record of a single patient,[16] a man who had had schizophrenia for 27 years, who had been treated four years in an institution, had received insulin therapy (60 comas) and electric shocks (20 convulsions) and had remained unimproved for four years thereafter, prior to the institution of direct analytic therapy.

Certain recognized psychiatric procedures are horrifying to persons

[16] The editor (of the Psychiatric Quarterly) was given the opportunity to examine this patient privately and is able to confirm the author's claim of recovery.

who hear of them for the first time; "shock" treatment may be interpreted as cruelty. And the reactions it brings on may be terrifying to the inexperienced onlooker. The coma of insulin "shock" resembles death; the convulsions caused by metrazol and electric shock may cause bone fractures. Yet the public in general and the next of kin of hospital patients have come to accept the presumed risk of injury or possible death when it is understood that apparent cures are often effected by these methods: indeed, relatives now often demand that "shock" treatments be used.

Treatment by direct analytic therapy will be as horrifying to some persons who hear of it for the first time as treatment by the shock therapies is, for direct analytic treatment is planned to meet psychotic patients on their own level — a very regressed level. All severe mental disorders involve regression, in one form or another, to early childhood or even infancy, regression in the way of individual acts or reactions in the neuroses and in a whole altered state of life and consciousness in the psychoses. This is particularly true in dementia praecox. We all know what the deteriorated schizophrenic may occasionally say or do. To point out that the A, B, C's of psychiatry — he often speaks of things in the "dirty words" which a child would use in a tantrum. It is sometimes necessary, if one is to meet the regressed schizophrenic on his own level, to employ words he hears in his hallucinations. These may comprise the only vocabulary that will make an emotional contact with his distraught self-absorption and gain a response.

All of us know what those words are. Most of us learned them as children. All of us have seen them in public or school toilets. Anybody so squeamish as to shudder at them or at the desires or actions toward which they point has no business in psychiatry and psychotherapy.

Throughout modern times the lot of the medical man, whenever sex "has reared its ugly head," has not been a happy one. The practice of obstetrics was hampered from the time the physician replaced the midwife and the bed the obstetrical chair, so that a sheet could be drawn to cover the genitalia of some high-placed lady during the business of birth. The first gynecologists, as witness the case of Dr. Marion Sims, were objects of intense suspicion, dislike and opprobrium. They were whispered about by the general public, denounced from the pulpit and by colleagues in the medical profession. Nobody in modern psychiatric work has forgotten the persecution and the vilification endured by Freud when he began his researches into the rôle of the sex instinct.

We think psychiatry should have attained at least near-adulthood by this time. It is somehow astonishing to see a modern psychiatrist reacting as a mental hospital chaplain did recently in discussing "Freudian filth."

We are quoting, without the author's permission (for we have no idea who the author is) from the same bawdy little poem, "Ode to the Four-Letter Word," with which we commenced this discussion:

> Let your morals be loose as an alderman's vest
> If your language is always obscure.
> Today, not the act, but the word is the test
> Of vulgar, obscene and impure.

ADDENDUM (Written for this volume by Dr. Rosen.)

The appearance of this paper sharpened the controversy between those who favored physical approaches to the therapy of the psychoses and those who favored psychological approaches based on the insights of Sigmund Freud. In the past ten years many words have appeared, both pro and con, with regard to direct analysis. For the most part the discussions have been strongly influenced by emotional bias. Some opponents of the method have suggested that when patients have recovered, the original diagnosis was in error. Other claimants have emphasized the faulty criteria and the unreliability of the "cure." More magnanimous critics have indicated that the treatment may be effective for those in "acute" psychotic states. Most of the proponents have seen and felt the dramatic changes that take place in a patient as a result of direct analytic intervention. These changes have been demonstrated in patients who were thought to be beyond the point of retrieve. Matters of fact, however, are not resolved by debate and so we have agreed to subject this method to empirical test.

At the present time direct analysis as a treatment for the psychoses is being investigated at the Temple University College of Medicine. This research supported chiefly by the Rockefeller Brothers Fund is investigating the principles upon which the treatment is based, its efficacy as a therapeutic method, and its communicability.

Every precaution is being taken to insure against the kinds of errors in research methodology suggested by previous critics. The selection of cases, the certainty of diagnosis, the evaluation of results, and the inclusion of control subjects are all handled by an impartial group who operate in complete independence of the therapist.

The fact that the ideas of direct analysis have survived these past fifteen years and are now the center of a large research effort is a source of no small gratification to the author. The ultimate value of this new approach to the psychoses will be decided on the basis of the evidence.

28

PSYCHOTHERAPY AND THE PLACEBO EFFECT

DAVID ROSENTHAL

National Institute of Mental Health

AND JEROME D. FRANK

School of Medicine, Johns Hopkins University

It is by now generally recognized that all forms of psychotherapy yield successful results with some patients and that these successes depend to an undetermined extent on factors common to many types of relationship between patient and therapist. This poses a knotty problem for proponents of various specific forms of psychotherapy who are convinced that their successes result from their particular theory or technique and wish to convince others of this. As a result, problems of research design in psychotherapy have been receiving more and more critical attention in recent years, especially with reference to controls (6, 11, 20, 23, 24, 25, 27, 31, 34, 35, 38, 39).

Certain general aspects of the psychotherapeutic relationship seem very similar to those responsible for the so-called placebo effect, which is well known to investigators of the therapeutic efficacy of medications. The purpose of this paper is to describe the placebo effect, discuss some of its implications for the evaluation of psychotherapy, and make some recommendations concerning research design in psychotherapy based on these considerations.

THE PLACEBO EFFECT

We have now participated in two separate investigations of the effectiveness of drugs on the symptomatic distress of psychiatric outpatients (14, 22). Both studies involved the administration of a placebo, an inert agent outwardly indistinguishable from the agent being tested, as well as drugs. The physician never knew whether he was giving the patient drug or placebo. The patients were told that a new medicine had become available which, it was thought, might help them. The physicians rated symptoms on a 4-point scale of distress, with high reliability. In both studies a significant reduction of distress accompanied the taking of placebos, as shown in Table 1.

From the *Psychological Bulletin*, 53: No. 4, 1956. © 1956 by the American Psychological Association.

This phenomenon occurs with great regularity, not only with respect to the kinds of symptoms usually associated with psychologic illness, but with others as well. For example, in a study of vaccines for the common cold, there was found a reduction in the number of yearly colds of 55 per cent among those given vaccine and of 61 per cent among a control group who received injections of isotonic sodium chloride solution (4). Hillis (15) found placebos as effective as other agents in inhibiting the cough reflex. Wolf and Pinsky (37) studied medical outpatients suffering from peptic ulcer, migraine, muscle tension, headache, and tight muscles in the extremities. All were also tense and anxious. Twenty to thirty per cent felt better while taking placebos. Lasagna *et al.* (19) gave 1 ml. of saline by subcutaneous injection to surgical patients suffering from steady, severe wound pains and found that 30 to 40 per cent reported a satisfactory relief of pain. In a study by Jellinek (18) 60 per cent of 199 subjects with chronic headaches received relief from a placebo on one or more occasions.

TABLE 1. SYMPTOM DISTRESS BEFORE EXPERIMENTS AND AFTER A
TRIAL ON PLACEBOS

| Study | N | Drug tested | Mean distress scores | | |
			Before experiment	After placebo	Significance of difference
1st study	17	Mephenesin	25.58	15.88	.01
2nd study	16	Reserpine	34.06	24.69	.02

The placebo effect is not always favorable, but may also result in undesirable, distressful reactions. As far back as 1933, Diehl (3) using lactose placebos as a control for a variety of medications taken by mouth, found that some of his subjects receiving placebos developed nausea, faintness, and diarrhea. Sometimes this "toxic response" to placebos may even attain major proportions. Wolf and Pinsky (37) tell of one patient who had "overwhelming weakness, palpitation, and nausea within 15 minutes of taking her tablets." In another, "a diffuse itchy erythematous maculopapular rash developed after ten days of taking pills. A skin consultant considered the eruption to be typical dermatitis medicamentosa. After use of the pills was stopped, the eruption quickly cleared." A third patient developed epigastric pain followed by watery diarrhea, urticaria, and angioneurotic edema of the lips within ten minutes of taking her pills. One of our own patients, who had been tolerating a chronic syphilophobia fairly well, became acutely agitated shortly after placebo ingestion, bemoaning what the pills had done to him, and required hospitalization shortly thereafter.

Wolf and Pinsky (37) found that placebos produced more improvement in subjective than objective manifestations of anxiety and tension, but objective changes also occur. In our second study (22), 69 per cent of our patients showed decreased blood pressure and pulse readings following placebo, 19 per cent showed increased blood pressure, and 25 per cent showed a rise in pulse rate. Wolf (36) demonstrated clearly and convincingly that actual end-organ changes can follow placebo administration. This demonstration was made in a series of studies on the now-celebrated Tom, a human subject with a large gastric fistula, in whom it was possible to observe directly the gastric mucous membrane, correlating changes in color and turgidity with simultaneous measurements of gastric secretion and motor activity.

The placebo effect may actually reverse the normal pharmacologic action of a drug. For example, Wolf reports that Tom was repeatedly given Prostigmine, which induced abdominal cramps, diarrhea, as well as hyperaemia, hypersecretion, and hypermotility of the stomach. Subsequently, the same response occurred not only to tap water and lactose capsules, but also to atropine sulfate which usually has an *inhibiting* effect on gastric function. A pregnant patient with excessive vomiting showed the usual response of nausea and vomiting to ipecac. These manifestations were accompanied by cessation of normal gastric contractions. When ipecac was given through a tube with strong assurance that it would relieve her vomiting, gastric contractions were resumed at the same interval after ingestion of the drug that they would normally have ceased, and her nausea and vomiting were relieved.

The placebo effect, in short, can be quite powerful It can significantly modify the patient's physiological functioning, even to the extent of reversing the normal pharmacological action of drugs; and, as will be discussed below, it may be enduring. Placebo effects cannot be dismissed as superficial or transient. They often involve an increased sense of well-being in the patient and are manifested primarily by relief from the particular symptomatic distress for which the patient expects and receives treatment. Thus, the relief of any particular complaint by a given medication is not sufficient evidence for the specific effect of the medicine on this complaint unless it can be shown that the relief is not obtained as a placebo effect.

IMPLICATIONS OF THE PLACEBO EFFECT FOR RESEARCH IN
PSYCHOTHERAPY

The giving of any medication may have certain meanings for a patient in terms of his relationship to his physician which may benefit his condition irrespective of the pharmacological action of the drug. For example, it may relieve the anxiety resulting from the distress caused by his illness (10). Wolf believes the effects of placebos on his patients "depended for their force on the conviction of the patient that this or that effect would result." The degree of the patient's conviction might be expected to be influenced by his previous experiences with doctors, his confidence in his physician, his suggestibility, the suggestibility-enhancing aspects of the situation in which the therapeutic agent is being administered, and his faith in or fear of the therapeutic agent itself. These attitudes are obviously relevant to psychotherapy.

Psychotherapists have theories of personality and psychotherapy and plan their therapeutic actions in the belief that these are the active agents which produce the desired results. Any favorable changes in patients consequent to a course of psychotherapy tend to be cited as evidence for the validity of the theory of personality and neurosis which underlie the rationale of the psychotherapy. In view of the above discussion it may well be that the efficacy of any particular set of therapeutic operations lies in their analogy to a placebo in that they enhance the therapist's and patient's conviction that something useful is being done. Patients entering psychotherapy have various degrees of belief in its efficacy, and this may be an important factor in the results of therapy, but this has not been studied, to our knowledge. We know that the authoritarian attitude of the physician can produce this conviction in some patients.

At first glance the attitudes found by Fiedler (8, 9) to characterize experienced psychotherapists, viz. feelings of empathy for and closeness to the patient, an undemanding attitude, security, and the ability to "understand" the patient, seem diametrically opposed to the authoritarian attitude. It may be, however, that the therapeutic efficacy of these attitudes lies primarily in their ability to increase the confidence of certain patients in the ability of the therapist to help them. Lack of such confidence may be one of the reasons why patients of lower socio-economic status fare less well in psychotherapy than patients higher in this scale (16, 29), a talking therapy seeming to be beyond their comprehension and contrary to their conception of the doctor-patient relationship.

In this connection, the role of suggestion in psychotherapy has been emphasized for years, especially in therapies utilizing hypnosis, but suggestion effects have been thought by many since Freud to be superficial and transitory. We know of no experimental study which demonstrates that therapeutic effects based on insights or perceptual reorganization, which may also be suggested, are less superficial or less transitory.

It may be pointed out parenthetically that conviction of the helpfulness of therapy need not be equated with "motivation for therapy," which was investigated by Grummon (13) and Dymond (5) and found to have little relationship to success in psychotherapy. Patients are often sufficiently distressed to be strongly motivated to receive help, yet have little faith that a procedure such as psychotherapy can help them.

The similarity of the forces operating in psychotherapy and the placebo effect may account for the high consistency of improvement rates found with various therapies, from that conducted by physicians without psychiatric training to intensive psychoanalysis (7). This explanation gains plausibility from the fact that reported improvement rates for various series of neurotics treated by different forms of psychotherapy hover around 60 per cent (1). This is the same as that reported for the placebo effect in illnesses in which emotional components may play a major role such as "colds" (3) and headaches (18).

To show that a specific form of treatment produces more than a non-specific placebo effect it must be shown that its effects are stronger, last longer, or are qualitatively different from those produced by the administration of placebos, or that it affects different types of patients. Our knowledge of all these matters is still fragmentary, but some beginnings have been made.

With respect to the strength and qualitative nature of the effects of therapy, one line of endeavor has been to study the physiological changes occurring during psychotherapy. Since physiological measures usually used to provide evidence of resistance or frustration (26, 33) or similar psychological states during psychotherapy (28) may also be influenced by the placebo effect, one cannot conclude that demonstration of such physiological changes implies a greater *depth* of therapy or a more profound reorganization of the personality, unless we are willing to equate the placebo effect with such reorganization.

With respect to the duration of improvement, if it could be shown that the placebo effect is of shorter duration than changes specific to a given psychotherapy, this would provide one kind of evidence favoring that theory of psychotherapy. As far as we know, no study of the limits of duration of the placebo effect has been made. Our experiment with mephenesin vs. placebo covered four two-week periods. Figure 1 shows the curves for both agents for the eight weeks.

Figure 1 shows that the greatest decrease in distress following placebos was felt during the first two-week trial period. After that, a slight but statistically insignificant rise in distress occurred; and, at the end of eight weeks, the placebo effect was about as great as after two weeks. Unfortunately, our data yielded no information on how much longer it might have endured. If the effect is analogous to the relief of pain by placebos in patients with surgical wounds, we should expect it eventually to diminish. Lasagna *et al.* (19) found that as placebo therapy of such patients continued the relief experienced decreased.

Although the number of patients is too small to justify any conclusions, it is intriguing that the first dose of mephenesin seemed to counteract the placebo effect. In the study with reserpine (22), the only patients who failed to show a placebo effect were those who had received reserpine previously. It may be that any discomfort produced by a pharmacologically active agent tends to counteract the emotional state responsible for a placebo effect in susceptible patients. Analogously, an activity by the psychotherapist which disturbs the patient may conceivably counteract the placebo effect of psychotherapy with certain patients.

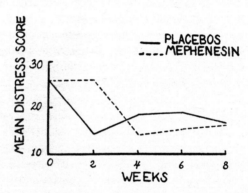

Fig. 1. Effects of mephenesin and placebo on symptomatic distress over an 8-week period. Total patients = 17. At the 2-, 4-, 6-, and 8-week intervals, N for placebo = 11, 6, 10, and 7 respectively, while N for mephenesin = 6, 11, 7, and 10 respectively. For the 2- and 4-week periods, the dosage of mephenesin was 3 gms. per day; for the 6- and 8-week periods, 9 gms. per day.

It would also be helpful to know if patients could be differentiated according to attributes which predisposed them to a positive or negative placebo effect. If patients who improved with a particular form of psychotherapy were all known to be positive placebo reactors, then the improvement could not be attributed to the specific form of treatment. If, however, they were known not to be positive placebo reactors, then any demonstrated improvement would constitute evidence of efficacy specific to the form of psychotherapy.

There is little known, however, with regard to the attributes of placebo reactors. Lasagna *et al.* (19) have made the first attempts to investigate this problem and report some attitudes and Rorschach categories which differentiated their reactors ($N = 11$) from their nonreactors ($N = 16$). However, only 14 per cent of their patients were consistent reactors, i.e., showed the effect with every placebo dose, and 31 per cent were consistent nonreactors, while 55 per cent showed the effect on some occasions but not on others. This contrasts with the findings of Jellinek (18) whose patients with headache were, for the most part, either in the always-relieved group or the never-relieved group, with only a small percentage of patients showing inconsistency of response. The apparent contradiction in findings may perhaps result from the difference in the cause of the pain in the two series or from other factors. In any case it indicates that the problem is a complex one needing much more study.

In the light of these considerations, any method of demonstrating the specificity of response to a given type of psychotherapy would have to provide an adequate control design. As far as we know, the study which has paid closest attention to the question of controls in research in psychotherapy is that of Rogers and his colleagues (31). They employed two different kinds of control groups. One was a group of nonclients who were simply given a battery of tests before and after specified time periods. The other was a group of clients who were required to wait a specified period of time before beginning therapy. This group was tested at the beginning and end of the wait period, at the end of therapy, and after a follow-up period.

These procedures do not control for the placebo effect since neither control group was being subjected to any special procedures which could produce a reasonable expectancy in control subjects that certain changes should occur. The experimental group, however, could be expected to anticipate certain effects merely as a consequence of participating in the client-therapist interviews. Therefore, even though favorable changes could be demonstrated in their clients, the question of whether these were placebo effects could not be answered from such research design unless additional information were provided.

If we do not control for nonspecific factors like the placebo effect, we cannot know whether effects predicted from a theory lead to or result from improvement based on the nonspecific effect. Butler and Haigh (2), for example, report an increased correlation of perceived self with ideal self following client-centered therapy. The implicit inference is that the specific therapeutic method leads to this increased correlation which, in turn, contributes to amelioration of disability and distress.

It is conceivable, though, that as a result of a nonspecific placebo effect the client feels less disabled and distressed which, in turn, leads him to describe himself as more like his ideal self. Rogers' (30) findings of greater emotional maturity in successfully treated cases may be similarly explained, clients feeling less disabled and distressed due to a nonspecific placebo response and behaving consequently in ways which are less anxiety-determined and which are seen as more mature by others.

We would propose that the following conditions are optimal in planning research in psychotherapy:

1. A theory of personality and psychological distress (neurosis, maladjustment, etc.).

2. Predictions of effects in the patient or client consequent to psychotherapy, in accord with the theory.

3. Demonstration of a relationship between the predicted effects and some criterion of improvement.

4. Demonstration that the predicted effects and their relationship to the improvement criterion are not due primarily to the patient's conviction that therapy will help him. This will permit greater confidence that the relationship found is specific to the therapeutic technique derived from the theory.

Ideally, these conditions should obtain both for process and outcome research. There seems to be general agreement with regard to the first two conditions although Mackinnon (21) has some reservations about beginning with a theory rather than a hunch. Gordon *et al.* (12) have come to question the third condition, at least with respect to a "global" criterion of improvement.

The fourth condition has not been met in any research of which we are aware. It is not possible to set up an experiment precisely analogous to comparison of a medication with a placebo because there is no such thing as inert psychotherapy in the sense that placebos are pharmacologically inert. However, it may be possible to study the possible specific effects of any particular form of therapy by the use of a matched control group participating in an activity regarded as therapeutically inert from the standpoint of the theory of the therapy being studied. That is, it would not be expected to produce the effects predicted by the theory. The "placebo psychotherapy" in this sense would be analogous to placebos in that it would be administered under circumstances and by persons such that the patients would expect to be helped by it.

Let us say that our theory is psychoanalytic and our predicted effect is an increased correlation between the moral values of the patient and the therapist (superego identification) and that we also expect an association between the increased correlation and a criterion of improvement (32). According to the theory, there is no reason to believe that control patients receiving, for example, relaxation therapy (17) will show the increased correlation of moral values with their therapist's moral values, nor should they show as much or as lasting improvement as the patients receiving psychoanalytic therapy of equal length. Such a design would constitute a fair test of the hypothesis based on the theory. In comparative studies where one type of psychotherapy is tested against another, differences found between them in predicted effects or amount, nature, and duration of improvement would not be explainable as placebo effects, if the condition could be met that patients had equal faith in the efficacy of the therapies and therapists to which they are assigned.

SUMMARY AND CONCLUSIONS

The literature on the therapeutic efficacy of drugs compared with placebos is briefly reviewed, and its relevance for research in psychotherapy considered. It is concluded that improvement under a special form of psychotherapy cannot be taken as evidence for: (*a*) correctness of the theory on which it is based; or (*b*) efficacy of the specific technique used, unless improvement can be shown to be greater than or qualitatively different from that produced by the patients' faith in the efficacy of the therapist and his technique — "the placebo effect." This effect may be thought of as a nonspecific form of psychotherapy and it may be quite powerful in that it may produce end-organ changes and relief from distress of considerable duration.

To show that a specific form of psychotherapy based on a theory of personality and neurosis produces results not attributable to the nonspecific placebo effect it is not sufficient to compare its results with changes in patients receiving no treatment. The only adequate control would be another form of therapy in which patients had equal faith, so that the placebo effect operated equally in both, but which would not be expected by the theory of therapy being studied to produce the same effects. We need to learn more about the nature of the placebo effect, the conditions giving rise to it, and the attributes of patients most susceptible or resistant to it so that we may obtain a better understanding of the role of nonspecific factors in psychotherapy.

REFERENCES

1. Appel, K. E., Lhamon, W. T., Myers, J. M., & Harvey, W. A. Long term psychotherapy. In *Psychiatric treatment. Proc. Ass. Res. Nerv. Ment. Dis.* Dec. 14, 15, 1951, New York. Baltimore: Williams & Wilkins, 1953, 21–34.
2. Butler, J. M., & Haigh, G. V. Changes in the relation between self-concepts and ideal concepts consequent upon client-centered counseling. In C. R. Rogers & Rosalind F. Dymond (Eds.), *Psychotherapy and personality change*, Chicago: Univer. of Chicago Press, 154. Pp. 55–75.
3. Diehl, H. S. Medical treatment of the common cold. *J. Amer. Med. Ass.*, 1933, 101: 2042–2045.

4. Diehl, H. S., Baker, A. B., & Cowan, D. W. Cold vaccines, further evaluation. *J. Amer. Med. Ass.*, 1940, 115: 593–594.

5. Dymond, Rosalind F. Adjustment changes in the absence of psychotherapy. *J. consult. Psychol.*, 1955, 19: 103–107.

6. Edwards, A. L., & Cronbach, L. J. Experimental design for research in psychotherapy. *J. clin. Psychol.*, 1952, 8: 51–59.

7. Eysenck, H. J. The effects of psychotherapy — An evaluation. *J. consult. Psychol.*, 1952, 16: 319–324.

8. Fiedler, F. E. The concept of the ideal therapeutic relationship. *J. consut. Psychol.*, 1950, 14: 239–245.

9. Fiedler, F. E. A comparison of therapeutic relationships in psychoanalytic, nondirective, and Adlerian therapy. *J. consult. Psychol.*, 1950, 14: 436–445.

10. Frank, J. D. Psychotherapeutic aspects of symptomatic treatment. *Amer. J. Psychiat.*, 1946, 103: 21–25.

11. Greenhill, M. H., Ford, L. S., Olson, W. C., Ryan, W. C., Whitman, S., & Skeels, H. M. *Evaluation in mental health*, Bethesda: National Institute of Mental Health, 1955.

12. Gordon, T., Grummon, D. L., Rogers, C. R., & Seeman, J. Developing a program of research in psychotherapy. In C. R. Rogers & Rosalind F. Dymond (Eds.), *Psychotherapy and personality change*, Chicago: Univer. of Chicago Press, 1954. Pp. 12–34.

13. Grummon, D. L. Personality changes as a function of time in persons motivated for therapy. In C. R. Rogers & Rosalind F. Dymond (Eds.), *Psychotherapy and personality change*, Chicago: Univer. of Chicago Press, 1954, 238–255.

14. Hampson, J. L., Rosenthal, D., & Frank, J. D. A comparative study of the effects of mephenesin and placebo on the symptomatology of a mixed group of psychiatric outpatients. *Bull. Johns Hopkins Hosp.*, 1954, 95: 170–177.

15. Hillis, B. R. The assessment of cough-suppressing drugs. *Lancet*, 1952, 1: 1230–1232.

16. Imber, S. D., Nash, E. H., & Stone, A. R. Social class and duration of psychotherapy. *J. clin. Psychol.*, in press.

17. Jacsobson, E. *Progressive relaxation*, Chicago: Univer. of Chicago Press, 1938.

18. Jellinek, E. M. Clinical tests on comparative effectiveness of analgesic drugs. *Biometrics Bull.*, 1946, 2: 87.

19. Lasagna, L., Mosteller, F., Felsinger, J. M., & Beecher, H. K. A study of the placebo response. *Amer. J. Med.*, 1954, 16: 770–779.

20. Lebo, D. The present status of research on nondirective play therapy. *J. consult. Psychol.*, 1953, 17: 177–183.

21. Mackinnon, D. W. Fact and fancy in personality research. *Amer. Psychol.* 1953, 8: 138–145.

22. Meath, J. A., Feldberg, T. M., Rosenthal, D., & Frank, J. D. A comparative study of reserpine and placebo in the treatment of psychiatric outpatients. (Unpublished manuscript.)

23. Morse, P. W. A proposed technique for the evaluation of psychotherapy. *Amer. J. Orthopsychiat.*, 1953, 4: 716–731.

24. Mosak, H. H. Problems in the definition and measurement of success in psychotherapy. L. W. Wolff & J. A. Precker: *Success in psychotherapy*, New York: Grune & Stratton, 1952, 1–25.

25. Mowrer, O. H. (Ed.). *Psychotherapy: theory and research*, New York: Ronald, 1953.

26. Mowrer, O. H., Light, B. H., Luriz, Z., & Zeleny, M. P. Tension changes during psychotherapy, with special reference to resistance. In O. H. Mowrer (Ed.), *Psychotherapy: theory and research*, New York: Ronald, 1953. Pp. 546–640.

27. Oberndorf, C. P., Greenacre, Phyllis, & Kubie, L. Symposium on the evaluation of therapeutic results. *Int. J. Psychoanal.*, 1948, 29: 7–33.

28. O'Kelly, L. I. Physiological changes during psychotherapy. In O. H. Mowrer (Ed.), *Psychotherapy: theory and research*, New York: Ronald, 1953, 641–656.

29. Redlich, F. C., Hollingshead, A. B., Roberts, B. H., Robinson, H. A., Freedman, L. Z., & Myers, J. K. Social structure and psychiatric disorders. *Amer. J. Psychiat.*, 1953, 109: 729–734.

30. Rogers, C. R. Changes in the maturity of behavior as related to therapy. In C. R. Rogers & Rosalind F. Dymond (Eds.) *Psychotherapy and personality change*, Chicago: Univer. of Chicago Press, 1954. Pp. 215–237.

31. Rogers, C. R., & Dymond, Rosalind F. (Eds.) *Psychotherapy and personality change*, Chicago: Univer. of Chicago Press, 1954.

32. Rosenthal, D. Changes in some moral values following psychotherapy. *J. consult. Psychol.*, 1955, 19, 431–436.

33. Thetford, W. N. An objective measurement of frustration tolerance in evaluating psychotherapy. In W. Wolff & J. A. Precker, *Success in psychotherapy*, New York: Grune & Stratton, 1952, 26–62.

34. Thorne, F. C. Rules of evidence in the evaluation of the effects of psychotherapy. *J. clin. Psychol.*, 1952, 8: 38–41.

35. Watson, R. I., Mensch, I., & Gildea, E. F. The evaluation of the effects of psychotherapy III. Research design. *J. Psychol.*, 1951, 32: 293–308.

36. Wolf, S. Effects of suggestion and conditioning on the action of chemical agents in human subjects — the pharmacology of placebos. *J. clin. Invest.*, 1950, 29: 100–109.

37. Wolf, S., & Pinsky, R. H. Effects of placebo administration and occurrence of toxic reactions. *J. Amer. Med. Ass.*, 1954, 155: 339–341.

38. Wolff, W., & Precker, J. A. *Success in psychotherapy*, New York: Grune & Stratton, 1952.

39. Zubin, J. Design for the evaluation of therapy. In *Psychiatric treatment. Proc. Ass. Res. Nerv. Ment. Dis.* Dec. 14, 15, 1951, New York. Baltimore: Williams & Wilkins, 1953. Pp. 10–15.

29

THE NEW PSYCHIATRIC DRUGS

HAROLD E. HIMWICH

Galesburg State Hospital, Illinois

We seem to be entering a new era in the study and treatment of mental illness — a biochemical era. Research on the chemistry of mental disease has recently brought forth several exciting new discoveries. One is the new information on the emotional effects of adrenalin and nor-adrenalin [see "The Physiology of Fear and Anger," by Daniel H. Funkenstein; *Scientific American*, May 1955]. Another is the finding that a psychotic state can be induced artificially by injections of lysergic acid ["Experimental Psychoses," by Six Staff Members of Boston Psychopathic Hospital; June 1955]. This article will review a third major development: the so-called "tranquilizing" drugs which psychiatrists are using with remarkable effect in treating psychotic patients. These drugs are chlorpromazine (trade name: Thorazine), reserpine (Serpasil) and azacyclonol (Frenquel).

It is well known that in dealing with a psychotic individual the psychiatrist's greatest problem is to make some kind of effective contact with the patient. This is particularly true of schizophrenia. The patient may be aloof and apathetic; he may be living in a world of hallucinations and grandiose delusions; he may fancy that the radio on the ward is directing insults to him personally. Some schizophrenics are so out of touch with their surroundings that even their speech is completely incomprehensible to others (doctors call it "word salad"). Naturally it is of no avail to attempt to argue or reason with such a patient. When he becomes violent, the hospital physicians usually have no recourse but to apply a drastic treatment such as electroshock or to quiet the patient temporarily with barbiturates.

The new tranquilizing drugs have introduced a new regime in the management of patients in mental hospitals. The drugs calm the patients without putting them to sleep. Their effects last longer than sedatives. They make it possible to keep severely disturbed patients in an open ward instead of locking them up. And most important, they make even "hopeless" patients accessible to psychotherapy by reducing their anxiety and removing some of the barriers between the patient and the psychiatrist.

From *Scientific American*, October 1955.

The new drugs promise to reduce the cost of caring for the nation's mentally ill, to decrease the number who must be kept in hospitals and to make mental hospitals more attractive places to work. Moreover, the drugs are becoming popular outside of hospitals. Physicians are prescribing them for mildly psychotic patients whom they now treat in their offices, for neurotic patients and even for entirely normal individuals who become tense under some temporary stress or crisis. A dose of one of these drugs relaxes an anxious person and enables him to deal with a trying situation more objectively.

How do the drugs produce their effects? Before we review the research on their mode of action in the body, let us look at the psychological effects in more detail.

At the Galesburg State Research Hospital in Illinois we have found that the drugs produce the most dramatic results in the most disturbed patients. They are particularly effective in quieting elderly psychotics who are apprehensive, irritable and aggressive. Most surprisingly, they show good results on many chronic psychotics who have been ill and hospitalized for a long time.

The three drugs differ in activity. Chlorpromazine seems to be most effective in suppressing the delusions of paranoid patients and in quieting patients who are restless, hyperactive and over-elated. Reserpine is most successful in helping hebephrenic patients (those whose speech is unintelligible) and catatonic ones (e.g., patients who keep a peculiar posture for long periods or turn only at right angles when they walk). Frenquel moderates various kinds of schizophrenic behavior, but its effect is less marked than those of chlorpromazine and reserpine. However, no one drug is uniformly successful against a given type of disorder, and it may be desirable to try another drug or a combination of the drugs in some cases.

There are drawbacks, unfortunately, to the use of some of the drugs. Substantial doses of chlorpromazine or reserpine may produce large reductions of blood pressure, tremors, gastric disturbances, skin eruptions and jaundice. These drugs therefore have to be administered with care. Frenquel has not shown any such undesirable side reactions so far.

The tranquilizing drugs temporarily banish symptoms of mental illness, relieve anxiety and make a psychotic patient more nearly normal. Thus they are a great boon to psychiatric medicine. And in addition the drugs afford a new instrument for exploring how the machinery of the body breaks down when a person has mental or emotional aberrations.

One obviously important site to investigate is the hypothalamus, a structure at the base of the brain which, as Walter B. Cannon showed, plays a key part in mobilizing reactions to an emergency. When an animal is threatened or under stress, it responds with a number of physiological changes which are triggered by mechanisms in the hypo-thalamus, particularly in its posterior part. In this portion of the brain are centers which correlate breathing and the heart rate with the indi-vidual's emotional state, raise the blood pressure, control basal metab-olism and the body temperature, rouse the body and put it to sleep.

Now experiments on animals indicate that chlorpromazine and reserpine inhibit the activities of the hypothalamus. Reserpine is an alkaloid extract from the snakeroot plant (named Rauwolfia for a 16th-century German physician), which has been used in India for centuries as a sedative and a treatment for epilepsy, snake bite and various other ailments. Chlorpromazine is a synthetic. Both of the drugs act on the hypothalamus to lower the rate of basal metabolism and the body temperature, reduce blood pressure and quiet agitated emotions. Chlor-promazine also seems to affect the nerve system outside the brain, caus-ing the nerves to relax and dilate the small blood vessels.

The hypothalamus is not the only part of the brain influenced by the two drugs. My colleague F. Rinaldi and I have detected effects of the drugs on other brain centers. Our method of research was to analyze electroencephalograms of brain waves.

When the body is touched or stimulated in some way, nerve impulses go from the site of stimulation by pathways called the lemnisci to the thalamus in the center of the brain [see Fig. 1]. From there the im-pulses are relayed to parts of the cerebral cortex which interpret the sensation — touch, pain, heat, cold or the like. But there is also a parallel mental system, so to speak, which is affected by the stimulus. In the central core of the brain is a structure known as the activating system; it is located in the "reticular formation." When stimulated, the activating system produces an arousal reaction. This reaction is clearly shown in an electroencephalogram by a sharp change in the brain-wave pattern [see top pattern in Fig. 2].

Chlorpromazine in small doses blocks the arousal reaction. If it is given in advance to an experimental animal, even a painful stimulus will not produce the brain-wave change indicating arousal [see bottom pattern in Fig. 2]. From this we deduce that in a human patient chlor-promazine inhibits the activating system, preventing some stimuli from rising to the level of the cerebral cortex. It thereby places a block be-tween the environment and its influence on the mind. The individual is rendered more aloof from his surroundings. A psychotic is insulated against the terrifying creations of his imagination. A normal person is made less sensitive to troublesome situations which would ordinar-ily arouse a strongly emotional response, and he can be more objective in evaluating the situation.

On the other hand, small doses of reserpine (or large doses of chlor-promazine) stimulate the activating system. The drug still has a calming

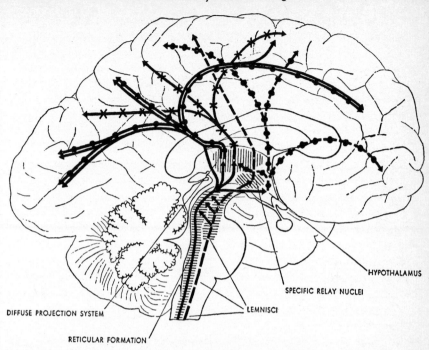

Fig. 1. Two pathways of stimulation in the human brain are shown in this diagram. Sensory impulses pass through the lemnisci to the specific relay nuclei of the thalamus in the center of the brain. From there they are relayed to the parts of the cerebral cortex concerned with the analysis of specific sensations. This system is shown by the broken line with arrows. The other set of pathways, called the activating system, begins with branches from the lemnisci. They carry impulses to the midbrain reticular formation, which in turn relays these impulses to the thalamus. From there the activating impulses are carried to the cerebral cortex by way of the diffuse projection system. These paths are indicated by solid lines with crosses. The reticular formation also sends impulses to the hypothalamus. Secondary impulses from the hypothalamus are suggested by broken lines with dots; from the thalamus, by solid dotted lines, paralleling the solid lines that leave the reticulum and end in the cortex. These lines represent the possibilities that some fibers of the reticular formation pass as far as the cerebral cortex without interruption, and others though interrupted transmit impulses other than those carried by the diffuse projection fibers.

effect upon a patient, because it depresses the hypothalamus, but it does not make him sleepy. Unlike a barbiturate, reserpine keeps the sedated patient wide-awake and at full efficiency.

It is clear that the action of the tranquilizing drugs is far from simple. The mystery of their action is deepened when we come to the third of the drugs. Frenquel does not depress the hypothalamus nor interfere with the usual functions of the activating system. How, then, does

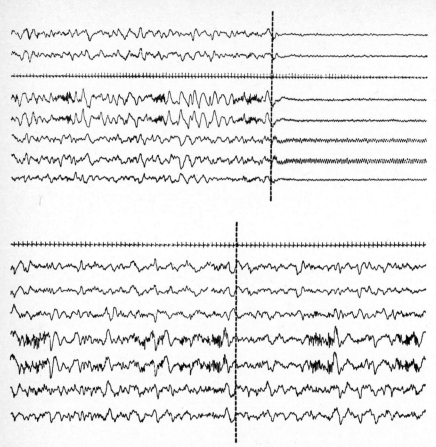

Fig. 2. Electroencephalograms are used to show the effect of a drug on the brain's activity. In the two patterns shown here each wavy line represents the electrical impulses recorded from distinct areas of a rabbit's brain. In the upper record the wave pattern at the left is the resting pattern. When a painful stimulus is applied it changes the brain-wave pattern to that on the right side of the dashed line. The lower record shows the effect of chlorpromazine: the pattern remains essentially unchanged after the stimulus.

it calm a psychotic patient? A hint came from some observations by Howard D. J. Fabing of Cincinnati. Dr. Fabing demonstrated that Frenquel could prevent the psychotic symptoms, including hallucinations, which are usually produced by the drugs lysergic acid and mescaline. We returned to our animal experiments to investigate this finding further. Experiments showed that lysergic acid and mescaline would induce the arousal reaction in animals, and that Frenquel would quench this experimentally induced reaction. In other words, Frenquel has

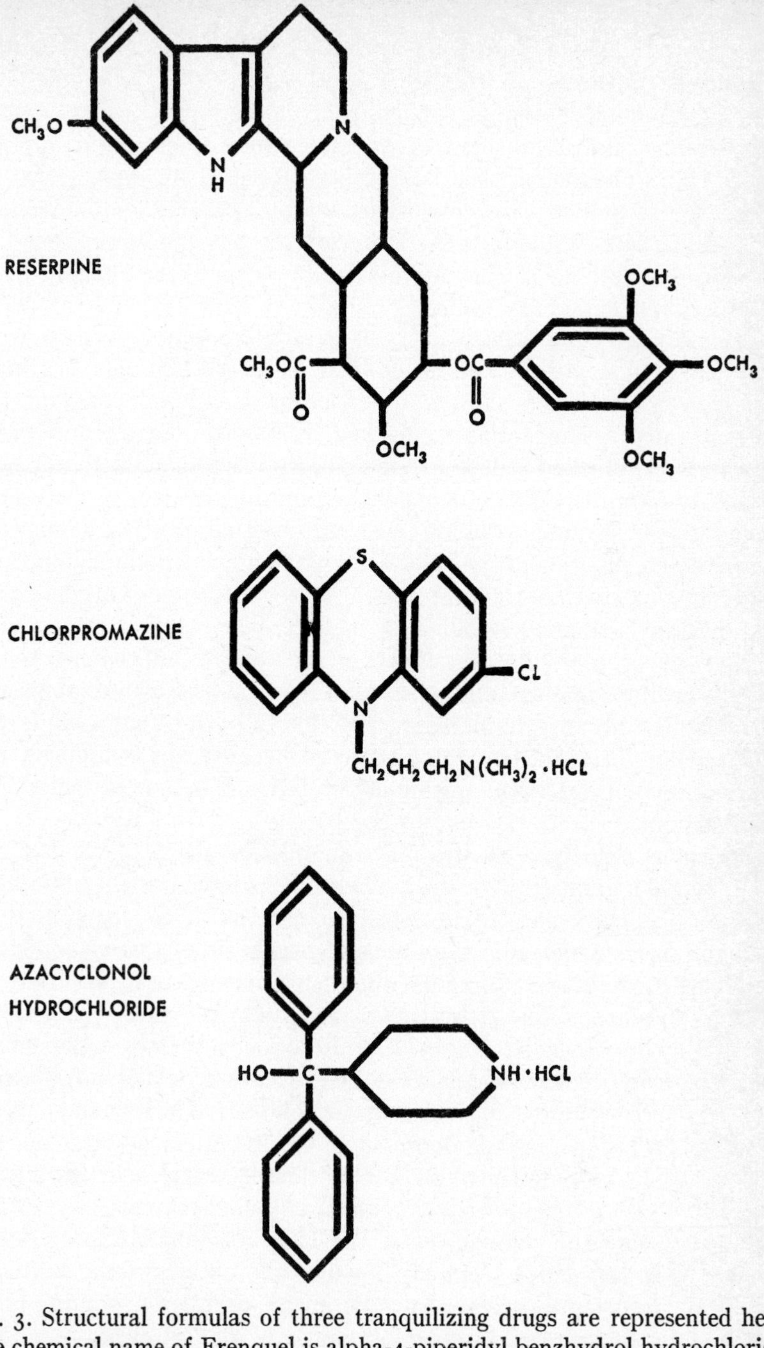

RESERPINE

CHLORPROMAZINE

AZACYCLONOL HYDROCHLORIDE

Fig. 3. Structural formulas of three tranquilizing drugs are represented here. The chemical name of Frenquel is alpha-4-piperidyl benzhydrol hydrochloride. Both it and chlorpromazine (Thorazine) are synthetics. Reserpine (Serpasil) is extracted from Rauwolfia.

an antagonistic effect against these drugs. But just how does it act on a psychotic patient?

The problem has been approached from another angle: the chemistry of the brain. Chlorpromazine and reserpine cause fundamental changes is the brain's chemistry; this has been established by experiments of Robert G. Grenell and his co-workers at the University of Maryland and by my wife Williamina A. Himwich, in our laboratory. And it now appears that an important role is played in these changes by a brain hormone called serotonin.

Serotonin, a neurohormone, acts as a sedative when given in large doses. Bernard B. Brodie and his co-workers at the National Institutes of Health in Bethesda showed in experiments on animals that the hormone's depressant action is blocked by chlorpromazine and Frenquel, and it is blocked still more strongly by lysergic acid. In our own laboratory Erminio Costa studied the action of serotonin in the uterus of the rat (the hormone is found in certain internal muscles). Serotonin causes the uterus to contract. Costa found that the tranquilizing drugs could prevent this contracting action of the hormone. On the other hand, lysergic acid and mescaline increased the contraction, intensifying the effect of serotonin. If these effects on muscle turn out to apply to the brain as well, we may be able to say that lysergic acid evokes abnormal mental states because it increases the effects of serotonin, while the tranquilizing drugs help mental patients because they diminish the effects of the hormone. An exciting investigation is being conducted into this question.

Physicians who have tested the tranquilizing drugs are convinced that they are a great step forward. Their effects have been corroborated widely in the U. S. and in Europe. Psychiatrists at last have at their command drugs which stop symptoms of psychosis just as insulin stops symptoms of diabetes. Moreover, the drugs may be used generally as sedatives in place of the barbiturates now commonly prescribed.

But chlorpromazine, reserpine and Frenquel are only a beginning. The first two produce undesirable side reactions which must somehow be avoided. None of the three drugs is effective in relieving melancholia (a profound, passive depression) or certain long-standing neuroses and psychosomatic troubles. Nor do the drugs help all schizophrenics. Yet they represent a beachhead which should be steadily extended during the coming years. We have a valuable basic clue in the fact that the drugs seem to influence the action of the hormone serotonin. Future progress seems to lie in the direction of finding other drugs which can act on the neurohormones of the brain to counteract disturbances and suppress mental illness.

30

PHARMACOTHERAPEUTIC EVALUATION AND THE PSYCHIATRIC SETTING

MELVIN SABSHIN, M.D. AND JOSHUA RAMOT, M.D.

Once again we are immersed in a period of intense interest in pharmacotherapy in psychiatry. The recent advent of chlorpromazine, reserpine, pipradrol (Meratran) and its derivatives, meprobamate (Miltown), etc., has catalyzed interest in the field, and our specialty journals are filled with enthusiastic reports. Physicians in diverse medical specialties frequently prescribe these drugs to patients with almost any variety of affective component in their symptom pattern. Such an intensely hopeful response once again reflects the unfulfilled therapeutic needs of the psychiatric profession, which potentiate the hope of quick closure for many problems. It is natural to empathize with those persons responsible for therapeutic programs in our state hospitals when they become enthusiastic over a new type of therapy. They have the greatest needs and the largest immediate responsibility of the profession. At present, as a group, they are very enthusiastic about the new drugs, and this is of profound social importance. It prompted Nolan Lewis at a recent meeting to use the old adage, "You should treat as many patients as possible with the drugs while the effects still last." At any rate, the field is afire with new interest, and this may be as important as the new drugs themselves.

At the Institute for Psychosomatic and Psychiatric Research and Training, however, no such enthusiasm has been generated. Six months ago we sent out a questionnaire to our staff in an effort to assess its experience with the newer drugs. Chlorpromazine had been prescribed for a total of 51 patients, two-thirds of whom were outpatients. The staff psychiatrists, as a group, reported quite poor results, and in general they were unimpressed with the effect of the drugs.

During the past six months we have evaluated the use of both chlorpromazine and reserpine on inpatients. Our present data comprise essentially anecdotal and descriptive material on 60 patients, 42 of whom received chlorpromazine and 18 reserpine. The nosological

From the Institute for Psychosomatic and Psychiatric Research and Training of the Michael Reese Hospital, and published in the *A. M. A. Archives of Neurology and Psychiatry*, April 1956. © 1956, by American Medical Association.

grouping of the patients includes a fairly representative sample of our patient population; thus, 38% were depressive patients, of whom two-thirds were of the agitated variety, and 29% were schizophrenic; in 20% the diagnosis indicated high degrees of anxiety, 8% had organic brain diseases, and 5% were manic. In terms of agitation, 5% of the patients showed none, 36% mild, 42% moderate, and 17% severe. The highest dosage of chlorpromazine was 400 mg. a day, while the highest dosage of reserpine was 16 mg. a day. Only 5 of 42 patients on chlorpromazine received the treatment over 30 days. Of the 18 patients on reserpine, 7 received the drug over 30 days.

Since the differences between the effects of chlorpromazine and reserpine were indistinguishable, we shall present them as a composite group. Forty per cent of the patients showed no effects or side-effects alone. Another 40% showed a minimal to moderate sedative effect. Twenty per cent had moderate sedative effects, which were deemed by their therapist to have played an important role in the patient's recovery. Of these 12 patients, 10 had intensive psychotherapy. Of the entire group, about 35% had intensive psychotherapy concomitantly. The factor of concomitant therapy is further illustrated by the fact that 40% of the patients receiving the drugs were also given electroshock at one time or another during the hospitalization. Thirty-five per cent of the patients depended regularly on additional daytime sedation, and it was the rare case that did not require additional night-time sedation. Eight patients with Grade 3 (severe) agitation were included in the series. Six of these showed moderate quieting effects with a definite reduction of their agitation, but of the eight, seven required electroshock during the hospitalization. Of the six agitated patients who responded to the medication with moderate sedation, three were subsequently sent to state hospitals.

Many of our staff have been struck by the similarity of the present period of drug enthusiasm with that at the introduction of insulin, pentylenetetrazol (Metrazol), corticotropin (ACTH), histamine, mephenesin (Tolserol), the barbiturates (especially amobarbital), carbon dioxide, ergotamine, and the amphetamines. The first reports tended to be enthusiastic. They emanated, primarily, from institutions with the greatest need for immediate results. After several years the limitations for use became more apparent, and some of the above-named drugs have been relegated to limbo in psychiatry.

We have been struck by the extent of the contrasting attitudes and findings of our own staff and those of others reporting on the new drugs. We felt that an exploration of the effects of the variations of milieu upon the new drug treatment might explain the discrepancies. Hence the main purpose of this paper is to contrast our hospital with other psychiatric settings with special reference to the use of the newer drugs.

Our assumptions may be stated in this way: At the present time the vast majority of psychiatric illnesses have no specific treatment in the traditional medical sense, i. e., such as penicillin for Pneumococcus infections. Integration and improvement are accomplished by several transacting processes, and require social reinforcement through time for maintenance. We believe that this concept is valid, irrespective of the types of psychiatric therapy employed. Even for lobotomy success of therapy is conditional on the attitude of persons in the same environment to which the patient is discharged. Hence it seems fallacious to shift frames of reference when somatotherapies are used. By this we mean that the concentration on the neuropharmacological level and the minimizing of other processes when one prescribes drugs may bring about distortions in the evaluative judgment. Paradoxical effects occur, depending on the prior state of the patient receiving the drug. Additional shifting effects occur when the milieu is varied. We feel that it is a rare type of somatotherapy that transcends the milieu and produces consistently independent clinical improvement. Drug effects seem much less specific, even though on very high dosage the toxic signs are fairly uniform irrespective of environment. To give one illustration of this point, Wolf and Wolff (1) have shown that their gastrostomy patient, Tom, had varied gastric responses in different situations. He showed paradoxical responses to drugs, depending upon the moment-to-moment relationship with the examiner. We are aware that many of these statements seem self-evident, but the implications of these assumptions are not accepted in the day-to-day use of somatotherapy in psychiatry.

Let us now contrast the setting in our hospital, which will be abbreviated in the paper as P&PI, derived from Psychosomatic & Psychiatric Institute, with that of certain typical state hospitals. P&PI is part of a general hospital but is housed in a separate building. There are 80 beds, of which 80% are private. About 750 patients are admitted each year, and they are treated by a large attending staff of psychiatrists. The latter have been trained primarily with a psychoanalytical orientation. There is an additional courtesy staff of physicians whose training background varies. There are 15 psychiatric residents and a relatively large staff of nurses, O. T. workers, aides, and other ancillary therapeutic personnel.

PATIENT POPULATION

Patients admitted to psychiatric sections of general hospitals are qualitatively different from those seen in the state hospitals. Irrespective of the nosological groupings, patients who enter general hospitals tend to be in a more acutely disruptive phase of illness. The vast majority of state hospital patients have reached a steady state of illness even if their behavior remains bizarre, agitated, or querulous. Our knowledge of the long-term aspects of psychiatric illnesses is limited, and we know very little about what processes maintain the patients in a psychotic steady state for a long time. Nevertheless, there may be a host of paradoxical responses to drugs, dependent upon the different phases of the same nosological entity.

Other elements in patient population besides the phase of illness are crucial in assessing the effect of any new therapeutic variable. As a group, the patients at P&PI are more conversant with psychotherapy as a process, although they are not as homogeneous in this respect as patients in some other centers. Stanton and Schwartz (2) point out that at Chestnut Lodge treatment is equated by the patients with psychotherapy. In the patient's value system somatotherapies rank quite low. At P&PI there have been several examples of patients who became angry with their doctors when they were placed on drug treatment. They thought that this was deprecatory to them. For example, the 55-year-old wife of a local physician was recently admitted in an agitatedly depressed state. She had had intensive psychotherapy 10 years previous to the admission. When she was placed on chlorpromazine, she was bitterly resentful. This implied to her that she had a poor prognosis and that she was being treated in a "second-class way." On the other hand, P&PI and general hospital patients tend to differ from patients at places that are considered more as homes, foundations, schools, or lodges. A large number of our patients see us clearly as part of a hospital, and some have a strong expectancy of the more traditional type of medical treatment. This, of course, facilitates the use of drugs.

Our patients stem from good economic circumstances, and the great majority pay for their psychiatric care. Redlich (3) has clearly illustrated how the type of therapy employed may be related to the class background or economic circumstances of the patient. Economic pressure may force the psychiatrist to choose a quicker form of therapy if the hospital stay must be curtailed. In this context, it should be noted that chlorpromazine and reserpine often require a lengthy clinical trial. At times the necessary length of treatment cannot be maintained at the private hospital.

There are several other aspects about our patients that facilitate the use of psychotherapeutic methods. The patients in general hospitals and at P&PI tend much more frequently to be hospitalized for the first time. They differ from state hospital patients in possessing superior reality testing, ego flexibility, internal resources, and previous successful adaptive modes. Consequently, they possess greater social communicability, which allows them to participate more in psychodynamically oriented therapy.

As our patients are treated closer to their homes than are most state hospital patients, the relatives may be better integrated in the total treatment plan. This facilitates the use of psychotherapeutic methods if the chances for alteration of the home surroundings of the patient are good.

ENVIRONMENTAL FACTORS

Each psychiatric treatment center has a therapeutic aura which is a concatenation of many factors. The milieu at P&PI is more complex than usual, in that we stand at the crossroads of several divergent approaches. At the roots of our organization we are medically grounded, and there is much in our structural organization which reflects general hospital attitudes. On the other hand, we possess a larger measure of autonomy than is usual for a psychiatric section of a general hospital. This permits the infusion of psychodynamic principles, and also permits the utilization of types of inpatient policy novel for general hospitals. In effect, the multiplicity of approaches has allowed a rather wide base of therapeutic alternatives.

For many people on our staff, however, there is a distasteful aspect to the utilization of somatotherapy. As an example, one of the nurses said that the only somatotherapy that she felt positive toward was insulin therapy. She elaborated by saying that it was not the insulin per se that was approved, but the fact that the patient had eight hours of close contact with another person during the treatment. This staff attitude is communicated through the various levels of personnel to the patients and affects the drug responses. The attitude of a particular staff defines its position in reference to many conflictual areas in the field of psychiatry. It is clear that both subtle latent conflict and more overt problems emerge when new treatments are discussed. People identify strongly with modes of therapy. Let us now look at the attitudes at P&PI and compare them point by point with some state hospital values.

1. Activity Rate of Staff-Patient Interaction

At P&PI the average patient has an active daily program. He sees his therapist and unit personnel quite often. He goes to occupational therapy frequently and participates in a host of activities and interpersonal relationships. The addition of a drug into this complex field makes it difficult to isolate the specific effect of the drug. In the state hospital the introduction of a new drug is often made into a vacuum of relative inactivity. The patient has achieved a certain steady state, and there is lack of personnel to provide a variety of activities. Hence drug changes are more easily ascribed to the drug per se, as it is deemed the only new variable. We say "deemed," as it is our contention that the attitude of the staff toward the drug is an equally important variable. The addition of a new drug at P&PI is often looked upon unenthusiastically as a questionable and unimportant addition to an already full schedule, and to many on our units it seems like a chore. This contrasts with many state hospitals, where the drugs have markedly raised the hopes of therapeutic success.

2. Staff Tolerance of Agitated Behavior and Immediate Goals of Treatment

In the state hospital the lack of adequate personnel and the presence of large numbers of extremely disturbed patients make it imperative that immediate limits be placed on various types of hyperactivity. The implicit and explicit goals of treatment are to keep the unit as near to tranquility as possible. Drugs which tend to diminish psychomotor activity are utilized by the staff as a means to maintain order. At P&PI there is a much greater individualization, with the realization that for many patients "tranquility" may be markedly deleterious. In this context, Spinka,[1] at another hospital, reports better results in female patients on chlorpromazine. He suggests that male patients may equate tranquility with passivity and a threat to masculinity. Agitatedly depressed patients may respond with increased painful affect to a reduction of the agitated defense. In addition, several reports[2] have indicated that up to 15% of hypertensive patients have responded to reserpine therapy with depressive reactions. On the whole our patients are encouraged to keep an optimum rate of activity, and such signs as lethargy and withdrawal are not regarded in the same light as they are in the state hospitals.

It is clear that evaluation of a patient's response to a drug would be affected by the goals of the unit as a whole. These goals shift a great deal. To give an illustration: Often when a single manic patient enters a unit there is a tendency for a period of disequilibrium to occur. During this time the immediate goals of the unit may change quite a bit. Peace and quiet may be more at a premium. We are stressing the shifting goals of our units, in contrast to many state hospital units, where the goals tend to be more constant. Of course, the attitudes of the

---

[1] Spinka, I.: Personal communication to the authors.
[2] References 4 to 6.

personnel to specific patients affect individual goals for all the patients. Thus, with certain patients they would be very alarmed at lethargy. In other patients they would very much welcome this sign. Occasionally, the personnel respond to patients with either overt or covert belief that increased dependency gratification would be quite helpful. The giving of a drug, with the attendant procedures accompanying its administration, provides a vehicle to afford such gratification where other channels are blocked. The personnel may then welcome the fact that patients on chlorpromazine and reserpine tend to become lethargic, often requiring bed care. Several of our best results of drug administration occurred in this context.

3. Tolerance for Delayed Effect and Toxicity

Both chlorpromazine and reserpine have a large number of toxic signs. The expectation for a drug plays an important role in the toleration of toxic signs. It is clear that our staff is quite concerned over those toxic signs that we have seen already. Before one will utilize a drug with this kind of potentiality, one must have a positive impression that beneficial effects will be forthcoming. In addition, the less dangerous, but still annoying minor toxic signs are engrafted upon a low frustration tolerance which our personnel possess in this area. Their feelings are readily communicated to the patients. Of course, the way in which these procedures are carried out connotes many things to patients. This has varied from anxiety lest something be seriously wrong with them to the conception of blood-pressure recordings as a highly erotic experience. For example, one female patient had frequent dreams revolving about the administration of reserpine by a male nurse. The dreams were filled with sexual symbolism relating to the frequent blood-pressure recordings. In contradistinction, the state hospital personnel tend to see the minor toxic signs as indicators that they are approaching or have exceeded effective dosages. At a meeting of the Illinois Psychiatric Society, one speaker, Steinfeld,[3] indicated that he greets the development of Parkinson's syndrome with enthusiasm in that he feels that this indicates that the drug has finally achieved effective levels.

Both chlorpromazine and reserpine are often quite slow in producing effective responses. Reserpine especially may take weeks to act. As a matter of fact, in most patients reserpine is said by Barsa and Kline[4] to produce a state of turbulence, accompanied often by a florid

---

[3] Steinfeld, L.: Personal communication.

[4] Kline, N. S.: Clinical Applications of Reserpine, presented before the American Psychiatric Association, Section of Medical Sciences, American Association for Advancement of Science, Berkeley, Calif., Dec. 30, 1954.

exacerbation of symptoms. Needless to say, it takes a great deal of faith to ride through such stormy periods, unless one looks at the response as an indicator of positive things to come. In our hospital it is a rarity to find a patient who has gone through the gamut of all the available therapies and failed — in marked contradistinction to the state hospital, where such cases are quite common. Hence, at P&PI the tendency is to have hopeful expectation that one of a number of possible alternatives can work, especially psychotherapy.

4. Exploration with Higher Dosage Level

It is clear that at P&PI we have been very conservative with the dosages employed in the newer drugs. This reflects the quantity and quality of the alternative choices of therapy. It also reflects our unwillingness to risk toxic signs from a drug about which we are doubtful. We started with a dosage of 0.25 mg. of reserpine t. i. d. and 25 mg. of chlorpromazine t. i. d. More recently we have gone up to daily doses of 16 mg. of reserpine and 450 mg. of chlorpromazine. We know that other institutions have gone up to doses ten times as high as our maximum doses, i. e., 4 gm. of chlorpromazine and 130 mg. of reserpine a day. In the higher ranges of reserpine doses the toxic signs increased sharply. Some people would explain our lack of dramatic findings on "inadequate dosage." Although we believe that this is only a small part of the picture, we would agree that we have lagged behind some other hospitals in stepping up the dose. We feel that this is a reflection of our attitude toward our patients and the drugs. We do not wish to risk untoward signs when we are surer of the alternative ways to treat outpatients.

5. Intrastaff Relationship and Effect on Therapy

Caudill and associates (7) and Stanton and Schwartz (2) have well illustrated how the patient's course in a mental hospital may be affected by problems in intrastaff relationships. While their frame of reference is largely the effect on the psychotherapeutic processes, we feel that this is also true of the somatotherapies. At P&PI the large staff and multiple lines of communication increase this problem in many ways; this situation is in marked contradistinction to that in the state hospitals, where there are fewer people treating the patients. At P&PI the unit personnel tend to be disappointed if somatotherapies are carried on without an active psychotherapeutic approach. If the psychotherapeutic plan is explicit in defining the roles of the unit personnel, the patient is liable to benefit from more positive feeling about the therapy. This is also dependent on the working relationships of the various people involved in treating the patient, if there is friction, the patients will feel it in one way or another. These working relationships are important in the responses of patients to pharmacotherapy. One of the nurses thought that reserpine was more effective than chlorpromazine. Her opinion stemmed from the fact that two of the patients placed on reserpine on her unit were treated by doctors who worked intensively and effectively with the unit personnel. While the more "objective" evidence of the positive effect of the drug was lacking, both patients received a good deal of extra care. Another physician with extensive drug experience, at a different hospital, has prescribed chlorpromazine for three patients at P&PI. His results were uniformly poor. He tended to explain this difference on the fact that the three patients at P&PI were all depressed. This doctor used much higher doses of chlorpromazine than did the rest of our staff, in view of his previous experience. The nurses reported being alarmed by this dosage. In addition, the doctor involved was not well known by them. We feel that the intrastaff relationships may have been equally important in the results as the type of patient treated here.

COMMENT

In this paper the emphasis has been placed on certain transactional factors between the individual patient and his environment which raise problems in drug evaluation. This emphasis has largely by-passed the more specific psychophysiological area of drug effects and, in so doing, may have distorted the perspective by relative omission. It is clear that both chlorpromazine and reserpine are not inert drugs. Both drugs seem to have the property of producing a measure of tranquility without some of the more untoward signs of the barbiturates. If this finding is maintained, both the drugs will have found a definite place in psychiatric utilization.

Claims for the drugs, however, have gone far beyond the sedative stage. There have been statements which indicated that the drugs have certain intrinsic curability. We feel that these claims are premature in several ways. In the broadest sense, the evaluation of the therapeutic effect in any new treatment in psychiatry is subsumed under the question of the methodology of the evaluation. Although, at times, we feel that our techniques for evaluation of results are good, our empirical evidence for this is surprisingly poor. For this reason, of course, the evaluation of any new therapy can be no better than the older available evaluations in the field. The physiological processes involved in the drug therapies are quite obscure. Certainly, we are a long way from an understanding of the neurophysiological correlates of behavior. It is our opinion that the psychodynamic understanding of when to use a drug in the course of therapy is also quite limited. It is the major contention of this paper, however, that special social factors would have to be taken into consideration, even if we had much greater knowledge of both the neurophysiological correlates of the psychiatric disorders and the psychodynamic principles important in the utilization of the drugs. There is a great deal of recent evidence to indicate that other branches of medicine have recognized the importance of some of these concepts. Quite recently, Lasagna and associates [5] have shown that morphine, heroin (diacetylmorphine), the amphetamines, etc., have varying effects, depending upon the population studied. He gave normal volunteers, chronically ill patients, and postaddicts randomized samples of these drugs and placebo. In normal volunteers the morphine and heroin were experienced as quite unpleasant drugs. In contradistinction, the postaddicts found the morphine quite pleasant. Lasagna illustrated that the addicts are unusual in responding with euphoria to a wide variety of agents, such as analgesics, amphetamines, antihistaminic agents, and even Coca-Cola. We believe that he has clearly illustrated how the prior personality is an important variable in the response to drugs.

Gold (10), in a recent Cornell conference on drug therapy, illustrated that the effect of a drug varied greatly with a patient's mood. He showed how unconscious bias of the physician can affect the results of even so-called objective measurements, such as iron in anemia, and anticoagulants in thrombotic diseases. Lasagna and Gold have emphasized the interaction of the previous personality with the drug being given.

In this paper, we are highlighting another dimension, i. e., the social field in which the patient interacts with the drug. The social factors are not merely added variables but also integral parts of the transactional field of drug response. We agree with both Gold and Lasagna when they call for more rigorous methods in an attempt to eliminate the bias of the observer in the evaluation. We would like to point out, however, that the use of double-blind studies has certain limitations. Thus, when one compares active drugs like chlorpromazine or reserpine with a relatively inert preparation such as saline, problems may develop which stem from the instructions to the personnel and the patients as to what to expect from the drugs. If on a particular psychiatric unit some patients are placed on placebo and other patients on the active drug, the personnel is instructed as to what autonomic signs may occur. The patients, too, are often instructed in a similar

[5] References 8 and 9.

fashion. In view of the fact that both chlorpromazine and reserpine affect many systems, these signs become the cue, both to the patient and to the personnel, that these patients are receiving the active drug and not placebo. It is here that interaction may take place among the tester, the attending personnel, and the patient. Often the patient may interpret a change in his internal milieu in the context of being a change in the expected direction. It is thus possible for a subtle type of communication to take place among the various participants, and this may potentiate the drug effect. Hence a relatively nonspecific effect can be geometrically increased. Thus, the hopeful expectancy or lack of expectancy plays a role even in the double-blind studies. It is necessary to compare drugs such as reserpine and chlorpromazine with very active placebos that stimulate some of the reserpine and chlorpromazine action.

The most rigorous experimental designs hitherto used do not entirely control special factors in the evaluation of drugs in psychiatry. A special problem is the particular criteria that one uses for change; i. e., we have indicated that diminution in agitation is not necessarily an adequate prognostic indicator. Length of hospitalization is not adequate, either. Thus, in many of our patients, long-term hospitalization signifies the most intensive treatment, and the goals for therapy may be closer to a basic reconstruction of character patterns. Simple statements of improvement or lack of improvement on discharge and follow-up sometimes may be useful, but have definite limits.

The problem merges into the broader question of how to judge the effect of hospitalization upon the patient's course of illness. We believe that the evaluation of somatotherapy will lag behind the broader problem. We do not mean to imply by this a nihilistic attitude toward the pragmatic utilization of somatotherapy. Nor do we mean to imply that we must have a measure for change that approximates the blood sugar for insulin effect or an EKG for digitalis effect; however, we are emphasizing the need for better criteria than those currently available.

While the major theme in this paper has emphasized caution in terms of the evaluation of the newer drugs, another theme has run through it. It is clear that we feel that a negative attitude toward somatotherapy plays a role in hindering the proper utilization of such treatment. Thus, we have presented relatively negative results from the use of both chlorpromazine and reserpine at our hospital. We have not controlled for our negative attitude, however, and we are just as liable to criticism for saying that our results prove the inefficacy of the drugs as are those people who were overenthusiastic. The phenomenon of negative attitudes toward somatotherapy needs amplification, and we have attempted to illustrate it. We have also illustrated that this attitude is communicated to all levels of personnel at psychiatric hospitals and plays a role in the entire therapeutic aura. We have shown that each inpatient center has its distinct milieu which in a complex way facilitates or inhibits drug usage. Extreme facilitation occurs at places with the greatest immediate needs and the most intense expectations from the drug. The greatest inhibition occurs when there exists strongly negativistic attitudes toward its use, for a variety of reasons.

We believe that the present role of pharmacotherapy in psychiatry is undefined, but perhaps some of the intense response to chlorpromazine and reserpine can be channelized into a fuller understanding of the area.

Summary

Data are presented illustrating the effects of chlorpromazine and reserpine prescription to patients at the Institute for Psychosomatic and Psychiatric Research and Training of the Michael Reese Hospital. The results have been less positive than most studies reported elsewhere. An attempt is made to analyze factors in the specific psychiatric setting and patient population that might account for these findings. One factor appeared to be the relatively negative attitude of our hospital personnel toward the prescription of drugs as compared with alternative modes of therapy. This attitude seemed to be the antithesis of enthusiasm regarding drug effects seen elsewhere. "Double-blind" studies of drug effects do not entirely preclude the communication of such attitudes, especially when "active drugs" are compared with relatively inert preparations.

We conclude that the social context within which pharmacotherapy is undertaken has importance in the over-all evaluation of therapeutic effect. It appeared as relevant as the specific pharmacological action of the drug and the psychodynamic meaning to the patient of receiving the drug. An attempt has been made to explore some of the implications of these conclusions for evaluation of results in other psychiatric therapies.

References

1. Wolf, S., and Wolff, H. G. *Human Gastric Function: An Experimental Study of Man and His Stomach*, New York, Oxford University Press, 1943.

2. Stanton, A. H., and Schwartz, M. S. *The Mental Hospital*, New York, Basic Books, Inc., 1954.

3. Redlich, F. C., Hollingshead, A. B., and Bellis, E. Social Class Differences in Attitudes Toward Psychiatry. *Am. J. Orthopsychiat.* 25: 60, 1955.

4. Wilkins, R. W. New Drug Therapies in Arterial Hypertension. *Ann. Int. Med.* 37: 1144, 1952.

5. Genest, J., Adamkiewicz, L., Robillard, K., and Tremblay, G. Clinical Uses of Rauwolfia: I. In Arterial Hypertension. *Canad. M. A. J.* 72: 483, 1955.

6. Locket, S. Oral Preparation of Rauwolfia in Treatment of Essential Hypertension, *Brit. M. J.* 2: 844, 1955.

7. Caudill, W., Redlich, F. C., Gilmore, H. R., and Brody, B. Social Structure and Interaction Processes on a Psychiatric Ward. *Am. J. Orthopsychiat.* 22: 314, 1952.

8. Lasagna, L., von Felsinger, J. M., and Beecher, H. K. Drug Induced Mood Changes in Man: 1. Observations on Healthy Subjects, Chronically Ill Patients and "Postaddicts," *J. A. M. A.* 157: 1006, 1955.

9. von Felsinger, J. M., Lasagna, L., and Beecher, H. K. Drug-Induced Mood Changes in Man: 2. Personality and Reactions to Drugs. *J. A. M. A.* 157: 1113, 1955.

10. Gold, H., in Conference on Therapy: How to Evaluate a New Drug. *Am. J. Med.* 17: 722, 1954.

Part IV

SOMATIC FACTORS IN PSYCHOPATHOLOGY

31

ON GOING BERSERK: A NEUROCHEMICAL INQUIRY

HOWARD D. FABING, M.D.

Cincinnati, Ohio

Berserk was a mighty hero in Norse mythology. Legend states that he was the grandson of the mythical 8-handed Starkadder. He was renowned for his consummate bravery and for the fury of his attack in battle. He had 12 sons who were his equal in courage. He never fought in armor but in his *ber sark*, which means "bearskin" in the Nordic languages. Thus the term berserk became synonymous with reckless courage. During the Saga Time (1) in Iceland and in the Scandinavian countries (870–1030 A.D.), and for some time prior to that period of careful historical recording, the Berserks, bearing the same name as the legendary warrior, arose as a predatory group of brawlers and killers who disrupted the peace of the Viking community repeatedly. Today in the United States we would probably use such slang terms as "mobsters" and "hoodlums" in classifying them.

There is a fascinating theory that *Berserksgang*, or the act of "going berserk," which was the hall-mark of their discordant behavior, may not have been a psychogenically determined habit pattern, but may rather have been due to the eating of toxic mushrooms. This idea, fantastic though it may appear at first glance, has won general acceptance among Scandinavian scholars according to Larsen (2). It is the purpose of this communication to review this theory in the light of present-day studies on hallucinogenic drugs which have chemical similarities with mescaline and LSD-25 (lysergic acid diethylamide) and which are capable of producing model psychoses.

Certain members of the vast botanical family of mushrooms have been among the most widely used "phantastica" throughout history to produce temporary psychoses. Among these are the *Amanita muscaria* and *A. pantherina* of Eurasia. The muscaria species[1] is the more com-

From *The American Journal of Psychiatry*, November 1956.

[1] This beautiful fungus crowned by a vivid red cap dotted with white spots was depicted by Walt Disney in the "Dance of the Mushrooms" with Tschaikowsky's *Nutcracker Suite* music in *Fantasia*.

mon. These are distinct from those species of the genus Amanita which kill the eater (*phalloides, verna* and *virosa*), and which contain a deadly hemolysin (3).

The muscaria fungus is commonly known as fly-agaric. Albertus Magnus (4) noted before 1256 A.D. that when it was freshly cut and placed in a dish of milk or water it killed flies (muscae) when they ingested its juice, and Linnaeus reported that it had been advocated for killing bedbugs (5). It has long been used orgiastically by Siberian tribes of the Kamchatka peninsula. The first European to describe the practice was von Strahlenberg (6) in 1730. Prodigious feats of physical strength are reported under its influence. Vanderlip (7) wrote, "Curiously enough, after recovering from one of these debauches, they claim that all the antics performed were by command of the mushroom." The myths of the Koryaks contain the belief which is held to this day that a person affected with fly-agaric is guided by the spirits of the Wapaq which live in the mushroom. If an old man would eat agaric and the Wapaq within the agaric should whisper, "you have just been born," the old man would begin to cry like a baby. If the Wapaq should say, "go to the afterworld," then the old man would die, according to their belief (8).

Jochelsen (9) who travelled among the Koryaks in 1900–01, wrote:

Fly-agaric produces intoxication, hallucinations, and delirium. Light forms of intoxication are accompanied by a certain degree of animation and some spontaneity of movements. Many shamans, previous to their seances, eat fly-agaric to get into ecstatic states. . . . Under strong intoxication the senses become deranged; surrounding objects appear either very large or very small, hallucinations set in, as do spontaneous movements and convulsions. So far as I could observe, attacks of great animation alternate with moments of deep depression. The person intoxicated by fly-agaric sits quietly rocking from side to side, even taking part in conversations with his family. Suddenly his eyes dilate, he begins to gesticulate convulsively, converses with persons whom he imagines he sees, sings, and dances. Then an interval of rest sets in again. However, to keep up the intoxication additional doses of fungi are necessary. . . . There is reason to think that the effect of fly-agaric would be stronger were not its alkaloid quickly taken out of the organism with the urine. The Koryak knows this by experience, and the urine of persons intoxicated with fly-agaric is not wasted. The drunkard himself drinks it to prolong his hallucinations, or he offers it to others as a treat.

The drinking of the Siberian mushroom eater's urine during these amanita debauches has been noted by many other travellers (10). An early satirical comment on this practice was made by Oliver Goldsmith (11) in 1762. It is reported such urine can be drunk successively by as many as 5 people, passing in and out of one into the next, so that all of them can gain the hallucinogenic effect from one dose of mushrooms. It would be most revealing to know the chemical composition of the hallucinogen which is passed around in the urine of these tribesmen, but this fact is not known. Studies looking toward the solution of this problem have been undertaken by Evan Horning and his associates at the National Institutes of Health, Bethesda, Maryland. In 1953 Wieland and Motzel (12), employing paper chromatographic analysis, determined that this mushroom, *Amanita muscaria*, as well as *A. mappa*, and *A. pantherina*, all contained bufotenine, or n-n-dimethyl serotonin, an indole compound first isolated and defined chemically by Handovsky (13) in the skin of poisonous toads.

I am indebted to Dr. Arthur Drew (14) of the Department of Neurology of the University of Michigan for his account of a modern version of *A. muscaria* poisoning.

Dr. Drew reports that the patient, a middle-aged tavern keeper, picked some wild mushrooms and ate them at 10 o'clock one night in October 1955. These mushrooms were later identified by the botany department as *A. muscaria*. Two hours after ingestion the patient had an explosive onset of diarrhea, profuse sweating, excessive salivation and vertigo. He fell asleep and wakened at 2 a.m. completely disoriented, irrational, and violent. On admission to University Hospital, Ann Arbor, Michigan, his nail beds were dusky and he appeared cyanotic, B.P. was 150/90, pulse 120, respirations 24/min., and the temperature 98.4°. He did not react to deep pain stimulation, but responded to pinprick. He was disoriented in all 3 spheres. Somnolence alternated with periods of excitement. He thought that he was in hell and identified the interne, nurses, and attending physicians as Christ, Satan, God, or angels. Nursing notes on admission indicate that he was threshing about in bed, talking constantly and irrationally.

As the day wore on the content of his hallucinatory and illusional output remained almost entirely religious. He constantly misidentified a tall resident physician as Christ. He kept referring to nurses and other attendants as God or angels. He felt that he was in the Garden of Eden, and then in hell. As evening came he cleared up mentally, lost his motor excitement, and felt relaxed. All laboratory tests were within normal limits. He appeared to be recovered on the following morning and was discharged.

Another mushroom eating practice deserves mention. Ever since the time of the conquest of Mexico by the Spaniards in 1522 there have been references (15) to a sacred fungus, *teonanacatl*, employed by the Aztecs and other Mexican Indians. Schultes (16) identified this as the *Panaeolus campanulatus, var. sphinctrinus* mushroom in 1938. This "fungus of the devil," as the early Spanish priests called it, is now under study by Mr. R. Gordon Wasson (17), and his wife, Dr. Valentina P. Wasson, of New York City. The Wassons have eaten the mushrooms and report visual hallucinations in brilliant colors, an ecstatic state of heightened perception, loss of time and space perception and a serene feeling of inward peace while being drawn into an "other-worldly detachment" during dissociation periods of at least 6 hours' duration.

Mr. Wasson reports that there are many colloquial names for the mushrooms at the present time. He writes:

Every Indian language in Mexico has its own name for the divine mushrooms, and, as you would expect with sacred growths, every village is apt to use evasive or euphemistic names as well. In Nahuatl (the language of the Aztecs) the name was teonanacatl, 'God's flesh,' but we find in a village where classic Nahuatl is still used today that the word is *apipiltzin*, "little children of the waters."

He has also noted the terms *nti-si-tho, tum'uh, mbeydo*,' etc., used by other ethnic groups. He has identified species of 4 genera of Mexican mushrooms in use at this time for their hallucinatory properties — *panaeolus, stropharia, conocybe*, and *drosophila* (also called *psathyrella*). Species identification among the genera has not been completed. The chemistry of these mushrooms is not known. It would be interesting to determine whether or not they contain bufotenine. There is no report of urine drinking among Mexican ritual mushroom eaters.

Other evidence suggests the use of bufotenine as an hallucinogenic substance. Fra Ramon Pane, who came to America with Columbus on his second voyage, described the ceremonial use of cohoba (18), a snuff derived from the seeds of the *piptadenia peregrina* tree, as early as 1496, reporting that "it intoxicates them to such an extent that when they are under its influence they know not what they do." This inhalant was so potent in producing temporary dissociation states that it became tribal custom for the women to tie up the Otomaco Indians when they used it. Stromberg (19) determined that bufotenine was the active indolic principle of cohoba. Recently Horning et al. (20) were able to find a few milligrams of the snuff in the bottom of a Piaroa ceremonial snuff box in the Smithsonian Institution. Paper chromatographic analysis showed that this snuff contained large quantities of bufotenine. Evarts (21) and Fabing (22) have also found that the effect of bufotenine in experimental animals is reminiscent of LSD-25. It would appear, then, that there is chemical, experimental, and anthropologic evidence that bufotenine is one of the hallucinogenic indoles, that it is distributed widely in nature, and that one of its chief sources of supply is the mushroom.

Turning to the Viking hoodlums, a vivid description of their behavior is given by Schübeler (23), who relies on the renowned Norse historian, Munch, in his account:

In the old Norwegian historical writings it is mentioned, in many places, that in olden times there was a specific kind of giants who were called *Berserks*, that is, men who at certain times were seized by a wild fury, which, at the moment, doubled their strength and made them insensible to bodily pain, but which also deadened their humanity and reason, and made them like wild animals. This fury, which was called "Berserksgang," occurred not only in the heat of battle, but also during laborious work. Men who were thus seized performed things which otherwise seemed impossible for human power. This condition is said to have begun with shivering, chattering of the teeth, and chill in the body, and then the face swelled and changed its color. With this was connected a great hotheadedness, which at last went over into a great rage, under which they howled as wild animals, bit the edge of their shields, and cut down everything they met, without discriminating between friend or foe. When this condition ceased, a great dulling of the mind and feebleness followed, which could last for one or several days (24).

One of the curious aspects of *Berserksgang* is that it disappeared abruptly in the twelfth century A.D., after plaguing Viking sociopolitical life for more than 3 centuries. In 1784, Samuel Lorenzo Ødman (25), a theologian at the University of Uppsala, undertook to explain the phenomenon of *going berserk*. He reviewed the Sagas for descriptions of the state. He found King Halfdan's Berserks depicted in Rolf's Saga in this manner:

On these giants fell sometimes such a fury that they could not control themselves, but killed men or cattle, whatever came in their way and did not take care of itself. While this fury lasted they were afraid of nothing, but when it left them they were so powerless that they did not have half of their strength, and were as feeble as if they just came out of bed from a sickness. This fury lasted about one day.

Ødman also recounted a tale from the Hervarar Saga. There were 12 brothers who lived on the island of Samsoe in Denmark. Orvar-Odd sailed to the island with his Viking ships, debarked and went inland to visit his cousin, Hjalmar. The 12 Danish brothers went berserk and killed his crews to a man. When he returned to the shore with his cousin, then encountered the Berserks who were now in the enfeebled state after their fury. Hjalmar killed one and Orvar-Odd killed the other 11. Ødman saw in this fury followed by a state of exhaustion a paroxysm, and stated:

I am not of the opinion that these ecstasies can be explained as effects of a peculiar temperament or of auto-suggestion because . . . they were not able to keep up their hated arrogance between paroxysms.

He argued further:

Since the vegetable kingdom gives us various means to bring our power of imagination into chaos and to induce the most ferocious excesses of courage, I am inclined to believe that the Berserks had knowledge about such an intoxicating means, and that they made use of it and kept it secret so that their prestige would not be reduced by the general populace's knowledge of the simplicity of the technique.

He then reviewed the possible botanical products indigenous to Scandinavia which might have been used in this manner, and decided that "flugswamp," the *Amanita muscaria* mushroom, was the one which solved the riddle of the Berserks.

He then compared the accounts of *Berserksgang* in the Sagas to the "amanita debauches" of the Koryaks and other far-Eastern Siberians, and found them to be almost identical behavior patterns. In furtherance of his contention he turned to theological history. He stated:

What in particular seems to me to argue for flugswamp is the fact that to partake of it is a custom from that part of Asia from which the pagan god Odin, with his pantheon, made their migration to our North. . . . Its [the mushroom's] use was spread by these hordes who used them and travelled northward. The history of the Berserks in our North begins with Odin's coming. Not only this, but it fits so well with the intentions of a conqueror who . . . could make himself feared and safe among foreign people.

More than a century later, in 1885, F. C. Schübeler, a physician and Norway's great botanist, arrived at the same conclusion. He wrote (26):

I still have a vivid remembrance that, on confronting all the symptoms that appeared under the so-called "Berserksgang," I came to the conviction that this paroxysm hardly could be anything but a kind of intoxication, the symptoms of which reminded me of the effects of taking fluesop [2]. . . . Some time after I had come so far in this matter, I happened to find, while looking for something else, that the Swedish professor, Samuel Ødman had uttered the same opinion a hundred years ago.

Schübeler agreed with Ødman concerning the similarity between *Berserksgang* and the behavior of Siberian mushroom-eaters. He added

----

[2] Norwegian equivalent for the Swedish "flugswamp."

that he could not agree with Munch that the condition was a "periodically returning insanity," because the symptoms were of a peculiar sort not ordinarily seen by physicians, and because they were the same each time a man went berserk. He argued that the effects could not be those of malted beverages because they produced quite different behavior patterns, and that distilled spirits were not known in Norway before 1531 A.D. In addition, opium and cannabis were unknown to the Nordics in Saga times. He argued too, in favor of secrecy concerning mushroom eating among the Berserks, and that for this reason no accounts of the practice were written down. He wrote:

The Berserks were feared by everyone, and they could, in a certain sense, enforce their pleasure. It is therefore in the nature of the case that they tried as best they could to keep this peculiar reputation in the eyes of the people. Hence, the knowledge of the intoxicant was probably transferred as a secret from individual to individual.

It is worthy of note that the Wassons find a similar attitude of secrecy in the Mexican peons who use sacred mushrooms today.

Schübeler pointed out, too, that the more enlightened Viking leaders soon learned that the state was one which could be prevented, and therefore could be legislated against. He wrote:

Before Erik Jarl left Norway he called together (in 1015 A.D.) the feudatories and the mightiest peasants in order to deliberate with them about the lawgiving and the rule of the country. At this meeting camp-fighting (holmgang) was abolished, and Berserks and robbers were outlawed. In Thorlak's and Ketil's Icelandic Christian Law, which was adopted in 1123 A.D., there is the following decree: "If someone goes berserk, he is punished with three years of banishment (fjorbaugsgard), and the men who are present are also banished if they do not bind him; but if they bind him, none are punished. If this is repeated, then the punishment occurs."

Schübeler regards this as proof that the Vikings came to know that the paroxysm was temporary and preventable. *Berserksgang* ceased after this law was passed.

Fredrik Grön (27) reviewed the subject of the fury of the Berserks in 1929, and did not agree with the Ødman-Schübeler hypothesis. He points out that because of the general reliability of the historical Icelandic family sagas, none of the authors who have written about *Berserksgang* have raised any doubt about the reality of the phenomenon, but the explanations for it have varied over a wide range. Even in the more fantastic prehistoric sagas there are enough common traits in their descriptions to establish a background of reality for the phenomenon. He feels, however, that the best explanation would be that of ecstatic fury psychogenically determined in a group of aggressive psychopathic personalities.

Recently we (28) have had the opportunity to study the effects of the intravenous injection of bufotenine [3] in the human during the course of our inquiries into possible chemical factors in the causation of schizophrenia (29). The subjects were healthy young long-term convicts at the Ohio State Penitentiary (30). All were well above the normal intelligence level, all had been college students, none were recidivist criminals, and all were considered to be relatively stable emotionally. Injections of one part bufotenine base in 1.8 parts creatinine sulfate were given steadily over a 3-minute period. A dose of 1.0 mg. bufotenine produced only a sensation of tightness in the chest and paraesthesias of the face. Two mg. produced a "tightness in the stomach" plus flushing and a purplish hue of the skin of the face. Four mg. produced a sensation of tingling in the face and neck, a sense of chest oppression, a subjective report that "a load is pressing down from above and my body feels heavy," and a "very pleasant Martini feeling." This was followed by visual hallucinations of vivid red and black blocks moving before the visual field, inability to concentrate, and a feeling of great placidity and less anxiety than before the onset of the experiment. The face of the subject appeared lividly purple for 13 minutes.

Eight mg. produced an immediate sensation of light-headedness, burning in the face, hyperpnea, deep purple facial color, and a sense of calm. At the end of the injection, the subject blurted, "I see white straight lines with a black background. I can't trace a pattern. Now there are red, green and yellow dots, like they were made out of fluorescent cloth, moving like blood cells through capillaries." Six minutes later he reported that he felt relaxed and languid. In retrospect he said, "Even at the height of this, my mind felt better and more pleasant than usual."

Sixteen mg. produced severe purpling of the face and facial sweating, tingling sensation throughout the body, a feeling that his chest was crushed, and the onset of hallucinations of purple spots on the floor, all in rapid succession before the injection was completed. Three minutes later the visual phenomena were gone, but space perception was impaired. He complained of difficulty in concentration, and could not subtract serial 7's from 100, saying that he was "all loused up." During the next hour his face remained deeply purple, he was unable to express

[3] The drug was kindly supplied by the Research Department of the Upjohn Co., Kalamazoo, Mich.

himself in words, stating that his mind felt crowded, and he showed motor restlessness, stating that he wanted to "walk it off" and that "my body feels nervous." Time and space perception were grossly impaired, and he expressed depersonalization feelings with such statements as "I am here and not here."

Nausea was an initial accompaniment of the syndrome as the injection began, and proceeded to retching in the 16 mg. dose. Nystagmus and mydriasis occurred in all cases, and increased in magnitude and duration as the dose increased. Pulse and blood pressure changes were minimal throughout. Another noteworthy finding was that of relaxed placidity and languor which all subjects reported for as much as 6 hours after injection. They lay contentedly in bed, feeling pleasantly relaxed, stating that they felt a lack of drive rather than a sense of fatigue.[4] These observations were repeated on a later date (31) using 6 other convicts as subjects. The results were of similar type, except that lesser symptoms occurred if the injection was slowed to a 10-minute period rather than a 3-minute one.

It would appear then, that intravenous bufotenine is hallucinogenic for man, that its action is rapid and the duration of effects is fleeting except in higher dosages. As the dose increases distortion of time and space perception occurs, as does depersonalization and bodily restlessness. Mydriasis and nystagmus make one think that at least a portion of this drug's action is in the brainstem tegmentum. The picture which remains most vividly in the memory of the observers is the purple faces of these subjects. If the color of an eggplant were diluted, it would approximate the hue which they assumed. An artist could describe the color more accurately, but he would have to use the word "purple" in his description.

Students of model psychoses are confronted constantly with the general "schizophrenic" response of subjects despite wide individual variations in behavioral activity. Much of this case-to-case variation may be due to personality differences or may be culturally determined. In many Orientals, for instance, the use of cannabis provokes erotic ideation and behavior for the most part, whereas in our culture it is used primarily by devotees of music who do not become sexually stimulated by the drug in most cases.

Within the dimensions of such variations there seems to be much in common between amanita mushroom-eating experiences and the response to intravenous bufotenine. When the purpling of the faces, as

---

[4] E. L. Kropa and R. D. Morin of the Battelle Memorial Inst. kindly assisted in making these observations.

well as the hallucinations, the motor restlessness, the time and space distortion, the depersonalization, and the terminal languor of our experimental subjects are placed in juxtaposition with the accounts of the rage of the Berserks, the mushroom debauches of the Siberians, and Drew's recent case, the general similarity is striking.

It would appear, then, that recent observations on the human tend to support the Ødman-Schübeler hypothesis that the Norse giants ate the *Amanita muscaria* mushroom to produce the ecstatic reckless rage for which they are renowned, and which was a culturally accepted temporary psychotic aberration in their group. *Berserksgang* on a hill in Iceland in 955 A.D. might well have had the same neurochemical basis as an injection of bufotenine under experimental conditions in Columbus, Ohio, a thousand years later and three thousand miles away.

SUMMARY

The ingestion of hallucinogenic mushrooms by Siberian tribes of the Kamchatka peninsula and by Indians of the Mexican highlands has been carried out in ritual and orgy for centuries. Ødman and Schübeler have advanced the hypothesis that the furious rage of the Berserks in the heyday of Viking culture a thousand years ago was brought about by the same agency, specifically the *Amanita muscaria* mushroom. A few years ago it was found that these fungi contain bufotenine, or n-n-dimethyl serotonin, a substance which is under scrutiny at this time for its possible neurochemical role in the causation of schizophrenia. Recent observations on the intravenous injection of bufotenine in man disclose that it is an hallucinogen, and that its psychophysiological effects bear a resemblance to the *Berserksgang* of the Norsemen in the time of the Sagas. These observations appear to offer support to the Ødman-Schübeler contention that the famed fury of the Berserks was what we would call a model psychosis today.

REFERENCES

1. Vicary, J. F. *Saga Time*, London: Kegan, Paul and Trench, 1887.
2. Larsen, Henning. Provost, University of Illinois, Urbana, Ill., personal communication.
3. Schlesinger, H., and Ford, W. W. *J. Biol. Chem.*, 3: 279, 1907.
   Ford, W. W. *J. Pharmacol. & Exp. Ther.*, 2: 285, 1911.
   Ford, W. W., and Clark, E. D. *Mycologia*, 6: 167, 1914.

4. Magnus, Albertus. De Vegetabilibus, quoted by Ramsbottom, J. *Mushrooms and Toadstools*, London: Collins, 1953.

5. Linnaeus, Carl P. 430 in *Skansa Resa*, Stockholm, 1751.

6. von Strahlenberg, P. J. *An Histori-geographical Description of the North and Eastern Part of Europe and Asia* (English tr.), London, 1736.

7. Vanderlip, S. P. 212 in *In search of a Siberian Klondike*, 1903.

8. Leach, M. (Ed.). P. 26 in *Standard Dictionary of Folklore, Mythology and Legend*, New York: Funk & Wagnalls, N. Y., 1949.

9. Jochelsen, W. *Mem. N. Y. Amer. Mus. Nat. Hist.*, 10: 1, 1906.

10. Bourke, John. *Scatologic Rites of All Nations*, Lowdermilk, Washington, D. C., 1891. See Ch. XI for a large collection of these accounts.
   Kennan, G. *Tent Life in Siberia*, London, 1870.

11. Goldsmith, Oliver. *Citizen of the World*, Letter No. 32, 1762.

12. Wieland, T., and Motzel, W. *Liebig's Ann. Chem.*, 581: 10, 1953.

13. Handovsky, H. *Arch. Exp. Path. Pharmakol.*, 86: 158, 1920.

14. Drew, A. Personal communication.

15. Bourke, John. Cf. Ref. 10.
   Guerra, F., and Olivera, H. *Las Plantas Fantasticas de Mexico*. Diario Espanol, Mexico, D.F., 1954.

16. Schultes, R. E. *Anthrop.*, 42: 429, 1940.

17. Wasson, R. Gordon. Personal communication. (A monograph on ethnomycology by the Wassons is now in preparation.)

18. Stafford, W. E. *J. Wash. Acad. Sci.*, 6: 547, 1916.

19. Stromberg, V. L. *J. Am. Chem. Soc.*, 76: 1707, 1954.

20. Fish, M. S., Johnson, N. M., and Horning, E. C. Piptadenia alkaloids. Indole bases of P. peregrina (L.) Benth, and related compounds. *J. Am. Chem. Soc.* (in press).

21. Evarts, E. *Medicinal Chem. Symp.*, Am. Chem. Soc., Syracuse, N. Y., p. 145, 1954.

——— Landau, W., Freygang, W., Jr., and Marshall, W. *Am. J. Physiol.*, 182: 594, 1955.

——— *A.M.A. Arch. Neurol. Psychiat.*, 75: 49, 1956.

22. Fabing, H. D. The abnormal production of indoles as a possible cause of schizophrenia, *A.P.A. Research Report* (in press).

23. Schübeler, F. C. *Viridarium Norvegicum* (Norges Vaextrige et Bidrag til Nord-Europas Natur- og Culturhistorie) Fabritius, Christiania, Bind I, p. 224–226.

24. The translation of this passage and others from the Norwegian and Swedish were kindly done by Jakob Meloe, Chas. P. Taft Fellow, Dept. of Philosophy, University of Cincinnati.

25. Ødman, Samuel Lorenzo. Forsok at utur naturens historie forklara de nodiska gamla Kampars berserka-gang (an attempt to explain the old Nordic giants' berserka-gang from natural history), *Kongl. Vetenskaps Academiens nya Handlingar*, Tom. V, 1784, pg. 240 et seq.

26. Schübeler, F. Cf. Ref. 23.

27. Grön, F. Berserksgangens Vesen og Arsaks forhold, (the nature and causes of Berserksgang), *Kgl. Norsk. Videnskabers Selskabs Skrifter*, IV, 1929.

28. Fabing, H. D., and Hawkins, J. R. Intravenous bufotenine injection in the human. *Science*, 123: 886, 1956.

29. Fabing, H. D. *Neurology*, 5: 603, 1955.

———— *Drug and Cosm. Ind.*, 78: 32, 1956, also *J. Clin. Exper. Psychopath.*, 17—, 1956.

———— Cf. Ref. 22.

30. Dr. John Porterfield, Director, Div. of Mental Hygiene and Correction, State of Ohio; Mr. R. H. Alvis, Warden of the Penitentiary, and Dr. R. H. Brooks, Prison Physician, kindly permitted these observations to be made.

31. Fabing, H. D., Kropa, E. L., Hawkins, J. R., and Leake, C. D. *Fed. Proc.* 15: 421, 1956, part 1.

32

INFLUENCE OF AMYGDALECTOMY ON SOCIAL BEHAVIOR IN MONKEYS

H. ENGER ROSVOLD, ALLAN F. MIRSKY, AND KARL H. PRIBRAM

Department of Psychiatry and Laboratory of Physiology, Yale University, and Department of Neurophysiology, Institute of Living

Several authors (2, 4, 5) have reported that temporal lobe lesions result in changes in social behavior of monkeys. Since these investigators were only incidentally interested in social behavior, they reported only summary descriptions of their methods or results. It is generally impossible to determine from their reports on what basis they arrived at their conclusions and what, in fact, they meant by social behavior. Therefore, a series of studies using a uniform method of observation has been undertaken to relate brain function to social behavior in monkeys.

Brody and Rosvold (1) reported in detail a method for studying the effects of frontal lobotomy on the social interaction in a colony of *Macaca mulatta*. A similar method was used in the present study of the effects of a temporal lobe lesion on social interaction among monkeys. In addition, the behavior of each monkey, when housed separately, was observed.

METHOD

Animals

Eight young male rhesus monkeys, ranging in weight from 2.90 to 3.85 kg, were housed for a total of 18 two-week periods alternately, either separately in individual cages or together in a large group cage, according to the temporal sequence designated in Table 1. The individual cages were 2 ft. by 2½ ft. by 2½ ft. The group cage was 7½ ft. by 4½ ft. by 6½ ft. and included a movable partition at the center, thus permitting the large cage to be divided into two smaller cages 3¾ ft. by 4½ ft. by 6½ ft. When the monkeys were housed individually, they were fed Rockland monkey pellets and peanuts, one at a time, through the wire mesh of the cage front. When the monkeys were in the group cage, either pellets or peanuts were introduced, one at a time, through a feeding device consisting of a length of 1½-in. pipe mounted obliquely on a stand so as to extend 1 ft. into the large cage. It was fitted at the animals' side with a can containing a small opening large enough to admit

From *The Journal of Comparative and Physiological Psychology*, June 1954.

only one monkey's paw. At the end of the observation hour, additional pellets were thrown into the group or individual cage, as the situation required, in amounts sufficient to make up the total daily ration of 80 cal/kg body weight per animal. This diet was supplemented three times a week with one-half orange per animal.

Observational: Group Cage

When the animals were together in a group cage, one E observed them at the same time each day for 1 hr. during the peanut-feeding situation. Four hours later another E observed while introducing the pellets. Food was also frequently offered directly to one or another of the animals, or placed between two monkeys of the group. Diary records were kept of group behavior, and when the typical group interaction had been reliably described, the most dominant — i.e., the highest animal in the hierarchy — was subjected to a two-stage bilateral amygdalectomy. Two other animals were operated on at two-month intervals. During the two weeks allowed for surgery and recovery, all animals were housed individually.

During the latter half of six of the two-week group-cage periods, alterations in group size and living space were instituted to increase interaction and to isolate those parts of the group in which the hierarchy was not clear for more intensive study. In addition, food was withheld from the colony at various times for 48 or 72 hr.

Observational: Individual Cages

At the same time on each day of the individual-cage periods, one E observed each monkey while offering it three peanuts. Four hours later, another E observed each animal while offering it five pellets. During period 1, diary records were kept of each animal's behavior. At the end of this period, and before placing the animals together for the first time in the group cage, the two Es independently ranked the eight animals in order of aggressiveness and/or fearlessness.[1] On each day of succeeding individual-cage periods the monkey's behavior was rated according to the categories listed in Table 2. The total score was used as a measure of the aggressiveness of each animal.

Surgical and Anatomical Procedures

A two-stage myoplastic craniotomy was performed on three of the animals; they were anesthetized with 0.8 cc/kg of a 5 per cent solution of Nembutal injected intraperitoneally. In each case, the left side was operated first and the right side a week later. A semilunar incision was made over the zygoma, curving forward over the orbit. Temporal muscle was split and the zygoma excised. After a burr hole had been enlarged to expose the orbit and temporal fossa, the dura was opened in a cruciate manner. The temporal lobe was

---

[1] Hereafter ratings of individual-cage behavior will be labeled "aggressiveness." They probably could equally well be labeled "fearlessness." The definition is according to the categories listed in Table 1. In the group-cage situation, however, "aggressiveness" has the objective behavioral referrant of one animal attacking or threatening another.

TABLE 1. TEMPORAL SEQUENCE OF OBSERVATION PERIODS

Description	Number (2-wk. periods)	Cage Situation
Preoperative period	1	I
	2 *	G
	3	I
	4	G
	5	I
	6	G
1st operation	7	I
1st postoperative period	8 *	G
	9	I
	10 †	G
2nd operation	11	I
2nd postoperative period	12	G
	13	I
	14 *, §	G
3rd operation	15	I
3rd postoperative period	16	G
	17	I
	18 *, †	G

Note: *I* refers to individual cage; *G* refers to group cages.
* Large cage divided in two, top four animals in one, bottom four in the other.
† Cage space reduced by one half.
§ Most submissive animal in the group removed from the colony.

TABLE 2. INDIVIDUAL-CAGE BEHAVIOR SCORING SCHEME

Categories	Rating and Description
Vocalization	Noisy-loud = + 2
	Soft noises = + 1
	Silent = 0
Position at start of feeding	At front of cage = + 3
	Goes from front to middle (back) = + 2
	At middle of cage = + 1
	At back of cage = 0
Pellet taking	One + for each taken, up to 5. If none taken = 0
Behavior after tak- pellets	Stays at front for all pellets = + 2
	Retreats after each to middle of cage = + 1
	Retreats after some but not all = + 1
	Retreats after each to back = 0
Threatening be- havior	Jumps at *E* during feeding = + 2
	Teeth baring or grimacing = + 1
	Neither = 0
Flight behavior	Animal makes as if to escape = − 1 for each time it occurs

Note: Aggressive toward *E* = high positive score (max. + 14); fearful of *E* = low positive or negative score.

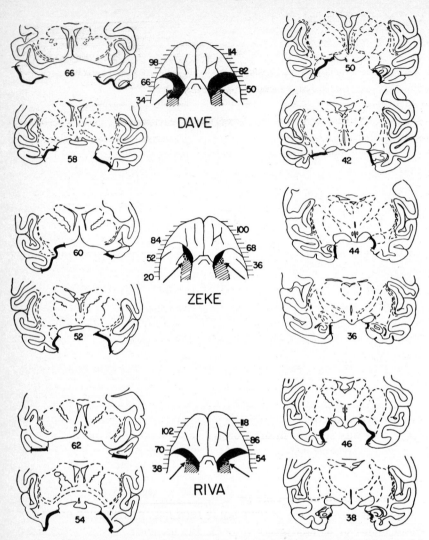

Fig. 1. Representative cross sections and reconstructions of brains of operated animals. Black indicates lesion, arrows indicate spared amygdala, oblique lines indicate spared Ammon's formation.

retracted, thus exposing the periamygdaloid region just medial and posterior to the Sylvian fissure. An 18-gauge sucker was inserted into the amygdala, and the entire formation removed subpially downward and backward as far as the temporal horn of the ventricle and medially as far as the brain stem. Bleeding was controlled by packing and cautery, and the wound was thoroughly irrigated before closing the dura. Fascia was closed in layers with interrupted silk technique and the scalp with continuous subcuticular stitch.

When the behavioral observations had been completed, the operated animals were sacrificed and their brains prepared for histological examination as described by Pribram and Bagshaw (4).

RESULTS

Anatomical

The reconstruction of the lesions is illustrated in Figure 1. The lesions in the three animals were approximately bilaterally symmetrical. In Dave's brain, in the right hemisphere, the medial portion of the temporal polar cortex, together with all of the amygdaloid complex except for a small portion of the lateral nucleus, was resected. Posteriorly, this lesion invaded the uncal extremity of Ammon's formation. In the left hemisphere, the lesion in the temporal polar cortex was slightly more extensive laterally, a little more of the basolateral amygdala was spared, and Ammon's formation barely touched on its ventromedial surface.

In Zeke the temporal polar cortex was barely invaded on either side. The corticomedial group of amygdaloid nuclei was completely resected bilaterally, but a small portion of the basolateral group remained intact. The posterior end of the lesion barely touched Ammon's formation.

In Riva the lesion invaded the temporal polar cortex bilaterally, and again the corticomedial nuclei of the amygdala were completely resected. However, the basolateral group of nuclei was fairly extensively spared on both sides. The uncal extremity of Ammon's formation was slightly injured on its ventromedial surface.

Group-Cage Behavior

By the second group-cage period a dominance hierarchy was firmly established on the basis of primacy in food getting and such other dominant behavior as aggressive chasing, biting, and threatening gestures. This hierarchy is portrayed in Figure 2.

Within five days after Dave had been operated on, he became submissive to all but Larry. Zeke now monopolized the feeding pipe, dominated the feeding situation, and occupied the preferred floor area of the cage once held by Dave. Toward the end of this period, when the group was divided into top and bottom four, Dave became completely submissive, even to Larry; he avoided other animals, made no attempt to get food, and even refused to accept food from E. Attempts to reach Dave's threshold for aggressive response by increasing group interaction were unsuccessful. Even though he would be bitten until

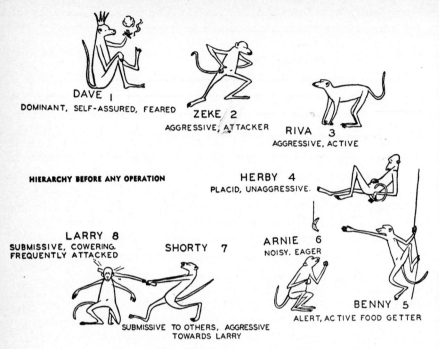

DAVE 1
DOMINANT, SELF-ASSURED, FEARED

ZEKE 2
AGGRESSIVE, ATTACKER

RIVA 3
AGGRESSIVE, ACTIVE

HIERARCHY BEFORE ANY OPERATION

HERBY 4
PLACID, UNAGGRESSIVE.

LARRY 8
SUBMISSIVE, COWERING.
FREQUENTLY ATTACKED

SHORTY 7

ARNIE 6
NOISY, EAGER

BENNY 5
ALERT, ACTIVE FOOD GETTER

SUBMISSIVE TO OTHERS, AGGRESSIVE
TOWARDS LARRY

Fig. 2. Hierarchy before any operation.

blood flowed, he exhibited no aggressive or retaliatory reaction toward the animal that had attacked him.

On the twelfth day after his second operation (the fifth day of group interaction), Zeke became submissive to all but Larry and Dave. Riva now dominated the feeding situation and the food pipe, sharing with no one. Zeke continued to be dominant over Larry and Dave until shortly after the colony was separated into the top and bottom four, when Larry began attacking Zeke. Coincident with this reversal in the Larry-Zeke relationship, Zeke exhibited a tremendous increase in his aggression toward Dave, attacking him almost continuously during the feeding situation. By way of increasing interaction with Zeke, in an attempt to reach his threshold for aggressive response against the other animals in the group, Dave was removed from the colony. This had the effect, *not* of eliciting aggression on Zeke's part, but of eliminating it completely. He now behaved much as did Dave, cringing and fleeing from all, and adopted the tactic of sitting in the corner of the cage and facing the wall.

In contrast to the other two operated animals, Riva did not fall in dominance at any time during the two-month postoperative period. Manipulations of cage space and food deprivation up to 72 hr. were

effective only in increasing Riva's aggressiveness. The hierarchy at the
end of the experiment is depicted in Figure 3.

Individual-Cage Behavior

The two *E*s agreed significantly better than chance (rho = .95, *p*
< .01) on the ranking of the monkeys according to their aggressive
behavior in individual cages during the first individual-cage period.
This order correlated negatively (rho = − .595; *p* = .16) with the

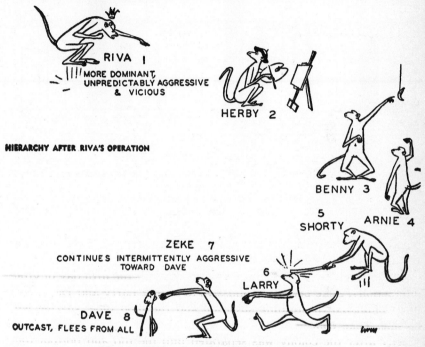

RIVA 1
MORE DOMINANT,
UNPREDICTABLY AGGRESSIVE
& VICIOUS

HERBY 2

HIERARCHY AFTER RIVA'S OPERATION

BENNY 3

5
SHORTY   ARNIE 4

ZEKE 7
CONTINUES INTERMITTENTLY AGGRESSIVE
TOWARD DAVE
6
LARRY

DAVE 8
OUTCAST, FLEES FROM ALL

Fig. 3. Hierarchy after Riva's operation.

hierarchical arrangement that developed in the group cage. In subsequent individual-cage periods, the rating scheme described in Table 1
was used. Figure 4 shows the mean of the last three preoperative and
postoperative scores of each animal. The mean scores of a typical nonoperated control, obtained at the same time, are included for comparison. Two months separate the pre- and post-operative measures in
each case. A Mann-Whitney (3) *U* test of the significance of the differences in these comparisons indicates that there were no differences in
aggressiveness among the monkeys before surgery. Afterward, the
scores of the operates show an increase significant beyond the .01 level
of confidence, while that of the unoperated animals shows no change.

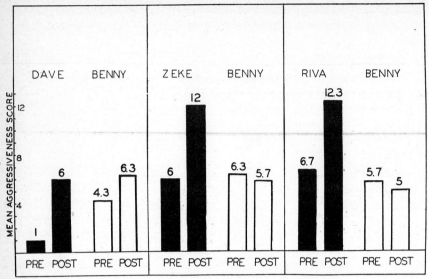

AGGRESSIVENESS IN INDIVIDUAL CAGE SITUATION
PRE AND POST AMYGDALECTOMY
BENNY'S SCORES AT SAME TIME INCLUDED FOR COMPARISON

Fig. 4. Aggressiveness before and after amygdalectomy.

DISCUSSION

The results of the present study indicate that following amygdalectomy there are marked changes in social behavior of monkeys. However, there are differences among the animals in the direction and degree of this change.

After surgery all operates, though appearing more aggressive in the individual-cage situation, appeared to be less dominant (in two of three cases) in the group-cage situation. In addition to this difference in direction of effect, there is uniformity of change in the individual-cage situation but not in the group-cage situation.

As evident in Figure 2, the differences in direction and degree of change cannot confidently be attributed to differences among the lesions. If variations in extent of damage to the temporal lobe determined the degree of change in behavior, then Dave should have changed most and Zeke least; this was not so either in the group- or individual-cage situation. It is probable, therefore, that one or more of the discrete structures in the temporal lobe are critical in bringing about the alterations in aggressiveness. Since the degree of change in the group-cage situation, i.e., most in Dave and least in Riva, was consistent only with the extent of damage to the basolateral nuclei, these nuclei may be critical for changes in aggressiveness in the group-cage situation.

The differences in direction and degree of change were consistent with the social environment confronting each operated animal after surgery. Upon return to the colony, Dave was confronted with aggressive and active Zeke and Riva; he fell in dominance. Zeke was confronted with Riva; he too fell in dominance. Riva was faced with relatively submissive nonaggressive animals such as Herby; Riva remained dominant.

The differences in direction and degree of change are also consistent with the length of time preoperatively that the dominance-submission relationships had existed. Dave, who changed immediately after his operation, had elicited submissiveness for only six weeks; Zeke, who maintained the No. 1 position for four days after being returned to the colony postoperatively, had elicited submissive responses for 10 weeks; while Riva, who did not change in status, had elicited submissive responses for 16 weeks.

This study, then, suggests that the pattern of social interaction within the group to which it is returned after surgery and the length of preoperative time the relationships had existed may be as important considerations as the locus and extent of a lesion in determining the effects of a brain operation on the social behavior of a monkey. It is meaningless, therefore, to speak of the effect of an operation on "emotional behavior," "social behavior," and the like, without specifying in detail the conditions in which the particular behavior is observed. And, unless the effect of an operation on behavior is studied in a variety of situations, the findings are at best of limited generalizability.

SUMMARY

1. Eight young male rhesus monkeys were studied in individual and group cages for a period of nine months; during this time, the three animals that were most dominant in the group situation were subjected to bilateral amygdalectomy.

2. There was found to be a negative relationship between aggressiveness in the individual-cage and dominance in the group-cage situation before surgery.

3. After amygdalectomy all animals appeared more aggressive in the individual-cage situation. In the group-cage situation, the same animals, in two of three instances, fell from top to bottom positions in the hierarchy. The third animal suffered no loss in dominance and appeared more aggressive in the group situation after operation.

4. The differences in changes in behavior appear to be related to the social environment confronting each animal upon return to the group after surgery and to the length of time the preoperative relationships had existed.

5. The differences in changes in behavior are not related to the differences in extent of lesions as a whole, though they are consistent with differences in damage to the basolateral nuclei of the amygdala.

REFERENCES

1. Brody, E. B., & Rosvold, H. E. Influence of prefrontal lobotomy on social interaction in a monkey group. *Psychosom. Med.*, 1952, 5: 407–415.

2. Klüver, H., & Bucy, P. C. Preliminary analysis of functions of the temporal lobes in monkeys. *Arch. Neurol. Psychiat.*, Chicago, 1939, 42: 979–1000.

3. Moses, L. E. Non-parametric statistics for psychological research. *Psychol. Bull.*, 1952, 49: 122–143.

4. Pribram, K. H., & Bagshaw, M. Further analysis of the temporal lobe syndrome utilizing frontotemporal ablations. *J. comp. Neurol.*, 1953, 99: 347–375.

5. Thompson, A. P., & Walker, A. E. Behavioral alterations following lesions of the medial surface of the temporal lobe. *Folia psychiat. neurol. neurochir. Neerl.*, 1950, 53: 444–452.

33

AN EXPERIMENTAL INVESTIGATION OF THE BLOCK DESIGN ROTATION EFFECT

An Analysis of a Psychological Effect of Brain Damage

M. B. SHAPIRO, M.A.

Department of Psychology, Institute of Psychiatry, Maudsley Hospital, London

The Block Design Rotation Effect is an effect produced by some subjects when they are doing the Block Design test, otherwise known as the Kohs Block. In this test the subject has to copy coloured patterns with diversely coloured one inch cubes. Some subjects, while reproducing the designs correctly, leave their blocks in an obviously rotated position. An example is seen in Fig. 1, which shows at the top a card with a pattern on it, and below the rotated blocks. The experimenter has asked whether the reproduction is correct and the subject has answered 'yes' to this question. The amount of rotation shown in the illustration is equal to 45 degrees. This amount of rotation, though very rarely exceeded, itself occurs frequently.

Data have been published showing that this effect occurs much more frequently among brain-damaged psychiatric patients than among non-brain-damaged psychiatric patients (Shapiro, 1952). By 'brain-damaged' are meant patients who, at the time of the study, were considered by their doctors to be probably suffering from an anatomical lesion of the brain. Non-brain-damaged patients are those who, at the time of the study, were considered by their doctors as probably not suffering from such a lesion.

Data so far collected indicate that the rotation effect may be associated with lesions occurring in any part of the brain, including the basal ganglia.

The purpose of this paper is to present an explanation of the association of the rotation effect with brain damage, to explain the explanation, and to describe in some detail one experiment carried out to test that explanation.

The essence of this explanation is that one of the general dysfunctions sometimes produced by brain damage is the inhibition of a large number of incoming sensory cues which are usually at the disposal

From the *British Journal of Medical Psychology*, 27: 84, 1954, published by Cambridge University Press.

of normal persons. So much so that it is presumed that the perceptions of a brain damaged person can be similar in quality to those of
a normal person in a dark room in which only the perceived object
is illuminated.

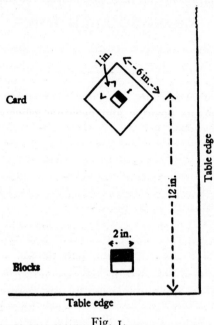

Fig. 1.

This explanation was based first of all on a consideration of the
nature of attention. The nervous system is subjected to a continuous
barrage of simultaneous stimulation of various kinds and intensity.
A small and ever changing portion of this stimulation finally develops
the quality of consciousness. The rest is prevented from doing so.
Thus attention has both positive and negative aspects.

This double character of attention is similar to certain observations
of Pavlov (1927). He showed in his dogs that if one reflex was soon
followed by another the strength of the second one could be considerably diminished. Pavlov called this phenomenon negative induction.
His definition of it was that an excitatory process in one part of the
brain could be followed by an increase or development of inhibitory
effects in other parts.

When we come to consider the psychological effects of brain damage
we find that the negative or inhibitory aspects of attention are often
intensified in brain-damaged subjects. As an example, imagine a case
in which the part of the brain that is especially concerned with the

experience of touch on the right leg has been damaged. If the right leg is stimulated, the subject will perceive it and localize it, though perhaps imperfectly. If, however, the face is stimulated at the same time as the leg, then the sensation from the leg will disappear. As soon as the stimulation of the face is removed the sensation from the leg will reappear. This phenomenon can be produced while the subject is actually looking at the affected limb. A similar phenomenon has been demonstrated in visual perception. We have here an exaggeration of the phenomenon of negative induction to be found in normals. Bender (1951) has given this phenomenon, which he has described in detail, the name of extinction. To name it thus obscures the double nature of attention, its positive and negative aspects. It is therefore less accurate, and of less use as an explanatory concept from which precise deductions can be made. It would seem to be more accurate to say that brain damage can result in the intensification of inhibitory processes. Therefore the negative or inhibitory aspects of attention will be exaggerated. An inhibitory process is defined as one which removes or diminishes a psychological effect.

From these considerations one can deduce the proposition that when a brain-damaged subject is looking at an object, all the surrounding cues available to the normal subject will be less available to him. Now, there are indications that in this second situation the quality of a person's perceptions is influenced by the character of the available stimulation. For example, Asch & Witkin (1948a, b) have shown that if, in a dark room, a tilted illuminated rod is placed within the frame of an equally tilted illuminated square, the rod will tend to be seen as upright. Many examples of this fact can be found outside the laboratory. Thus the pilot flying at night through cloud could be flying at a steepily tilted position and still think he is flying upright, because the only positional cues of a visual nature available are those provided by the cockpit.

With this conception in mind let us go back to the block design test situation. Let us imagine a normal person in a dark room in which only the card is illuminated. (See Fig. 1.) First of all the card as a whole would tend to be seen as a square: at this stage, which of the upper sides of the square would be taken as the top it is impossible to say. Secondly, the *design* on the card would tend to be seen as a square: again there is at this stage no way of predicting which side is seen as the top. This is finally determined by the line of symmetry. The line of symmetry is the line which divides the design into two mirrored halves as in K and L in Fig. 2. This we have found provides a powerful and unambiguous positional cue. In our example this would mean that the right-hand side marked *t* in Fig. 1 would then be regarded as the top of our perceived square. Thus our subject would probably end up by perceiving a square in which side t was the top and it would be 45 degrees to the right of the actual top.

This phenomenon is similar to that of the pilot in the tilted aeroplane who thinks that he is flying upright.

Now, what happens when the subject has to manipulate the blocks to reproduce the design on the card above? In our test procedure he

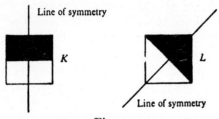

Fig. 2.

is forced to work near the table edge with the card 12 inches above the blocks. To continue our analogy of the normal person in the dark room, we would have to switch off the light round the blocks and turn it on round the table edge where the subject is made to work. The visual positional cues here will consist of the table edge, a limited area of the subject's body, and the wood graining. The perceived top will be exactly the same as the actual top: the perceived top in this situation is therefore 45 degrees to the left of the perceived top in the previous situation. The subject now begins to reproduce the design with the Kohs blocks. He makes, within this new positional framework, what he saw in the first one, a square. In fact the copy will have rotated about 45 degrees. (See Fig. 1.)

An important clue leading to this explanation was the actual laws determining the appearance and non-appearance of the block design rotation effect. Three laws have so far been established and the findings published (Shapiro, 1951, 1952).

The first of these laws is that when the line of symmetry of a design is at an angle to the vertical axis of the visual field, subjects will tend to rotate their blocks more. For examples, look at c and d in Fig. 3. When the line of symmetry is parallel to the vertical axis of the visual field the tendency to rotate will be decreased. (See a and b in Fig. 3.) All subjects who rotate do so according to this law.

The second law is also concerned with the design. When the design is in a diamond orientation, as in c and d of Fig. 3, the tendency to rotate will be increased. When the design is in a square orientation, as in *a* and *b* of Fig. 3, the tendency to rotate will decrease. Nearly all subjects who rotate do so according to this law.

The third law concerns the orientation of the whole card. This is exactly the same as that of the design. When the card is in a diamond orientation the tendency to rotate will be increased (*b* and *d* in Fig. 3). When it is in a square orientation, the tendency to rotate will decrease (*a* and *c* in Fig. 3). This law does not operate as consistently as the first two. When the directions of their influence are in conflict, the effect of the angle of the line of symmetry is greatest, design orientation next, and that of card orientation least. These laws are now based on results from over 100 subjects.

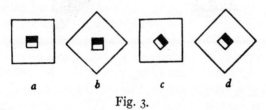

a   b   c   d

Fig. 3.

A brief recapitulation is necessary at this point. We have two main findings to consider about the block design rotation effect. The first is that it tends to be produced more by brain damaged persons; the second is that it is produced according to three laws of organization of the visual field — the angle of the line of symmetry, figure orientation and ground orientation.

The explanation put forward links these findings together in the following way. Brain damage is supposed to produce an exaggeration of the negative induction effects which normally characterize attention. The subject is therefore deprived of positional cues which are not at the centre of attention, but which are normally available. The three laws are in fact characteristics of the organization of the remaining space which have positional value for us. For example, if there is only a square available to perception, it is one of the sides and not one of the corners which will be seen as the top: that is why the three laws determine the amount of rotation.

Now we come to the experimental testing of the explanation of the block design rotation effect. The most obvious deduction was that normal people would rotate on the block design test if we could in some way deprive them of their visual directional cues which they were doing the test. I shall now go on to describe an experiment which was made to test this deduction (Shapiro, 1953).

The material in this experiment consisted of a specially designed version of the block design test. This consisted of forty cards. Ten different designs were used, each design appearing four times in the manner shown by Fig. 3, *a*, *b*, *c* and *d*.

For the removal of directional cues two arrangements were made. First of all a mask was constructed which deprived the subject of all stimulation except that provided by a hole of about ¼ in. in diameter. The subject, when wearing the mask, could see only the card and some part of the surface of the table; or some part of the table edge, his own hands and part of his body.

The second arrangement was the provision of a piece of black felt which was placed on the table to complete the elimination of positional cues coming from the graining around the cards and the blocks.

A camera was used to photograph the product of each trial so that the amount of rotation could be objectively measured.

The special Block Design test was given to two groups of subjects. The first group was given the test with the special mask on and the black felt on the table. This group was called the 'pseudo-brain-dam-aged' group. The second group, the control group, was equated with the experimental group for age and sex. This group was given the Block Design Rotation test under normal conditions, i.e. without the special mask and without the black felt on the table.

There were twenty subjects in each group and they were between the ages of eighteen and thirty. None of them had a weighted Wechsler Vocabulary score below 6.

The results were consistent with expectation. The 'pseudo-brain-damaged' rotated slightly more than the original real brain-damaged group of patients. The difference was, however, not statistically significant. The control group rotated less than the 'pseudo-brain-dam-aged' group, the difference being significant at the 0·025 level. The second main requirement of the deduction tested by this experiment was also fulfilled in that the effects of the three factors, the angle of line of symmetry, design orientation, and card orientation, were all operating significantly in both the control and the pseudo-brain-damaged group in the required direction. (For detailed data, see Shapiro, 1953.)

Now for discussion and conclusions. It should be pointed out that the exaggerated negative induction effect does not apply only to perception, but to the total behaviour of the patient. For example, Eugen Bleuler (1911) made some observations of patients suffering from G. P. I. He says of such a patient: 'he will want to appropriate some object in his ward; he will steal it with a sly expression on his face and hide it carefully under his clothes, all this before the very eyes of the attendants and the other patients who, at the moment, have ceased to exist for him. The old man wants to satisfy his sexual drives. He sees in a little girl only the woman. He does not stop to consider the moral reasons which forbid sexual intercourse with children; he abuses the first child he happens to meet.' Then Bleuler actually ends up by saying of the paretic that 'he peeps at the world through a small hole.' This passage was found after the experiment was started.

It is now necessary to consider possible alternative explanations of the findings. The Goldstein-Scheerer (1941) theory that brain damage results in the disorder of figure-ground relations does not seem to explain the finding. The experimental situation implies, not a disorder between figure and ground, but that a large part of the available percepts have been totally removed. The remaining figure-ground relations continue to behave in a perfectly orderly fashion.

The theory of Werner & Thuma (1942) that brain damage results in dissociation, in a separation of mental activities, appears to be inconsistent with the facts. Bender's work on simultaneous stimulation above shows just the opposite, the excitation of one part of the brain has an over-intense inhibitory effect on other parts.

Finally, a theory of disturbed set or attention seems not to account for the experimental conditions which could, if anything, be argued to have the effect of concentrating the attention of the subject on the task in hand. The results can only be explained in terms of the removal of positional cues which are normally available.

The main outcome of this paper is that the theories have been both sufficiently general and sufficiently precise to enable us to deduce the conditions under which normal persons were made to behave, in a limited respect, like brain-damaged subjects.

While there are many psychological effects of brain damage which cannot be explained by such theories, one can say that the possibility has been confirmed of laying the basis of an experimentally founded theory of the psychological effects of brain damage. Such a theory should permit a rational and systematic approach to the problems of treatment, training, and adjustment of brain-damaged subjects.

References

Asch, S. E. & Witkin, H. A. (1948a). Studies in space orientation. I. Perception of the upright with displaced visual fields. *J. Exp. Psychol.*, 38: 325.

Asch, S. E. & Witkin, H. A. (1948 b). Studies in space orientation. III. Perception of the upright in the absence of a visual field. *J. Exp. Psychol.*, 38: 603–14.

Bender, M. B. (1951). *Disorders of Perception.* Amer. Lecture Series. No. 120. Ch. Thomas, Springfield.

Bleuler, E. (1911). *Dementia Praecox and the Group of Schizophrenias,* New York: Int. University Press (1950).

Goldstein, K. & Scheerer, M. (1941). Abstract and Concrete Behavior. An Experimental Study with Special Tests. *Psychol. Monogr.*, 53: no. 2.

Pavlov, I. P. (1927). *Conditioned Reflexes*, London: Oxford University Press, 1946.

Shapiro, M. B. (1951). Experimental studies of a perceptual anomaly. I. Initial experiments. *J. Ment. Sci.*, 97: 90–110.

Shapiro, M. B. (1952). Experimental studies of a perceptual anomaly. II. Confirmatory and explanatory experiments. *J. Ment. Sci.*, 98: 605–17.

Shapiro, M. B. (1953). Experimental studies of a perceptual anomaly. III. The testing of an explanatory theory. *J. Ment. Sci.*, 99: 394–409.

Werner, H. & Thuma, A. (1942). A deficiency in the perception of apparent motion in children with brain injury. *Amer. J. Psychol.*, 55: 58–67.

34

CORTICAL CONDUCTIVITY IN THE BRAIN-INJURED

GEORGE S. KLEIN, *The Menninger Foundation*
AND
DAVID KRECH, *University of California*

THEORETICAL CONTEXT AND PROBLEM

Every model of cortical integration must deal with the problem of transmission of excitation through the neural and surrounding media. With respect to one of these problems — the resistance to or ease of transmission — one of two general assumptions can be made. We can assume that rate of transmission of *excitation patterns* is a constant for all individuals of any one species and is homogeneous over the entire cortical area. In this case, transmission of excitation, being a constant, cannot be appealed to for an understanding of inter- or intra-individual differences in cortical integration. Alternatively, we can assume that transmission-rate of excitation patterns varies from individual to individual, from time to time within the same individual, and from area to area within a single cortical field at any time. With this assumption it is possible to appeal to *differential cortical conductivity* as a parameter which will help us understand inter- and intra-individual differences in cortical integration and therefore in behavior.

Krech (7, 8) in his recent speculations toward a brain model has made the second of these assumptions and has suggested that differences in cortical conductivity may be critical in accounting for differences in cortical integration. In Krech's proposals cortical conductivity is seen as an important parameter which defines the cortical functioning of the individual and is used in connection with the problems centering around the functional communication among different cortical areas. For example, Dynamic Systems (in Krech's terminology) in order to interact or to reorganize must be in communication among themselves. Whether such communication can occur and the ease with which it can occur would depend, in part, upon the specific cortical conductivity of the individual. Certain forms of "behavioral rigidity,"

From *Journal of Personality*, September 1952. © 1952 by Duke University Press.

chaotic behavior, etc., are accounted for by Krech by appeal to this assumed attribute of cortical functioning.[1]

It is possible to generalize the effects of this postulated characteristic of cortical functioning and to propose that one might account for individual differences on a large variety of so-called perceptual, learning, and problem-solving tasks with the assumption that lowered cortical conductivity tends to isolate functional cortical areas. Since we are interested in exploring this very possibility, it becomes desirable (and necessary, if we are to exploit this toward the formulation of a brain model) to know something about the various attributes of the process of transmission of *activity patterns* in the cortex — its possible physiological mechanisms as well as its formal properties. In considering this latter problem it appeared to us that the theory and experimental techniques of Köhler (5) if applied to the study of brain-injured patients might contribute to its solution. This paper represents our initial study in this direction.

The electrical-field theory proposed by Köhler and Wallach (6) suggests a possible mechanism of cortical conductivity, as well as a method which might permit us to measure cortical conductivity. However, at certain points, we find it necessary to deviate somewhat from the Köhler-Wallach analysis and to postulate mechanisms which, while having much in common with their suggestions, cannot fairly be laid at their door. In the Köhler-Wallach view the current flow (differences in electrical potential) initiated by stimulation of a defined cortical area creates a condition of electrotonus. Electrotonus involves immediate polarization of tissue surfaces and a more gradual change of polarizability due to these counter forces initiated by the current flow; thus, electrotonus affects the pattern of current flow and subsequent transmission across the affected region. Continued local excitation is assumed to increase the duration of electrotonic aftereffects and therefore to alter further the pattern of current flow in the polarized medium. In the electrotonic condition the local area is said to be "satiated." Now, if the satiated area is restimulated (before the electrotonic condition has been dissipated), the new current introduced into this area is "distorted" or "deflected" and the behavioral consequences of this

---

[1] "Finally, I will assume that the physiological states of the tissue and fluids which make up the substrata of the specific Dynamic System can vary with respect to the ease with which they will permit a change in the redistribution of electrical-chemical activities (e.g., an analogy might be the physiological state which determines the speed of neural impulses, or the permeability of nervous tissue, or the electrical conductance of the fluids, etc.). Such a postulated physiological variable could, most reasonably, be a general factor. A change in the general physiological condition of the entire brain (or, indeed, of the entire organism) could therefore show up as a change in the rigidity of all systems. Presumably the behavior units coordinated with Dynamic Systems would reflect this 'rigidity' characteristic of the Dynamic Systems" (8).

distortion or rerouting is seen in the so-called "figural aftereffect." Translated in terms of our present hypothesis, "satiation" is a state of lowered cortical conductivity in a *localized cortical area* (here we are equating electrotonus and resistance), and we may thus regard the figural aftereffect as a behavioral measure of this temporary and localized lowered conductivity.

However (and here is where we depart somewhat from the Köhler-Wallach analysis), for them satiation is a phenomenon involving *boundary*-current. In their view, the stronger the *figure* current, the stronger the counter forces (electrotonus) engendered, and the stronger the figural aftereffect. Thus Köhler and Wallach restrict satiation to the set of events issuing from the isomorphic impression which a stimulus (described as a *figure*) has on the brain. We would hold to a less restrictive conception. We would maintain, merely, that *any neural activity induces heightened resistance within the area stimulated* and that the degree of resulting distortion of a new stimulation pattern would not necessarily depend upon strong figure-ground differentials. Thus we would rephrase the argument as follows: The current flow initiated by stimulation of a defined cortical area results in a heightened resistance, *within that area*, to further electrical activity. Should further stimulation occur, the resulting pattern of electrical activity would, as a consequence of this increased resistance, be "dampened," distorted, or rerouted. In this event we can then speak of *reactive* or a temporary condition of decreased cortical conductivity; i.e., in one specific area and for a finite time cortical conductivity is reduced. For this temporary and localized condition we would assume that the degree of decrease in cortical conductivity is a function of the amount of original stimulation, such that the more stimulation, the greater the drop in cortical conductivity (within certain limits). However, we would postulate another factor which contributes to the extent of drop in cortical conductivity: we would assume that the *over-all state of the cortex* helps to determine the initial or *basal* value of cortical conductivity and the degree of drop *possible*. For example, individuals may be thought of as having high or low cortical conductivity *prior to any stimulation*, i.e., the basal or characteristic level of cortical conductivity. A person with high basal conductivity may be thought of as one whose neural substratum will offer relatively little resistance to the transmission of neural patterns from one area to another and who will suffer a relatively small drop in conductivity as a consequence of a given amount of local stimulation; a person with low basal conductivity may be thought of, conversely, as one whose neural substratum will offer relatively greater resistance to the transmission of neural patterns from one area to another, and who will suffer a relatively large drop in conductivity as a consequence of the same given amount of local stimulation.

This postulated relationship between *reactive* and *basal* cortical conductivity permits us, of course, to get some indication of an individual's "basal" level of cortical conductivity by measuring his "reactive" cortical conductivity, i.e., by measuring his reaction to localized stimulation or his *satiationability*. More specifically, we can postulate that people with high basal cortical conductivity will differ from people with low basal conductivity in the following satiationability characteristics: (1) *rate* of satiation, (2) *degree* of satiationability, (3) *rate of dissipation* of satiation. That is, people with high basal cortical conductivity will approach satiation more slowly, will not suffer as large a drop of cortical conductivity for the same amount of stimulation, and will recover from whatever satiation does occur more quickly.

The above attributes of satiationability depend, then, upon the immediate and local nature of stimulation (e.g., upon the length and, perhaps, strength of stimulation) and upon the basal or characteristic level of cortical conductivity of the specific cortex in question. Various observations — experimental and clinical — suggested to us that one very important condition which may in part determine the basal level of cortical conductivity of an individual is gross injury to the cortex. Of particular interest in hitting upon this suggestion were data collected by Klein (4) in studies of afterimage duration among the brain-injured. Klein found that where persistence of afterimage was measured as a function of the duration of stimulus-exposure, it appeared that for longer exposures the duration of the afterimages in brain-injured fell off significantly as compared with non-brain-injured. This could be interpreted to mean that among brain-injured neural activity in regions which had previously been exposed to prolonged excitation is "dampened" as compared to "normals," i.e., consequent upon the same amount of original excitation there is a greater degree of satiation in the brain-injured than in the non-brain-injured. That satiation in the brain-injured is not only greater in extent than in "normals," but that it also persists for a longer time is suggested by another finding of Klein's: the *rate of decrease* in after-image duration upon repeated exposures was more rapid in the brain-injured than in the controls. In general, then, Klein's studies are congruent with the hypothesis that in the brain-injured successive, prolonged exposure to stimulation induces *satiation* attributes which we have postulated to be characteristics of individuals with a lowered basal cortical conductivity.

Similar reasoning makes it possible to subsume under the coordinating concept of "cortical conductivity" certain clinical observations of changes in integrative behavior among brain-injured patients. Here we are not concerned with "satiation" consequences of brain-injury but, rather, with the general behavioral consequences of a lowered *basal* cortical conductivity. The behavior patterns described by Goldstein (1) as characteristic for the brain-injured and which for him are evidences of a "concrete attitude" might be viewed as concomitants of gross impairment of cortical conductivity. For if we assume that one outcome of a gross cortical assault is a correspondingly large-scale general alteration in cortical tissue whereby redistribution of electrochemical activity becomes more difficult or grossly deflected (lowered cortical conductivity), then a "functional isolation" among localized areas may result. The effect of lowered conductivity would then have wholesale consequences on integrative functioning resulting in a "narrowing of experience," "unavailability of experience,' "rigidity" in behavior, "perseverativeness" — conditions in which only immediacies of experience are effectively grappled with.

As has already been indicated, the present experiment was designed to investigate the validity and usefulness of the concept of cortical conductivity and its possible role in the development of a brain model. Because of the various considerations listed above, it appeared to us that cases of brain-injury offered a promising approach to such an investigation. It should, of course, be possible to investigate our major problem in the noninjured. Obviously our interest in the brain-injured, per se, is secondary to spelling out the properties of our postulated cortical conductivity as a parameter of a brain model, i.e., as an organismic process to which we could refer certain differences in behavior. However, it was felt that brain-injury may bring into relief any such relationships (if they exist) and make our initial approach easier. But our choice of the brain-injured as our subjects does *not* mean that we believe the cortical conductivity process to be explainable in terms of local conditions of the cortex alone. Excitability and satiation-ability, we assume, are influenced by events throughout the organism. For instance, our results, as we shall see later, suggest that changes in conductivity are in some respects more extensive in the presence of a tumor than where there is an externally produced focal lesion. The likelihood that a tumor is a *local* consequence of more extensive metabolic changes in the organism, as compared to a sharply delineated injury, may very well be the important consideration here.

Let us summarize briefly our various arguments and assumptions in order to see more clearly the rationale of the present experiment:

(1) Variation in cortical conductivity is proposed as a central variable which contributes to individual differences in cortical integration and, therefore, to individual differences in "cognitive" behavior.

(2) Differences in cortical conductivity can express themselves in differ-

ences in rate of satiation, degree of satiation, and persistence of satiation, such that the lower the conductivity the faster the rate, the greater the degree, and the slower the dissipation of satiation.

(3) The figural aftereffect affords a possible behavioral measure of cortical conductivity, such that the lower the conductivity, the greater the figural aftereffect.

(4) It is finally proposed that one consequence of severe injury to cortical tissue is reduced cortical conductivity. (The mechanism for this is not specified.)

We are now in a position to state the specific experimental question to be dealt with in this paper. From the above assumptions and derivations certain specified differences in figural aftereffect behavior should appear between brain-injured and control subjects. These predictions are:

(1) The brain-injured should show figural aftereffects after less prolonged stimulation than would be required for controls.

(2) The brain-injured should show a more pronounced figural aftereffect than the controls — where stimulation is constant.

(3) The figural aftereffects should persist longer in the brain-injured than in the controls.

The specific purpose of the present experiment was to test these predictions.

APPARATUS AND PROCEDURE

The figural aftereffect has been observed in two modalities by Köhler and his coworkers: the visual and kinesthetic. For the present experiment the kinesthetic, rather than the visual, figural aftereffect test was chosen for two major reasons. In the first place the kinesthetic figural aftereffect lends itself more easily to reliable quantification than do the available visual tests. Since our predictions are phrased in "more than," "quicker than," etc., terms, it was essential that we be able to describe the observed figural aftereffects quantitatively. In the second place, the visual figural aftereffect testing situation seemed too complicated and too demanding a task for patients with extensive brain injuries, whereas we were able to devise a simple and not too demanding kinesthetic figural aftereffect test. This test — both the apparatus and the procedure — was adapted from that described by Köhler and Dinnerstein (5). However, in choosing the kinesthetic figural aftereffect we were fully aware of the fact that the justification for the kinesthetic figural aftereffect as a measure of "satiation" was not as clear cut as that for the visual figural aftereffect. The discussion of the validity of the kinesthetic figural aftereffect as a measure of satiation will be postponed until after we have described the testing situation, in the hope that our discussion will be clearer at that point.

Apparatus

The testing apparatus consisted of a "Standard Test Object," a "Stimulus Object," a "Comparison Scale," and stands and tables upon which these various objects were mounted. The Standard Test Object was a block of unpainted, smoothed hardwood, six inches in length, one and one-half inches wide, and one inch deep. The Stimulus Object was made of the same wood but with corresponding dimensions of six inches by two and one-half inches by one inch. The Comparison Scale was a wooden block (similar to the other objects) which tapered in width from a half inch at the narrow end to four inches at the wide end. The scale was thirty inches long and one inch deep. Scale readings were calibrated to one thirty-second of an inch. The scale was permanently fixed on a mount while the Standard Test Object and Stimulus Object could easily be inserted into the second mount. To aid accuracy in measurement all three objects were equipped with a sliding "rider" which fixed the position of thumb and forefinger as the subject held the sides of the objects. The apparatus was so arranged as to present the Comparison Scale to the left of the seated subject, the Test and Stimulus Object (as the case might be) to the right of the subject. The stimulus situation and apparatus are shown in Figure 1.

Procedure

The subject was blindfolded before he had any opportunity to view any of the apparatus or equipment. After he was seated in front of the apparatus, he was carefully told what his task was to be and he was given a demonstration of what was required of him. For this demonstration the Standard Test Object was used. The thumb and forefinger of the subject's right hand were inserted into the sliding rider of the Test Object and the thumb and forefinger of his left hand into the rider on the Comparison Scale. The subject was then shown that he could move the rider of the Comparison Scale back and forth and that as he moved the rider the width of the Comparison Scale changed. He was told that his task was to move the rider until he felt that the distance between his thumb and forefinger of his left hand felt equal to the distance separating the thumb and forefinger of his right hand. When that point was reached, he was to announce "Here." [2]

[2] The question arose early whether the figural aftereffect varied with stimulation of the preferred and nonpreferred hand. This was independently tested on a group of 18 subjects (Harvard students) and no differences were found. Consequently, for all subjects in the present experiment the right hand was used for the "rubbing" period and scale judgments were made with the left.

Instructions regarding the requirement of judgment of width had to be carefully drawn and elaborated specifically for each individual subject. Finally, checks were made after the testing was all done to make certain that the subject had understood the task. This was especially important with some of the injured who occasionally misunderstood the instructions to mean that they were required to move their arms until the finger tips of both arms extended an equal distance from the body.[3]

A. **Comparison Scale**
B. **Fixed Stand for Standard Test Object and Stimulus Object**
C. **Standard Test Object (1 ½" wide)**
D. **Stimulus Object (2 ½" wide)**

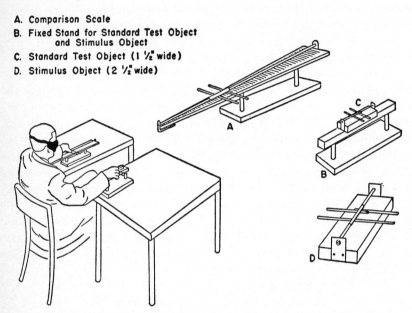

Fig. 1. Diagram of kinesthetic figural aftereffect test.

After we had satisfied ourselves that the subject understood what was required of him, four control judgments were taken on the Standard Test Object. After each judgment the subject removed his fingers from the equipment, and the rider of the Comparison Scale was brought back to its initial position. These control judgments (and all succeeding ones) were all taken with the rider of the Comparison Scale at the narrow end; i.e., all judgments were in the "up" direction. To guard against the possibility that with repeated trials the subject would tend to rely upon position cues of the extended arms rather than in terms of the felt width between the thumb and forefinger, the position

---

[3] This specific misunderstanding of the instructions (early in the experiment) equivocated the entire test series of one of the brain-injured subjects, and his results were thrown out.

of the Comparison Scale mount was irregularly shifted approximately four inches from its initial position on the table.

Immediately after these four judgments were taken, the Standard Object was removed from the mount and replaced with the Stimulus Object. The thumb and forefinger of the subject's right hand were then placed in the rider of the Stimulus Object (his left hand resting in his lap) and he was instructed to rub the sides of the Stimulus Object at an even rate (determined by the subject himself) for 30 seconds. Immediately after this "rubbing period" or "stimulation period," the subject withdrew his fingers from the rider, the Stimulus Object was replaced by the Standard Test Object in the mount, and then four more judgments with the Standard Test Object were taken — under the same conditions as had held for the control judgments. This was followed by another stimulation period of 60 seconds of rubbing the Stimulus Object, following which judgments were again taken on the Standard Test Object. Stimulus periods of 90 seconds and 120 seconds then followed. After the last judgment of the 120-second stimulation period, the apparatus was hidden from sight, the blindfold was removed from the subject, and a five-minute rest period intervened. During the rest period the subject was allowed to smoke, converse, etc. Then he was again blindfolded and four more judgments of the Standard Test Object were taken. The same procedure was followed after a ten-minute rest period; four more judgments were taken with the Standard Test Object. This concluded the experiment. The testing sequence may be summarized as follows:

1. 4 Control Judgments.
2. 30 Seconds Stimulation; 4 Test Judgments.
3. 60 Seconds Stimulation; 4 Test Judgments.
4. 90 Seconds Stimulation; 4 Test Judgments.
5. 120 Seconds Stimulation; 4 Test Judgments.
6. 5 Minutes Rest Period; 4 Test Judgments.
7. 10 Minutes Rest Period; 4 Test Judgments.

Subjects

A total of 28 hospitalized male patients, divided into two groups, were tested in the foregoing manner. Twelve of these subjects comprised the Experimental or Brain-Injured group, and sixteen the Control or normal group.

The 12 experimental subjects were cases in which, at the time of referral to us, there was a presumption of cortical lesion as gleaned from actual operative reports or clinical signs at admission to the hospital. These cases were selected by staff members of the Neurological Service. As it turned out, the group proved to be extremely heterogeneous as regards extent of injury and verification of lesions through subsequent examinations. In seven cases, surgical procedures had been tried, ranging from burr-hole incisions for exploratory probing to full-scale operations for removal of tumor tissue. However, not less than five months intervened before the experimental testing occurred in any of these cases. In one case, to which we will have occasion to refer later, there had been at first a strong suspicion of an astrocytoma, but the subsequent history of the case proved this diagnosis erroneous; no definitive evidence of a cortical lesion was ever found. The essential diagnostic status of the twelve experimental subjects is given in Table I.

The sixteen controls were selected from the Surgical Service. These cases had been hospitalized for formal disturbances (mostly for hemorrhoids and hernias) and, so far as could be ascertained, none of these control cases had a history of neurological complication. Development of a control group for studying brain-injured is at best a hazardous affair because of the improbability of an exclusive correlation between any behavioral index and brain injury. One cannot rule out the possibility of correlation of behavior, varying over an extremely wide range, with the more or less intangible variables called "personality factors." Even where some clear-cut presumptions are made about the latter, it is difficult to introduce appropriate controls except with sizable populations and special selection of brain-injured cases. Matching — admittedly the procedure of choice — is exceedingly difficult where brain-injured patients are concerned, because it is obviously impossible in a short-term study to gather a sufficient number of brain-injured cases with the requisite qualities. The most to be hoped for, then, is equivalence between groups as a whole — using some of the presumed salient and most easily controlled variables as a basis for comparison. In the present instance it was practical to take into account only the most obvious of the probably important variables: Sex, age, schooling, and occupation. The sixteen control subjects — in both range and averages — were similar to the experimental subjects in these respects, as can be seen from Table II. The average age of the controls was 33.13 years and of the brain-injured 33.75 years.

RESULTS

The available data lend themselves to two different kinds of analyses. We can compare the brain-injured as a group with the non-brain-injured with respect to various figural aftereffect indices, and we can analyze the behavior of individual subjects within the brain-injured group alone to determine correspondences between nature of the lesion and figural aftereffect behavior.

TABLE I. Diagnostic Summary of Brain-Injured Group and Clinical Ratings of Degree of Functional Disturbance

Code Designation of Subjects	Clinical Rating *	Diagnostic Summary	Code Designation of Subjects	Clinical Rating *	Diagnostic Summary
E-10	1	*Admission diag.*: Posterior fossa tumor; no confirmation in later examinations; complete clinical remission.	E-9	5	*Admission diag.*: Right-sided hemiparesis. *Final diag.*: Cerebral thrombosis of branches of right middle cerebral artery. Steady clinical improvement.
E-8	2	*Admission diag.*: Subarachnoid hemorrhage, probably traumatic. *Final diag.*: post-traumatic encephalopathy, grand mal seizures, cerebellar symptoms, ventricular enlargement. Steady clinical improvement, with residual cerebellar symptoms.	E-1	6	*Admission diag.*: Closed head injury following auto accident. Left hemiplegia and aphasia symptoms. *Final diag.*: Post-traumatic encephalopathy with hemiplegia.
E-7	3	*Admission diag.*: Left frontal tumor; slight clinical signs. Confirmed on operation, Feb., 1951.	E-12	7	*Admission diag.*: Frontal-parietal, parasagittal meningioma. Left side tumor removed April, 1950; right side tumor removed Oct., 1950. Clear-cut excisions.
E-3	4	*Admission diag.*: Psychomotor epilepsy. Operation August, 1949: extirpation inferior temporal gyrus, small portions middle temporal and fusiform gyri.	E-2	8	*Admission diag.*: Glioma, right parietal-temporal. Exploratory operation June, 1950 indecisive. Clinical signs progressively more decisive. *Final diag.*: June, 1950, same. Inoperable tumor.
E-4	9	*Admission diag.*: Hemiplegia and speech loss, sudden onset. *Final diag.*: Operation, Nov., 1949. Thrombosis and embolism, left middle cerebral artery with concomitant softening.	E-11	11	*Admission diag.*: Accident resulting in right hemiplegia and aphasia. Operation spongy blood clot 3 cm. below cortex, left hemisphere, frontal-temporal. *Final diag.*: Thrombosis left middle cerebral artery. Continued aphasia, alexia.
E-5	10	*Admission diag.*: Sept., 1950. Head trauma in auto accident with skull fracture, cerebral lacerations in right occipito-parietal region. Moderate sensory aphasia. Poor clinical improvement.	E-6	12	*Admission diag.*: Trauma of unknown origin. Decerebrate rigidity and bilateral damage. Unconscious 17 days. *Final diag.*: Generalized cortical atrophy, bilateral pyramidal tract weakness.

* Rank order of 1 refers to least functionally impaired; a rating of 12 refers to most impaired.

GROUP COMPARISONS

Indices of Satiation

The control measures for each subject prior to the "rubbing periods" served as his base line for computing the figural aftereffect induced by the various stimulation periods. *Decrease* in judged width of the Test Object was considered evidence of "satiation." This interpretation is in accord with the formulation by Köhler and Dinnerstein (5) in their study of the kinesthetic figural aftereffect and is also congruent

TABLE II. DESCRIPTIVE SUMMARY OF CONTROL AND EXPERIMENTAL GROUPS

	Controls (N 16)				Brain-Injured (N 12)		
S	Age	Schooling	Occupation	S	Age	Schooling	Occupation
C-1	23	8th grade	laborer	E-1	22	7th grade	laborer
C-2	24	8th grade	laborer	E-2	23	9th grade	laborer
C-3	25	11th grade	shipping clerk	E-3	25	9th grade	truck driver
C-4	25	2 yrs. coll.	student	E-4	26	4 yrs. coll.	journalist
C-5	27	6th grade	laborer	E-5	28	grad. H.S.	clerk, laborer
C-6	28	1 yr. coll.	prof. baseball	E-6	30	2 yrs. coll.	student
C-7	29	grad. H.S.	asst. mgr. dept. store	E-7	32	8th grade	tailor
C-8	30	10th grade	laborer	E-8	40	8th grade	plasterer
C-9	29	grad. H.S.	clerical worker	E-9	41	3 yrs. coll.	teacher
C-10	34	9th grade	weaver	E-10	42	10th grade	machinist
C-11	37	7th grade	chauffeur	E-11	42	6 mos. coll.	carpenter
C-12	38	8th grade	machinist	E-12	54	8th grade	janitor
C-13	41	9th grade	truck driver				
C-14	42	8th grade	carpenter				
C-15	44	9th grade	laborer				
C-16	54	8th grade	laborer				

Average age, controls: 33.12 yrs.
Age range, controls: 23–54 yrs.

Average age, brain-injured: 33.75 yrs.
Age range, brain-injured: 22–54 yrs.

with the original interpretation developed by Köhler and Wallach (6) for visual figural aftereffects. In the latter case the argument is made that satiation due to the figure currents aroused by a stimulus object results in a *recession* from the areas previously occupied by that object. Thus, when an enclosed stimulus figure is large and is followed by a smaller test object which occupies the same region, the perceived width of the smaller object decreases.[4] However, as has already been

[4] For a detailed description of the assumed processes involved, the reader is referred to their original article (6) (see especially pp. 335–341).

indicated, their proposed mechanism is not directly pertinent to predictions of the same effect in kinesthesis, although Köhler and Dinnerstein are of the opinion that much the same sort of theory holds in both cases. The following formulation of a possible mechanism for the kinesthetic figural aftereffect may warrant consideration: we can assume that in the perception of the width of the Test Object, the *intensity* of sheer "amount" of the pattern of current flow consequent upon stimulation is a determinant factor. That is, the *more intense* the patterned neural activity resulting from stimulation when a subject grasps the Test Object, the *greater the perceived width* of the object. Now if, as we have assumed earlier, local stimulation tends to "dampen" neural activity in a particular area, it is reasonable to expect that perceived width of the Test Object will diminish when such dampening has taken place. This postulated sequence of events requires only that the neural activity resulting from grasping the Test Object takes place within the same cortical locus where the neural activity resulting from the "rubbing period" occurred. In either case, whether the Köhler and Wallach analysis be extended to the kinesthetic situation, or whether the mechanism here proposed be the acceptable one, a decrease in judged width of the Test Object may be considered as evidence of localized satiation.

As we have indicated, it is important that the prestimulation measures be used as base lines for this expected decrease in the perceived width of the Test Object. To measure merely the difference between the *objective* width and the *experienced* width would be quite misleading. Many subjects underestimated the width of the Test Object even *prior* to the rubbing experience. Only three of the subjects overestimated the Test Object initially.[5] In any event, the presence of this constant error and the differences among subjects in respect to the degree of this constant error (initial underestimation) necessitated the use of *individual* base lines for evaluating the effects of the rubbing stimulation.

Four different indices of "intensity" of figural aftereffect were computed. Of these, three may be considered independent measures, while the fourth (Average Poststimulation Figural Aftereffect) includes within it one of the first three (Maximal Figural Aftereffect).

The first of these indices, *Average Poststimulation Figural Aftereffect*, was computed in the following manner: Since a set of four judgments was taken after each stimulation period, and since there were

---

[5] In the case of one brain-injured subject (No. E-1) the degree of initial underestimation was such as to make it difficult to assess the effects of the stimulation periods since he was already close to the limiting extreme of underestimation (and the apparatus) prior to stimulation.

four stimulation periods, there was a total of four sets of four judgments each for every subject. Each set of four judgments was averaged, and this average was converted from absolute values into a percentage score. Taking the *average* of the person's four control measures as 100, each set of his test judgments was expressed as a percentage of that base line. This would mean that any figural aftereffect would express itself as a value of something less than 100 (decrease in judged width). These four sets of percentages were then averaged to give us, for each subject separately, an *Average Poststimulation Figural Aftereffect*. The average of these individual averages could then be taken as the *group Average Poststimulation Figural Aftereffect*.

The second index, *Maximal Figural Aftereffect*, refers to the lowest percentage score received on any one set of four poststimulation judgments. This presumably indicates the limit to which a stimulation period of 30, 60, 90, or 120 seconds (or any segment of this *sequence*) could depress the subject's felt width of the Test Object.

The third index, *Recovery Period 1*, is based on the average (again expressed as percentage of the control base line) of the four judgments taken immediately after the five-minute rest period.

The fourth index, *Recovery Period 2*, is similar to *Recovery Period 1* but refers to the judgments taken after the ten minutes' rest period (or, after a total of fifteen minutes, i.e., after the first and second rest periods).

Intensity of Figural Aftereffects

It is clear in Table III that the differences are in the direction predicted, i.e., the brain-injured group shows a greater figural aftereffect than do the controls. The *average* size of the over-all figural aftereffect was 12.08 per cent for the brain-injured, 6.25 per cent for the controls; the *maximum* degree of effect for the brain-injured averaged 19.50 per cent, for the controls, 13.00. Because the direction of the differences was predicted a priori, and because the found differences conform to this direction, the significance of the resulting *t*'s are evaluated by the one-tail test. Both differences are significant at better than the 10 per cent level.

In summary, then, these first two measures are consistent with the hypothesis that the brain-injured, as a group, show a greater magnitude of figural aftereffect than do the controls. While the probability values for these comparisons are outside the conventionally accepted limits of significance,[6] the consistency of these measures, *and all other*

[6] For a further evaluation of the significance of these differences the reader is urged to read footnote 9.

TABLE III. COMPARISON OF DEGREE OF FIGURAL AFTEREFFECT IN BRAIN-INJURED
AND CONTROLS
(Expressed in percentage points decrement from control judgments)

	Average Poststimulus Aftereffect	Average Max. Figural Aftereffect	Average 1st Recovery Period	Average 2nd Recovery Period
Brain-Inj. ($n = 12$) ..	12.08	19.50	15.25	11.58
Controls ($n = 16$)	6.25	13.00	5.19	5.94
Difference	5.83	6.50	10.06	5.64
t	1.39	1.41	1.95	1.11
p	<.10	<.10	<.05	<.15

measures (which we will consider in the following pages) with our theoretical expectations warrants some degree of confidence in these conclusions.

Rate of Satiation

It was also our prediction that the brain-injured would show the figural aftereffect after less prolonged stimulation than would be required for the controls. Another way of putting this would be to say that the rate at which the brain-injured approached the maximum level of effect would be appreciably faster than would be the case for the controls. In Figure 2 we see the development of the figural aftereffect in each group. Figural aftereffect is shown in relation to the control values which are indicated in the figure as "zero aftereffect." There is a relatively rapid development of the aftereffect in the brain-injured, e.g., the effect quickly develops after 30 seconds of stimulation, and a leveling-off (level of maximal aftereffect) seems also to be reached fairly early. The controls show a slower approach to their maximal aftereffect. To test this apparent difference in rate, we computed the regression line of each subject's curve based on the first three points (zero, 30", 60" tests) and the corresponding slope constant. We then estimated the significance of the difference between the average slope constants of each group.[7] This difference was significant at the 1 per cent level. These data, then, are consistent with our second prediction: brain-injured approach maximal level of figural aftereffect after less prolonged stimulation than is required for controls.

Persistence of the Figural Aftereffect

It is evident from Figure 2 that there are marked differences between the two groups in degree of recovery after rest. Controls reached max-

[7] Derived from a procedure described by Johnson (3).

imal recovery after five minutes of rest; in the brain-injured, however, recovery became substantial only after 10 minutes additional rest (i.e., after a total of fifteen minutes following the last "rubbing period"). Indeed, Table III shows that at the five-minute rest point, the differences between the two groups is greater than at any other point of comparison. At that point the brain-injured showed a figural aftereffect of 15.25 and the controls, 5.19 — a difference which is significant at better than the 5 per cent confidence level.

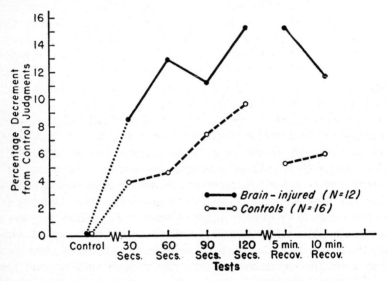

Fig. 2. Comparisons of rate of development of figural aftereffect in brain-injured and controls.

The differential extent of recovery in the two groups can be evaluated by several methods — all of which tell the same story. We can compare, for instance, the degree of figural aftereffect remaining at each rest point expressed as a proportion of the maximum effect which had occurred over the four sets of stimulation trials. If recovery has occurred, the difference between the maximal effect previously achieved and the value of the effect at the rest point should be considerable. This is in fact the case for the control group. From a maximum effect of 13.00 the control group falls to 5.19 after five minutes of rest, a difference of 7.81 percentage units. The brain-injured, however, show much less recovery. From a maximum of 19.50 they drop to 15.25, a difference of 4.25. The difference between the groups in this decrement is significant at less than the 10 per cent level. By the ten-minute rest period, the brain-injured group had begun to catch up with the control. Now the corresponding drops for the control and brain-injured groups are 7.06 and 7.92 respectively (t = .32).

Still another way of analyzing the different recovery rates is to determine the recoveries of individual subjects of the two groups. Again there are at least two ways of doing this. First we can ask the question: How many subjects of each group showed *complete* recovery after five, and after ten minutes? Or we can ask: What was the average value of the figural aftereffect of subjects who did *not* show complete recovery after five and after ten minutes? The answer to the first question appears to be as follows: For the Control Group seven of the sixteen subjects showed zero figural aftereffect after five minutes (i.e., 43.8 per cent of the subjects had recovered *completely* by that time); for the Brain-Injured Group, only one of the twelve subjects (i.e., 8.3 per cent) had recovered completely. But it must be noted that this one "brain-injured" subject who showed complete recovery was E-10, *the subject who had been misdiagnosed* and who, according to all available evidence, never did have a brain lesion. (See footnote 9.) If we were to omit him from our analysis, the results would then indicate *43.8 per cent complete recovery for the controls and zero per cent recovery for the brain-injured.* By the end of an additional ten minutes this value of 8.3 per cent (or 0 per cent) had risen slightly to 25 per cent or 18 per cent (i.e., three subjects now showed complete recovery, but again this includes E-10, and without him, the 25 per cent shrinks to 18 per cent, i.e., 2 out of 11 subjects). Thus, after fifteen minutes fewer brain-injured subjects had shown complete recovery than was true of the Control Group after *five* minutes.[8] The answer to the second question (the degree of figural aftereffect for those subjects who did *not* show complete recovery) is as follows: For the Control Group the average after five minutes of rest was 14.2 per cent; for the brain-injured, 17.5 per cent. After ten more minutes of rest, the average for the Controls had dropped to 10.5 per cent, for the brain-injured, the average remained at 17.9 per cent. Thus again, for those subjects who did *not* show complete recovery, the average value of the figural aftereffect for the brain-injured was greater after fifteen minutes of rest than it was after five minutes for the controls.

Our prediction, then, that rate of dissipation of the figural aftereffect would be slower in the brain-injured seems to be adequately supported.

[8] That fewer Control subjects showed 100 per cent recovery after the second rest period than after the first rest period merely reflects, in our opinion, variability in measurement. With such a rigid criterion of "complete recovery" (i.e., 100 per cent), a score of 98 per cent recovery, for instance, removes the subject from the "complete recovery" category. Actually that is exactly what happened in two of the Control subjects.

Possible Vitiating Effects of Differential Fatigue and Learning

Conceivably many of the above differences between the two groups may have arisen either from differential fatigue induced by the experimental procedure or from differential practice effects, i.e., learning. It could be argued that with each successive rubbing period the brain-injured subjects fatigued more easily than did the controls. At the same time the controls, while fatiguing less, "learned" to be more accurate. These two divergent tendencies could then be appealed to to account for the disparate trends in figural aftereffects as the experiment progressed, since the larger the deviation (in the negative direction) from the objective value, the greater the figural aftereffect. But if this were so — if the brain-injured subjects' judgments were disintegrating due to fatigue and the normals growing more efficient through learning — then the absolute error of judgment should increase in the brain-injured at a greater rate than would be true for the controls, who, indeed, should show improvement in judgment, or at the very least remain constant. Figure 3, which shows the absolute error of

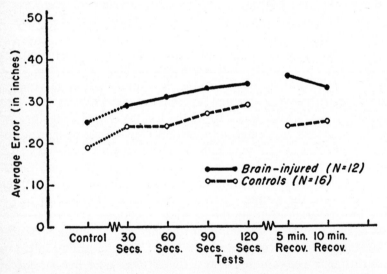

Fig. 3. Comparison of average errors in brain-injured and controls.

judgment (disregarding signs) at each series of test trials, dispels these possibilities. If fatigue were operating in the one group and learning in the other, the two groups should steadily diverge as exposure time lengthens. Clearly this is not the case: the two curves run perfectly parallel courses, with error in both groups steadily increasing with longer exposure periods. Neither differential fatigue nor learning seems adequate to account for the group differences.

INDIVIDUAL COMPARISONS

Relationship between figural aftereffect and degree of functional impairment: If cortical conductivity is an essential variable to which to refer observed variations in behavior, it is reasonable to expect that the degree of functional impairment should be correlated with variations in conductivity. *Independent* ratings of degree of impairment of the brain-injured group were made by Dr. Fred A. Quadfassel, Director of the Neurological Service of the hospital. Using all the clinical materials available in a case, including reports of operations, EEG's, and neurological examinations, he rank-ordered the group with respect to pervasiveness of malfunctioning. This ranking, it should be noted, did not necessarily parallel extent of known cortical damage if the behavior observed clinically did not indicate extensive functional loss. *The ranks were highly correlated with extent of damage,* even though cortical pathology took its place as only one aspect of the total clinical picture which contributed to the rank. For instance, one of the cases (E-7) was known to have an extensive parasagittal frontal tumor but showed relatively *less behavioral* disturbances upon neurological examination than did other members of the group; this case was therefore given a relatively high rank (less impaired). The ranks represent, then, an evaluation of the over-all, organismic loss of functioning which accompanied the injury.

The neurologist's rankings were correlated with the figural aftereffect indices and are summarized in Table IV. The correlations range from +.63 (second recovery period) to +.92 (maximal aftereffect). Three are significant at the 1 per cent level and the fourth at the 5 per cent level.[9] Evidently depth of satiation and slowness of recovery are especially reliable indices of clinically observable disturbances of

---

[9] A particularly dramatic instance of this correlation occurred in one patient of the brain-injured group (Subject E-10). Upon admission to the Neurological Service, this man had shown diagnostic signs of a malignant posterior fossa tumor, and his referral to us was based upon this diagnostic impression. In our test he showed very little figural aftereffect. Unknown to us, however, follow-up neurological procedures disclosed no signs whatever of a tumor nor were there any signs of behavioral disturbance. It was then presumed that the earlier symptoms were transitory and attributable to another source, probably a virus infection which had since disappeared completely. Nevertheless, we have kept this case in our "brain-injured" group. Had we excluded him from the group, the average values for the "brain-injured" group given in Table III would have shown the following changes: *Average Poststimulus Aftereffect,* 14.63 (instead of 12.08); *Average Max. Fig. Aftereffect,* 21.30 (instead of 19.50); *Average 1st Recovery Period,* 17.55 (instead of 15.25); *Average 2nd Recovery Period,* 13.37 (instead of 11.58). *In every instance this would have increased the differences between the brain-injured group and the*

TABLE IV. Rank Order Correlations between Neurologist's Rankings and Figural Aftereffect Indices

	Average Poststimulus Aftereffect	Maximal Aftereffect	1st Recovery Period	2nd Recovery Period
RHO	.78	.92	.79	.63
P	.01	.01	.01	.05

function. The particularly high correlation with maximum depth of the figural aftereffect and a relatively lower one with second recovery period illustrate the likelihood that different properties of the cortical conductivity process may be differentially impaired. Pervasive disturbance in all properties of the process is, however, reflected in correspondingly severe functional impairment.

Is conductivity related to *extent of cortical pathology?* Accurate information regarding actual extent of cortical involvement was not available for every case in our group but, as has been pointed out, there is some basis for assuming that the clinical ranks are also highly correlated with extent of injury; therefore, the ranks can be used for an approximate answer to our question. From these considerations there certainly appears to be a fairly close relationship between rank and extent of injury.

Importance of nature of pathological process: Our experimental group was heterogeneous as to type of injury. It is therefore appropriate to ask whether there are any indications that cortical conductivity is particularly impaired in certain *types* of cortical disturbance and less so in others. Because of the relatively few cases in our experimental group a definitive answer is not possible. However, within the rough breakdown of cases permitted by our small numbers suggestive trends do appear.

Excluding the one case in which no clear evidence of cortical pathology was discovered (E-10), the cases fall into three main categories of onset of disturbance: cases of hemorrhaging and thrombosis; severe cortical assaults from without (accident, blows, etc.); and proliferating cellular processes (tumors). Eight cases were in the first two categories, three in the third. Since we are assuming that the tumor process implies an etiological picture which includes a more extensive involvement of bodily processes than is the case with local injuries or assaults, it is of special interest to see whether these cases differ from the rest in cortical conductivity. A more refined breakdown of types and locus

---

controls and would also have increased the reliability of these differences. Thus, where the *t*'s as presented in Table III are 1.39, 1.41, 1.95, and 1.11, the corresponding corrected *t*'s would be 2.01, 1.81, 2.49, and 1.45.

of tumor would of course be desirable and essential, but the cases in the present study were insufficient. The three tumor cases were subjects E-2, E-7, and E-12, described in Table I. In the case of E-12 a parasagittal meningioma had been cleanly excised; he made a good postoperative recovery. He was the only one of the three who was tested after the final operation (five months). In E-2 a glioma was located predominantly in the right parietal-temporal region; E-7 had a tumor in the left frontal region. These three cases were compared with the other eight on the magnitude of the figural aftereffect at each stage of the experiment and the results are plotted in Figure 4.

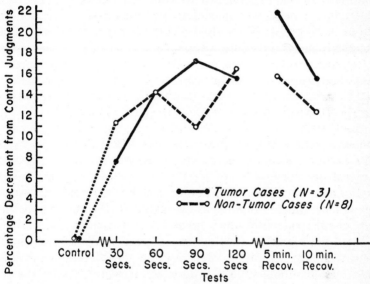

Fig. 4. Comparison of tumor cases and other cases of experimental group.

There is little to choose between the groups as to over-all *magnitude* of the effects. But the most striking difference appears in the *recovery* portion of the curve. In the tumor group not only has recovery not occurred at the five-minute point but there is indication of a continuing build-up of satiation so that the figural aftereffect at the five-minute point is *greater* than at any other point in the experiment. At the very least, then, we can conclude that recovery is exceedingly slowed in the tumor group.

Putting side by side the relations found between figural aftereffect and the variables of functional impairment, extent of damage, and the trend in tumor cases, what can we conclude regarding the effects of nature of injury? (1) It is unlikely that there is any simple relation between brain injury and cortical conductivity which is independent of, on the one hand, *pervasiveness* of cortical pathology and nature of pathology (tumors vs. "extreme" assaults, focal lesions), and on the other, of *particular properties* of the conductivity process (e.g., magnitude of figural aftereffects, rate of satiationability, recovery). (2) Our limited groups offer suggestive leads regarding these relationships: (a) the single most sensitive indicator of presence of a lesion seems to be variation in *recovery* rate. (b) The more *extensive* the lesion the more severely affected are degree of satiation, speed of satiation (development of figural aftereffect), and speed of recovery. (c) Our limited evidence suggests that tumors produce effects which are exceeded only by those seen in cases of extensive damage. Whether a distinction should be drawn between benign tumors (e.g., meningiomas) and more malignant ones in this respect awaits further study. The tumor cases we studied showed especially anomalous disturbance in the recovery phase, to an extent not even approximated by otherwise comparable extensively damaged, nontumor cases.

DISCUSSION

The data tend to support our hypothesis that one effect of massive cortical lesions is marked alterations in general cortical conductivity. This now poses the question of what *behavioral qualities* can be linked with such altered conductivity. The correlations with clinical estimates of over-all functional impairment suggests that the concept of differential cortical conductivity may be useful in accounting for individual differences in cognitive functioning in general. While we did not directly verify it, it seems a likely assumption that clinical estimates of functional loss implicitly relied upon a clinical appraisal of cognitive status. The next research step is to spell out in more specific detail the relations between cortical conductivity and varying form of cognitive behavior.

In what ways can cortical conductivity influence the course of cognitive functioning? For one thing we may suppose that conductivity through the neural medium helps determine *functional communication* among localized cortical regions (Dynamic Systems in Krech's terms), and therefore helps determine the possibility and rate of cognitive reorganization. In general we believe that it may prove useful to account for individual differences in performance in a large variety of perceptual, learning, memory, and problem-solving tasks in terms of the conductivity process. We have said that reduced conductivity implies reduced potential for communicability among cortical areas. Consequently, tasks which involve functional integration or communication among cortical loci (as, for example, problem-solving, retroactive or proactive interference, etc.) may show wide differences between brain-injured and controls. It is possible that behavioral correlates of heightened conductivity may well be such experiences as "alertness" or hypersensitivity to multiple stimuli. Behavioral correlates of low conductivity (especially in the brain-injured) may be a "narrowing of awareness" and "isolation of effective stimuli," conditions usually alluded to in the concept of "rigidity." Future reports will deal with some of these behavioral consequences.

The present results do not allow simple application to the diagnostic problem of detecting brain injury. Of the three properties of conductivity studied here only *rate of recovery* promises an especially efficient indicator of mere *presence* of a lesion. Variations in other properties — magnitude and speed of satiation — seem to parallel extent of the lesion, the results also suggesting that tumors result in extensive effects in conductivity which approach those of extensive nontumor lesions, especially with respect to speed of recovery. With more focal lesions, unilateral effects in these two properties are much less drastic; results overlap the normal range to a considerable degree. In general, the major differences between the controls and brain-injured group arose from cases with more inclusive pathology — diffuse bilateral lesions or tumors.

The analogous effects of *diffuse* nontumor (e.g., "externally caused") lesions and areal tumors is especially suggestive. On what basis can we account for the similarity of effects of tumors and extensive injuries? One possibility is that a tumor, even though it may be relatively segregated (to a specific cortical area), signals the presence of a more extensive organismic disturbance (e.g., metabolic?). The effect of the tumor is then not so much to be evaluated in terms of its locus but in terms of the organismic imbalance or physiological changes of which it is only a symptom. The key to understanding the effects of the tumor would be as much the more general disturbance as the locus of its particular symptom — the tumor — itself. It may be this more general imbalance which may result in equivalent effects arising from a tumor and those of diffuse cortical injury. Similarly, we may reason that the gravity of extensive brain-injuries of nontumor variety lies not merely in the loss of particular cortical loci and associated functions, but in the more general organismic imbalances of physiological processes which come about in their wake; injuries may have consequences beyond the brain itself. Perhaps it is in the more general *organismic* consequences rather than in local cortical effects alone that tumors and diffuse lesions are analogous. (Of course, locus and type of tumor need more systematic study to see how much qualification this interpretation requires.) It is possible that more focal lesions of external origin (e.g., unilateral gunshot wounds) may not have the extensive organismic consequences of bilateral diffuse lesions or imply the disintegrative changes that are symptomatically revealed in a tumor. The present study provides a further basis for evaluating the relation between cortical conductivity and brain injury. Since we assume cortical conductivity to reflect the status of the total neurophysiological economy, it would be significantly altered by brain injury *only to the extent that the latter induces or reflects a more general physiological change.* It is possible to conclude tentatively that the more extensive is the organismic involvement in a cortical disturbance (e.g., metabolic changes resulting from extensive damage or those of which presence of a tumor may be symptomatic), the greater will be the effects upon the conductivity process.

The latter principle seems to us a key one in gaining true perspective to the relation of cortical conductivity to brain injury. We have seen that the more focal lesions are probably less extensive in their effects on conductivity; overlap with normals is considerable. Now if we consider cortical conductivity as a parameter of organismic control, we would expect it to reflect the more general imbalance more than the purely *local* cortical changes. Thus, local lesions need not result in significant changes in properties of cortical conductivity (though the slowed rate of recovery is possibly the one property which is more sensitive to relatively slight disturbances in the physiological balance). This may account for the failure of Jaffe and Teuber (2) to find any significant deviations of figural aftereffects in cases of unilateral somatosensory impairment. Evidently, none of their experimental cases involved tumors or diffuse bilateral lesions of the type which contributed to the considerable deviations seen in our study.

The present study suggests, then, an interesting direction in research: that tumors and lesions should be regarded not as local events but as reflecting wider organismic changes. It would of course be a necessary first step to compare impairments accompanying tumor cases and those with focal externally caused lesions where both occupy similar *cortical* extents; then it would be desirable to compare the effects of more or less well localized tumor cases with more *diffuse nontumor* lesions. Such studies would promote clear understanding of the significance of tumors and other lesions for the total physiological economy as well as for local cortical functioning alone.

The specification of cortical conductivity as one parameter of a brain model suggests two general directions for further research. In the first place, a physiological or chemical basis of differences in cortical conductivity can be sought. Also, the suggested work with tumor cases may provide clues as to metabolic factors affecting conductivity. If tumors do involve a more general imbalance, and if conductivity is especially impaired by tumors, then much may be learned from them regarding the physiological mechanism of conductivity. Furthermore, future work should explore the possibility of *direct* physiological measurements of conductivity to replace the indirect psychological measures used in the present study. Secondly, as was suggested earlier, the concept points also to further *behavioral correlates* in cognitive functioning.

The individual differences in conductivity observed within the brain-injured group impel us to comment briefly on the general problem of diagnosis of brain-injury. Previous approaches have sought to detect brain-injury on the basis of particular behavioral signs which then were considered to be *specific* to cortical lesions. This avenue of psychological approach has been relatively unproductive: only the grosser lesions have been found to have such "specific" signs. Evidently, almost every behavior deviation found in the brain-injured can be found in some portion of the non-brain-injured population. The range of behavior of which non-brain-injured are capable *includes* behaviors found in brain-injured. Especially in the case of more subtle, localized lesions does the search for a "pure diagnostic test" of brain injury seem to be a chimera; almost every behavioral "indicator" in such cases can be found in large portions of control populations. One problem encountered by previous approaches has been the difficulty of reconciling the assumption of *specific effects* of brain injury with the finding of wide individual differences among brain-injured. Now, in non-brain-injured the occurrence of such differences is attributed to "personality factors." If so, then in the brain-injured the occurrence of behavior similar to that found in non-brain-injured is also presumably of "personality origin." All of this highlights still further the contradictions inherent in the "sign" approach. For if certain behaviors are at one time due to "personality" and at another due to brain lesions, in what meaningful and consistent way are we to explain the wide individual differences among brain-injured?

The most reasonable assumption upon which to anchor an approach to the effects of brain injury seems to be this: Personality is itself a series of neurophysiological events; brain injury is an "interruption" or "intrusion" upon this usual pattern of cortical integration. The effects of brain-injury, therefore, necessarily depend upon the personality constellation (i.e., the neurophysiological constellation), which will qualify, exacerbate, or modulate the trauma of a particular lesion and thereby determine its effects in part. Stated simply, this expresses the view that brain injury occurs within a context of personality organization; it is, as it were, "handled" or "responded to" by an existing neurophysiological structure (the personality) which partly determines its effects.

The principal stumbling block for this approach, however, has been the absence of a workable model of personality organization which would provide definitions of personality organization that would be suitable to the brain-injury problem. Effective research on the brain-injured must then face two ways: toward a formulation of neurophysiological principles of organization (personality structure) and their relation to modes of cognitive behavior; and secondly, toward specifying the relations between these variables and the extent, degree, and locus of cortical injury. The brain model would then account for variations in cognitive behavior and provide a systematic means for representing behavioral changes that accompany cortical pathology. The present study has postulated one central parameter of personality organization — cortical conductivity — and has proposed, first, that it may have possible value as a means of accounting for certain qualities of cognitive behavior and, secondly, that the effects of brain injury on behavior may be better understood via the effects of the injury on this physiological parameter of personality.

Summary and Conclusions

1. Assumptions proposed for a brain model suggested the hypothesis that if prolonged exposure to stimulation results in decreased conductivity (satiation) of cortical tissue, this effect will be particularly marked where there exist severe brain lesions. The present experiment compared brain-injured and controls on degree and rate of satiation after exposure to a kinesthetic stimulus, and on the extent and rate of recovery (dissipation of satiation).

2. Hospitalized male patients (N = 12) with cortical lesions of varying severity and locus were compared with equated hospitalized controls (N = 16). Subjects were blindfolded and rubbed the sides of a 2½-inch wide standard for 30-second, 60-second, 90-second, and 120-second periods; after each period they judged the width of a 1½-inch test object by adjusting a tapering scale. Persistence of the effect was measured 5 minutes and 10 minutes after the last satiation period. Control measurements taken prior to satiation trials provided individual baselines. The brain-injured were rated for severity of disturbance by the hospital's chief neurologist.

3. Consistent trends were: (a) frequency and intensity of satiation effects were significantly greater in the brain-injured; (b) the brain-injured reached maximal satiation more quickly; (c) the satiated state persisted longer in the brain-injured, recovery being less pronounced

and slower (ancillary findings ruled out "fatigue" and "learning" factors as sources of these differences); (d) correlations of satiation indices with neurological ratings ranged from +.63 to +.92, clearly suggesting a relation between extent of clinically observed disturbance and figural aftereffect measures. These results offer support to the "cortical conductivity" concept and the suggestion that a generalized effect of *severe* brain injury is lowered conductivity.

4. Tumor cases showed alterations which approximated those of diffuse nontumor lesions, especially in rate of recovery, which was excessively slowed. This suggested that a broader organismic imbalance rather than merely the local changes in specifically affected regions may be an important source of variations in conductivity.

REFERENCES

1. Goldstein, K. *The organism.* New York: American Book Co., 1939.
2. Jaffe, R., and Teuber, H. L. Influence of cerebral trauma on kinesthetic aftereffects. *American Psychol.*, 1951, 6: 264 (abstract).
3. Johnson, P. O. *Statistical methods in research.* New York: Prentice-Hall, 1949.
4. Klein, G. S. Studies of duration of negative after images: effect of brain-injury. (Unpublished.)
5. Köhler, W., and Dinnerstein, D. Figural after-effects in kinesthesis. In *Miscellanea psychologica Albert Michotte.* Louvain: Institut Superieur de Philosophie, 1947.
6. Köhler, W., and Wallach, H. Figural after-effects. An investigation of visual processes. *Proc. Amer. Philos. Soc.*, 1944, 88.
7. Krech, D. Dynamic systems, psychological fields, and hypothetical constructs. *Psychol. Rev.*, 1950, 57: 283–290.
8. Krech, D. Dynamic systems as open neurological systems. *Psychol. Rev.*, 1950, 57: 345–361.

35

PSYCHOLOGICAL CONSEQUENCES OF BRAIN LESIONS AND ABLATIONS

SEYMOUR G. KLEBANOFF, JEROME L. SINGER, AND
HAROLD WILENSKY

Franklin D. Roosevelt Veterans Administration Hospital, Montrose, New York

In a previous paper, the senior author (164) reviewed the literature dealing with the psychological consequences of organic brain lesions and ablations through the year 1941. The intervening period of over ten years has witnessed considerable research in this area. In addition to the need to scrutinize and systematize the new and extensive literature relative to the problem of therapeutic psychosurgery, it is also important to observe significant trends in the development of new psychological evaluative techniques. Also, there have been notable modifications in the use and application of existing test methods in organic brain disease.

In the previous review of the literature by Klebanoff (164), effort was made to formulate certain basic generalizations. It appears appropriate now to examine critically these conclusions in the light of the extensive research of the last decade. One is impressed by the striking development of new specialized test techniques. It seems important to evaluate these new techniques in terms of their potential clinical value. Research of the last decade has stressed the potential importance of such variables as the patient's age and the quality of interaction with the environment in producing differences in deficit in patients with apparently similar disease processes.

In the light of all the above considerations, the present review has been undertaken. The general attitude underlying this survey is one of critical appraisal rather than mere review; the basic objectives are to organize, integrate, clarify, and extract significant generalizations. Such an approach appears to be indicated if the basic conclusions in the area of psychological testing in organic brain disease and psychosurgery are to be evaluated in terms of essential contribution to scientific and clinical knowledge.

From the *Psychological Bulletin*, January 1954. © 1954, by the American Psychological Association.

BRAIN INJURY IN CHILDREN

Psychological studies of persons who have suffered congenital brain injury, encephalitis, or other types of cerebral damage early in life have proven an increasingly fertile area of research. The significance of research with brain-injured children, in addition to its practical value for rehabilitation, lies in the possibilities of obtaining valuable understanding of the developmental aspects of brain function or dysfunction. Theories of normal mental development (135, 180, 286) have stressed the fact that psychological functioning and cerebral organization show an increase in differentiation and integration with age through adolescence. Although the less differentiated structure in the child leads to a more diffuse effect of injury if it occurs early, it also makes possible maturation with compensatory development of function. This negates the influence of an injury which would frequently have serious long-term sequelae in adults.

Probst (222) followed up a group of 95 children with skull fractures occurring between ages one and fifteen. After seven to fourteen years there was no evidence of impairment in school or vocational achievement, social adjustment, or intellectual development. Several investigators (50, 64, 84, 126, 163, 297) obtained varied results in brief case studies of functions disturbed by brain injury in rather young children. French (84) studied ten children who were operated upon for cerebellar tumors with an extensive battery of generalized intelligence and specialized tests and found no evidence of impairment on deterioration-sensitive tests. Some children showed superior performance. On the other hand, Cotton (64), employed a control group in studying the thought processes of spastic children and found striking differences between them and the normal control group. It is possible that differences in severity of injury may well account for these divergent findings. An unusual case study described by Klapper and Werner (163) compared three children with cerebral palsy with their normal identical twins, using a large battery of tests sampling a wide variety of functions. The brain-injured children were impaired in every area when compared with their normal twins.

The major portion of research on brain injury in children has emerged in the extensive work on the distinction between endogenous and exogenous feeblemindedness. This distinction has proven of great heuristic value in stimulating an intensive study of the various dysfunctions consequent upon brain injury. As a result of this research, it has been possible to develop fairly adequate criteria for distinguishing these two types of defective children (32, 176, 247, 256). This has resulted in the addition of a number of fairly sensitive and important techniques to the repertory of the clinician for measuring basic functions likely to be impaired in early brain injury.

Motor Functions

The brain-injured child is generally subject to motor disturbances, since either cerebellar injuries or disturbances in the motor cortex are common (32, 176, 247). Even when obvious motor disturbance is not present, the brain-injured child shows awkwardness and incoordination in performance. Heath (130, 131), comparing exogenous and endogenous feebleminded children of comparable mental age in their performance on a simple rail-walking test, found that the exogenous children proved strikingly inferior. Descriptive studies of the motor performance of these exogenous feebleminded characterize them as hyperkinetic, overactive, restless, impulsive, and incoordinated (247, 283). The impression gained from such descriptive studies suggests that motor difficulties are as much a function of fairly subtle disturbances in the integration of behavior and the inhibition of overt responsiveness as they are of specific damage to motor areas of the cortex. The use of the Van Der Lugt Scale (270) seems to offer potential for major research in the area of motor development and defect in the future.

Perceptual Functions

The most extensive and definitive studies of brain-injured children have been in the area of perception. This work has been of theoretical as well as of practical importance since it has demonstrated striking relations between perceptual and motor functioning that has led to suggestions for a sensory-tonic theory of perception (248, 282). Thus, Strauss (255), in summarizing three case histories, described perceptual and thought processes which mirror the forced responsiveness, hyperkinesis, and incoordination of the brain-injured child in his motor performance. Bender and Silver (33) describe the case of a brain-injured child with a severe modification in perception of the body. They conclude that the body image of the brain-damaged child is disturbed by "tonus pulls," equilibrium problems, and perceptual and integrative difficulties which heighten his social inadequacy.

Werner and Strauss (292) studied normal children equated for mental age with endogenous and exogenous mentally defective children without gross motor or central visual defects. They used tachistoscopic presentation of marred figures and copying of patterns of marble boards or reproduction of the patterns by drawing. Although the endogenous children were generally inferior to the normal group, they differed strikingly in mode of response from the exogenous children.

The latter made a great many errors that suggested failure to discriminate between figure and ground.

Subsequent reinforcement of these findings has come from the investigations of Lord and Wood (186) and Dolphin and Cruickshank (70). The latter studied perception of embedded figures and mosaic reproduction by matched normal and cerebral-palsied children of low-average intelligence. They attributed the significant inferiority in perceptual performance of the children with cerebral palsy to forced responsiveness and meticulosity. Bensberg (42), in a careful study, compared familial mental defectives and brain-injured defectives using the marble-board procedure. The brain-injured group proved significantly inferior in accuracy and tended more often to show "jumps" to new lines in their drawings. The results continue to point to pathological figure-ground perception as a basic difficulty consequent on brain injury. Werner (283), studying the performance of the two feebleminded types on the Rorschach, noted significantly more white space responses (S) for the exogenous group. Case studies by Strauss and Werner (257, 258), and Werner and Carrison (289), demonstrate ingeniously the interrelationships of defective figure-ground formations in brain-injured children and other symptoms such as finger agnosia and arithmetic disability.

Similarly, these brain-injured children showed inability to grasp and retain visual patterns made up of discrete elements. The authors attributed this to a basic difficulty in integrating several aspects of a visual stimulus. This is a defect similar to that reported for a brain-injured adult by Nichols and Hunt (205) and considered a basic consequence of severe brain pathology by Hunt and Cofer (145) in their review of psychological deficit. A case study by Schilder (243) has similar possibilities for interpretation of this deficit.

Brief mention may be made of additional perceptual difficulties manifested by brain-injured children. Werner and Thuma (295) compared equated groups of feebleminded representing the two etiological types on performance in critical flicker fusion perception. Results showed the exogenous feebleminded fell significantly below the familial group in critical flicker frequency at all three brightness levels. This finding is quite important in view of extensive research on adults reported by Teuber (263) and Halstead (120). Similarly, a marked defect in the perception of apparent or illusory motion, the phi phenomenon, and tachistoscopic presentation of stick figures in imbalance was found among the exogenous feebleminded by Werner and Thuma (294). These children also showed fewer movement percepts on the Rorschach than an equated group of endogenous feebleminded. In one of the few studies involving auditory perception in brain pathology,

Werner and Bowers (288) found that the brain-injured feebleminded were deficient in discriminating melodic patterns, revealing much the same disturbance in figure-ground pathology noted above.

Thought Processes

Sorting tests have proven increasingly useful in studying thought in process and in its effect. Strauss and Werner (259) employed the Halstead sorting test to determine if the findings with brain-injured adults were comparable to those obtained with brain-injured children. Twenty pairs of exogenous and endogenous feebleminded children were matched for mental age and intelligence. The brain-injured children formed more relationships between objects in the voluntary sorting but accomplished this by forming "singular and unusual combinations." In choosing objects to go with rather unambiguous pictures, the brain-injured children also selected uncommon objects. They deviated more from standard names, organized objects into circumscribed units, overstressed orderliness, and showed extreme concreteness. In contrast with the endogenous children and particularly with a group of healthy children, the brain-injured children were attracted to "properties of objects apt to elicit motor responses." The latter finding seems important in view of the hyperkinetic tendencies ascribed to brain-injured children.

In a further study of thought processes, Werner and Carrison (290) employed a standard procedure for studying animism or the tendency to perceive natural events of objects as living. The results, based upon levels of thought development derived from the work of Piaget, showed significantly more animistic responses by the exogenous children. In keeping with certain concepts of Goldstein (93) and Werner (286), the animistic tendencies of brain-injured children may be looked upon as functions of a greater ridigity and concreteness which prevent them from detaching themselves from objects and events. They are thus unable to differentiate between their own feelings and those of the surrounding world. Evidence that these tendencies are a result of impairment due to brain injury rather than merely representing a particular type of intellectual limitation is forthcoming in a study by Cotton (64), who compared physically normal children with spastic children of average intelligence. Results on a series of sorting, verbal completion, and patterning tests showed a decided inferiority for the spastics whose responses were more stereotyped and who were less inclusive in sortings and more given to highly personal associations and other signs of concreteness. These findings were particularly associated with speech difficulties and were found less often when the congenital injury was restricted to motor areas.

The problem of the rigidity or perseveration of brain-injured or feeble-minded generally has been discussed theoretically by Lewin (180) and Kounin (173). The latter carried out several significant studies demonstrating differences in rigidity patterns as a function of chronological and mental age. It is not clear whether the subjects used by Kounin were exogenous or endogenous feeble-minded, although apparently they were physically normal as determined by medical examination. Werner (284), summarizing four experiments comparing rigidity patterns of brain-injured and familial feebleminded, observed more perseveration in the former group. He characterized the rigidity of the brain-injured as *abnormal*; it involved a trend away from the global approach toward isolation of elements of a series which became self-contained and were repeated monotonously or "jumped" suddenly into the foreground. The familial feebleminded, on the other hand, showed *subnormal* rigidity related to a relative lack of differentiation. They showed predominantly global behavior, perception, or action, organized as undifferentiated wholes so that situations not sharply set apart were easily fused, resulting in stereotyped responses.

Personality

There have been comparatively few attempts at extensive personality evaluations of brain-injured children. Werner (283) studied the Rorschach test performance of brain-injured feebleminded and found that they showed a restriction of creative fantasy activity, strong tendencies toward explosive emotionality, negativism, and the disintegrative behavior described above. Colm (62), employing the Lowenfeld Mosaic Test, compared normal and brain-injured children. She described the brain-injured children as "stimulus bound," with an inability to shift and a repetitiveness which indicated an impairment in abstraction. Thus, these children showed simple additive placement of the mosaic pieces using side-by-side or color-by-color patterns and showed difficulty in formulating and executing a plan for a design. Colm indicated an important distinction between the exogenous children and compulsive or autistic children who also showed repetitiousness. The latter perseverated chiefly on words with strong emotional content while the brain-injured children repeated almost any phrase regardless of the emotional tone.

In conclusion, the extensive research on brain-injured children indicates defects that are generally like those described for brain-injured adults. The children show inability to develop abstract functions, pathological rigidity, lack of creative imagination, stimulus bondage, and disintegrative behavior in all areas. Brain-injured children also show strikingly unequal development of capacities, suggesting some cerebral localization of damage, but the basic defects in abstraction hinder any possibility of really integrated development for many.

Organic Psychoses and Degenerative Diseases of the Nervous System

Despite the increased interest in problems of the aged in the past decade, there has been little extensive research dealing with psychological deficit or emotional changes concomitant with senescence. A major trend in the past decade has been an awareness of some decline in intellectual functioning with increased age (151, 274). There has been little attempt, however, at precise analysis of the nature of this decline and its relationship to emotional stability and the psychological milieu.

Fortunately, some studies on the organization of mental life in organic psychoses are beginning to appear. Botwinick and Birren (49), for example, compared the intellectual performance of hospitalized seniles with that of normal persons of the same age range (60 to 70 years) and with that of a matched group of young normals. They used the Wechsler-Bellevue and Babcock-Levy Revision to test for deterioration. These investigators concluded that while differences between the two aged groups existed, the older persons were far more like each other than were the normal aged and the younger group.

Of greater theoretical interest, perhaps, are studies attempting to delineate the pattern of mental change consequent on the fairly diffuse degenerative brain changes that seem to occur with cerebral arteriosclerosis and similar diseases. Thus, in studies comparing 100 male senile dements with an average age of 73, and employing such tests as Raven's Progressive Matrices, Eysenck (72, 73) found considerable deterioration in the patients in terms of healthy adult and child norms. A factor analysis of the results showed a general factor and three factors relating to speed, memory, and physical strength which could be identified fairly readily. Tests of abstract reasoning proved most sensitive to deterioration in contrast to tests involving memory and stable knowledge. A differential deterioration in abilities appeared to occur along the lines suggested many years ago by Hughlings Jackson (149) in which the diffuse cerebral damage leads to initial loss of the most complex functions which develop most recently in the evolution of the nervous system. In this connection, Halstead (115) studied senile dements over 70 with an extensive battery of psychological tests. There were two groups in different stages of dementia. Tests discriminating between the two groups involved the more complex functions. The tests included Porteus Mazes, Knox Cubes, Block Designs, and various recent memory tests.

The impoverishment of functioning in senile psychotics was brought out in a study by Cleveland and Dysinger (57). These investigators studied the performance of institutionalized seniles, whose average age was 75, with the Wechsler-Bellevue scale and an object-sorting test. The patients manifested decided difficulties in assuming an abstract attitude and could not sort on a conceptual basis. That even verbal behavior suffers impairment in senile dementia was demonstrated by Feldman and Cameron (75) and Ackelsberg (3). The former investigators compared the speech of senile psychotics with that of normal adults and children. Although based on rather small samples, this study does suggest that seniles have difficulty in dealing with abstract terms and rely most heavily on concrete nominal forms or words of action to the neglect of adjectives which involve imaginative processes. Ackelsberg (3) obtained comparable findings in vocabulary studies of seniles. Recent studies by Pinkerton and Kelly (217) and Hall (113) contrasted deteriorated seniles with children and depressives by the use of various sorting tests and supported the thesis that a loss of conceptual ability occurs early in the course of brain degeneration while more general intellectual test performances remain relatively intact.

Diffuse degeneration of the cortex, particularly in the frontal areas, occurs in general paresis. The behavior of paretics in the classic description of the disease, while more flagrantly psychotic, does resemble that of the older senile dementia or arteriosclerotic patients. With the improved methods for treating syphilis and arresting general paresis, a re-evaluation of the description of the disease may well be necessary.

Psychological studies of patients with general paresis have been fairly frequent in the past decade and have provided suggestive findings. Studies with the Wechsler-Bellevue scale (88, 195) as well as with the CVS abridgment (198) have suggested the usefulness of these tests in delineating the intellectual performance of paretics. While there were individual differences in the degree of impairment on the various subtests, the general findings suggested lowered concentration ability, greater difficulty in new learning, verbal comprehension, and concept formation in the case of the paretic group. Trist, Trist, and Brody (269) used a large battery of cognitive tests in comparing normals, neurotics, and paretics and observed that the paretics found it difficult to ignore irrelevant detail, and a flowing together of figure and ground was evident in their performance.

A somewhat novel approach to the psychological study of paresis is offered in studies by Rashkis, Cushman, and Landis (225) and Rashkis (224). The former study involved the administration of a word-sorting test to normal adults, normal children, general paretics, and schizophrenics equated for educational achievement. On the basis of an analysis of the sortings, only the normal adults were able to assume the abstract attitude. Children and schizophrenics functioned at the complex, "pseudo-conceptual" level, while the paretics were unable to reach even that degree of attainment. From the standpoint of volitional attitude, the schizophrenics more closely resembled the normal adults while the paretics resembled the children. Rashkis (224), employing more careful controls, amplified and extended these findings. Rashkis studied three groups consisting of schizophrenics, general paretics, and cerebral arteriosclerotics. The schizophrenics proved somewhat better "coordinated" and more capable of accounting for their performance. The arteriosclerotics, although "uncoordinated," also attempted to account for their performance, in contrast to the paretics who were "uncoordinated" and offered no excuse or apology.

In one of the few attempts to study the personality characteristics of general paretics, Klebanoff (165) employed the Rorschach inkblots to compare findings between a homogeneous group of paretics and a normal control group matched for age and education. The paretics lacked sufficient intellectual drive to function at an abstract level. They showed concrete mental activity which lacked accuracy, conformity, and "fundamental adaptivity to environmental needs."

A promising and somewhat different approach to this problem is suggested by the preliminary study of Wittenborn, Bell, and Lesser (300) who carried out a factor analysis of symptom ratings along various scales for deteriorated organics, hebephrenics, and young patients with functional psychoses. Different symptom clusters emerged with only anxiety and paranoid factors coinciding for the groups. Deterioration was most marked among the organic patients.

Research is just now beginning to appear in connection with presumably subcortical neurological degeneration such as is found in multiple sclerosis. Although somewhat contradictory results have emerged with respect to possible mental deterioration concomitant with multiple sclerosis (25, 53, 68), differences in the populations studied and in the duration of the disease may account for these discrepancies. Canter (53), for example, found definite evidence of deterioration among patients in the early phases of the disease when compared with both their own military induction test scores and a control group of clinic employees. Diers and Brown (68) reported no evidence of decline, while Baldwin (25) reported loss of abstract ability in some patients and no apparent decline for many others.

It is in the area of personality that a striking uniformity emerges in three separate studies. A brief report by Harrower (127) was based on comparisons of Rorschach and Szondi findings for multiple sclerotics, control groups of normals, emotionally unstable psychosomatic patients, and patients with poliomyelitis and Parkinson's disease. It was found that the multiple sclerotic patients differed from the other groups in showing *least* concern with bodily symptoms, extreme dependency, resignation, denial of conflicts, and a need to excite sympathy. This general similarity to the classical picture of the hysteric patient with *belle indifference* also emerged in Rorschach studies by Blatt and Hecht (48) and an intensive study by Baldwin (25) of family background, premorbid factors, and data from Minnesota Multiphasic Personality Inventory patterns. The general similarity of the multiple sclerotic and neurotic hysteric is particularly striking in the early phases of the disease (25) and suggests the importance of a premorbid personality factor. In view of similar findings with idiopathic epileptics (91), an important area of research in the psychosomatic implications of neurological disease appears to require extensive exploration.

BRAIN TUMOR, SURGICAL ABLATION, AND CEREBRAL TRAUMA IN ADULTS

Disturbances in Perception

The majority of studies have been restricted to the field of visual perception. For excellent reviews of material on the borderline of visual sensation and perception, the reader is referred to Bender and Teuber (40) and Teuber and Bender (267). Halstead (120) has ascribed important theoretical significance to the critical flicker fusion frequency as a result of factor analyses of the test performances of normal individuals. On the basis of intercorrelations between the critical flicker frequency and performance and other techniques. Halstead (120) has tentatively defined a power factor (P) which indicates the kinetic capacity of the individual, not unlike the "central vigilance" described by Head (128) in his studies of aphasia. Halstead (117, 119) has reported evidence that individuals of equal IQ may differ markedly in the P factor, which is sensitive to disruption by the presence of relatively small lesions in the brain and under conditions of low-grade anoxia or fatigue. Since Halstead indicates that a lowered critical flicker frequency is one of the prime indicators of a depressed level of the P factor of biological intelligence, the value of this simple laboratory procedure for psychological evaluation of the consequences of brain lesions is greatly enhanced.

Unfortunately, the findings of Halstead have not been fully confirmed. Battersby (27, 28) and Battersby, Bender, and Teuber (29) obtained negative results in studies of veteran patients with frontal lobe head wounds. These patients failed to show any significant differences in critical flicker frequency level when compared with an equated control group. On the other hand, a series of studies (28, 29, 38, 40, 265, 266, 303) has shown definite lowering in critical flicker frequency after occipital lobe lesions. This impairment was detected in areas that appeared normal under routine perimetric examination. Bender and Teuber (38, 40) have reported that defects emerged more strikingly when critical flicker frequency was tested in the periphery of vision rather than in the macular region. These results, while confirming those of Halstead (120) in raising doubts concerning the significance of an anatomic point-to-point projection in visual structures, are difficult to reconcile with his observations on frontal lobe patients. The differences may be a function of procedural variations or, as Battersby (28) has suggested, the result of differing patient groups.

Case studies comprise the bulk of the studies on perceptual response following brain injury. Rather challenging for general theories of perception are observations of a phenomenon tentatively labelled "extinction," in which patients confronted with an object in their left-half field report that it disappears as soon as another object is shown in their right-half field (34, 36, 303). As Hebb (136) has noted, these phenomena are difficult to assimilate into current perceptual theories. Bender and Furlow (34) describe the manner in which tendencies to reorganize a psychological field of vision about a subjective center make it difficult for a patient with occipital lobe damage to recognize that he has lost central vision.

Problems of unusual spatial reorganizations brought out only by special testing devices are described in a number of cases of occipital injury. Paterson and Zangwill (211) observed in two cases of right parieto-occipital lobe injuries a tendency to overestimate the distance of very near objects and to underestimate the distances of far objects, although the ability to appreciate depth and distance and the "implicit awareness of space" were not affected. Analysis of spatial structure was difficult, and various spatial relations tests and the Kohs Blocks brought out the defects in the patient. Drawings of complex objects were carried out piecemeal with poor articulation of subwholes. Temporal disorientation, also found by Coheen (58) with a larger number of patients and various control groups, was also present. Since most case studies in this group represent traumatic injuries, a report by Stengel (254) of consequences of vascular lesions with an eclampsia in a 40-year-old woman is interesting since quite severe spatial reorganization occurred. Extensive testing revealed that for this subject the complex spatial organization of the outside world had been replaced by a most primitive organization in which "nearness" served as the only measuring scale.

A series of cases of parietal and occipital lobe injuries reported by Bender and Teuber (38, 40) is particularly valuable because of the careful attempts by the authors to relate findings to a general theory of brain function. On the basis of an intensive sampling of increasingly complex perceptual performances, the authors report such defects as disturbance (limited to the lower left quadrant for some patients) in localizing objects, teleopsia with a tendency toward an excess of depth in the subjective field, higher threshold for phi, lowered critical flicker frequency, and tendency to enlarge unfamiliar objects. For some patients the subjective coronal plane was rotated as a whole, away from them on the left, toward them on the right. This shifting could be compensated for by one patient in daily life, while for another, subjective visual space no longer coincided with his tactile or locomotor space and led him into many constant errors in pointing. The authors feel that these results argue against associational theories and in favor of "vector" theories generally related to Köhler's (170) views of brain function.

In an experimental attempt to test certain hypotheses concerning cerebral function related to Köhler's theories, Klein and Krech (166) and Jaffe (150) independently carried out recent studies of the kinesthetic figural aftereffects in matched brain-injured and control groups. Jaffe, using patients with traumatic head wounds, found no differences between controls and patients. Klein and Krech tested the hypothesis that both concreteness and figural aftereffects in the brain-injured were functions of reduced "cortical conductivity" (174). They predicted more pronounced figural aftereffects that would appear sooner and last longer for subjects of varied degrees of brain pathology than for equated controls. Results supported the hypotheses and, in addition, high positive correlations were found between neurologists' ratings of extent of damage and the vividness and duration of the effect. The differences in results of the two studies may be in part a function of different patient populations, traumatic head wounds as against surgical ablations, a persisting obstacle to the reconcililation of data in this field.

There has as yet been little effort to relate perceptual defects in brain-injured patients to more general areas of functioning such as motivation and personality. Critchley (66) has stressed the relation of body image to alteration in cerebral functioning following parietal lesions. Halstead (118) has shown a possible relationship of lowered and fairly rigid critical flicker frequency and poor performance on the Dynamic Visual Field test to severe judgmental defects in a man following unilateral lobectomy. More recently, Weinstein and Kahn (278, 279, 280) have investigated motivational and interpersonal aspects of the perceptual response of 50 patients with bilateral lesions of neoplastic or vascular origin. These patients showed distortions not only in body image, but in self-concepts and manifested tendencies to deny illness or impairment and to misperceive stimuli related to their disability or hospitalization. The denial of affective involvement sometimes reported following lobotomy may represent a similar phenomenon and quite a serious threat to future adjustment since it substitutes an equally unrealistic self-orientation for the previous "tortured self-concern."

Summarizing results in psychological studies of perceptual functioning following brain lesions and ablations, it is apparent that the movement toward specialized testing techniques pointed out by Klebanoff (164) has progressed rapidly. Perceptual research with brain-injured patients suggests that the repertory of the clinical psychologist in the examination of neurological patients may soon be augmented by the use of specialized laboratory methods such as tachistoscopic presentation, critical flicker fusion frequency testing, apparent movement thresholds, and other so-called "brass instrument" techniques. The value of these perceptual techniques in localization of lesions remains equivocal. It seems clear, nevertheless, that subtle perceptual impairments or reorganizations following cerebral injury are most clearly brought out by intensive laboratory examination rather than by the widely used global clinical methods like the Rorschach, Bender-Gestalt, Wechsler-Bellevue, Hunt-Minnesota, etc. These laboratory techniques or those outlined by Goldstein (95) are now chiefly available in only a few research centers (120, 263, 307). Before long, with the aid of these new techniques, the clinical psychologist may be in a position to play an ever more vital role in a neurological setting.

Memory and Attention

The past decade has provided comparatively little intensive research on specific memory or attention disturbances in brain-injured patients. The emphasis, rather, has been on incorporation of these functions within broader categories such as perception or general intelligence. Certainly, many disturbances of immediate memory may actually reflect difficulties in attention to presented material. The distractibility and stimulus bondage which are reported to be characteristic of both brain-injured adults and children (93, 94, 291, 293) would naturally impede original learning of material. Hall and Crookes (114) compared a heterogeneous brain-injured group with normals and schizophrenics in learning ability and found some qualitative suggestion of impairment in the organic patients, although differences between the organic patients and the schizophrenic patients were not definitive. Ruesch and Moore (234) studied 190 patients immediately following head injury and reported that the serial subtraction test ("100–7") proved most sensitive, suggesting that the ability to maintain sustained effort is particularly sensitive to cerebral dysfunction, whether momentary or persistent. Similarly, other investigators have found evidence of memory loss dependent largely upon failures in attention and immediate retentiveness (4, 10, 20). Tests such as Halstead's Formboard Retention and Dynamic Visual Field (120), Teuber's Field of Search (263), and Benton's Visual Retention (43) have revealed fairly clear evidence of attention and immediate memory defects in cases of brain trauma or surgical ablation. Definitive standardization of these procedures in the future should prove them valuable clinical aids. The major problem of devising laboratory and clinical procedures capable of discriminating between certain schizophrenic patients and individuals with various kinds of brain pathology remains a difficult methodological consideration.

Mention should be made of some tests designed to detect brain damage by memory techniques (69, 102, 144). Hunt (144) has developed an extensive battery employing as a base the 1937 Stanford-Binet with verbal and nonverbal learning and recall tests. The test was developed on patients with diffuse brain injury, but subsequent research (4, 20, 154, 196) suggests that the test does not discriminate well.

Employing an omnibus memory test approach, Graham and Kendall (102), while reporting significant differences between a brain-damaged group and a neurotic group, found impairment present in only half of the organics. In a careful study by Cohen (59) no measures of the Wechsler Memory scale discriminated between neurotics and patients with intracranial pathology. These negative findings do not necessarily indicate that memory defects are uncommon among patients or that memory scales are without value in neurological testing. These scales have undoubted usefulness as part of an individual testing battery in the hands of an experienced clinician. It is clear, however, that the complexity of brain functioning and the subtlety of psychological sequelae of organic brain impairment severely limit any research or clinical studies with omnibus memory scales.

General Intelligence

Although reports on general intellectual consequences of brain injuries or diseases are considerable in quantity, the past decade has seen little progress in the treatment of this issue. Critical case studies (129, 132, 202, 207) have suggested that general intelligence as measured by standard scales may be normal or actually improve following large but clean excisions of previously pathological brain tissue. Concern in employing intelligence tests has been, with certain exceptions, limited to the Wechsler-Bellevue Intelligence Scale and various measures of deficit derived from this test. Recognizing that intelligence in general may not show a change after brain lesion, investigators, following the clinical suggestions of Wechsler (275), have attempted to tease out patterns of test performance capable of differentiating the brain-injured or diseased from normal individuals. Unfortunately, as Rabin and Guertin (223) have noted in their review of Wechsler-Bellevue research, the Mental Deterioration Index (MDI), originally developed on the basis of decline in scores with increasing age among normals, has been translated too hastily to indicate decline following organic brain damage.

A brief report on clinical cases by Levi, Oppenheim, and Wechsler (178) indicated, for example, the practical usefulness of the MDI in differentiating patients with organic lesions from patients with hysterical and other psychogenic disturbances. Although cautious in their generalizations, these authors did raise an important principle for use in studying deterioration. The concept of tests that "hold up" with age and hence may conceivably be less resistant to the inroads of brain damage is a challenging one. The question remains, however, as to the specific nature of "hold" and "don't hold" tests and to the quantitative relationships necessary to suggest pathological deterioration. In its purely quantitative form, the MDI has not been shown to be sufficiently discriminating in individual determinations of brain-injured and normals (8, 15, 47, 110, 156).

It should be noted, however, that the general principle of the contrast of "hold" and "don't hold" tests seems to be operative and that the majority of brain-injured are properly diagnosed by its use. For individual prediction, however, reliance on quantitative scores alone seems relatively futile. Anderson (15, 16) compared clinically substantiated cases of focal lesions in the dominant hemisphere with comparable cases of lesions in the nondominant hemisphere. He found that while the MDI did not yield very reliable quantitative discrimination, differences were in the expected direction. Brain-injured patients with focal lesions of the dominant hemisphere were more easily picked up by the use of the index than were those with nondominant lesions. On the basis of several studies and a comparison of brain-injured and brain-diseased patients, Allen (7, 8, 9, 10, 11) suggested a modification of the index, but other studies have provided data which suggest that this modification is not significantly more discriminating than the original (4, 47, 230). Other attempts at developing deterioration indices (138, 227) have been evaluated by Gutman (110), who found that a rather complex method developed by Hewson (138) agreed fairly well with clinical diagnoses of brain damage.

Far more significant perhaps than the empirical derivation of complex indices (which are not very discriminating and have not been cross-validated by the investigators) is evidence that certain functions appear again and again in the list as particularly susceptible to impairment by brain injury. Almost all investigators have noted that Digit Symbol, representing disciplined psychomotor learning, is most clearly affected. Also easily impaired by brain injury are Digit Span, a test of recent memory or attention (7, 9, 227, 233, 234); Block Design, testing analytic and synthetic capacities (4, 7, 9, 92, 107, 183); and Arithmetic (4), testing concentration and simple numerical facility. Since these subtests are most easily affected by anxiety or other emotional disturbances, a great deal of overlap between various clinical groups (223) is almost inevitable.

Too much of the research in this field has been excessively test-bound and empirical, relying heavily upon omnibus scales of general intelligence. New concepts like Cattell's "crystallized" and "fluid" abilities (54), similar views of Hebb (135) related to his physiological rationale, and Halstead's four factors as components of "biological intelligence" (120) should provide useful theoretical bases for more precise explorations.

Halstead provided some data to suggest a differential influence of brain lesions on his four factors of biological intelligence, with the P factor considered the most sensitive and disturbed, particularly in prefrontal lobe lesions, in his data. Halstead's results also suggest a gradient of impairment in biological intelligence with the frontal areas most sensitive. This hypothesis needs extensive testing since somewhat contradictory data are available from other studies (29, 40). Nevertheless, Halstead's work poses a challenge to clinical psychologists to reconsider their techniques and their excessive reliance upon omnibus tests or techniques standardized for other purposes.

Disturbances in Thought and Language

In the past decade, research has continued to suggest that a major consequence of brain lesions and ablations is a disturbance in thought and language, classified as a loss of abstract or conceptual ability in the viewpoint popularized by Goldstein (94, 100). The directions taken by research in this period have involved (*a*) more precise exploration of this basic defect by the use of refined procedures (100, 113, 120, 121, 141, 264); and (*b*) attempts to ascertain whether the loss of abstract ability was particularly a consequence of frontal lobe pathology.

Extensively studied cases of both frontal and diffuse brain pathology have been reported (2, 44, 118, 123, 205, 306) in which patients manifested fairly general signs of impairment in abstract behavior as measured by procedures like the Weigl color-form sorting, the object-sorting tests, the Shipley-Hartford Conceptual Quotient, the Kohs Blocks, etc.

A striking well-studied negative case was presented by Hebb (134) in which the patient was operated upon for removal of frontal scar tissue that had led to near-psychotic behavior. This patient improved subsequent to a fairly clean but extensive bilateral frontal lobectomy. He showed no clear signs of unusual disturbance in abstract behavior when presented with a host of psychological tests, many of which tapped conceptual processes. Differences. between Hebb's case and cases discussed by Goldstein (98) may lie in the nature of the injury and the possible persistence of pathological tissue in some instances.

The value of various tests of abstraction in clinical neurological testing has been brought out in a number of studies (95, 97, 108, 139, 307). Greenblatt, Levine, and Antwell (108) found that, in comparing patients with known heterogeneous types of brain damage and patients without brain damage, abstraction tests like the Kohs Block, Weigl form-color, and Shipley-Hartford were extremely successful in differentiation, and, in combination with the somewhat less accurate EEG, they could discriminate almost perfectly between groups. The tests were used clinically and the specific contribution of each is not presented, unfortunately. Similarly, Hoedemaker and Murray (139) noted almost perfect discrimination of 16 brain-injured from 16 schizophrenics and 16 neurotics by the use of a battery including the Wechsler-Bellevue, Rorschach, Szondi, Ellis Visual Designs, and B.R.L. Sorting tests. Inspection of their breakdown of the various functions tapped reveals that thought process disturbance (tapped chiefly by the sorting tests) and memory were most consistently found and most accurate in differentiating. Electroencephalograms were less accurate, but the test battery combined with EEG and routine neurological examination led to perfect discrimination.

Although originally devised as a nonverbal intelligence test, the Kohs Block test has proven a valuable and interesting technique in diagnosis of brain-injured patients. Wechsler (275) reported it to be one of the most useful subtests in his intelligence scale for this purpose, while almost all the investigators using the Wechsler-Bellevue scale with brain-injured patients indicate severe impairment on the Block Design subtest (4, 7, 9, 92, 107, 183). To the extent that a combination of analytic and synthetic capacities is demanded of the subject by this test, it may measure the primarily abstract components of general intelligence. Thus, a study by Lidz, Gay, and Tietze (183) has shown a significant difference in mental age scores obtained from Vocabulary tests and the Stanford-Binet and the mental age scores obtained from the Kohs Blocks. A comparable group of 15 schizophrenics showed no significant differences between the three types of tests.

Significant attempts to devise more elaborate and subtle tests of conceptual or abstraction ability have been reported recently (103, 113, 120, 121, 141, 241, 264). A basic need in this area is a far more extensive study of the role of abstract processes in normal human behavior, and studies like those of Heidbreder (137) or Hanfmann (122) represent only tentative beginnings.

A second major problem in the area of abstract processes following brain lesion has been the question of localization. In the studies summarized by Klebanoff (164) the predominant trend suggested that lesions of the frontal areas in particular led to disturbance in abstract behavior. Studies by Rylander (236) and Halstead (120) particularly have supported this view. The latter investigator presented a small number of cases demonstrating greater loss of abstract ability on the category test in patients with frontal ablations than in patients with lesions in other lobes. Using a study of 147 cases of traumatic head injury, Halstead reported that the tendency these patients showed for impairment, as compared with controls, suggests again the greater effect of frontal injury, since mechanical and autopsy studies (65, 140) indicate that frontal injury is most likely to follow any type of head trauma. Lacking neurotic controls for his head injury group, Halstead's results are of limited generality, in view of the findings of Ross and Ross (231) which suggest difficulties in differentiating between these groups. The fact is that Halstead's patients with nonfrontal lesions also obtained scores considerably below those of the controls. This suggests impairment which, in view of the small number of subjects, may not be, practically speaking, less significant than findings for the frontal lobe patients. Finally, the age differences of the groups indicate that the frontal lobe patients were, on the average, seven years older than nonfrontal patients, who, in turn, tended to be somewhat older than the controls, so that age differences rather than location of lesion might account for the results. It would appear, therefore, that Halstead's views are in need of further validation.

A series of well-executed studies (30, 264, 268) has attempted to test the hypothesis that abstract thinking and fairly complex visual functions are most readily impaired by frontal lesions. These authors studied three well-matched groups of veterans, patients with anterior lobe traumatic lesions, patients with parieto-occipital traumatic lesions, and patients with peripheral nerve injuries who served as nonbrain-injured controls. Lesions were localized by wound of entrance. From a varied series of complex visual tasks, including the Gottschaldt "hidden figures," the Wisconsin Sorting test (103), a visual-choice reaction test, and an adaptation for humans of Maier's reasoning situation, these authors concluded that test performance of groups of brain-injured was significantly below that of control subjects, despite fairly equal motivation for solution. On some tasks, the occipital lobe patients were inferior to the frontal patients. The authors feel that these results suggest that complex visual performance involving aspects of abstraction is at least as difficult for patients with posterior lesions as for patients with frontal lobe lesions.

While these results cannot be compared directly with those of Halstead (120) because of the difference in the nature of the pathology (trauma versus tumor), they do point up the serious consequences of any type of brain injury, particularly when it is recalled that the patients, unlike most tumor patients, were tested four to seven years after injury. On the other hand, since both the studies of Halstead (120) and Teuber and Bender (268) lack any anatomical or pathological data definitely localizing the injuries, the results have only limited value for theories of brain function. In view of the findings of Holbourn (140) and Courville (65), Halstead might well argue that the trauma of the impact of high velocity missiles in any area of the brain would most likely involve the frontal lobes in any case, thus questioning the conclusions of Teuber and Bender.

An interesting contribution to the problem of localization comes from results presented by McFie and Piercy (192), who studied 74 patients, largely tumor cases, with unilateral lesions. Employing the Weigl form-color sorting test, they found that patients with left-sided lesions proved significantly inferior to patients with lesions located in the so-called nondominant right side, *irrespective of location in the frontal, parietal, or occipital lobes.* This finding prevailed even when the aphasic patients were excluded. These results somewhat contradict those of Anderson (16) whose studies with the Wechsler-Bellevue subtests showed opposite results for patients with dominant and nondominant hemisphere lesions. Here the former patients proved inferior in verbal tests and superior in performance tests. Difficulty in comparing these results, a persistent problem because of brief reporting, makes conclusions necessarily tentative.

Personality Following Brain Lesions and Ablations

Research on personality functioning following brain lesions and ablations has been based chiefly upon the use of the Rorschach test. A major difficulty arises in conclusions drawn from the Rorschach since it is apparent that the critical factors leading to differentiation of organic patients from others derive not from general personality characteristics as much as from disturbances in thinking and perception of the types described above.

The practical usefulness of the Rorschach in studies of brain injury is emphasized in a number of studies. Aita, Reitan, and Ruth (5) compared 60 patients with posttraumatic brain injury with 100 controls representing a heterogeneous group of hospital patients. While quantitative analysis of Rorschach records yielded no consistent picture, use of certain of Piotrowski's qualitative signs (218), e.g., impotence, perplexity, repetition, and color-naming, in addition to other signs suggesting extreme concreteness, catastrophic reactions, inflexibility, and vagueness, proved helpful. Many neurotic-like signs, depression, anxiety, and hypochondriasis were also found among the organics. Insufficient data are presented for more definitive evaluation of the discriminability of these signs, but it is clear that disturbance in the capacity for abstract thinking manifested by rigidity and extreme concreteness emerged primarily.

Koff (168) similarly reports the usefulness of the Piotrowski (218) signs in differentiating postconcussion neurotics from patients with spinal tap evidence of brain involvement. Again, differentiation is based chiefly upon those aspects of Rorschach performance which may well reflect thought and perceptual disturbances as the primary impairment. Further evidence which supports the value of a related technique calling for subjects to draw impressions from the Rorschach cards comes in a series of papers (51, 104, 179). Using both the Rorschach and the Graphic Rorschach, Grassi (104) reports ten signs generally similar to those of Piotrowski which proved most discriminating between organics and other syndromes. A distinction between blot and concept dominance in performance is made by these authors who point out the extent to which brain-injured patients are blot-dominated.

The general trend of results suggests again primarily primitive thinking and concreteness rather than a basic personality disturbance.

Similar indication of a perceptual and thinking impairment is suggested by the work of Hughes (143), who derived a new list of Rorschach signs to differentiate organics from other groups of patients and normals by factor analysis. Another study by Ross and Ross (231) evaluated a number of different clusters of signs and, after extensive manipulation, developed a fairly complex scoring system of "instability" and "disability" ratings that differentiated normals from neurotics and brain-damaged patients.

The "sign" approach, as seen in these studies, seems to work fairly well with brain-injured patients, but extensive cross-validation seems essential. There has been little effort to establish the reliability of various "signs." In general, qualitative analyses of the Rorschach protocols seem to be most successful in selecting brain-injured patients. The sign approach, excessively empirical, gives little real feeling for the basic personality factors that emerge as a consequence of brain injury. It should be noted that signs described, such as impotence, perplexity, inflexibility, etc., are not intrinsic, specifically called forth by the Rorschach blots. They merely represent behavioral evidences of slowed reaction times, abnormal concreteness, perceptual disturbances, and awareness of impaired functioning. It seems that the Rorschach has thus far offered little that is new toward our understanding of the personality of the brain-damaged. However, the value of intensive Rorschach studies of individuals with brain damage is brought out by several case studies (2, 71, 207, 306).

Somewhat unique in the field of personality studies of the brain-injured is a research by Anderson and Honvik (17) comparing Minnesota Multiphasic Personality Inventory profiles of patients with frontal lobe lesions and with parietal involvement. The frontal lobe patients approximated the clinical picture of the "hysteriod reaction type" while the parietal patients more closely resembled that of the "anxiety neurosis." Since this study lacked any normal or neurotic control groups and since no estimate of the degree of overlap is presented, conclusions remain tentative.

Summarizing the results of the meager personality studies of brain-injured patients, it would appear that in general these patients manifest abnormal concreteness, diffuse and overly generalized modes of organizing their experiences, uncontrollable emotional outbursts, diffuse anxiety ("catastrophic reactions"), and a profound sense of personal inadequacy (1, 5, 104, 148, 155, 179, 306). Lacking in the studies of the personality of the brain-injured has been any attempt to consider the personality dynamics and the adequacy of interpersonal relationships following brain damage of various types. Comparatively little effort at systematically observing social interaction patterns of the brain-injured has been reported, although some authors (6, 94, 203, 278) have referred to problems of this sort.

Psychological Concomitants of Epilepsy

Psychological studies of patients with conclusive seizures diagnosed as epileptics have sought generally to answer two questions: Is there evidence of psychological deficit or deterioration in patients with epileptic seizures? Are there distinctive personality types or patterns of traits characteristic of epileptic patients? Since epilepsy has generally been considered a physiochemical disease (177), treatment has been largely by chemical means. For many years, it was felt that the chemical disturbance in the brain led necessarily to mental deterioration. By 1943, sufficient data had appeared in a variety of studies to lead Lenox (177) to conclude in his review that mental deterioration was by no means a concomitant of idiopathic epilepsy. A number of studies employing psychometric intelligence tests, usually the Stanford-Binet, failed to find any signs of deterioration (18, 74, 245, 252).

Concern in the past decade has centered not only upon evidence of deterioration but upon exploring characteristic performance patterns of idiopathic epileptics with standard intelligence scales. Collins and Lenox (61) studied a large, heterogeneous group of epileptic outpatients with the Wechsler-Bellevue and found that the group was of better than average intelligence, probably the result of a socioecomonic selective factor in the group studied. A somewhat better controlled study by Sands and Price (239) compared Wechsler-Bellevue patterns of idiopathic epileptics with and without "personality problems." The groups showed average intelligence with only slight differences in their patterns.

Somewhat more definitive findings based on better controlled studies have been reported by Goldman (91) and Winfield (298). The former compared Wechsler-Bellevue patterns of equated groups of idiopathic epileptics, patients with hysterical seizures, and patients with brain lesions but without seizures. In general, the epileptic patients and neurotics showed a similar pattern and both groups differed strikingly from the patients with organic damage, whose performance was generally impaired in the areas of concentration and abstract thinking. No impairment in intellectual functioning was observed in the idiopathic epileptics.

In a similar study Winfield (298) compared intellectual performances of well-equated groups of idiopathic ("cryptogenic") epileptics, symptomatic epileptics with known lesions, posttraumatic brain-injured patients without seizures, and normal controls. Where possible, school IQ or military test scores were used to insure matching of premorbid intelligence levels. Brief tests of verbal meaning, spatial relations, reasoning, associate learning, and abstraction were employed. Results indicated no significant differences between the controls and the idiopathic epileptics, while the two groups with known brain damage showed significantly lower scores in all areas. As in the study of Goldman (91), the seizure symptom seemed less significant than the factor of structural brain damage in relation to intellectual impairment.

In general, results of recent studies of the intellectual performance of idiopathic epileptics do not provide any evidence of intellectual deterioration or of any clear-cut characteristic pattern of performance unique to these patients. The importance of distinguishing between the clearly idiopathic or cryptogenic epileptics and those who show seizures following traumatic head injury or tumor has been indicated, since in the latter group intellectual impairment does seem to occur.

 A more complex problem in the psychological study of epilepsy has been the attempt to delineate a personality pattern characteristic of epileptic patients. Psychological research in this area has largely been restricted to Rorschach studies, following the original descriptions by Rorschach of a number of signs observed in epileptics. Rorschach's signs suggest a general lowered mental functioning level, poor emotional control, and difficulty in abstraction. These findings, partially confirmed by Guirdham (109), may, however, be a function of the use of heterogeneous, institutionalized epileptics, many of whom may have been symptomatic cases. Rorschach studies (19, 125, 169) revealed no peculiarly epileptic patterning, although tendencies toward poor emotional control were frequently observed. Lisansky (185), in a comparison of idiopathic epileptics and diabetics, while yielding no clear-cut pattern, pointed to slower responsivity and a greater evidence of "neurotic signs" among the epileptic population. The findings of these studies agree chiefly in the long response time observed, poor form quality, emotional constriction, and poor emotional control. In view of the heterogeneous nature of the epileptic samples, however, the findings, which strongly resemble those for brain-injured patients on the Rorschach, are difficult to interpret.

The study by Goldman (91) is one of the few employing well-matched groups. Goldman found no clearly defined personality pattern for the idiopathic epileptics. They did, however, show quantitative and qualitative manifestations in the Rorschach of greater drive for achievement, poorly controlled emotionality, immaturity, lowered "inner control and poise," inward turning of affect, and sexual disturbance. In general, the epileptics resembled the hysterical seizure patients more closely than the brain tumor patients in these personality characteristics. These results, while somewhat limited because of the absence of normal controls, point to a strong emotional involvement in epileptics.

PSYCHOSURGERY

Attempts to determine the functions of the frontal lobes in man, based upon studies of individuals with brain pathology, have been hampered by the lack of evaluations of premorbid behavior, the uncontrolled destruction of brain tissue, and the frequent difficulty in localization of areas affected. The various psychosurgical procedures developed may avoid these problems to some extent, but not without many seriously limiting complications. While individuals with presumably anatomically intact brains are subjected to relatively deliberate brain damage, these persons necessarily are in the midst of great emotional upheaval whether they suffer from excruciating pain, severe neuroses, or psychoses. In many cases, preoperative measures of specific functions are not obtainable. Limiting the population to accessible patients introduces a sampling bias of unknown direction and degree. When examination is possible, the reliability of the obtained data, particularly with psychotic patients, is open to question. The assessment of postoperative impairment of changes in functioning is additionally hampered by the fact that many of these persons were impaired intellectually as a result of emotional factors prior to the introduction of a brain lesion.

Essentially, frontal lobe tissue can be rendered nonfunctioning by three methods: (*a*) direct attack on the thalamus, a technique called thalamotomy or stereoencephalotomy; (*b*) cutting into the white matter and destroying varying numbers of fibers connecting the cortex and the thalamus — lobotomy, leucotomy, cortical undercutting, etc.; (*c*) excision or destruction of the cortex — prefrontal lobectomy (215), topectomy (199), gyrectomy (212), and thermocoagulation and venous ligation (200). These diverse techniques have been developed in attempts to improve upon surgical procedures and to avoid some of the undesirable personality changes accompanying the techniques as employed initially. Surgical precision, however, appears to lag far behind the specificity of the hypotheses underlying these variations. In postmortem studies Meyer and McLardy (201) reported great variability in the anatomical lesions produced in lobotomized patients regardless of the intentions of the neurosurgeon. In direct attacks upon the cortex, accuracy generally is not increased because of individual differences in human brains and the lack of clear differentiation among areas. Even in thalamotomy, which in theory appears to be a most precise method, additional damage may result from the gases generated during electrolysis and interference with blood vessels (200). The large variety of pyschosurgical techniques plus the possibility of considerable variation in the extent of the lesions produced by means of any one operative procedure contribute to the difficulty of evaluating experimental findings in terms of altered functions.

Many uncontrolled factors are also at play after surgery which obscure and confound changes in functioning. Social improvement or at least increased cooperativeness is a frequently reported concomitant along with altered attitudes of clinical personnel and relatives. Attempts to organize the many and apparently contradictory findings of various investigations are difficult because of inadequate experimental designs. Samples are generally small; adequate control subjects are rarely available; the time of testing, both pre- and postoperatively, varies considerably within as well as among studies; practice effects are generally ignored; and statistical evaluation of data is frequently omitted or inadequate. In an attempt to bring some structure into this confusion, the present review will deal as much as possible with data from specific techniques rather than with the interpretations made by the various authors.

Standardized Intellectual Tests

Table 1 presents a summary of the data in a number of studies in which standardized intellectual tests (Stanford-Binet and Wechsler-Bellevue) were administered pre- and postoperatively with quantitative data reported. Examination of the postoperative changes reveals that most of these studies show a decrement in IQ for operated patients, which in several instances in quite large or statistically significant (172, 197, 214, 238, 304). Nonsignificant changes are reported in the others (191, 199, 200, 262, 272).

Before evaluating these findings, practice effects must be assessed. In the first Columbia-Greystone report (199), Form I of the Wechsler-Bellevue was administered once preoperatively and twice postoperatively. In the second investigation (200), Form I was given twice preoperatively and twice postoperatively and Form II at the fifth session. While both operated and control groups manifested fairly consistent increases in IQ, the operated groups gained less (statistically not significant) than the control groups. The apparent increment in intellectual ability can thus be attributed to other factors, most likely practice. This effect also is evident in Form II of the Wechsler-Bellevue test, although to a lesser extent than in Form I. The question now arises as to the possibility that the decrements reported in the other studies might be of greater magnitude had control groups been available for comparison. Information concerning possible practice effects are practically necessary to evaluate the McCullough (191) and Rylander (238) studies, which involved more than one retest. In retesting the same patients nine months postoperatively, Petrie (213) reports that the significant loss in IQ persisted, suggesting that with sufficient time interval between retests, practice effects may be minimized.

Notwithstanding the possible practice effects, all but two of the studies in which data are presented, show some decrement in postoperative performance in comparison to preoperative IQ or control group scores. Some investigators who employed other intelligence test batteries also report postoperative losses in IQ (13, 24, 172). These studies, while not entirely conclusive, strongly suggest that intellectual impairment measurable by means of standardized test techniques does occur following therapeutic destruction of frontal lobe tissue.

With regard to preoperative level and severity of illness, several factors stand out which should be considered in further studies. The higher the preoperative intellectual level, the more likely a large or significant decrease postoperatively (197, 214, 238, 304). In testing a hypothesis dealing with increased variability in the behavior of post-topectomy patients, Wittenborn and Mettler (299) found that ten psychotic patients with relatively high preoperative Wechsler-Bellevue scores tended to decrease more than four controls with similar initial scores. Fernandes (76), although giving no data, mentions that patients obtaining higher preoperative scores tended to drop while those with low scores tended to increase. In Table 1, the patients who obtain the higher IQ's are, for the most part, diagnosed as neurotic rather than psychotic. It seems likely that more accurate and valid estimates of intellectual ability can be obtained with neurotics, so that the impairment that occurs following psychosurgery is more readily observed in these patients. The investigation of patients lobotomized for relief from pain, moreover, reveals a large postoperative decrement (172). To what extent the severe pain interfered with optimal functioning is not known, but the postoperative relief apparently was not sufficient to overcome the loss due to brain lesion. A complicating factor in studying such populations is the fact that many of these patients are approaching death rapidly. A nonoperated control group or at least repeated examination seems essential.

With regard to the Verbal and Performance scales of the Wechsler-Bellevue, higher Verbal than Performance losses have been reported (153, 172, 214, 304). The differential effects on Verbal and Performance tasks, however, cannot be evaluated without a control group for comparison. Abilities measured by performance tests may be as impaired as verbal functions following psychosurgery, but the impairment may be obscured by improvement due to differential practice

TABLE I. SUMMARY OF STUDIES PRESENTING PRE- AND POSTOPERATIVE IQ's FOR PSYCHOSURGERY PATIENTS

Author	N	Diagnostic Category	Surgical Technique	Test	Mean Preoperative IQ	Time of Post-test	Mean IQ Change	Remarks
Porteus & Kepner (220)	18	Psychotic	lobotomy	SB	83.9	varied	—3.2	modified Stanford-Binet
Rylander (238)	5	Neurotic	lobotomy	SB	116.2	varied	—11.6*	calculation by these authors
Strom-Olsen et al. (262)	11	Psychotic	lobotomy	SB	94.3	6 wks.	—2.2	calculation by Crown (67)
Yacorzynski et al. (304)	1	Psychotic	lobotomy	SB	118	3 mos.	—21	pt. received two preoperative WB's
				WB	104.5	3 mos.	—17.5	
Koskoff et al. (172)	5	Normals with intractable pain	lobotomy	WB	87.2	3 mos.	—20.4*	
Malmo (197)	6	Neurotic	5 lobotomy 1 gyrectomy	WB	107.8	1–3 mos.	—8.3*	WB Form II on retest
McCullough (191)	10	Psychotic	lobotomy	WB	83.4	2 mos.	2.9	mean IQ change calculated from 2nd postoperative test
Petrie (214)	20	Neurotic	lobotomy	WB	105.8	2–3 mos.	—5.0*	
Vidor (272)	21	Neurotic & Psychotic	lobotomy	WB or SB	111.5	varied	0.6	16 pts. received SB 5 pts. received WB
King (199)		Psychotic	topectomy	WB	101.7	3 wks.	3.9	surgical group gained 3.7 points less than control group
Sheer et al. (200)	20	Psychotic	misc.	WB	79.3	6 mos.	3.4	WB Form II on retest. Surgical group gained 4.5 points less than control group

* Significant at .05 level of confidence.

effects. Such improvement also makes it difficult to evaluate the permanence of any changes, although Petrie's study (213) does suggest the possibility of permanent impairment. Social improvement does not seem to bear a relationship to intellectual change as measured by standardized intellectual tests (199, 200).

Miscellaneous Cognitive Functions

In dealing with the more specific aspects of cognitive ability, such as planning ability, abstract ability, memory, learning, attention, etc., the reported findings become considerably more difficult to evaluate because of the variety of tests employed which presumably measure these functions. In examining these functions by means of the specific tests employed rather than the purported specific functions, the confusion is alleviated somewhat, and it is possible to suggest trends.

Porteus Mazes

Despite the susceptibility to practice effects of a performance test such as the Porteus Mazes, impairment below the obtained preoperative level is revealed in many studies on the *first* postoperative examination (197, 199, 200, 214, 220, 221). The time of the first postoperative test varies considerably among and occasionally within studies, but the immediate effects of surgery probably are not involved. Crown (67), reanalyzing Porteus and Kepner's and Porteus and Peter's (220, 221) data, reports that 23 patients whose first postoperative tests took place after three or more months show a highly significant decrement. Preoperative tests were not administered by Robinson (83), but a significant 3.3-year difference in favor of a socially improved nonoperated psychotic control group over the lobotomized group was found. Two studies (153, 262) show insignificant improvement following psychosurgery. The group Jones (153) employed, however, obtained almost a minimal score preoperatively.

A summary of the data of several studies in which the Porteus Mazes were administered pre- and postoperatively is presented in Table 2. Only the changes in the first postoperative examinations are given. Generally, additional examinations result in gains which eventually reach or exceed the preoperative level, but Sheer *et al.* (200) point out that the operated group gained less from practice than did the nonoperated controls. In the first Columbia-Greystone study (199), one year posttopectomy the surgical group had attained the same mental age level as the nonoperated controls. In Petrie's nine months postoperative study (213), the lobotomized patients did not regain the immediate postoperative loss completely, but the difference was no longer significant. Possibly the practice effect was reduced by the six-month interval between tests.

Porteus and Peters (221) and King (199) believed that a pattern of distinct loss on immediate postoperative testing followed by gains up to or beyond the preoperative level in subsequent examinations is

TABLE 2. SUMMARY OF STUDIES GIVING PORTEUS MAZES TO PSYCHOSURGERY
PATIENTS PRE- AND POSTOPERATIVELY

Author	N	Diagnostic Category	Surgical Technique	Preoperative Mean MA	Time of Posttest	Mean MA Change	Remarks
Jones (153)	24	Psychotic	lobotomy	5.0	3 wks.	3.0	
Koskoff et al. (172)	3	Normals with intractable pain	lobotomy	not given	3 mos.	− 4.1	
Petrie (214)	20	Neurotic	lobotomy	not given	3 mos.	− 1.8 *	
Porteus & Peters (221), Porteus & Kepner (220)	72	Psychotic	lobotomy	11.3	varied	− 1.7 *	combined data analyzed by Crown (67)
Strom-Olsen et al. (262)	11	Psychotic	lobotomy	12.0	6 wks.	0.1	calculated by Crown (67)
King (199)	19	Psychotic	topectomy	13.2	3 wks.	− 1.2	surgical group mean MA is 2.2 yrs. below control
Sheer et al. (200)	23	Psychotic	misc.	10.8	10 days	− 1.5	immediate preoperative MA (2nd pretest) is presented

* Significant at or beyond .05 level of confidence.

related to social recovery. This observation merits further investigation.

Abstract Thinking

Studies which report impairment on standardized intellectual tests also find impaired abstract ability (197, 214, 238, 304). Rylander (238) gained this impression from interpretation of proverbs and fables and the definitions of certain abstract words. Petrie (214) similarly supports this view through the use of the Stanford-Binet proverbs. In addition, however, several studies which report no over-all intellectual impairment do report some decrement in ability to think abstractly (78, 105, 160, 199, 200).

Studies employing the Capps Homograph test consistently report a decrement in the ability to shift. Malmo (197) reports a slight but definite impairment. The first Columbia-Greystone project (199) found a statistically significant decrease ten days posttopectomy. While most patients regained the original loss, the decrease in the ability to make verbal shifts was not regained after one year in six of the 19 subjects. In the second Columbia-Greystone investigation (200) the definite loss was confirmed at the ten-day postoperative test. The loss was regained at the end of 30 days owing to reacquisition of identical definitions originally given but lost postoperatively. Such studies suggest that psychosurgery results in a definite, but probably transient, deficit in verbal ability to shift.

Various sorting, grouping, and block design tasks are less consistently reported to reveal loss due to frontal lobe surgery. Employing the Goldstein-Scheerer tests with 42 lobotomized patients, Atwell (23) found only slight impairment. Grassi (105) found that patients who showed no general intellectual impairment, evinced a temporary reduction in achievement on his Block Substitution Test. This decrement was almost completely eliminated at the end of a year. Practice effects were not considered. Freudenberg and Robertson (85) report a significant postoperative loss on the Kohs Blocks. The operatees also gained significantly less than did controls on a sorting test. With the modified Kohs Blocks, Weigl color-form, and the Halstead Object-Sorting tests, Kisker (160) concluded that some impairment does occur postoperatively.

While King (199), employing a wide number of measures of abstraction, failed to show any posttopectomy group changes, certain patients did show abstraction difficulties postoperatively which suggested the possibility that such deficit might be related to specific areas of the cortex excised. In the second project (200), postoperative deficit on a modified Weigl test at the ten-day retest was evident, with the loss regained by most patients at the three-month retest.

Some improvement on the color-form sorting test is reported by Jones (153), but no controls were used to determine the amount of gain attributable to practice. Hunt (81) and Strom-Olsen et al. (262) report no change in pre- and posttesting with the Kohs Blocks while studies employing the Shipley-Hartford consistently report no impairment postoperatively (14, 79, 228, 262).

Memory, Learning, Attention

Although memory and related functions have been found to be extremely sensitive to impairment associated with brain pathology in clinical situations, the reported investigations of individuals undergoing psychosurgery have not been fruitful. The gross attention and concentration difficulties characteristic of emotionally disturbed persons probably interfere markedly with preoperative assessment of these functions. Some studies simply report no gross or permanent changes postoperatively (13, 14, 194, 238). Extremely varied results on rote memory tasks are reported by many investigators (24, 153, 191, 197, 228). Thus, Freudenberg and Robertson (85) report significant memory loss postoperatively in a group of 24 lobotomized patients on paired associates and recall of the Bender-Gestalt figures, but no impairment in memory for objects, perhaps because of the greater concreteness of the latter task. A fairly comprehensive investigation of memory and learning was undertaken by Stauffer (199). Control and topectomy groups learned semimeaningful and meaningful paired-associate lists and a paragraph of verbal directions preoperatively. In general, retention of previously learned material and the ability to learn new material was unaffected by topectomy.

King (199) also included in his study of intellectual functions, a continuous-problem task which utilized an instrument intended for selection of pilots by the Army Air Forces. The test involved a complicated choice reaction which permitted obtaining a measure of "the patient's ability to perform on a task requiring close attention and sustained effort over a period of time." While the topectomy group suffered no marked impairment on this task, the control group manifested a greater trend in the direction of more problems solved and fewer errors than did the operated group. Robinson (83, 228), testing the capacity for prolonged attention and deliberation by means of simple arithmetic problems, rhyming, and three of the Downey Will-Temperament Tests, reports clearcut deficit in the lobotomized group as compared to nonoperated controls. Malmo (197) also found that deliberation was reduced postoperatively as indicated by more rapid performance on Raven's Progressive Matrices Test. Reduction in time and score on the Matrices Test as well as very rapid performance on the MMPI postoperatively was observed by Vidor (272). In the Columbia-Greystone project the topectomized group showed a trend toward poorer performance in addition tests, but not significantly different from the controls. A subtraction test showed significant changes in variability attributable to the operation. On a cancellation test, Rylander (238) reports a decrease one month postoperatively with subsequent gains to preoperative level. Hunt (81), however, reports postoperative increased time with improvement in accuracy on a cancellation test, as well as improvement in immediate memory.

Sensory Functions

The relief of intractable pain by means of psychosurgery is apparently afforded without increasing the threshold for pain. Using ordinary clinical tests in neurological examination of such patients, Watts and Freeman (274) failed to disclose any evidence of impaired sensation. Indeed, Chapman, Rose, and Solomon (55) report increased withdrawal reactions to pin prick are not uncommon in lobotomized patients. Following up this clinical impression and employing the Hardy-Wolff-Goodell apparatus for more accurate evaluation, they found that postoperatively their group of 23 psychiatric patients withdrew their heads from the apparatus at less intense levels of stimulation than before lobotomy. Over a two-year period, consistent trends toward a return to preoperative threshold levels were revealed (56). Malmo (197) also found a much higher rate of withdrawal after lobotomy. King *et al.* (158) supported these findings in a study of five patients operated unilaterally for relief of pain. In the second Columbia-Greystone study (200), slightly reduced thresholds were observed in only two of the nine operated patients. In this study, the radiant heat was applied to the forearm rather than the forehead.

Extensive psychophysiological studies were employed in both Columbia-Greystone projects. No marked losses or consistent changes were found in auditory acuity, visual acuity, peripheral vision, brightness discrimination, color vision, time judgment, autokinetic effect, critical flicker frequency, recognition of tachistoscopically exposed stimuli, or various motor tasks.

Personality

In his review of the clinical studies of lobotomized patients Crown (67) points out that "almost invariably . . . *personality changes* have followed the operation." These changes are in the direction of increased cheerfulness, complacency, apathy, restlessness, shallowness of affect, indifference to criticism and feelings of others, and decreased self-consciousness, reserve, and tact. Kolb (171) also points out that there is little difference of opinion among clinicians as to the nature of the personality changes following lobotomy.

Rating scales have been employed in several studies (153, 226, 244), which generally found improved ward behavior. Cooperativeness, sociability, and tidiness are increased; anxiety, depression, and bizarre behavior are decreased. Affect and feeling are adversely affected in the direction of greater apathy (226). Lack of initiative is also noted (244). In a series of ratings, Jones (153) indicates that for the group, over-all behavior did not improve after the eighth week postoperatively. A time sample of behavior was obtained for surgical patients alone and in pairs by Kinder and Willenson (200) with no changes in patterns of behavior apparent following surgery. Patients under 40 showed some increase in activity while those over 40 manifested a decrease. Bockoven and Hyde (106) observed 16 patients pre- and postlobotomy in groups, recording sociograms of the patients' interactions. Improvement in psychiatric cases was generally accompanied by increased socialization and development of a friendly democratic attitude toward other patients. It is possible that increased familiarity with observers and examiners and the additional attention may lead to improvement and reduction in anxiety.

The necessity for control groups is suggested by the findings of Wittenborn and Mettler (299). Employing symptom rating scales, no significant differences between the topectomized and control groups were found; both groups manifested a reduction in symptomatology. Indeed, a return of certain pathological symptoms was noted in some surgical patients who had been free from such pathology prior to topectomy.

Noticeable lessening of psychotic symptomatology is reported for lobotomized patients in studies employing personality inventories (14, 81, 199, 272, 304). Standardized interviews, utilized to obtain attitudes dealing with feelings of guilt, religion, sex, and prejudice failed to reveal any over-all attitudinal changes (200). Employing a sensibility questionnaire to measure degree of concern with one's past and future and with the opinions of others and a self-regarding span (a measure of the time spent talking about oneself), Robinson (83) compared a lobotomized group with a nonoperated control group and found that the operated patients showed less self-preoccupation, less concern with the past, future, and opinions of others Thus, for the most part the feelings and attitudes expressed by patients undergoing psychosurgery are in accord with the clinical observations and ratings made of their behavior.

In summarizing the Rorschach data for the first Columbia-Greystone project, Zubin (199) points out that some subjects showed altered personality trends, but that no definite patterns of changes emerged. Analysis of group changes revealed a pronounced decline in reaction time for the operated patients. Suggested trends were post-topectomy decreases in number of responses and factors primarily associated with anxiety, ambitiousness, conflict, introspection, and perceptual accuracy. Atwell (23) also reports increased constriction, perseveration, and stereotypy along with less spontaneity, initiative, and fantasy. The most marked postoperative change in Atwell's study was the patient's carefree and unconcerned approach to the Rorschach. Similar changes in Rorschach factors also emerged in studies employing fewer subjects (86, 304). Jones (153) found an increase in responses, but taking into account the initially constricted record and possible practice effects of repeated testing, these results do not contradict the above-mentioned studies.

Some retest changes apparently may occur regardless of surgery according to Wittenborn and Mettler (299). Employing a novel Rorschach measure (lack-of-perceptual-control score), revealed by responses in which form is absent or secondary to color or shading, they found a significant difference between topectomized patients and controls. <u>Topectomy patients increased in "lack of perceptual control" postoperatively while control patients showed a decrease in this measure.</u>

In a comparison of pre- and postlobotomy Rorschach records of 40 patients, Hunt (81) reports greater constriction two weeks postoperatively. Somewhat contradictory to the other studies are findings of increased populars and testing time and decreased perseveration and self-references. The patients also manifested less reluctance in their approach to the task, less self-criticism and concern over performance. Amaral (13) reports an almost identical picture postoperatively for 18 patients.

In a study on creative ability, Hutton and Bassett (147) indicate that the Rorschach, the Harrower-Erickson Multiple-Choice Rorschach, a story-telling, and a drawing test reveal a lessening of creative ability in leucotomized patients. Few patients, however, manifested a creative urge prior to the operation. In a later study, Ashby and Bassett (21) employed a drawing test and found no difference between operatees and psychotic controls. Both patient groups did worse than normal control subjects.

Ashby and Bassett (22) studied that psychogalvanic response of 21 lobotomized patients and 21 controls to real and symbolic (unfulfilled) threat. Six patients were also studied pre- and postoperatively. No uniform postoperative trends emerged; the symbolic threats retained the power of eliciting the psychogalvanic response. Thus, the authors conclude that <u>emotional drive is not diminished by lobotomy.</u> ✳

Petrie (214) report<u>s a postoperative decrease in neuroticism as manifested by reduced body sway suggestibility and a smoother work curve in a neurotic group. Diminished introversion was also evident as revealed by loss in persistence, a tendency to go for speed rather than accuracy, reduced self-blame, greater reality adjustment on level-of-aspiration tests, and a tendency to live in the present.</u>

<u>In general, personality studies do suggest a decrease in depression</u> ✳ <u>and anxiety following psychosurgery.</u> These changes seem to occur at the expense of greater personality constriction, decreased critical standards and regard for others. Evaluation of the presence of "organic" indicators is obscured by their presence in preoperative Rorschach records (161, 271) or by the overlap with postoperative psychotic residuals.

CONCLUSIONS

The last decade has witnessed a significant change in the orientation of research in the field of organic brain dysfunction. Klebanoff (164), in his earlier review, had concluded that psychological studies in this field had been concerned primarily with relating mental functions to localized areas of the brain, the determination of the presence of brain pathology on the basis of psychological test performance, and the definition of an "organic psychological syndrome." Methodologically, essential reliance had been placed upon the use of omnibus test techniques such as the Stanford-Binet and Rorschach. However, the beginning of a trend toward the use of more specialized test techniques had been observed.

 The period covered by the present review reveals decreased emphasis upon localization and diagnosis and a concomitant increase of interest in the developmental aspects of brain injury, emphasis upon patterns of functioning through the use of specialized tests including laboratory methods, and an overly hasty concentration of effort upon the psychological consequences of psychosurgery.

During the past ten years, increased theoretical sophistication and research findings have served to dispel the earlier optimism concerning the ability of psychological test techniques to contribute toward localization of brain pathology. The correlation of psychological test performance with specific areas of brain damage has been found to be limited by vast differences in brain pathology caused by different types of injury or disease as well as by serious limitations in the techniques of anatomical localization. In general, psychological instruments have proven incapable of differentiating patients with presumptive injury to specific cortical areas. Indeed, the limited number of studies which do report such differentiation merit repetition or cross-validation, an apparent constant necessity in this field of research.

The continued development of specialized test methods reflects the inability of conventional psychometric techniques to reveal clear pictures of organic impairment. Thus, the considerable research employing the Wechsler-Bellevue scale reveals that although the test as a whole proves relatively insensitive for diagnostic purposes in patients with brain injury, certain of the subtests appear to be quite discriminating in numerous studies. In addition, the trend toward the use of laboratory perceptual techniques, such as the critical flicker fusion, the phi phenomenon, and the tachistoscopic presentation of stimuli, have opened additional horizons for study and merit concerted research exploration. These methods do reveal promise, but one is not yet able to evaluate their ultimate significance as differentiating techniques.

A further significant development in recent years has been the rather extensive research upon children with organic brain disease. Analysis of the deficit findings in children with brain damage reveals that the impairment tends generally to parallel that observed in adults with brain damage. There is, however, the definite suggestion that children with brain pathology manifest marked unevenness and inconsistency in the development of their intellectual capacities, and this may indicate more generalized cerebral localization of function in children. The research directed toward differentiating endogenous and exogenous feebleminded children has suggested promising new psychological approaches and techniques in addition to making interesting theoretical contributions.

Finally, it is felt that subsequent research in this field should recognize the importance of the interaction of such related variables as environment and premorbid personality of patients with organic brain damage. It is apparent that intellectual deficit must be evaluated in relation to the richness and complexity of past and present environmental situations. Indeed, the tempo and degree of so-called deterioration in certain senile and organic conditions may be determined significantly by the nature of social and other environmental factors. In addition, numerous questions arise that emphasize the need for additional research dealing with the matter of personality changes believed to be associated with organic brain disease. For example, do existing intellectual limitations present the appearance of fundamental personality alteration or are there basic qualitative changes in the premorbid drives, motives, and basic personality dynamics of patients following organic brain insult?

It is unfortunate that most studies of personality changes in organic brain disease have utilized the Rorschach test and reliance upon test signs which have not been adequately cross-validated. A more fruitful evaluation might involve an approach aimed at an analysis of the particular social, familial, and personal demands made upon the patient with organic brain damage. Following such an analysis of expected and desired behavior, specialized psychological techniques might be employed to evaluate the capacities required to fulfill these environmental demands. Such an approach would appear to offer extremely vital information concerning the consequences of brain injury or ablation. At the present time, there is a striking absence of psychological research designed to understand the altered dynamic field of the adult with brain injury. Similarly, there is a need for scientific investigation of the relationship between such variables as premorbid personality and socioeconomic and cultural milieu in relation to mode of adjustment to brain disease.

When one considers the literature dealing with psychosurgery, the results prove generally to be disconcerting. Although inconsistent and paradoxical results are observed when identical test techniques are employed, there are some trends in the results reflected in Tables 1 and 2. The varied conclusions in this area of research appear to be a consequence of numerous kinds of errors. First, psychosurgery is an extremely broad term and subsumes a large number of different surgical procedures involving varying degrees of destruction of brain tissue. Second, when psychometric and psychological test techniques are utilized with severely psychotic patients, the reliability or representativeness of the results may be questioned. Third, the results in the majority of the studies are not comparable since different or heterogeneous diagnostic groups of patients were employed. Finally, a large number of studies dealing with the effects of psychosurgery have been marked by faulty experimental design, particularly by absence of the use of adequate control groups.

Despite the difficulties cited above, it is possible to extract some generalizations regarding the impact of therapeutic psychosurgery. For example, in those patients whose preoperative test performance was not markedly disturbed, there is some suggestion of impairment in general intelligence, abstract thinking ability, memory functioning, learning ability, and sustained attention. Qualitative evaluation of personality changes appears to indicate a more apathetic, less complex, and constricted individual who shows less introspective concern with himself and less depression of mood following lobotomy. It is clear, however, that experimental knowledge of the sequelae of psychosurgery remains restricted and conflicting. Continued research is necessary in this field with subsequent emphasis upon experimental design and the use of control groups.

The present review has attempted to organize and integrate the extensive literature dealing with organic brain damage over the past decade. The voluminous body of literature covered reflects adequately the degree of scientific preoccupation with this area of research. It appears that the change in emphasis from mere diagnosis and localization in the direction of the study of related variables represents a scientifically healthy reorientation. The introduction of laboratory test methods represents significant continued exploration of the utility of specialized techniques. It is felt, finally, that future research upon the patient with organic brain disease should regard him as a complex individual whose social, economic, and intellectual environmental demands must be considered in order to attain total understanding of the specific consequences of brain pathology.

REFERENCES

1. Abbot, W. D., Due, F. O., & Nosik, W. A. Subdural hematoma and effusion as a result of blast injuries. *J. Amer. med. Ass.*, 1943, 121: 739–741.

2. Ackerly, S. S., & Benton, A. L. Report of case of bilateral frontal lobe defect. *Res. Publ. Ass. nerv. ment. Dis.*, 1950, 27: 479–504.

3. Acklesberg, S. B. Vocabulary and mental deterioration in senile dementia. *J. abnorm. soc. Psychol.*, 1944, 39: 393–406.

4. Aita, J. A., Armitage, S. G., Reitan, R. M., & Rabinowitz, A. The use of certain psychological tests in the evaluation of brain injury. *J. gen. Psychol.*, 1947, 37: 25–44.

5. Aita, J. A., Reitan, R. M., & Ruth, Jane M. Rorschach's test as a diagnostic aid in brain injury. *Amer. J. Psychiat.*, 1947, 103: 770–779.

6. Alexander, L. The element of psychotherapy in the treatment of organic neurologic disorders. *J. nerv. ment. Dis.*, 1951, 114: 283–306.

7. Allen, R. M. The test performance of the brain injured. *J. clin. Psychol.*, 1947, 3: 225–230.

8. Allen, R. M. A note on the use of the Bellevue-Wechsler Scale Mental Deterioration Index with brain-injured patients. *J. clin. Psychol.*, 1948, 4: 88–89.

9. Allen, R. M. The test performance of the brain diseased. *J. clin. Psychol.*, 1948, 4: 281–284.

10. Allen, R. M. A comparison of the test performance of the brain-injured and the brain-diseased. *Amer. J. Psychiat.*, 1949, 106: 195–198.

11. Allen, R. M. An analysis of the comparative evaluation of Allen's brain-injured patients and of normal subjects. *J. clin. Psychol.*, 1949, 5: 422–423.

12. Allen, R. M., & Krato, J. C. The test performance of the encephalopathic. *J. ment. Sci.*, 1949, 95: 369–372.

13. Amaral, M. A. Comparative results with Moniz's prefrontal leucotomy and Freeman's lobotomy. *First int. Cong. Psychosurg.*, Lisbon, 1949, 173–184.

14. Anderson, A. L. Personality changes following prefrontal lobotomy in a case of severe psychoneurosis. *J. consult. Psychol.*, 1949, 13: 105–107.

15. Anderson, A. L. The effect of laterality localization of brain damage on Wechsler-Bellevue indices of deterioration. *J. clin. Psychol.*, 1950, 6: 191–194.

16. Anderson, A. L. The effect of laterality localization of focal brain lesions on the Wechsler-Bellevue subtests. *J. clin. Psychol.*, 1951, 7: 149–153.

17. Anderson, A. L. & Hanvik, L. J. The psychometric localization of brain lesions; the differential effect of frontal and parietal lesions on MMPI profiles. *J. clin. Psychol.*, 1950, 6: 177–180.

18. Arieff, A. J., & Yacorzynski, G. Deterioration of patients with organic epilepsy. *J. nerv. ment. Dis.*, 1942, 96: 49–55.

19. Arluck, E. W. A study of some personality characteristics of epileptics. *Arch. Psychol.*, 1941, No. 263.

20. Armitage, S. G. An analysis of certain psychological tests used for the evaluation of brain injury. *Psychol. Monogr.*, 1946, 60: No. 1 (Whole No. 277).

21. Ashby, W. R., & Bassett, M. The effect of leucotomy on creative ability. *J. ment. Sci.*, 1949, 95: 418–430.

22. Ashby, W. R., & Bassett, M. The effect of prefrontal leucotomy on the psychogalvanic response. *J. ment. Sci.*, 1950, 96: 458–469.

23. Atwell, C. R. Psychometric changes after lobotomy. *J. nerv. ment. Dis.*, 1950, 111: 165–166.

24. Babcock, Harriet. A case of anxiety neurosis before and after lobotomy. *J. abnorm. soc. Psychol.*, 1947, 42: 466–472.

25. Baldwin, M. V. A clinico-experimental investigation into the psychological aspects of multiple sclerosis. *J. nerv. ment. Dis.*, 1952, 115: 299–343.

26. Barnes, T. C. Electroencephalographic validation of the Rorschach, Hunt, and Bender-Gestalt tests. *Amer. Psychologist*, 1950, 5: 322. (Abstract)

27. Battersby, W. S. Critical flicker frequency in patients with cerebral lesions. *Amer. Psychologist*, 1950, 5: 271–272. (Abstract)

28. Battersby, W. S. The regional gradient of critical flicker frequency after frontal or occipital lobe injury. *J. exp. Psychol.*, 1951, 42: 59–68.

29. Battersby, W. S., Bender, M. B., & Teuber, H. L. Effects of total light flux on critical flicker frequency after frontal lobe lesion. *J. exp. Psychol.*, 1951, 42: 135–142.

30. Battersby, W. S., Teuber, H. L., & Bender, M. B. Problem-solving behavior in men with frontal or occipital brain injuries. *Amer. Psychologist*, 1951, 7: 264–265. (Abstract)

31. Bender, Lauretta. Psychological principles of the Visual Motor Gestalt Test. *Trans. N. Y. Acad. Sci.*, 1949, 11: 164–170.

32. Bender, Lauretta. Psychological problems of children with organic disease. *Amer. J. Orthopsychiat.*, 1949, 19: 404–415.

33. Bender, Lauretta, & Silver, A. Body image problems of the brain-damaged child. *J. soc. Issues*, 1948, 4: 84–89.

34. Bender, M. B., & Furlow, L. T. Visual disturbances produced by bilateral lesions of the occipital lobes with central scotomas. *Arch. Neurol. Psychiat.*, 1945, 53: 165–170.

35. Bender, M. B., Shapiro, M. S., & Teuber, H. L. Allesthesia and disturbance of body schema. *Arch. Neurol. Psychiat.*, 1949, 62: 222–236.

36. Bender, M. B., & Teuber, H. L. Phenomena of fluctuation, extinction, and completion in visual perception. *Arch. Neurol. Psychiat.*, 1946, 55: 627–658.

37. Bender, M. B., & Teuber, H. L. Ring scotoma and tubular fields: their significance in cases of head injury. *Arch. Neurol. Psychiat.*, 1946, 56: 200–226.

38. Bender, M. B., & Teuber, H. L. Spatial organization of visual perception following injury to the brain. *Arch. Neurol. Psychiat.*, 1947, 58: 721–739; 1948, 59: 39–62.

39. Bender, M. B., & Teuber, H. L. Disorders in the visual perception of motion. *Trans. Amer. neurol. Ass.*, 1948, 73: 191–193.

40. Bender, M. B., & Teuber, H. L. Disorders in visual perception following cerebral lesions. *J. Psychol.*, 1949, 28: 223–233.

41. Bender, M. B., & Teuber, H. L. Psychopathology of vision. In E. A. Spiegel (Ed.), *Progress in neurology and psychiatry*. New York: Grune & Stratton, 1949. Pp. 163–192.

42. Bensberg, G. J. A test for differentiating endogenous and exogenous mental defectives. *Amer. J. ment. Def.*, 1950, 54: 502–506.

43. Benton, A. L., & Collins, Nancy T. Visual retention test performance in children, normative and clinical observations. *Arch. Neurol. Psychiat.*, 1949, 62: 610–617.

44. Benton, A. L., & Howell, L. I. The use of psychological tests in the evaluation of intellectual function. *Psychosom. Med.*, 1941, 3: 138–151.

45. Berliner, F., Mayer-Gross, W., Beveridge, R. L., & Moore, J. N. P. Prefrontal leucotomy: report on 100 cases. *Lancet*, 1945, 249: 325–328.

46. Bijou, S., & Werner, H. Language analysis in brain injured and nonbrain injured mentally deficient children. *J. genet. Psychol.*, 1945, 66: 239–254.

47. Blake, R., & McCarty, B. A comparative evaluation of the Bellevue-Wechsler Mental Deterioration Index distributions of Allen's brain-injured patients and normal subjects. *J. clin. Psychol.*, 1948, 4: 415–418.

48. Blatt, B., & Hecht, I. The personality structure of the multiple sclerosis patient as evaluated by the Rorschach psychodiagnostic technique. *J. clin. Psychol.*, 1951, 7: 341–344.

49. Botwinick, J., & Birren, J. E. The measurement of intellectual deterioration in senile psychosis and psychosis with cerebral arteriosclerosis. *Amer. Psychologist*, 1950, 5: 364–365. (Abstract)

50. Bridgman, O. A case study of gross brain damage. *Amer. J. ment. Def.*, 1941, 46: 195–197.

51. Brussel, J. A., Grassi, J. R., & Melniker, A. A. The Rorschach method and postconcussion syndrome. *Psychiat. Quart.*, 1942, 16: 707–743.

52. Busemann, A. Demenz als Dauerfolge von Hirnverletzungen. *Schweiz. Z. Psychol. Anwend.*, 1950, 9: 119–128.

53. Canter, A. H. Direct and indirect measures of psychological deficit in multiple sclerosis. *J. gen. Psychol.*, 1951, 44: 3–50.

54. Cattell, R. B. The measurement of adult intelligence. *Psychol. Bull.*, 1943, 40: 153–193.

55. Chapman, W. P., Rose, A. S., & Solomon, H. C. Measurement of heat stimulus producing motor withdrawal reaction in patients following frontal lobotomy. *Res. Publ. Assoc. nerv. ment. Dis.*, 1948, 27: 754–768.

56. Chapman, W. P., Rose, A. S., & Solomon, H. C. A follow-up study of motor withdrawal reaction to heat discomfort in patients before and after frontal lobotomy. *Amer. J. Psychiat.*, 1950, 107: 221–224.

57. Cleveland, S. E., & Dysinger, D. W. Mental deterioration in senile psychosis. *J. abnorm. soc. Psychol.*, 1944, 39: 368–372.

58. Coheen, J. Disturbances in time discrimination in organic brain disease. *J. nerv. ment. Dis.*, 1950, 112: 121–129.

59. Cohen, J. Wechsler Memory scale performance of psychoneurotic, organic, and schizophrenic groups. *J. consult. Psychol.*, 1950, 14: 371–375.

60. Cole, E. M., Baggett, Miriam P., & MacMullen, Marjorie R. Mental and performance testing of neurologic patients. *Arch. Neurol. Psychiat.*, 1947, 58: 104–107.

61. Collins, A. L., & Lennox, W. G. The intelligence of 300 private epileptic patients. *Res. Publ. Ass. Res. nerv. ment. Dis.*, 1947, 26: 583–603.

62. Colm, Hanna. The value of projective methods in the psychological examination of children: the Mosaic Test in conjunction with the Rorschach and Binet tests. *Rorschach Res. Exch.*, 1948, 12: 216–237.

63. Colom, G. A., & Levine, M. H. Self-inflicted prefrontal lobotomy: report of a case. *J. nerv. ment. Dis.*, 1951, 113: 430–436.

64. Cotton, C. B. A study of reactions of spastic children to certain test situations. *J. genet. Psychol.*, 1941, 58: 27–35.

65. Courville, C. B. Coup-contrecoup mechanism of cranio-cerebral injuries: some observations. *Arch. Surg.*, 1942, 45: 19–43.

66. Critchley, M. The body-image in neurology. *Lancet*, 1950, 1: 335–340.

67. Crown, S. Psychological changes following prefrontal leucotomy: a review. *J. ment. Sci.*, 1951, 97: 49–83.

68. Diers, W. C., & Brown, C. C. Psychometric patterns associated with multi-

ple sclerosis. I. Wechsler-Bellevue patterns. *Arch. Neurol. Psychiat.*, 1950, 63: 760–765.

69. Di Nolfo, A. A simple screening device for and in detection of brain damage. *J. Amer. osteop. Ass.*, 1947, 47: 244–247.

70. Dolphin, J. E., & Cruickshank, W. N. The figure background relationship in children with cerebral palsy. *J. clin. Psychol.*, 1951, 7: 228–231.

71. Elonen, Anna S., & Korner, Anneliese, F. Pre- and post-operative psychological observations on a case of frontal lobectomy. *J. abnorm. soc. Psychol.*, 1948. 43: 532–543.

72. Eysenck, M. D. A study of certain qualitative aspects of problem solving behaviour in senile dementia patients. *J. ment. Sci.*, 1945, 91: 337–345.

73. Eysenck, M. D. An exploratory study of mental organization in senility. *J. Neurol. Psychiat.*, 1945, 8: 15–21.

74. Falk, R., Penrose, L. S., & Clar, S. The search for intellectual deterioration among epileptic patients. *Amer. J. ment. Def.*, 1945, 49: 469–471.

75. Feldman, F., & Cameron, D. E. Speech in senility. *Amer. J. Psychiat.*, 1944, 101: 64–67.

76. Fernandes, B., *et al.* A clinical and psychological study in leucotomy. *First int. Congr. Psychosurg.*, *Lisbon*, 1949, 147–165.

77. Fischer, Liselotte K. A new psychological tool in function: preliminary clinical experience with the Bolgar-Fischer World Test. *Amer. J. Orthopsychiat.*, 1950, 20: 281–292.

78. Fleming, G. W. T. H. Some preliminary remarks on prefrontal leucotomy. *J. ment. Sci.*, 1942, 88: 282–284.

79. Fleming, G. W. T. H. Prefrontal leucotomy. *J. ment. Sci.*, 1944, 90: 486–500.

80. Frank, J. Clinical survey and results of 200 cases of prefrontal leucotomy. *J. ment. Sci.*, 1946, 92: 497–508.

81. Freeman, W., & Watts, J. W. *Psychosurgery.* Springfield, Ill.: Charles C. Thomas, 1942.

82. Freeman, W., & Watts, J. W. Psychosurgery: an evaluation of two hundred cases over seven years. *J. ment. Sci.*, 1944, 90: 532–537.

83. Freeman, W., & Watts, J. W. *Psychosurgery.* (2nd Ed.) Springfield, Ill.: Charles C. Thomas, 1950.

84. French, L. A. Psychometric testing of patients who had brain tumors removed during childhood. *J. Neurosurg.*, 1948, 5: 173–177.

85. Freudenberg, R. K., & Robertson, J. P. S. Investigation into intellectual changes following prefrontal leucotomy. *J. ment. Sci.*, 1949, 95: 826–841.

86. Furtado, D., Rodrigues, M., Margues, U., Alvins, F., & De Vasconcelos, A. Personality changes after lobotomy. *First int. Cong. Psychosurg.*, *Lisbon*, 1949, 35–49.

87. Gelb, A., & Goldstein, K. *Psychologische Analysen hirnpathologischer Fälle.* Leipzig: Barth, 1920. (Partially translated in Ellis, W., *A source book of Gestalt psychology.* New York: Harcourt, Brace, 1938.)

88. Gilliland, A. R., Wittman, P., & Goldman, M. Patterns and scatter of mental abilities in various psychoses. *J. gen. Psychol.*, 1943, 29: 257–260.

89. Glik, E. E. A comparison of recall and recognition types of measurement on verbal items, and their implications for deterioration testing. *J. clin. Psychol.*, 1951, 7: 157–162.

90. Goldensohn, L. N., Clardy, E. R., & Levine, K. N. Schizophrenic-like reactions in children. *Psychiat. Quart.*, 1945, 19: 572–604.

91. Goldman, G. D. A comparison of the personality structures of patients with

idiopathic epilepsy, hysterical convulsions, and brain tumors. Paper read at East. Psychol. Ass., Atlantic City, 1952.

92. Goldman, R., Greenblatt, M., & Coon, G. P. Use of the Bellevue-Wechsler scale in clinical psychiatry with particular reference to cases with brain damage. *J. nerv. ment. Dis.*, 1946, 104: 144–179.

93. Goldstein, K. *The organism*. New York: American Book Co., 1939.

94. Goldstein, K. *Human nature in the light of psychopathology*. Cambridge, Mass.: Harvard Univer. Press, 1940.

95. Goldstein, K. *After-effects of brain injuries in war*. New York: Grune & Stratton, 1942.

96. Goldstein, K. Some experimental observations concerning the influence of colors on the function of the organism. *Occup. Ther.*, 1942, 21: 147–151.

97. Goldstein, K. Brain concussion: evaluation of the after-effects by special tests. *Dis. nerv. Syst.*, 1943, 4: 325–334.

98. Goldstein, K. Mental changes due to frontal lobe damage. *J. Psychol.*, 1944, 17: 187–208.

99. Goldstein, K. *Language and language disturbances*. New York: Grune & Stratton, 1948.

100. Goldstein, K., & Scheerer, M. Abstract and concrete behavior: an experimental study with special tests. *Psychol. Monogr.*, 1941, 53: No. 2 (Whole No. 239).

101. Gomez del Carro, J. El test del arbol in clinica psyquiatrica; Koch's Baumtest. (The tree test in the psychiatric clinic: Koch's tree-test). *Acta med. hispanica*, 1950, 8: 53–59.

102. Graham, F. K., & Kendall, B. S. Performance of brain-damaged cases on a memory-for-designs test. *J. abnorm. soc. Psychol.*, 1946, 41: 303–314.

103. Grant, A. D., & Berg, Esta A. A behavioral analysis of degree of reinforcement and ease of shifting to new responses in a Weigl-type card-sorting. *J. exp. Psychol.*, 1948, 38: 404–411.

104. Grassi, J. R. The Graphic Rorschach as a supplement to the Rorschach in the diagnosis of organic intracranial lesions. *Psychiat. Quart. Suppl.*, 1947, 21: 312–327.

105. Grassi, J. R. Impairment of abstract behavior following prefrontal lobotomy. *Psychiat. Quart.*, 1950, 24: 74–88.

106. Greenblatt, M., Arnot, R., & Solomon, H. C. (Eds.) *Studies in lobotomy*. New York: Grune & Stratton, 1950.

107. Greenblatt, M., Goldman, R., & Coon, G. P. Clinical implications of the Bellevue-Wechsler test (with particular reference to brain damage cases). *J. nerv. ment. Dis.*, 1946, 104: 438–442.

108. Greenblatt, M., Levine, S., & Atwell, C. R. Comparative value of electroencephalogram and abstraction tests in diagnosis of brain damage. *J. nerv. ment. Dis.*, 1945, 102: 383–391.

109. Guirdham, A. The Rorschach test in epileptics. *J. ment. Sci.*, 1935, 81: 870–893.

110. Gutman, Brigette. The application of the Wechsler-Bellevue scale in the diagnosis of organic brain disorders. *J. clin. Psychol.*, 1950, 6: 195–198.

111. Haffter, C. Der Labyrinth-Test von Rey bei Oligophrenen, Epileptikern und Organisch Dementen. (Rey's maze test in mental defectives, epileptics, and organic dements). *Mschr. Psychiat. Neurol.*, 1942, 106: 1–10.

112. Hall, K. R. L. The testing of abstraction, with special reference to impairment in schizophrenia. *Brit. J. med. Psychol.*, 1951, 24: 83–150.

113. Hall, K. R. L. Conceptual impairment in depressive and organic patients of the pre-senile age group. *J. ment. Sci.*, 1952, 98: 257–264.

114. Hall, K. R. L., & Crookes, T. G. Studies in learning impairment. I: Schizophrenic and organic patients. *J. ment. Sci.*, 1951, 97: 729–737.

115. Halstead, H. Mental tests in senile dementia. *J. ment. Sci.*, 1944, 90: 720–726.

116. Halstead, W. C. Preliminary analysis of grouping behavior in patients with cerebral injury by the method of equivalent and non-equivalent stimuli. *Amer. J. Psychiat.*, 1940, 96: 1263–1294.

117. Halstead, W. C. A power factor (P) in general intelligence: the effect of brain injuries. *J. Psychol.*, 1945, 20: 57–64.

118. Halstead, W. C. Brain injuries and higher levels of consciousness. *Res. Publ. Ass. nerv. ment. Dis.*, 1945, 24: 480–506.

119. Halstead, W. C. A power factor (P) in general intelligence: effects of lesions of the brain. *Arch. Neurol. Psychiat.*, 1946, 56: 234–235.

120. Halstead, W. C. *Brain and intelligence*. Chicago: Univer. of Chicago Press, 1947.

121. Halstead, W. C., & Settlage, P. H. Grouping behavior of normal persons and of persons with lesions of the brain. *Arch. Neurol. Psychiat.*, 1943, 49: 489–506.

122. Hanfmann, Eugenia. A study of personal patterns in intellectual performance. *Charact. & Pers.*, 1941, 9: 315–325.

123. Hanfmann, Eugenia, Rickers-Ovsiankina, Maria, & Goldstein, K. Case Lanuti: extreme concretization of behavior due to damage of the brain cortex. *Psychol. Monogr.*, 1944, 57: No. 4 (Whole No. 264).

124. Hanvik, L. J., & Andersen, A. L. The effect of focal brain lesions on recall and on the production of rotations in the Bender-Gestalt test. *J. consult. Psychol.*, 1950, 14: 197–198.

125. Harrower-Erickson, M. R. Personality changes accompanying cerebral lesions: II. Rorschach studies of patients with focal epilepsy. *Arch. Neurol. Psychiat.*, 1940, 43: 1081–1107.

126. Harrower-Erickson, M. R. Personality changes accompanying organic brain lesions: III. A study of preadolescent children. *J. genet. Psychol.*, 1941, 58: 391–405.

127. Harrower, M. R. The results of psychometric and personality tests in multiple sclerosis. *Res. Publ. Ass. nerv. ment. Dis.*, 1950, 28: 461–470.

128. Head, H. Aphasia and kindred disorders of speech. Cambridge: Cambridge Univer. Press, 1926.

129. Heath, R. G., & Pool, J. L. Bilateral frontal resection of frontal cortex for the treatment of psychoses. *J. nerv. ment. Dis.*, 1948, 107: 411–429.

130. Heath, S. R. Clinical significance of motor defect, with military implications. *Amer. J. Psychol.*, 1944, 57: 482–499.

131. Heath, S. R. A mental pattern found in motor deviates. *J. abnorm. soc. Psychol.*, 1946, 41: 223–225.

132. Hebb, D. O. Intelligence in man after large removals of cerebral tissue: report of four left frontal lobe cases. *J. gen. Psychol.*, 1939, 21: 73–87.

133. Hebb, D. O. The effect of early and late brain injury upon test scores, and the nature of normal adult intelligence. *Proc. Amer. phil. Soc.*, 1942, 85: 275–292.

134. Hebb, D. O. Man's frontal lobes. *Arch. Neurol. Psychiat.*, 1945, 54: 10–24.

135. Hebb, D. O. *The organization of behavior*. New York: Wiley, 1949.

136. Hebb, D. O. Comparative and physiological psychology. *Annu. Rev. Psychol.*, 1950, 1: 173–188.

137. Heidbreder, Edna. Toward a dynamic psychology of cognition. *Psychol. Rev.*, 1945, 52: 1–22.

138. Hewson, L. The Wechsler-Bellevue scale and the substitution test as aids in neuro-psychiatric diagnosis. *J. nerv. ment. Dis.*, 1949, 109: 158–183, 246–265.

139. Hoedemaker, E., & Murray, M. Psychological tests in the diagnosis of organic brain disease. *Neurology*, 1952, 2: 144–153.

140. Holbourn, A. H. S. Mechanics of head injuries. *Lancet*, 1943, 2: 438–441.

141. Howson, J. D. Intellectual impairment associated with brain-injured patients as revealed in the Shaw Test of abstract thought. *J. Psychol.*, 1948, 2: 125–133.

142. Hoyt, R., Elliot, H., & Hebb, D. O. The intelligence of schizophrenic patients following lobotomy treatment. *Queen Mary Vet. Hosp. Serv. Bull., Montreal*, 1951, 6: 553–557.

143. Hughes, R. M. Rorschach signs for the diagnosis of organic pathology. *Rorschach Res. Exch.*, 1948, 12: 165–167.

144. Hunt, H. F. A note on the problem of brain damage in rehabilitation and personnel work. *J. appl. Psychol.*, 1945, 29: 282–288.

145. Hunt, J. McV., & Cofer, C. N. Psychological deficit. In J. McV. Hunt (Ed.), *Personality and the behavior disorders*. New York: Ronald, 1944. Pp. 971–1032.

146. Hutton, E. L. Results of prefrontal leucotomy. *Lancet*, 1943, 1: 362–366.

147. Hutton, E. L., & Bassett, M. Effect of leucotomy on creative personality. *J. ment. Sci.*, 1948, 94: 332–350.

148. Ingham, S. D. Head injuries in relation to psychoneurotic symptoms and personality changes. *Bull. Los Angeles neurol. Soc.*, 1944, 9: 61–64.

149. Jackson, J. H. *Selected writings of J. Hughlings Jackson*. London: Hodder & Stoughton, 1931–1932.

150. Jaffe, R. Influence of cerebral trauma on kinesthetic after-effects. *Amer. Psychologist*, 1951, 7: 265. (Abstract)

151. Jeffress, L. A. (Ed.) *Cerebral mechanisms in behavior. The Hixon Symposium.* New York: Wiley, 1951.

152. Jones, H. E., & Conrad, H. S. The growth and decline of intelligence. *Genet. Psychol. Monogr.*, 1933, 13: 223–298.

153. Jones, R. E. Personality changes in psychotics following prefrontal lobotomy. *J. abnorm. soc. Psychol.*, 1949, 44: 315–328.

154. Juckem, H., & Wold, J. A. A study of the Hunt-Minnesota Test for organic brain damage at the upper levels of vocabulary. *J. Psychol.*, 1948, 12: 53–57.

155. Karnosh, L. J., & Gardner, W. J. An evaluation of the physical and mental capabilities following removal of the right cerebral hemisphere. *Cleveland clin. Quart.*, 1941, 8: 94–106.

156. Kass, W. Wechsler's Mental Deterioration Index in the diagnosis of organic brain disease. *Trans. Kansas Acad. Sci.*, 1949, 52: 66–70.

157. Kendall, B. S., & Graham, F. K. Further standardization of memory-for-designs test. *J. consult. Psychol.*, 1948, 12: 349–354.

158. King, H. E., Clausen, J., & Scarff, J. F. Cutaneous thresholds for pain before and after unilateral prefrontal lobotomy: a preliminary report. *J. nerv. ment. Dis.*, 1950, 112: 93–96.

159. Kisker, G. W. Remarks on the problem of psychosurgery. *Amer. J. Psychiat.*, 1943, 100: 180–184.

160. Kisker, G. W. Abstract and categorical behavior following therapeutic brain surgery. *Psychosom. Med.*, 1944, 6: 146–150.

161. Kisker, G. W. The Rorschach analysis of psychotics subjected to neurosurgical interruption of the thalamo-cortical projections. *Psychiat. Quart.*, 1944, 18: 43–52.

162. Kisker, G. W. The behavioral sequelae of neurosurgical therapy: bilateral prefrontal lobotomy. *J. gen. Psychol.*, 1945, 33: 171–192.

163. Klapper, Zelda S., & Werner, H. Developmental deviations in brain-injured members of pairs of identical twins. *Quart. J. Child Behav.*, 1950, 2: 288–313.

164. Klebanoff, S. G. Psychological changes in organic brain lesions and ablations. *Psychol. Bull.*, 1945, 42: 585–623.

165. Klebanoff, S. G. The Rorschach test in an analysis of personality changes in general paresis. *J. Pers.*, 1949, 17: 261–272.

166. Klein, G. S., & Krech, D. "Cortical conductivity" in the brain-injured. *Amer. Psychologist*, 1951, 7: 264. (Abstract)

167. Klein, R. Loss of written language due to dissolution of the phonetic structure of the word in brain abscess. *J. ment. Sci.*, 1951, 97: 328–339.

168. Koff, S. A. The Rorschach test in the differential diagnosis of cerebral concussion and psychoneurosis. *Bull. U. S. Army med. Dep.*, 1946, 5: 170–173.

169. Kogan, K. L. The personality reactions of children with epilepsy, with special reference to the Rorschach method. *Res. Publ. Ass. nerv. ment. Dis.*, 1947, 26: 616–630.

170. Köhler, W. Relational determination in perception. In L. A. Jeffress (Ed.), *Cerebral mechanisms in behavior.* New York: Wiley, 1951. Pp. 200–230.

171. Kolb, L. C. An evaluation of lobotomy and its potentialities for future research in psychiatry and the basic sciences. *J. nerv. ment. Dis.*, 1949, 110: 112–148.

172. Koskoff, Y. D., Dennis, W., Lazovik, D., & Wheeler, E. T. The psychological effects of frontal lobotomy performed for alleviation of pain. *Res. Publ. Ass. nerv. ment. Dis.*, 1948, 27: 723–753.

173. Kounin, J. S. Intellectual development and rigidity. In R. Barker, J. S. Kounin, & H. F. Wright (Eds.), *Child development and behavior.* New York: McGraw-Hill, 1943. Pp. 179–197.

174. Krech, D. Dynamic systems as open neurological systems. *Psychol. Rev.*, 1950, 57: 345–361.

175. Krol, V. A., & Dorken, H. The influence of subcortical (diencephalic) brain lesions on emotionality as reflected in the Rorschach color responses. *Amer. J. Psychiat.*, 1951 107: 839–843.

176. Krout, M. H. Is the brain-injured a mental defective? *Amer. J. ment. Def.*, 1949, 54: 81–85.

177. Lenox, W. G. Seizure states. In J. McV. Hunt (Ed.), *Personality and the behavior disorders.* New York: Ronald, 1944. Pp. 922–967.

178. Levi, J., Oppenheim, S., & Wechsler, D. Clinical use of the Mental Deterioration Index of the Bellevue-Wechsler scale. *J. abnorm. soc. Psychol.*, 1945, 40: 405–407.

179. Levine, K. N. A comparison of graphic Rorschach productions with scoring categories of the verbal Rorschach record in normal states, organic brain disease, neurotic and psychotic disorders. *Arch. Psychol.*, 1943, No. 282.

180. Lewin, K. *A dynamic theory of personality.* New York: McGraw-Hill, 1935.

181. Lewinski, R. J. The psychometric pattern in epilepsy. *Amer. J. Orthopsychiat.*, 1947, 17: 714–722.

182. Liberson, W. T. Abnormal brain waves and intellectual impairment. *Inst. of Living*, 1944, No. 12, 234–248.

183. Lidz, T., Gay, J. R. & Tietze, C. Intelligence in cerebral deficit states and schizophrenia measured by Kohs Block test. *Arch. Neurol. Psychiat.*, 1942, 48: 568–582.

184. Lindberg, B. J. On the question of psychologically conditioned features in the Korsakow syndrome. *Acta psychiat., Kbh.*, 1946, 21: 497–542.

185. Lisansky, E. S. Convulsive disorders and personality. *J. abnorm. soc. Psychol.*, 1948, 43: 29–37.

186. Lord, E., & Wood, L. Diagnostic values in a visuo-motor test. *Amer. J. Orthopsychiat.*, 1942, 12: 414–429.

187. Lovtskaia, A. J. The functions of the occipital lobe. *Neuropat. Psikhiat.*, 1944, 13: 78–80.

188. Lutz, J. Zur psychischen Symptomatologie eines Schadebruches bei einem 1:1 alten Kinde. (Concerning the psychical symptomatology of skull fracture in a 13-month-old child.) *Z. Kinderpsychiat.*, 1949, 15: 173–185.

189. Lutz, J. Psychische Symptome und Rekonvalesenz nach Contusio Cerebri bei einem 6 Jahre alten Madelein. (Psychical symptoms and convalescence after cerebral concussion in a six-year-old girl.) *Z. Kinderpsychiat.*, 1949, 16: 97–109.

190. Lynn, J. G., Levine, K. N., & Hewson, L. R. Psychologic tests for the clinical evaluation of the late "diffuse organic," "neurotic," and "normal" reactions after closed head injury. *Res. Publ. Ass. nerv. ment. Dis.*, 1945, 24: 296–378.

191. McCullough, M. W. Wechsler-Bellevue changes following prefrontal lobotomy. *J. clin. Psychol.*, 1950, 3: 270–273.

192. McFie, J., & Piercy, M. F. The relation of laterality of lesion to performance on Weigl's sorting test. *J. ment. Sci.*, 1952, 98: 299–305.

193. Machover, Karen. A case of frontal lobe injury following attempted suicide. *Rorschach Res. Exch.*, 1947, 11: 9–20.

194. McKenzie, K. G., & Proctor, L. D. Bilateral frontal leucotomy in the treatment of mental disease. *Canad. med. Ass. J.*, 1946, 55: 433.

195. Magaret, Ann. Parallels in the behavior of schizophrenics, paretics, and presenile non-psychotic patients. *J. abnorm. soc. Psychol.*, 1942, 37: 511–528.

196. Malamud, Rachel F. Validity of the Hunt-Minnesota Test for organic brain damage. *J. appl. Psychol.*, 1946, 30: 271–275.

197. Malmo, R. B. Psychological aspects of frontal gyrectomy and frontal lobotomy in mental patients. *Res. Publ. Ass. nerv. ment. Dis.*, 1948, 27: 537–564.

198. Metarazzo, J. D. A study of the diagnostic possibilities of the C.V.S. with a group of organic cases. *J. clin. Psychol.*, 1950, 6: 337–343.

199. Mettler, F. A. (Ed.) *Selective partial ablation of the frontal cortex.* New York: Hoeber, 1949.

200. Mettler, F. A. (Ed.) *Psychosurgical problems.* New York: Blakiston, 1952.

201. Meyer, A., & McLardy, T. Leucotomy as an instrument of research. Neuropathological studies. *Proc. Roy. Soc. Med.*, 1947, 40: 145.

202. Mixter, W. J., Tillotson, K. J., & Weis, D. Reports of partial frontal lobectomy and frontal lobotomy performed on three patients: one chronic epileptic and two cases of chronic depression. *Psychosom. Med.*, 1941, 3: 26–37.

203. Napoli, P. J., & Sweeney, L. Hostility in the chronic neurological patient. Paper read at East. Psychol. Ass., Atlantic City, 1952.

204. Nathanson, M., & Wortis, S. B. Severe rigidity in performance and thought in a case of presenile degenerative disease. *J. nerv. ment. Dis.*, 1948, 108: 399–408.

205. Nichols, I. C., & Hunt, J. McV. A case of partial bilateral frontal lobectomy. *Amer. J. Psychiat.*, 1940, 96: 1063–1083.

206. Oltman, Jane E., Brody, B. S., Friedman, S., & Green, W. F. Frontal lobotomy. *Amer. J. Psychiat.*, 1949, 105: 742–751.

207. Ostrander, Jessie M. Rorschach record from a patient after removal of a tumor from the frontal lobe. *Amer. Psychologist*, 1947, 2: 406. (Abstract)

208. Parsons, F. H. Modifications of design block performance before and after corpus callosum section. *Psychol. Bull.*, 1942, 39: 494. (Abstract)

209. Parsons, F. H. Eight cases of section of corpus callosum in individuals

with a history of epileptic seizures: psychological tests. *J. gen. Psychol.*, 1943, 29: 227–241.

210. Partridge, M. *Prefrontal leucotomy*, Springfield, Ill.: Charles C. Thomas, 1950.

211. Paterson, A., & Zangwill, O. L. Disorders of visual space perception associated with lesions of the right cerebral hemisphere. *Brain*, 1944, 67: 331–358.

212. Penfield, W. Symposium on gyrectomy. Part I: Bilateral frontal gyrectomy and postoperative intelligence. *Res. Publ. Ass. nerv. ment. Dis.*, 1948, 27: 519–534.

213. Petrie, A. Personality changes after pre-frontal leucotomy. *Brit. J. med. Psychol.*, 1949, 22: 220–207.

214. Petrie, A. Preliminary report of changes after pre-frontal leucotomy. *J. ment. Sci.*, 1949, 95: 449–455.

215. Peyton, W. T., Noran, H. H., & Miller, E. W. Prefrontal lobectomy. *Amer. J. Psychiat.*, 1948, 104: 513–523.

216. Pflugfelder, G. Intellektuelle Storungen nach schweren Schadeltraumen. *Mschr. f. Psychiat. Neurol.*, 1949–1950, 118–119: 288–304, 378–404.

217. Pinkerton, P., & Kelly, J. An attempted correlation between clinical and psychometric findings in senile arteriosclerotic dementia. *J. ment. Sci.*, 1952, 98: 244–255.

218. Piotrowski, Z. The Rorschach inkblot method in organic disturbances of the central nervous system. *J. nerv. ment. Dis.*, 1937, 86: 525–537.

219. Porteus, S. D. Thirty-five years experience with the Porteus Maze. *J. abnorm. soc. Psychol.*, 1950, 45: 396–401.

220. Porteus, S. D., & Kepner, R. DeM. Mental changes after bilateral prefrontal lobotomy. *Genet. Psychol. Monogr.*, 1944, 29: 3–115.

221. Porteus, S. D., & Peters, H. N. Maze test validation and psychosurgery *Genet. Psychol. Monogr.*, 1947, 36.

222. Probst, H. Über psychische Folgen des Schadelleruches im Kindesalter. *Z. Kinderpsychiat.*, 1949, 15: 186–192.

223. Rabin, A. I., & Guertin, W. H. Research with the Wechsler-Bellevue test: 1945–1950. *Psychol. Bull.*, 1951, 48: 211–248.

224. Rashkis, H. A. Three types of thinking disorder. *J. nerv. ment. Dis.*, 1947, 106; 650–670.

225. Rashkis, H., Cushman, J., & Landis, C. A new method for studying disorders of conceptual thinking. *J. abnorm. soc. Psychol.*, 1946, 41: 70–82.

226. Reiner, E. R., & Sands, S. L. Lobotomy and psychopathology. *Arch. Neurol. Psychiat.*, 1951, 65: 48–53.

227. Reynell, W. R. A psychometric method of determining intellectual loss following head injury. *J. ment. Sci.*, 1944, 90: 710–719.

228. Robinson, Mary F. What price lobotomy? *J. abnorm. soc. Psychol.*, 1946, 41: 421–436.

229. Rogers, L. S. A comparative evaluation of the Wechsler-Bellevue Mental Deterioration Index for various adult groups. *J. clin. Psychol.*, 1950, 6: 199–202.

230. Rogers, L. S. A note on Allen's index of deterioration. *J. clin. Psychol.*, 1950, 6: 203.

231. Ross, W. O., & Ross, S. Some Rorschach ratings of clinical value. *Rorschach Res. Exch.*, 1944, 8: 1–9.

232. Rosvold, H. E., & Mishkin, M. Evaluation of the effects of prefrontal lobotomy on intelligence. *Canad. J. Psychol.*, 1950, 4: 122–126.

233. Ruesch, J., & Bowman, K. M. Prolonged post-traumatic syndromes following head injury. *Amer. J. Psychiat.*, 1945, 102: 145–164.

234. Ruesch, J., & Moore, B. E. Measurement of intellectual functions in the acute stage of head injury. *Arch. Neurol. Psychiat.*, 1943, 50: 165–170.

235. Rust, R. M. Some correlates of the movement response. *J. Pers.*, 1948, 16: 369–401.

236. Rylander, G. *Personality changes after operations on the frontal lobes.* London: Oxford, 1939.

237. Rylander, G. Mental changes after excision of cerebral tissue. A clinical study of 16 cases of resections in the parietal, temporal, and occipital lobes. *Acta Psychiat. Neurol.*, 1943, Suppl. 20.

238. Rylander, G. Psychological tests and personality analyses before and after frontal lobotomy. *Acta Psychiat. Neurol.*, 1947, Suppl. 47, 383–398.

239. Sands, H., & Price, J. C. A pattern analysis of the Wechsler-Bellevue Adult Intelligence Scale in epilepsy. *Res. Publ. Assoc. nerv. ment. Dis.*, 1947, 26: 604–615.

240. Scheerer, M. Problems of performance analysis in the study of personality. *Ann. New York Acad. Sci.*, 1946, 46: 653–678.

241. Scheerer, M. An experiment in abstraction; testing form-disparity tolerance. *Confinia Neurol.*, 1949, 9: 232–254.

242. Scheerer, M., Rothmann, E., & Goldstein, K. A case of "idiotsavant." An experimental study of personality organization. *Psychol. Monogr.*, 1945, 58: No. 4 (Whole No. 269).

243. Schilder, P. Congenital alexia and its relation to optic perception. *J. genet. Psychol.*, 1944, 65: 67–88.

244. Schrader, P. J., & Robinson, M. F. An evaluation of prefrontal lobotomy through ward behavior. *J. abnorm. soc. Psychol.*, 1945, 40: 61–69.

245. Sheps, J. G. Intelligence of male noninstitutionalized epileptics of military age. *J. ment. Sci.*, 1947, 93: 82–88.

246. Shorvon, H. J. Prefrontal leucotomy and the depersonalization syndrome. *Lancet*, 1947, 253: 714–718.

247. Silver, A. A. Diagnosis and prognosis of behavior disorder associated with organic brain disease in children. *J. insurance Med.*, 1951, 6: 38–42.

248. Singer, J. L., Meltzoff, J., & Goldman, G. Rorschach movement responses following motor inhibition and hyperactivity. *J. consult. Psychol.*, 1952, 16: 359–364.

249. Sloan, W., & Bensberg, G. J. The stereognostic capacity of brain injured as compared with familial mental defectives. *J. clin. Psychol.*, 1951, 7: 154–156.

250. Smith, K. U. Bilateral integrative action of the cerebral cortex in man in verbal association and sensori-motor coordination. *J. exp. Psychol.*, 1947, 3: 367–376.

251. Smith, K. U., & Akelaitis, A. J. Studies in the corpus callosum: I. Laterality in behavior and bilateral motor organization in man before and after section of the corpus callosum. *Arch. Neurol. Psychiat.*, 1942, 47: 519–543.

252. Somerfeld-Ziskind, E., & Ziskind, E. Effect of phenobarbital on the mentality of epileptic patients. *Arch. Neurol. Psychiat.*, 1940, 43: 70–79.

253. Spiegel, E. Physiologic and psychologic results of thalamotomy. *Arch. Neurol. Psychiat.*, 1950, 64: 306–307. (Abstract)

254. Stengel, E. Loss of spatial orientation, constructional apraxia, and Gerstmann's syndrome. *J. ment. Sci.*, 1944, 90: 753–760.

255. Strauss, A. A. Ways of thinking in brain-crippled deficient children. *Amer. J. Psychiat.*, 1944, 100: 639–647.

256. Strauss, A. A., & Lehtinen, L. Psychopathology and education of the brain-injured child. New York: Grune & Stratton, 1947.

257. Strauss, A. A., & Werner, H. Deficiency in the finger schema in relation to arithmetic disability. *Amer. J. Orthopsychiat.*, 1938, 8: 719–724.

258. Strauss, A. A., & Werner, H. Finger agnosia in children. *Amer. J. Psychiat.*, 1939, 34: 37–62.

259. Strauss, A. A., & Werner, H. Disorders of conceptual thinking in the brain-injured child. *J. nerv. ment. Dis.*, 1942, 96: 153–172.

260. Strauss, A. A., & Werner, H. Comparative psychopathology of the brain-injured child and the traumatic brain-injured adult. *Amer. J. Psychiat.*, 1943, 99: 835–838.

261. Strecker, E. A., Palmer, H. D., & Grant, F. C. Study of prefrontal lobotomy. *Amer. J. Psychiat.*, 1942, 98: 524–532.

262. Strom-Olsen, R., Lost, S. L., Brody, M. B., & Knight, G. C. Results of prefrontal leucotomy in 30 cases of mental disorder. *J. ment. Sci.*, 1943, 89: 165–181.

263. Teuber, H. L. Neuropsychology. In *Recent advances in diagnostic psychological testing: a critical summary*. Springfield, Ill.: Charles C. Thomas, 1950.

264. Teuber, H. L., Battersby, W. S., & Bender, M. B. Performance of complex visual tasks after cerebral lesions. *J. nerv. ment. Dis.*, 1951, 114: 413–429.

265. Teuber, H. L., & Bender, M. B. The significance of changes in pattern vision following occipital lobe injury. *Amer. Psychologist*, 1946, 1: 255. (Abstract)

266. Teuber, H., & Bender, M. B. Alterations in pattern vision following trauma of occipital lobes in man. *J. gen. Psychol.*, 1949, 40: 35–57.

267. Teuber, H. L., & Bender, M. B. Neuro-ophthalmology: the oculomotor system. In E. A. Spiegel (Ed.), *Progress in neurology and psychiatry*. New York: Grune & Stratton, 1951. Pp. 148–177.

268. Teuber, H. L., & Bender, M. B. Performance of complex visual tasks after cerebral lesions. *Amer. Psychologist*, 1951, 7: 265–266. (Abstract)

269. Trist, E. L., Trist, V., & Brody, M. B. Discussion on the quality of mental test performance in intellectual deterioration. *Proc. Roy. Soc. Med.*, 1943, 36: 243–252.

270. Van Der Lugt, M. J. A. *The V. D. L. Psychomotor Scale*. Springfield, Mass.; Meed Scientific Apparatus Co., 1951.

271. Van Waters, R. O., & Sacks, J. G. Rorschach evaluation of the schizophrenic process following a prefrontal lobotomy. *J. Psychol.*, 1946, 25: 73–88.

272. Vidor, Martha. Personality changes following prefrontal leucotomy as reflected by the Minnesota Multiphasic Personality Inventory and the results of psychometric testing. *J. ment. Sci.*, 1951, 97: 159–173.

273. Watts, J. W., & Freeman, W. Intelligence following prefrontal lobotomy in obsessive tension states. *Arch. Neurol. Psychiat.*, 1945, 53: 244–245.

274. Watts, J. W., & Freeman, W. Psychosurgery for the relief of unbearable pain. *J. int. Coll. Surg.*, 1946, 9: 679.

275. Wechsler, D. *The measurement of adult intelligence*. Baltimore: Williams & Wilkins, 1944.

276. Wechsler, D. A standardized memory scale for clinical use. *J. Psychol.*, 1945, 19: 87–95.

277. Weigl, E. On the psychology of the so-called processes of abstraction. *J. abnorm. soc. Psychol.*, 1941, 36: 3–33.

278. Weinstein, E. A., & Kahn, R. L. The syndrome of anosognosia. *Arch. Neurol. Psychiat.*, 1950, 64: 772–791.

279. Weinstein, E. A., & Kahn, R. L. Patterns of disorientation in organic brain disease. *J. Neuropath. clin. Neurol.*, 1951, 1: 214–225.

280. Weinstein, E. A., & Kahn, R. L. Nonaphasic misnaming (paraphasia) in organic brain disease. *Arch. Neurol. Psychiat.*, 1952, 67: 72–79.

281. Weisenberg, T., & McBride, Katherine. *Aphasia*. New York: Commonwealth Fund, 1935.

282. Werner, H. Motion and motion perception: a study in vicarious functioning. *J. Psychol.*, 1945, 19: 317–327.

283. Werner, H. Perceptual behavior of brain injured mentally deficient children. *Genet. Psychol. Monogr.*, 1945, 31.

284. Werner, H. Abnormal and subnormal rigidity. *J. abnorm. soc. Psychol.*, 1946 41: 15–24.

285. Werner, H. The concept of rigidity: a critical evaluation. *Psychol. Rev.*, 1946, 53: 43–52.

286. Werner, H. *The comparative psychology of mental development*. Chicago: Follett, 1948.

287. Werner, H. Thought disturbance with reference to figure-background impairment in brain-injured children. *Confina Neurol.*, 1949, 9: 255–263.

288. Werner, H., & Bowers, M. Auditory-motor organization in two clinical types of mentally deficient children. *J. genet. Psychol.*, 1941, 59: 85–99.

289. Werner, H., & Carrison, D. Measurement and development of the finger schema in mentally retarded children. *J. educ. Psychol.*, 1942, 33: 252–264.

290. Werner, H., & Carrison, D. Animistic thinking in brain-injured mentally retarded children. *J. abnorm. soc. Psychol.*, 1944, 39: 43–62.

291. Werner, H., & Strauss, A. A. Problems and methods of functional analysis in mentally deficient children. *J. abnorm. soc. Psychol.*, 1939, 34: 37–62.

292. Werner, H., & Strauss, A. A. Pathology of figure background relations in the child. *J. abnorm. soc. Psychol.*, 1941, 36: 236–248.

293. Werner, H., & Strauss, A. A. Impairment in thought processes of brain-injured children. *Amer. J. ment. Def.*, 1943, 47: 291–295.

294. Werner, H., & Thuma, B. D. A deficiency in the perception of apparent motion in children with brain injury. *Amer. J. Psychol.*, 1942, 55: 58–67.

295. Werner, H., & Thuma, B. D. Critical flicker frequency in children with brain injury. *Amer. J. Psychol.*, 1942, 55: 394–399.

296. Wertham, F. The Mosaic Test: technique and psychopathological deductions. In L. E. Abt, & L. Bellak (Eds.), *Projective psychology*. New York: Knopf, 1950. Pp. 230–256.

297. Wexberg, E. Testing methods for the differential diagnosis of mental deficiency in a case of arrested brain tumor. *Amer. J. ment. Def.*, 1941, 46: 39–45.

298. Winfield, D. Intellectual performance of cryptogenic epileptics, symptomatic epileptics, and post-traumatic encephalopaths. *J. abnorm. soc. Psychol.*, 1951, 46: 336–343.

299. Wittenborn, J. R., & Mettler, F. A. Some psychological changes following psychosurgery. *J. abnorm. soc. Psychol.*, 1951, 46: 548–556.

300. Wittenborn, J. R., Bell, E. G., & Lesser, G. S. Symptom patterns among organic patients of advanced age. *J. clin. Psychol.*, 1951, 7: 328–330.

301. Woltmann, A. G. The Bender Visual-Motor Gestalt Test. In L. E. Abt., & L. Bellak (Eds.), *Projective psychology*. New York: Knopf, 1950. Pp. 322–356.

302. Worchel, P., & Lyerly, J. G. Effects of prefrontal lobotomy on depressed patients. *J. Neurophysiol.*, 1941, 4: 62–67.

303. Wortis, S. B. Bender, M. B., & Teuber, H. L. The significance of extinction. *J. nerv. ment. Dis.*, 1948, 107: 382–387.

304. Yacorzynski, G. K., Boshes, B., & Davis, L. Psychological changes produced by frontal lobotomy. *Res. Publ. Ass. nerv. ment. Dis.*, 1948, 27: 642–657.

305. Yacorzynski, G. K., & Davis, L. Modification of perceptual responses in

patients with unilateral lesions of the frontal lobes. *Psychol. Bull.*, 1942, 39: 493–494. (Abstract)

306. Zangwill, O. L. Observations on the Rorschach test in two cases of acute concussional head-injury. *J. ment. Sci.*, 1945, 91: 322–336.

307. Zangwill, O. L. A review of psychological work at the Brain Injuries Unit, Edinburgh, 1941–1945. *Brit. med. J.*, 1945, 2: 248–250.

36

MODEL PSYCHOSES INDUCED BY
LSD-25 IN NORMALS

I. Psychophysiological Investigations, with Special Reference to the Mechanism of the Paranoid Reaction

NICHOLAS A. BERCEL, M.D., LEE E. TRAVIS, Ph.D.,
LEONARD B. OLINGER, Ph.D., AND ERIC DREIKURS, Ph.D.

With the Technical Assistance of Marilyn G. Polos

INTRODUCTION

Experimental psychosis has a long history. It might have started with the administration of Cannabis indica boiling in wine to the ancient Hun warriors, resulting in mental obfuscation, as they were prepared for surgery because of wounds sustained in battle. Scientific experimental psychiatry began toward the end of the last century, in the Kraepelinian era — when the organic theory of psychoses was in its fullest vogue. Beringer's experiments with mescaline (1) marked a milestone in research in that many of the symptoms induced were highly similar to those encountered in schizophrenia and the drug seemed to have a selective affinity for the brain. The discovery of LSD-25 [1] by Stoll and Hoffman (2) was an even more exciting event, because the drug worked similarly in infinitesimal-trace amounts. Stoll (3) (1947) suggested the pharmacological designation *Phantastium* for this substance, and he classified the resultant model psychosis as that of the acute exogenous reaction type. Such psychoses are said to exaggerate and caricature the underlying personality of the subject.

Some toxic-organic psychoses, however, have some symptoms all their own. Thus, regardless of the personality structure, the "perception" of moving small animals, in abundance and of vivid coloring, is

From the University of Southern California, Department of Physiology, and published in the *A. M. A. Archives of Neurology and Psychiatry*, June 1956. © 1956, by American Medical Association.

[1] *d*-Lysergic acid diethylamide is a semisynthetic derivative obtained by condensation of *d*-lysergic acid, an extract of ergot, with diethylamine, a secondary amine. LSD-25 thus belongs to the ergonovine group. The drug was generously supplied to us by Prof. E. Rothlin, of the Sandoz Pharmaceutical Co., Basel, Switzerland, and its West Coast representative, Mr. Harry Althouse, San Francisco.

the stereotype feature of delirium tremens, and confabulations filling in the memory gaps is characteristic of Korsakoff syndrome as part of a cerebral metabolic deficiency state associated with specific involvements in the brain. Those who aver that all psychoses have a biological basis were for a long time on the lookout for a broader foundation, and the drug-induced models were quickly incorporated in this search. No biological theory of psychosis, however, can be held valid if it fails to identify the anatomical area involved or the physiological and biochemical mechanism responsible for dysfunction. The discussion that follows clearly demonstrates how very far psychiatry is from the biological theory; it will attempt to summarize the ever-increasing pieces of a theoretical mosaic which represent contributions from many related disciplines, such as psychiatry, psychology, clinical neurology, neurophysiology, neuropathology, biochemistry, neuropharmacology, neurosurgery, and biophysics. Finally, a few working theories will be submitted for critical analysis.

There are excellent surveys available in the literature on the effects of LSD-25 on normal (3–12), psychotic (13, 15–20), and neurotic (14, 21–25) humans and on animals. It might be important to point out the differences among the authors in their approach to the study of the effects of this drug. Since the original publication of Stoll (1947) many authors have more or less completely confirmed his findings, employing mostly subjects trained in the biological sciences, and through self-experimentation. Some of the salient features of this intoxication become quickly obvious to even the untrained observer, who, while maintaining a state of self-scrutiny and detachment, is quick to point out particularly his perceptual anomalies. The majority of changes, however, strangely enough, first become noticeable only upon questioning, and it is then that the wide range of variation from one experimental sample to another becomes clear. Self-scrutiny varies in degree from one person to another, and the meaning of the test is conceivably different to each one; even so, the richness of the description and the very difficulty in trying to report often vague changes of the mind itself are distinguishing features of the LSD effect.

It would appear, therefore, of value to relate the personality structure of the subject to his LSD state. One suspects that differences in reaction to the drug might depend partly on the scientific sophistication of the subject, which could account for some of the discrepancies found in the literature as one tries to reconcile the various descriptions. Abramson (23) even called attention to the element of suggestibility of the subject and to the suggestive influence of the investigator, for which there appeared to be a good deal of evidence in the present series.

SELECTION OF MATERIAL

LSD-25 was administered to 25 presumably normal subjects, none of whom, to our best knowledge and in their own admission, suffered from any psychiatric disturbance. The age level varied from 20 to 35 years, and by profession they were classified as follows: four students in physiology, three students in psychology, one medical student, one graduate in theology, six actresses in television, one insurance salesman, one physicist, one car salesman, one ski instructor, two housewives, one grammar school teacher, one girl without any occupation, one filling station attendant, and one laboratory attendant. There were 17 men and 8 women.

At the beginning of our experiments, in the summer of 1951, LSD-25 was generally unknown to the public — in fact, even to many in the psychiatric professions. In the selection of our cases, therefore, we did not have the problem of overcoming artificial prejudices; on the other hand, a great deal more explanation was necessary in convincing the subjects to submit to the test than was the case later on, when several reports appeared, not only in medical journals but in magazines and newspapers, about the strange effects of this drug. Selection of the candidates was done with extreme care.

Usually a prospect was approached by one member of the team, who told him that scientific investigation of the effect of certain drugs on the working mechanism of the mind was in progress at our university. We were in need of volunteers who were considered normal. As a result of the ingestion of a tasteless and harmless liquid, they were going to experience something akin to alcoholic intoxication. They would be required to cooperate in describing whatever changes occurred; they would lie comfortably on a cot; they would be fed lunch at a certain time, and transportation would be provided to and from the place where these experiments were to take place. They were reassured that disturbing after-effects were not expected, that in all probability they would be free to do whatever they wished the evening of these experiments, and that self-scrutiny and insight would never be lost at any time.[2]

Only in two instances were our requests turned down because of fear. Three other candidates tried to get out of the experiments by giving all kinds of excuses, which, while quite plausible, left us to suspect that they were covering up their fears. No attempt was made to insist beyond this point.

As a general rule, most of the subjects were quite satisfied, interested, and even delighted by what went on, and, judging from their eagerness in trying to line up for subsequent control tests, it appeared that they were very intrigued about the outcome of the test. Some of them later asked to read the verbatim transcription of the experiment in order to satisfy this curiosity, also because exact recollection of the happenings was often obscure. They related occasionally during the experiment that they felt uncomfortable, anxious, or scared, but in retrospect they were quick to point out that they never regretted

[2] By now, several hundred subjects have been submitted to the LSD test, and from personal communication we know of four instances in which the drug precipitated a psychosis, one with a suicidal tendency. The law of averages will inevitably assert itself as the number of experiments increases, but the correctness of the above reassurance essentially prevails.

having undergone this experiment. The feeling was general that most subjects of this series considered their having undergone this test as a sign of valor. Many were eager to recruit other volunteers, and, at times, it was established that they did so out of sadistic-hostile motivation. Whenever such a subject volunteered to bring a friend, he was closely questioned about his relationship with the prospect. That this was justified was demonstrated by the refusal of a good number of the prospects to comply, indicating, at least on the surface, that the motives of the inducer were doubted or else that his qualifications for giving reassurance were not found quite satisfactory. This was admitted by those who, upon our own intervention and repetition of the reassurance, finally consented to come. There was one instance in which a husband was eager to convince his wife to volunteer and its was later established that he harbored a great deal of resentment against her.

Six subjects in this series were entertainers on radio and television. They were motivated by an unusual amount of curiosity, and they expressed a wish to read the four-hour-test protocols to one another in a group. They were exhibitionistic in the test, as they were in their own profession. There were more specific motivations to induce others to volunteer. One member of this group contemplated marrying one of our prospects, but he was not able to satisfy his sense of uncertainty about her qualifications. He frankly admitted that he would like to learn something about "what really makes this girl tick."

Whether the senior author of this article was the one who made the first step in trying to recruit volunteers or not, there was never any doubt about his being the leader. The subject's relationship with him during the height of the LSD effect often contained the irrational elements of his relationship to important authority figures, as determined by questioning his friends, relatives, and himself, and by examining the personality tests. In paranoid states the senior author was always the supreme target.

In spite of all the precautions taken to select subjects from the normal population, the control Rorschach test not infrequently brought out latent neurotic, and even schizophrenic, trends which appeared potentially disturbing. It was striking that these were the subjects who were most insistent in urging the author to live up to his promises and to deliver the Rorschach results to them as soon as possible. It would appear to be strongly advisable to be on the lookout for incipient schizophrenia during the process of selection, as the test (in reality a form of stress) could conceivably lead to decompensation.

During the second half of this study, articles appeared in national magazines and in newspapers about experiments with LSD-25 in other institutions. It seemed to us that this preexisting knowledge about LSD-25 had a double effect in our selections. There was an increased amount of curiosity and willingness to experience the bizarre effects of this drug, which were rather sensationally treated in the press, and the prospects required more reassurance about the safety and reliability of these experiments than their earlier colleagues. Fortunately, by that time more than half of our subjects had had their tests, so that we had a certain degree of authority with which to underscore our verbal assurances.

One member of the investigating team was a woman. Only one male subject, who was her acquaintance, showed signs of sexual stimulation toward her at the height of his euphoria. This would confirm the prevailing opinion(3) debated by few (20) that sexual drive in the LSD state is, if anything, decreased.

METHOD

The average amount of LSD-25 (given by mouth in distilled water) varied from 30γ to 100γ; but only two subjects had less than 40γ, and the majority received 1γ per kilogram of body weight. The experiments started at noon, the subject having had nothing to eat since breakfast. Lunch, which uniformly consisted of minced meat, bun, and malted milk, was served approximately three hours after the start. The subject would lie comfortably on a padded cot in a Faraday cage lined with a plastic board and provided with a window and a door, which was closed only when the EEG was recorded. Conventional needle electrodes were inserted in the scalp in the frontal, motor, temporal, and parietaloccipital areas and left in place during the experiment. A Grass III eight-channel apparatus was used, and the electrode combinations were both monopolar and bipolar. Each channel was fed into the input of an Offner differential automatic analyzer, which recorded six individual 10-second epochs per channel, and the frequency distribution from each area of the brain was quantitated in the form of a mean histogram on graded paper. The control EEG was recorded during the 10 minutes following the administration of LSD-25, when no effects could be expected, and none were observed or reported by the subject. Only during the few minutes of EEG recording was the subject left alone, though he was still watched through the window.

The first sign of LSD effect consisted of dilatation of the pupil, which occurred from 20 to 30 minutes after ingestion of the drug. Rarely were the subjects conscious of any particular change by that time. Subsequent recordings were made just prior to the administration of the Rorschach tests, one hour after the beginning, and also at two, and even in some instances three, hours after administration of the drug, when the effect reached maximal proportions. In almost every instance, at the end of the experiment (four hours) the EEG was back where it was in the beginning. Rarely, departure from this rigid schedule was made to record the EEG at such times as the subject reported particularly interesting or intensive delusional or hallucinatory phenomena. The effect of single-light-flash stimulation was studied with each sample. This was done in a darkened room with the subject's eyes closed. In some instances air blast through a rubber hose applied to the skin, usually on the leg, operated by an electronic valve, was also used both before and during the LSD effect.

At the height of the intoxication, which usually fell between the second and the third hour, in rapid succession serial seven-digit and test-word retention and recall tests were given, followed by tapping-rate determination of both hands. Tendon reflexes and coordination were tested according to a routine neurological survey of the central nervous system, in turn followed by a two-line writing test and a drawing test that was supposed to gauge ability to judge distance and parallelism and to draw circles. Remote and recent memory was tested in the conventional manner before and during the LSD effect. All these tests were finally repeated several weeks later, when the control Rorschach test was administered.

Throughout the four hours of testing, as nearly complete silence prevailed in the room as was possible. Movements of the members of the team in the neighboring rooms were reduced to an unavoidable minimum. The few standard auditory stimuli consisted of the monotonous drone of the paper drive of the EEG machine, the periodic clicking of the automatic analyzer, and the chimes of a nearby church at 15-minute intervals. All of these played a role and were commented upon during the experiments. In the hypomanic phase, the features of the examiner (at the time only one was in the cage), his clothes, pencil, and paper, were all included in the flighty, distracted verbalization of the subject. A Magnascriber wire recorder was set up in the neighboring room, with remote control and microphone attachments inside the cage. Not only the individual productions but also everything pertinent to the experiment was dictated into the sound track, and all the statements were time-marked. Whenever EEG recording was done simultaneously with the subject's description of his delusions and hallucinations, time markers were made on the EEG paper. The transcription was a phonetic one; not only were the patient's exact productions reproduced faithfully, but even his moanings and grunts were transcribed with as great a fidelity as was possible. Silences and hesitancy were marked on the transcription with dots.

It was felt that a compromise had to be reached between limiting the stimuli to the unavoidable minimum, keeping the environment as constant as possible, even though our set-up might have suffered from the impossibility of testing gait, station, and balance, and the possible distracting effects of objects and personnel that were outside the subject's visual field, under the conditions stated above. After the volunteers were taken home, they were invited to describe on paper whatever possible late effects the drug may have had upon them, but only in two instances were prolonged after-effects of significance reported. These experiments were done on Saturday, and no one was warned to change his usual plan for weekend activity. The subjects were guarded, however, from indulging in excessive amounts of alcohol, which was arbitrarily limited by us to two drinks. Even so, the majority of those who drank alcohol reported that their tolerance on that night was low, and it was exceedingly easy for them to get intoxicated. However, the form that this intoxication took was uniformly the same, namely, irresistible sleepiness. No one suffered major gastrointestinal disturbances either during or for the rest of the day after the experiments. One subject was a linotype setter for a local newspaper, who went to work two hours after the end of the experiment. He reported having heard several complaints of the many mistakes in spelling that he made that night. On the other hand, another subject, a student in physiology, who was preparing for an examination, was able to spend the evening and the following day in hard preparation without experiencing any difficulty in his efforts.

In all but the two first cases, the control Rorschach test was administered (no less than five weeks) after the LSD test. Owing to defects in retention and recall produced by LSD, the control test was less contaminated by the recollection of the drug Rorschach test than was true the other way around.

RESULTS

A. AUTONOMIC CHANGES

Dilatation of the pupil was present in each case; in fact, it was the first noticeable sign. It occurred on an average within 30 minutes, and in one hour the pupil reached its maximum diameter. Three and a half hours following administration it began to decrease in size, though even after four hours, when most of the experiments were concluded, the pupil was still not back to its original size. In four cases dilatation was noticed as late as seven hours after the start. In one instance, one pupil was dilated more than the other in a woman who used to complain of migraine headache and in whom a difference in the pupils during the headache had been noted previously.

Increased perspiration, particularly of the hands, was noted in three instances to a great excess and in six instances to a slight extent.

A feeling of general warmth occurred in one instance; it was of a definite, sharp onset and disappeared just as quickly, persisting for three minutes. In one instance a subject complained of a typical bolus hystericus. Five cases reported a mild degree of nausea.

The intensity of the autonomic changes did not seem to depend on the dose, which was maximally 1γ per kilogram.

B. PERCEPTUAL ANOMALIES

1. *Visual Sensations.* — Visual manifestations were most prevalent, as compared with other sensory changes (18 cases). There is no explanation for the comparative sensitivity of the visual system to LSD, though it never reached the predominance of eidetic phenomena described in mescaline-induced states. There was certainly no correlation with the high alpha index on the EEG, which some authors have related to great visual imagery in thinking.

Commonest were illusions, particularly noticeable with the eyes closed, of which examples are given.

Bright yellow coils that seem to jiggle like the lines of a poorly functioning television screen. These later on changed into a multicolored, painted turtle, with the colors flowing into one another rapidly.

Black slivers, in the shape of a diamond, the angles of which disappeared when someone clapped his hand close to the subject's ear.

In another case, light manual pressure over one eye caused a black-and-blue-colored, giant bug to appear in that eye, which quickly changed into multicolored flutes, then just as quickly into a spiral staircase, then into modern windows looking out on a pool and a house with the San Francisco Bay Bridge, with the rising sun behind it. This subject emphasized the extraordinary precision and vividness particularly of the last picture and insisted that one should let him enjoy this scenery a little while longer.

Another subject first saw Gothic windows with his eyes closed. Later on, however, searchlights appeared in the bottom of his visual field, with the beams directed upward in a vertical direction, making everything around them extremely dark.

Flickering flash bulbs spread out in a horizontal plane, oscillating and then quickly changing into multicolored ribbons, interrupted by spikes spaced at regular intervals.

Primitive masks of various colors with wings on them, changing into angular, crawling, filmy, feathery croppings, like a forest. In this instance, the change from the mask to the forest occurred upon clapping of the hands. At times, the images seen with eyes closed were very simple, like, for instance, gray-colored, muddy-looking curves, which, upon clapping of the hands, became suddenly elongated and then stayed that way.

One interesting feature of this set of symptoms was the fact that Gothic or cathedral windows, which some of the subjects were capable of reproducing with pencil and paper, were reported by seven subjects. Mayer-Gross also noted that under mescaline he had imageries of cathedrals.

With eyes open, one subject could see a crimson-colored glow around the edges of all kinds of objects placed before his eyes, upon which the light had fallen.

Visual hallucinations with the eyes open were reported by three subjects.

One subject, with eyes open, saw Mexican peons with sombreros, dancing or hopping around on donkeys.

Another subject saw, in a completely darkened room, light moving very slowly and deliberately from left to right, hitting only the subject's eyes in a cyclic fashion.

A third subject saw geometrical figures, half-purple and half-black in color, coalescing into a goldfish, and the goldfish then would dance on the wall with the hindfins moving rhythmically.

Anomalies of visual perspective, such as micropsia, metamorphopsia, and heteromegalometamorphopsia, were from time to time (usually for short periods) reported by 10 subjects. Some of these visual sensations were quite complex. For instance, one subject saw the cover of *Time* magazine, with eyes open, upon looking on the wall, with the faintly discernible photograph dilating and contracting in size at first, and later on coming out of the red frame and retracting into it in a rhythmic fashion. This he noted to be synchronous with his breathing. By holding his breath, for instance, he was able to hold the image quite close to his eyes.

The quick change-over from one image to another is illustrated by a subject who, at first with eyes closed, saw a stained Gothic window, the green colors of which began to peel off, turning quickly into autumn leaves, and by the time these autumn leaves had fallen to the ground they quickly changed over into peacock feathers, covering the ground in a random fashion.

It was interesting that the emotional reaction described by the subjects to these various strange occurrences varied from one order of sensation to another. Many subjects, up to the time when they were asked to close their eyes and to describe what they had seen, if anything, emphasized that they felt exactly as if they had taken two martinis and they were in no way in a position to detect anything novel about their state of intoxication. The moment they closed their eyes, however, and the above-described illusions appeared, they were quick to point out that this experience was a different one. Their reactions to the extraordinary variety of the illusions and images, whether they were looking upon them with eyes open or closed, was frequently one of exhilaration, and delight in some instances, and they were quite irritated when they felt that the observers would not allow them to continue to be absorbed and insisted on precise description. They would raise their hands and wave the observers away or, in some instances, very annoyedly ask them to be quiet for a minute, complaining that the kaleidoscopic images followed one another with such extraordinary variety that they were not able to give a proper verbal account.

The situation, however, became at times dramatically reversed when the subjects began to report shrinking or dilatation of images, or when walls were "breathing" in and out, or when various multicolored halos appeared around the lighted edges of certain objects placed in front of them. The prevalent emotional reaction now was one of apprehension. They admitted even a reluctance to describe them, and very frequently they had to be coaxed. It seems that dissolution of the familiar landmarks or spatial orientation was upsetting, and sometimes threatening to their reality control.

2. *Auditory Sensations.* — Nine subjects reported transient hyperacusis, and two noted sound reverberations. On the other hand, auditory stimuli frequently had a profound effect on other sensory experiences.

3. *Gustatory Sensations.* — In one case nausea was associated with a tobacco-like taste in the mouth in a subject who had never smoked, but the clarity suggested an actual hallucination. This appeared after

two hours and lasted two minutes; then in another half-hour it returned and lasted for one minute.

In another case, nausea and a metallic taste occurred each time that the subject had visual reverberations.

4. *Vestibular Sensations.* — This term is used because it involves in pure form the subject's relationship to space — reminiscent of, if not identical with, the vestibular aura common in psychomotor seizures.

In one instance a feeling of giddiness occurred, which quickly changed into a feeling of soaring off into space.

There were many visual anomalies with an alteration of perspective associated with feelings of propulsion and retraction — such an anomaly was a mixed visual-vestibular one.

5. *Bodily Sensations.* — Such changes occurred in 17 cases, and the descriptions of these anomalies are noteworthy for their great variety. It should, however, be noted that only rarely were changes spontaneously reported. These came out usually upon questioning, accounting perhaps for the fact that other authors have not reported a similarly high incidence of changes in body sensations.

The commonest occurrence was a difference in the way one part of the body felt as compared with the rest. The following descriptions will be given to indicate the range of abnormalities noted.

"I can't use my left arm, which feels strange; it has a disconnected feeling. It's flexible and it feels more elastic than the other, and it also feels busier. When the light shines on my limbs, the left looks bigger."

"It seems to me that my body feels different depending whether my mouth is open or closed, or whether my legs and arms are crossed or uncrossed. The left arm and leg feel different; their color is different and the right side appears to be more connected to my body. I also have a feeling as if I had a hole in the middle of my forehead."

"Both arms and legs feel detached. The right one more than the left. The left foot appears to be half as long as the right. I am not conscious of my throat between my head and body."

"My teeth feel numb. My right arm feels stronger, and my right eye definitely feels swollen every time that the light shines on it."

"The ulnar half of my left hand feels different, detached, and it gives me the feeling that I could not perform with it as well as with the rest of my arm."

"The right half of my body feels as if it were 6 o'clock in the evening, whereas the left one feels as if I had just gotten up early in the morning."

"I feel numb from my teeth up and it feels as if that small top part of my body would be completely covered by hair."

"The left arm feels numb, pulled into a knot. It appears thin when the light shines on it, more so than the right, and my whole left side is very suggestible. Whatever I think about it, I feel it right away."

"My body feels completely apart from my brain, and, incidentally, this is a very happy feeling. My abdomen feels disconnected from the rest of my body, and when I use my right hand to write with, it feels disconnected."

C. SYNESTHESIAE

This term will be used rather loosely in the text to describe phenomena characterized by one sensory experience influencing another. In 14 cases — as the complexity of these sensory cross influences increased — a paranoid type of schizophrenic reaction occurred, the evolution of which could be followed (and predicted) step by step. Hence, a detailed treatment of these experiences is deemed to be important.

As mentioned before, in every instance hand clapping, or some such noise as that, was able to change invariably the form of the images, and only seldom was it also capable of changing the color. When the kaleidoscopic illusions had sharp angles, hand clapping would smooth out the angles and turn the fingers into curved ones, which then stayed that way for a while. If the subjects happened to see, however, curved images at the time of hand clapping, these never turned into angular ones; but, rather, they began to coalesce and their color changed in some cases.

Optic sensations were most commonly influenced by auditory stimuli. It should again be emphasized that the emotional reaction of the subjects to the influence of random noises (including distant church bells) on their visual sensations was not considered disturbing, but when the auditory stimulus was the voice of the inquiring observer, the subjects began for the first time to become anxious, and from this point on usually anxiety increased, as illustrated by the following examples.

The subject (A) saw Mexican peons wearing sombreros on donkeys dancing on the wall, which after a while would vanish, but then the wall would "breathe" in and out at a rather rapid rate, not coinciding with the subject's own rate of respiration. When the observer, at this point, asked her to continue to describe what she was seeing, she began to complain that the examiner's voice was responsible for these changes; that the "breathing" of the wall followed exactly the examiner's voice, high sounds causing the wall quickly to retract and deep ones causing it to advance slowly forward. Random voices in the background were doing the same thing, causing the "breathing" of the wall to speed up and become extremely disorganized, and, at this point, the patient began to complain that the background voices were "talking terrible things about her." This, then, marked the beginning of a frank paranoid reaction, in which the members of the investigating team were placed in the category of "persecutors who have nothing else to do but to drive the subject out of [her] mind." When she was asked if she really believed that this was so, she admitted that she knew perfectly well that this was part of the experiment but she could not dissociate herself from this conviction. Her attitude became one of annoyance and negativism, which persisted during the rest of the experiment.

Another subject reported a series of experiences which started at the precise moment that Card 2 of the Rorschach test was shown to her. This rare case did not proceed, however, to feeling persecuted:

"As I look at this card I see cream-colored, long towers which, whenever I hear the church bell — like now, for instance — break up into ever so many little towers, but at the same time the color changes from cream to brown. At this moment, the towers coalesce (as you clapped your hand) into brown scrolls, and then everything on this card appears in a light-blue color. Now that you said 'Card #3,' I all of a sudden see music in the card which I can recognize as being a sequence from the "Bald Mountain Suite," but I don't hear the music — I see it in the form of mountain ranges interconnected by iron bridges." (This sort of experience obviously defies description.)

The influence exerted by the examiner's voice on the subject's body sensations likewise caused anxiety, often admitted to with reluctance, and this feeling apparently acted as the precursor of a subsequent reaction of paranoid coloring.

(Subject B) "I feel that my left arm is strange, disconnected, pliable, and it appears to be busier than the right side. When you talk about these sensations, however, these sensations leave me. I am frightened by the amount of influence that you have on my feelings, and I resent the fact that I am kept here against my will. I resent the fact that I am suggestible; I know you have fouled me up here, and I demand that you give me some ice that I could put in my left hand to get rid of that strange feeling. You are upsetting me by allowing people coming into this room, and they seem to come in only when I am talking. Why isn't there something done about this?"

The same subject had, at the conclusion of the experiment, reported that the left half of his body, including every organ, felt detached and entirely different from the right, as if he had been split into two and put back the wrong way. Even the left hemisphere of his brain felt different than the right. In addition, he had that feeling that up to the hip he had been suspended in a rubber tube. This split feeling persisted for 12 hours after the conclusion of the test, and it reportedly terminated suddenly, when, at that time, during a sexual act with his wife, he experienced an orgasm.

It was a short jump from complaining that the examiner's voice influences vision or illusion or body sensation to the more annoying complaint that the voice presently subjugates thinking and, finally, that the examiner's thoughts control the subject's thinking. Thought control was associated invariably with a hostile, conspiratorial trend.

When frankly persecutory ideas were admitted, the first target was the examiner; later on, however, all members of the team — in fact, everybody present in the room — was included. There has never been any doubt, however, that, of all the members of the investigating personnel, the No. 1 enemy was the senior author.

One subject, for instance, first complained that the interrogating psychologist was purposely irritating him. He then proceeded to admit that people whispering and walking around in the background were likewise in the league with an aim to annoy and upset him. When he was asked, however, how he felt about the senior author, this subject (C) snarled and spat out in space. It thus appeared that when synesthesiae led to ideas of thought control and influence, the referential ideas quickly went over into frank paranoid delusions. Insight, however, was never lost, but for the first time the subject had great difficulty in maintaining a detached objectivity about the experiment.

Another subject first noted that the psychologist's voice exerted an influence upon his thinking as he was presented the Rorschach cards, at which point he stated, using a language that became more and more reminiscent of that encountered in schizophrenia:

"I feel persecuted. I have no idea what goes on. I don't want to answer. I don't seem to be able to dissociate these cards. The color red means something that is interesting. I do not feel like answering. I already had suspicious feelings when you gave me a milk shake; I was not able to pull out the straw. I suspect some kind of a trick. I have a fear of losing control. I think you all want to confuse me. I resent that I am suggestible and that I can be talked into everything. I am getting fond of these cards the way one gets fond of one's mother. I think I simply learned to hate you all. I resent the way you talk to me; it's just a lot of 'ice cream' talk."

Another subject reported that the left leg felt lighter than the right; it also felt more excitable, and the excitement was directed and provoked by the examiner's questions. At this point the subject burst out with this:

"I suspect a trick. I have the feeling that what I say is unimportant and it's not going to be written down. Everything here seems to be up to the psychologist; what he thinks is important will be written down. I feel I am discriminated against."

Another subject admitted anxiety for the first time when he noted that his own words changed the Rorschach picture, and, after he had remained silent for a while, he stated that he was scared to admit this. At this point, while he was protesting against the examiner's allowing such strange influences to prevail, he also said that he was very uncomfortable and that "the place smells as it if would explode any minute."

One subject acted hypomanic and gave 25 to 30 responses to Rorschach Card 5. He then complained of feeling a hole in the middle of his forehead, and that the examiner, while talking, blew the cold air of his breath into ths hole, thus influencing the functioning of the subject's brain and his thinking. He suddenly became morose and taciturn, and when the usual lunch was presented to him, he refused to eat. When asked why, he gave a series of excuses. First, he objected to the straw in the milk-shake cup, claiming that it appeared to him about one mile long. Next, he claimed that he was not capable of eating in a lying-down position, even though he was propped up and covered with an oilcloth bib. He then "frankly admitted" that he was not hungry. It was only after the experiment was concluded that he stated the real reason, namely, that he had the feeling that the food was being poisoned. He gave only four responses to Rorschach Card 5, and all the subsequent responses remained under five per card.

In all instances save one, such a reaction was over at least within three and a half hours after the ingestion of the drug. This particular subject (C), one hour after the conclusion of the test, was standing in front of the building participating in a group discussion (not about the test) when the senior author noted that he kept a distance of approximately 6 ft. from the cluster of five people involved in the conversation. When he was asked about this, he came forward by 3 ft., drew an imaginery straight line with the heel of his shoe on the concrete, put the tip of his shoe on top of the line, and claimed that if he would push his foot one inch beyond the line in the direction of the senior author, he would immediately experience the feeling that he "hates [his] guts."

D. PERSISTENCE OF AFTER-IMAGE

The persistence of the after-image was very markedly increased in 15 instances. This increased coincided with a marked prolongation of the alpha perseveration time (the period during which alpha waves were blocked after visual stimulation). In one instance, the after-image persisted for two minutes. The average increase was 10 seconds. In all but one case it was the positive after-image that persisted. In one case, however, the negative after-image persisted for eight seconds.

E. DISTORTION OF TIME SENSE

Time sense was found to be distorted in 14 cases. In 5 of these 14 cases time appeared to be elongated. In six cases it was speeded up, and in the rest of the cases it appeared to be slowed down at first and then speeded up to the remainder of the experiment. This cyclic variation could not be correlated with a hypomanic-depressed emotional reaction cycle. Quite a few subjects were able to follow the passage of the time by counting the sound of a bell of a nearby church. When they were asked to give an opinion about the length of time that they had spent in the laboratory, they would say that, even though they knew exactly how much time had elapsed since they came in, it still appeared to them either much longer or much shorter on the basis of their own subjective experience of the duration.

F. DISTURBANCE OF EGO SENSE

The ego boundaries were disturbed in varying degrees, under various conditions, at various dosages, and this state persisted for various lengths of time. A feeling of depersonalization and estrangement of a vague character was noted in six subjects, while in another seven these disturbances occurred as an elaboration of the changes that interfered with their visual perspective, and, even more frequently, they were connected with anomalies of their bodily sensation. It seemed as if the ego boundaries were very sensitive to such subjective experiences, to which they reacted with anxiety. The subjects complained that when they were left alonge they feared "impending dissolution." Two other patients, however, became exhilarated, as a result of their "all-pervading expansion," and insisted on being left alone to enjoy this state of "floating," or "lightness." For short flashes many patients noted tendencies toward dissociation and self-observation, and one subject pictured himself as the statue "Thinker" by Rodin, with his head propped up in his palm, watching himself undergoing the strange reactions. Feeling of impending ego dissolution occurred mostly in subjects who had relatively large doses. In one subject various degrees of this distortion persisted for over 24 hours.

G. LANGUAGE CHANGES

Apart from a definite tendency toward playing with words in various ways, sometimes associated with forced laughter, instances of echolalia were common. The most characteristic language change, however, was condensation of words, consisting usually of uniting the first half of one word with the second half of its opposite. Sometimes a simultaneous feeling of opposite impressions was reported — for instance, "I feel as if I were going up and down in the elevator at the same time," or, "I feel as if I were lying down and standing up all at the same time." This sometimes was extended even to the description of images evoked by the Rorschach card — e.g., "I see the south side of a broad-beamed burlesque queen going north and I am standing in front of her."

Many examples of random condensation of words were picked up from the sound track. One example was "mopher," a condensation of mole and gopher. Instances of a tendency toward alliteration were likewise noted, as, for instance, when describing a Rorschach picture, "This looks like the late, lamented esophagus."

In general, the language changes were very similar to those that were reported by several authors, more particularly by Brickner (38) who studied the tape-recorded production of subjects who were under deep amobarbital (Amytal) sodium narcosis. Condensation and confusion over opposites and over choice between these opposites were not only expressed in language but were openly admitted in the thinking of the subjects. Most of them felt the simultaneous opposite feelings mildly annoying, though these were not limited to paranoid reaction cases.

There were only two subjects who used the typical peripheral circumlocutions noted in amnestic aphasia. The music coming from a Good Humor man's car was described as "church bells on wheels." Another called a cigarette "smoking stick."

H. MOTOR SYMPTOMS

Twitching of the muscles of the leg was reported in one instance; facial and eyelid twitches, in another instance. Choreiform hand movements were present in one case. Tremor without chill was present in one case; tremor with chill was noted in another instance, but the tremor outlasted for several hours the disappearance of the chill, and it was limited to the upper extremities.

All subjects were tested for reflexes before and during the test. In 10 instances hyperreflexia of a generalized character, without any pathological reflex activity or lateralization, was noted. Left hyperreflexia was noted in two instances. Since these subjects were lying in bed throughout the test, gait and station were not tested.

I. EMOTIONAL REACTION

A variety of emotional reactions occurred in every subject, to some extent. Euphoria throughout the experiment was the case in eight subjects, who spent a considerable amount of the time in giggling and in boasting about their wonderful feeling. In only two subjects was depression the prevailing mood throughout. In all the other subjects mood was variable from one time to another, usually starting out with euphoria, forced laughter, and giggling, and turning into anxious pre-occupation at the height of the experiment, especially when this was the forerunner of a frank, disturbed, suspicious, paranoid, dysphoric reaction. Anxiety was anticipatory in some; others, however, described the feeling as if their anxiety were an after-reaction to something terrible that had happened to them — as if they had undergone a big scare, which, however, was now over.

Without exception, the subjects who developed paranoid reactions admitted, not during the experiment but later on, that at the height of their reaction they had fear of losing self-control and of becoming violent. Even the euphoric subjects admitted to small annoyances which interfered with their "enjoyment" of their perceptual anomalies, or else they had the feeling that the variety of their subjective experiences were not taken too seriously. One such subject, for instance, resented the fact that his remarks were always written down on the margin of a white sheet of paper. Most of the subjects commented on the extraordinary redundancy of their perceptual anomalies or of their thoughts, and, while they protested that they were trying their best but could not keep up with words in their attempt to describe what they experienced, a few felt sorry for all the people who missed this extraordinary experience.

J. TAPPING RATE

The subject's ability to tap at maximum speed with both hands was part of the study. This was recorded on a wire recorder, and measurements were made at the height of action of LSD and compared with the control values. It was found that, on an average, in right-handed persons the tapping rate on the right side was 120 for a 10-second period, as compared with 110 on the left side. The control figures were 90 and 80, respectively. This would indicate, then, an increase in tapping rate while under the influence of LSD. No change in the pattern was noted.

K. HANDWRITING AND DRAWING

LSD produced insignificant distortions in handwriting, but ability to judge size, distance, parallelity, and angles in drawing was impaired as compared with the control samples.

L. RETENTION AND RECALL

Every subject, at the height of the test, was given 10 test words, with the explanation that the subject's speech was being examined.

In 14 instances, only 3 or fewer out of 10 test words were recalled after three minutes. In another six instances, 4 out of 10 words were recalled, which was considered borderline, while in the remainder, of five cases, recall was within the normal limits.

M. ELECTROENCEPHALOGRAPHIC CHANGES

In the spring of 1951, when our experiments began, the consensus was that, however pronounced the effect of LSD-25 was on the psyche, the EEG remained normal. In 1952 Delay and associates (27), however, injected LSD-25 into the veins of rabbits in amounts 25–600 times as large as the oral dose effective in man and reported a complete flattening of the record, with disappearance of the rhythmic elements of the animal's EEG. They, too, felt that in a few human cases the EEG remained unchanged.

The report of our experience with electroencephalography will be divided into several categories.

1. *Effects on Alpha Index* (22 cases). — Alpha index for our purposes is defined as the amount of alpha activity present in 100 seconds of record in a single channel (occipital) free from artifacts. As stated above, on occasions when the subject reported a particularly vivid or unusual hallucination, the EEG was recorded. Inasmuch as the experience described was sometimes anxiety-laden, there occurred, understandably, a more or less complete blocking of the alpha activity and its substitution by desynchronized low-voltage fast activity. When, however, the alpha index was determined at the time when the drug had its maximal effect and was compared with the control one, a strip of tracing was chosen when the patient was merely lying motionless in a darkened cage, not reporting any hallucination or delusion in particular. It was felt that such a strip would be more nearly representative of the background activity under maximal drug effect.

While the frequency of the background varied within the normal limits, alpha definition was affected in 18 out of 22 cases. Decrease in alpha index (11 cases) was 30% (range 20%–90%). Increase in alpha index (7 cases) was 50% (range 10%–70%).

In those cases in which decrease in the alpha index occurred two patterns were observable. In some cases the reduction of alpha activity was limited to the occipital areas, which remained that way throughout the experiment. More frequently, however, the normally present central (Rolandic) low-voltage beta pattern began to spread until finally the whole cortex became devoid of alpha waves. There was a time when the parietal alpha activity was gone while the occipital areas were still exhibiting synchronized alpha activity. Therefore, it would seem that we were not dealing with a sudden process of desynchronization, such as occurs in visual or mental stimulation — affecting the EEG in toto — as would be expected in anxiety. Rather, there was a gradual spread in the relative displacement of the alpha pattern, much as is seen after intravenous barbital administration, though without the characteristic monorhythmic fast activity seen in the latter.

2. *Abnormal Activity.* — In three cases large (up to $150\mu v$), 6 cps bursts swept through all the leads, in the absence of drowsiness.

3. *Paradoxical Activity.* — Gibbs has described the appearance rather than the blocking of alpha activity in response to light stimulation or opening of the eyes in drowsy subjects. This was seen in four of our cases, but drowsiness here could not be ascertained.

4. *Response to Single-Light Stimulation.* — Every subject was given 30 single-light stimuli in a darkened room with eyes closed. The perseveration time — the interval between disappearance and reappearance of alpha waves — following the 0.2-second light stimulus was determined before and two hours after the administration of the drug. Perseveration-time average before drug administration was 0.41 second; perseveration-time average after administration was 0.90 second. Alpha blocking was therefore over twofold prolonged. This might tie in with the clinical observation that the time of persistence of afterimage was frequently elongated — at times to two minutes.

5. *Deactivation in Response to Hallucination.* — It was known that during the visual hallucinations provoked by mescaline the well-synchronized alpha activity of relaxation was brusquely replaced by a deactivated low-voltage fast pattern. This observation was more than confirmed when working with LSD. In two subjects who had primary visual hallucinations in the right half-field only, the left occipital alpha was absent while the right one was prominent. This ceased immediately with the disappearance of hallucination.

Delay (27) and others were able to bring back bursts of normal rhythm in the flat, deactivated record of their rabbits under the LSD effect with the intracarotid administration of $40\gamma/kg.$ of acetylcholine. This would suggest that the mechanism to account for focal deactivation might be due to regional vasospasm.

6. *Response to Tactile Stimulation.* — In a previous work (34) we reported on the effect of tactile stimulation by graded air blast on the spontaneous electrical activity of the cortex. In some subjects, after a long latency (one second), bursts of fast activity (18–22 cps) appeared for 0.36 second (when the stimulus lasted 0.2 second) bilaterally without desynchronization of the occipital alpha waves. It was thought that this represented a secondary rapid after-discharge and

the rebound return of the central beta pattern. Four out of the six subjects originally used for these experiments, when given LSD, developed a delusion of body scheme involving the left side of the body, which they were unable to feel and which "did not belong to them." When the air blast was applied to that side, no change was noted on the EEG on either side. When, however, the tactile stimulation was applied to the uninvolved side, which they did feel, the fast bursts were clearly observable. This suggests that some blocking takes place in the proprioceptive feedback mechanism that operates in this area, which, as Gastaut has shown, is sensitive to proprioceptive, exteroceptive, and even associational, influences.

Findings such as this tend to emphasize that the EEG is related to the functional organization of the brain and is not merely a side-product of brain activity. More particularly, evidence appears to be present to the effect that the cortex has an ability to distinguish between internal and external stimuli in that it seems to be refracory to external stimulation when it is busy, as it were, for internal consumption.

In conclusion, it appears that LSD produces an alteration in the EEG, with only rare abnormalities outside the alpha range. It is to be expected that the widespread disturbances in mood, feeling tone, alertness, reality testing ability, and perceptional acuity are bound to influence the behavior of the spontaneous electrical activity of the brain, if only in response to various sensory stimuli.

N. RORSCHACH TESTS

All the subjects were tested, but, owing chiefly to the disruptive effect of LSD on test procedures, in only 13 cases was it possible to correlate the drug and control tests. The detailed description of our findings will be described in a later article. In general, there appeared to be potential indices in the control test that could predict a psychotic reaction — the kind of reaction, however, was considerably less precisely foretold. Paranoid and nonparanoid forms of schizophrenia reactions exhibited scores that were not widely differentiated. With one exception, however, the occurrence of complex synesthesiae in the 14 cases that developed paranoid-like reactions acted as a more reliable precursor of the feeling of being persecuted. Our impression was that both psychopathological and pathophysiological factors mattered in the development of the paranoid reaction.

COMMENT

At this point, we are in a position to inquire about the working mechanism of this drug.

A. BIOCHEMICAL ASPECTS

There is a general agreement among all the authors who have experimented with LSD–25 that the resultant psychosis model is of the acute exogenous type in the sense of Bonhoffer, as described in 1908. This author assumed in psychoses the existence of a toxic substance arising in an organ that is damaged, or even in the metabolism of the brain itself. He called such toxins "etiological intermediary products." Such an assumption had its starting point in the finding that in certain liver diseases and in some conditions associated with brain damage increased values of certain amino acids were detected in the cerebrospinal fluid. In a variety of psychoses tryptophan could be demonstrated in the spinal fluid with the help of glycoxylic acid as the reagent. The presence of tryptophan is believed to indicate cell damage in the cerebrum.

Blickenstorfer (37), who has made the most thorough analysis of this problem, postulates that acute exogenous reaction types may occur as a result of starvation, exhaustion, cachexia, fever, and cerebral circulatory embarrassment; and to the toxins due to tissue breakdown must be assigned an important role, besides the parts played by inherited constitution and by psychogenic factors. The question is whether the role of toxins is etiological or pathoplastic.

The infinitesimal amount of LSD sufficient to produce profound selective involvement of the central nervous system is meaningful. If no known measuring method can quantitate the LSD concentration in the body, it is hard to dismiss the possibility that in the psychoses some such substance in likewise small (tracer) amount might be the offending agent.

Fortunately, we do have of late a biological method that can at least affirm the presence — if not measure the amount — of LSD in the body. Witt (26) selected a spider (Zilla-X-notata) as the subject of standardization, because it has a central nervous system that is both complex and simple and presents negligible variation from one to the other. Also, the building of spider webs can be objectivated (photography), and the speed of formation can be recorded. The spider-web test has been used previously for the detection of Pervitin and strychnine. As compared with the effects of another *psychoticum*, such as mescaline, the regularity and symmetry of the angles of the web are pronounced with LSD, and the speed of its formation is increased. The latter factor is attributed to a better utilization of sensory stimulation. The marked differences between mescaline and LSD in their respective effects on the spider suggested to Witt a possible difference in point of pharmacological action, which is all the likelier as the effects of these drugs on the human also present definite differences. The suggestion is obvious that the body fluids of normals and psychotics should be compared as to their effects on the spider, a study which is one of our present projects.

Abramson and Evans (24) recently found a specific psychobiological effect of LSD on the Siamese fighting fish and set up nine criteria with respect to changes in posture and state of consciousness that would permit use of the fish for a biological assay. No mention is made, however, on the effect of other substances on the fish in their preliminary report.

There is general agreement that certain psychotics are relatively resistant to the effects of LSD. Resistance cannot be attributed to the negativism, dissimulative tendency, and fluctuating emotivity of the schizophrenic, for instance — which might interfere with the reporting of LSD changes — since resistance occurs in all forms of psychosis. Those who report on hallucinations are aware of an alien addition to their "customary" hallucinations. One reason for this refractoriness might be the existence of LSD or LSD-like substance in large quantities in the central nervous system of psychotics, so that the addition of a few micrograms of substance is ineffectual. The effective dose is 1γ/kg. for normals and 3γ–6γ/kg. for psychotics.

Reference is made to the presence of tryptophan and like amino acids in the spinal fluid after concussion and other conditions of brain damage.

Tryptophan is a waste product of protein catabolism, and it is incorporated into the formula of LSD–25. Blickenstorfer points out that, while this may be incidental, on the other hand, it may also be considered an indication that LSD somehow appears in human metabolism. It need not be an alien substance. LSD can be partially synthetized out of amino acids, such as tryptophan, two dipeptides, and two tripeptides, which are all normal metabolic products in the human.

There is evidence that some hallucinogens, such as mescaline, form bonds with liver proteins at the time of their maximal effect. Block (33) has shown the inclusion of radioactive mescaline in the liver protein of mice in vivo and adopted the working hypothesis according to which hallucinations found in men originated by mescaline are due to this union of mescaline with body proteins. The moment of appearance and the duration of hallucinations were in agreement with the formation, high-point, and destruction of mescaline-protein. He is of the opinion that it is possible that schizophrenics are suffering from an enduring intoxication by amine proteins, due either to the changes in the amine oxidase system or to the absence of an inhibiting agent. In normals, protection against such protein-amine unions is furnished by the aminoxidase system, an inhibiting factor, and the cell membrane.

Fischer (39) studied the affinity of mescaline, Methedrine, LAE (lysergic acid monoethylamide), and LSD–25 for wool, and found that wool absorbs them in the same ratio as the precipitate model psychoses in normal subjects (500 mg., 100 mg., and 100γ, respectively). All these substances produce initial sympathetic hypertonia, followed by peripheral adrenergic blockage, before psychotic symptoms appear. The higher the initial sympathetic overactivity (stress or the shock phase of the general adaptation syndrome of Selye, or administration of 1 mg. of atropine prior to LSD), the lower the dose of the drug needed to produce a model psychosis. Possibly, persisting stress, causing first sympathetic and later on parasympathetic overactivity, tends to increase the dosage of LSD necessary to produce psychotic symptoms (such as hallucinations) which may serve as an explanation for the resistance of psychotics to doses of LSD effective in normal subjects.

Besides bringing into play the adrenergic factor in the biochemical working mechanism of LSD, this study also points out the analogy between keratin of high sulfur content (wool) and the protein component of certain cell membranes which may be the structural target surface involved in psychoses.

According to Mayer-Gross (8), LSD–25 seems to interfere with carbohydrate metabolism as well. He found a transitory rise in blood sugar and blood hexose monophosphate in normal subjects subjected to LSD, while the other stages of carbohydrate metabolism were not modified. Although this finding is still awaiting confirmation, this author theorizes that LSD, by an antienzymatic action, interferes with the splitting of sugar to the hexose monophosphate stage. Intravenous injection of 33% dextrose suppressed the LSD effect, and large amounts of glutamic acid likewise acted as an LSD inhibitor. The effect of dextrose is significant in that, if glycogen metabolism is blocked at the hexose monophosphate stage by LSD, and if the psychotic state is related to this, the direct administration of dextrose, which would bypass the hexose monophosphate chain in order to be utilized, would be expected to have an inhibiting effect on the psychotic symptoms. Optic illusions, feelings of estrangement, euphoria, disturbance in concentration, and various perceptual anomalies did in fact become modified, and, to some extent, they tended to disappear. Since Mayer-Gross and associates did not consider clearly demonstrated a relation in time and severity between the psychological symptoms and the biochemical changes, they repeated their experiments on 13 hospitalized schizophrenics (41), in view of the fact that such persons have a considerably greater tolerance for the drug and, consequently, they may show only minimal psychological symptoms after the usual oral dose. Eighty micrograms of the drug produced slight psychological effects. Yet hexose monophosphate showed a rise of 1.46 mg. per 100/ml., whereas under control conditions, when water was given, the mean value fell by 1.17 mg. per 100/ml. Mescaline, when given to normals, has produced a psychotic picture rather similar to LSD without a similar rise in the blood hexose monophosphate level. In vitro experiments with tissue brei showed that LSD-25 stimulated the respiration of brain tissue, whereas this was not the case when the tissue was that of the liver of guinea pigs. The authors, therefore, concluded that LSD-25, both in vitro and in vivo, has a sparing effect on hexose monophosphate metabolism, which is greater in the brain than in the liver, and in this respect it reacts unlike mescaline hydrochloride, which has no effect on blood chemistry, even though it is just as capable of producing a psychotic state in normals.

Liddell and Weil-Malherbe (42) have studied the effect of LSD-25 on plasma epinephrine levels and blood sugar concentration in patients suffering from psychoses, as well as in patients with psychoneuroses, and found that there is an initial rise of the epinephrine level, followed by a drop below the starting point and, finally, a secondary rise in epinephrine. The moderate increase of the blood sugar concentration was not considered to be significant.

Rinkel and associates (43) are likewise of the opinion that LSD may interfere with a major enzyme system. They consider the epinephrine system the most important. This is suggested not only by the marked sympathicotonic effect of the drug but by the observations made by Witt (26), who, when feeding LSD to spiders, noted that each thread was much thinner than those in the control, leading to the speculation that this might be due to the exhaustion of the epinephrine supply of the spider, it being known that the spider web consists almost exclusively of epinephrine. Rinkel recalls the findings in animals by Heirman in 1938, according to whom a metabolite of epinephrine, called adrenoxin, had systemic effects similar to LSD, and an observation of Osmond and Smythies, who, in 1950, reported that an earlier epinephrine metabolite, adrenochrome, known for its hemostatic effects, which showed structural similarly with mescaline, produced dramatic psychotic phenomena in self-experiments. Rinkel was not able to duplicate this observation. However, he is of the opinion that the solution used by the above authors was deteriorating and thereby may have been contaminated by a further epinephrine oxidation product, namely, adrenoxin. He speculates that adrenoxin, a natural metabolite of the decomposition of epinephrine, may be operative in psychosis.

The recent findings of Marrazzi (32) further attempt to enlarge our knowledge about the behavior of epinephrine metabolites and similar substances with respect to their effect on the central nervous system. He found that in cats epinephrine, arterenol, and epinephrine preservatives cause synaptic inhibition, as measured by the decrease in the postsynaptic surface-negative wave, without affecting the presynaptic positive wave. This finding was obtained when stimulating one point of the cat's occipital cortex and recording from the symmetrical point on the other side, which two points are connected through the corpus callosum. He found a similar synaptic inhibition when using such hallucinogens as amphetamine, mescaline, LSD–25, adrenochrome, and serotonin, all showing structural similarity to epinephrine. An incidental observation of his was that serotonin, which was considered by Woolley and Shaw (31), on the basis of systemic antagonism in animals, as an LSD inhibitor, in his experience had the same effect as LSD on synaptic inhibition. He considered the effect of LSD and other hallucinogens on a group of synapses as typical of a more generalized effect and concluded "that the resulting pattern of overall activity would be a function of the variations in synaptic thresholds." If further experiments show that LSD affects the occipital cortical synapses differentially, then an explanation may be at hand for some findings which at the moment appear to be puzzling. It is well known that in LSD intoxication visual perceptual anomalies far outweigh the involvement of other sense organs. Alpha blocking following single flashlight stimulation is markedly prolonged in subjects receiving LSD, as compared with control experiments, when the stimulus is visual. Not so, however, when alpha blocking is achieved by other stimulation. Likewise, we have found that persistence of after-image, when the eyes were closed, very striking, whereas the echo-effect of other sensory modalities proved to be insignificant. The special affinity of LSD for the occipital cortex, which, incidentally, may apply also to mescaline, still has to be confirmed by comparison with the behavior of other synaptic systems.

From the first description of the marked psychotic effects of LSD and the observation that the threshold of psychotics to these drugs is much higher than that of normals, a widespread investigation was directed toward the discovery of LSD antagonists. It has been known that very large doses of barbiturates, or intravenous dextrose, had at least a partial or transitory LSD-blocking effect. In the hands of Hoch, chlorpromazine, as well as a combination of amobarbital sodium and metamphetamine, behaved similarly. Agnew and Hoffer (46) found the effect of intravenous nicotinic acid to be LSD-blocking, while Himwich showed that Frenquil (α-4-piperidyl diphenyl carbinol hydrochloride) has an antagonistic effect on the EEG of rabbits receiving large doses of LSD.[3] Serotonin, with a definite antagonistic effect systemically, failed to overcome the neurological effects of these drugs. Fabing (44) reported on the partially and transitorially antagonistic effect of pipradrol (Meratran) on LSD psychoses in men, while the same drug has a beneficial, euphoria-producing effect in patients who suffer from depression and thus is likely to exert its action on the hypothalamus. Hoff and Arnold (45) found that glumatic acid or succinic acid, which is found in the citric acid cycle, terminated the mental symptoms induced by LSD, and it has also been known that succinic acid temporarily relieved the acute symptoms of schizophrenics. These authors implicate the carbohydrate metabolism in schizophrenia and in conditions induced by LSD, being of the opinion that a disturbance in carbohydrate metabolism may exist in certain circumscribed areas of the brain, possibly in the posterior hypothalamus. It is of interest that patients with damage to this region of the brain were resistant to LSD.

From the available biochemical data, it appears that at the present time the widespread experimental and speculative findings cannot explain the action of LSD satisfactorily. The problem, however, is far greater than the biochemical working mechanism of a drug that is capable of producing psychosis. It ties in with the much more important problem of the biochemical foundation of at least some psychotic states. The ever-greater inclusion of an increasing number of disciplines in psychiatric investigations clearly points to the necessity of integration and synthesis of a great mass of scattered information.

B. NEUROPHYSIOLOGICAL ASPECTS

Comparison of the LSD state with intoxications produced by other, better-known agents shows similarity and, at the same time, a very definite measure of difference, which puts LSD in a class of its own among the experimental psychotic agents.

All the other agents except mescaline had in common the necessity of using relatively large amounts in order to produce a model psychosis.

In the mescaline state, psychic functions, more than any other, seem to be affected, and the resultant model psychosis appears to be more stereotyped and therefore more predictable. Eidetic phenomena

[3] Discussion on LSD Symposium, American Psychiatric Association, Atlantic City, May 12, 1955.

are very much in the foreground as compared with other systems. Catatonic-like schizophrenic states are more prevalent than the other forms. Mood is characterized by dysphoria and anxiety, the latter outlasting by as long a period as one week the administration of the drug. There is even a stereotyped response of the EEG in mescaline intoxication in that the substitution of synchronized alpha rhythm by desynchronized beta activity likewise may go on for several days in fairly good harmony with the state of anxiety which it reflects.

The peculiarity of the LSD model psychosis is the infinitesimal amount of drug necessary to produce a psychosis, which is approximately one-hundredth that of mescaline — an indication of a formidable degree of affinity. Considering the very profound psychotic-like changes produced by LSD, it is surprising how minimal is the interference with intellectual function, a fact which underscores its similarity with the undeteriorated schizophrenic reaction. The LSD psychosis is also noteworthy for its relative sparing of the corticospinal and of the cerebelloextra-pyramidal system.

In attempting to localize the possible site of origin of the various psychic manifestations of LSD, on the basis of anology, most of the symptoms reported are reminiscent of the sensory seizures or psychosensory seizures commonly seen in "psychomotor" epilepsy, and which were reproduced by cortical electrical stimulation by Penfield. This would suggest the primary involvement of the temporal lobe and its connection with the diencephalon. Very few of the phenomena noted in LSD psychosis would have to be localized elsewhere. Thus, for instance, the primary visual hallucinations, delusions, visions, and pareidolias bear a resemblance to the sensory seizures or sensory auras seen in that condition. Micropsia, metamorphopsia, and heteromegalopsia, which are so prominently displayed in the description of LSD psychoses, are elements of temporal lobe seizures, as are kaleidoscopic pictures, vertiginous attacks, and auditory and gustatory, as well as olfactory, perceptual anomalies. Auditory and visual reverberations, feelings of familiarity and unfamiliarity ("I had this test before"), based on both visual and auditory experiences, likewise fall into that category.

In psychomotor epilepsy, it can hardly be implied that the specific cell structures located in the temporal lobe gray matter, in and by themselves, are responsible for the reproduction of these phenomena when electrically stimulated. They merely mark the starting point of an excitation traveling down in a circuit of neuronal chains of various complexity.

Unlike the situation in epileptic phenomena, however — at least when recorded from the intact skull — in LSD psychosis no evidence of synchronized excessive electrical discharge could be detected. It has to be noted, however, that even in psychomotor epilepsy it is not always possible, when recording in this fashion, to find the electrical sign denoting excessive neuronal discharge. Recording directly from subcortical or poorly accessible areas in a human brain (rhinal fissure, undersurface of the temporal lobe) often discloses that, owing to the distance of the recording scalp electrode from the site of origin of the discharge, the spike may not always be picked up, or else, instead of picking up a spike, sharp waves appear, indicating the amount of distortion that takes place when the spike is conducted in distance. The complete absence of any abnormal electrical event in LSD psychosis, even when the site of origin is presumed to be the convexity of the temporal lobe cortex, has been uniformly confirmed. LSD may have a special affinity for these structures, but, because the neurons of these structures are intact, there is no excessive discharge and resultant electrical abnormality. Consequently, the activation and successive involvement of the neuronal chains responsible for the LSD phenomena must have a different mechanism than the one that prevails in seizures. The fact that sometimes these phenomena are enduring, and even rapidly changing back and forth, and that they can be influenced by introducing other stimuli operating in other sensory systems (synesthesiae), further underscores the difference between the mechanism of LSD-produced brain phenomena and seizure phenomena. Occasionally, psychomotor epileptics, recognizing the threat on the basis of a sensory aura, may produce voluntarily a reflex counter-stimulation, which, however, rather than changing the value of the sensory experience, merely terminates the aura, and, even so, not always.

The mood changes, which may vary from depression to elation in the same subject in the same experiment, may alternate from one to the other, along with such signs of emotional incontinence as seen in forced crying or forced laughter, suggest the activation of diencephalic circuits, possibly along the pathways of the two circuits for emotional expression originally described by Papez, although there may be many others.

These mood changes bring into mind the experimental findings by Foerster, Penfield, and Bailey, who were able to produce manic-like or depressive-like changes when mechanically stimulating the anterior or the posterior half of the floor of the third ventricle respectively.

The perceptual anomalies occurring in the somatosensory system, particularly those involving distortions and delusions of the body image, would implicate chiefly the postcentral parietal primary sensory receiving area, the surrounding associational strips, and the parietothalamic connections of the minor hemisphere, since most body-image distortions lateralized to that side.

The frequent complaints of numbness, particularly in the perioral area and in other midline structures, or the paresthesias prevailing in these same structures, are reminiscent of the sensory seizures, which are, in turn, localized to the secondary sensory receiving area.

In many cases a moderate defect in retention and immediate recall was noted, and it was also noteworthy that distortion occurred with respect to the correct appreciation of the duration component of time. There is a suspicion that the difficulty indicates interference with the recording element in the memory process, which, in turn, would suggest involvement of the amygdaloid complex. This structure may also be responsible for the reduction of sexual drive.

As mentioned under the heading of EEG changes, a marked increase in the average alpha perseveration time was observed in almost every instance. This means that, in response to a (visual) stimulus, the alpha blocking persisted for an inordinately long time. This finding has to be combined with another observation, namely, the markedly long persistence of the after-image, either positive or negative. Since here the occipital alpha rhythm is involved, there is reason to believe that the disturbance affects those cells responsible for occipital electrogenesis, and that some synaptic embarrassment is responsible for the prolonged alpha perseveration time and for the long persistence of the after-image.

The peculiarities of the LSD language, showing condensations of words, often of opposite meaning, suggest some conflict or confusion over twoness and an embarrassment over a choice. While this area has not been properly investigated, the similarity between these phenomena and what one commonly sees in schizophrenic states is not the least striking effect of the LSD psychosis.

A special chapter ought to be reserved to explain the modus operandi of the synesthesiae, especially because in a fair number of cases they occurred in a sequential order and so commonly ended by producing a paranoid state.

Ordinarily, sensory volleys travel in "closed conduits," even when the peripheral receptors of the various sense organs are simultaneously and maximally stimulated. Though collaterals reach such widely separated structures as the ascending reticular system in the brain stem, the hippocampus, and the cerebellum as the volley passes corticopetally, normally these impulses do not discharge into one another.

In the LSD state it was quite striking how often one form of stimulus influenced the perception of another form, suggesting some "cross-talk" mechanism between the individual sensory pathways. One can speculate about the level where this mutual penetration may take place. Sometimes the synesthesiae were quite primitive and quite simple, suggesting, in turn, that the confusion originates at a subcortical, for instance, a thalamic, level. A good example of this would be the disappearance of the illusion of angular-shaped designs and their instant metamorphosis to curved ones upon simply clapping the hands.

A far more complicated synesthesia, however, is the one in which the subject reports that his voice or his perceptual anomaly referable to the somatosensory system is influenced by the examiner's voice. Here, the correspondence, or, rather, abnormal correspondence, probably takes place on the cortical level between one sensory associational or recognition area and another, sensory primary receiving area, or its correspondent association and recognition components. In the most complicated instances, particularly when these sensory disturbances are associated with annoying emotional reactions, the frontal lobe and its connections both to the sensory associational areas lying more posteriorly and to the diencephalon will have to be implicated.

Another possibility is that the critical area is of one of cross talk in the hippocampus. Recent work indicates that the hippocampus is the recipient of afferent volleys coming in from all the sense organs, and it has earlier been established that the hippocampus is a very important link of the two primary emotional neuronal chains described by Papez. It is, therefore, conceivable that the distortion in sensory perception in the form of a synesthesia, entering in confusion in the form of afferent volleys into the hippocampus, may give rise to a strong discharge, which then will travel in the aforementioned two circuits of emotional expression, leading either to a fear or to anger or to both. Accordingly, the dysphoria of the paranoid state may originate at the hippocampal level.

Probing of the personality make-up of the subjects often furnished poorly reliable, and even contradictory, indices for the prediction of a subsequent paranoid reaction, so that the assumption gained momentum that the paranoid schizophrenic reaction need not be considered as a distortion of an underling personality so inclined, but, rather, may be the outcome of a perceptual overload to which priority ought to be assigned in the hierarchy of stresses that an individual can tolerate. The delusional hallucinatory experiences of a paranoid nature induced by LSD enabled one to break this reaction down into its elements, study its evolution, as it were, "in slow motion," and observe the sequence of events leading up to the ultimate break.

Where general knowledge of the subject and the Rorschach test suggested confusion over sexual identification and repressed homosexuality, delusions of thought control and control over body sensations emanating from an examiner of the same sex could conceivably have set the stage for a homosexual panic or acted as precursors of a flight into a paranoid state to keep homosexuality from breaking into awareness. Paranoid inclination of male subjects was not interfered with when the examiner was of the opposite sex, though it must be stated that one of the women subjects (C) was always aware that she was under the direction of the senior author, of the male sex. Then, again, examined by the (male) senior author, three of the "paranoid" subjects were women.

There is an individual variation in frustration- and anxiety-tolerance, and such factors as individual sophistication might also explain this type of personality reaction to mental stress. It comes to mind, however, that experiments have been devised before in which the frustration- and stress-tolerances of individuals were put to severe test. For instance, subjects who speak into a microphone and then hear their voice through earphones with a certain amount of fixed delay describe the resultant confusion as being exceedingly unpleasant, at times leading to stuttering and to a great deal of anxiety, but we are not aware that a paranoid state resulted.

Considerations of dosage had to be discarded. Some of our subjects who developed paranoid reactions have taken only 0.5γ per kilogram, which is half of the average dose given by almost every author to their normal subjects.

In toxic-organic psychoses, especially when the state of consciousness is interfered with, the EEG shows signs of diffuse slowing, while in functional psychotic reactions no abnormalities are seen. In this respect, the LSD-induced psychotic state shows greater analogy with functional conditions, which would permit the speculation at least that both share the same substrate in the brain for which LSD shows the greatest affinity. On the other hand, least affected are those systems which form the core of the routine neurological examination and which utilize long tracts, such as the corticospinal, ascending sensory, and cerebelloextra-pyramidal systems.

Many authors have emphasized the marked resistance of psychotic persons to such doses of LSD as are effective when given to normal subjects, though some observed such a resistance only in deteriorated cases. (9) This led some authors to assume that a LSD-like substance must already be present and in operation in psychotics; consequently, the addition of the infinitesimal amount which is effective in normal subjects, understandably, cannot possess any enhancing effect on the psychotic picture. As Condrau (13) has pointed out, the large doses merely increase the vegetative symptoms which set the limit of the amount of LSD anyone can tolerate. It is possible that in psychotics the same anatomicophysiological substrate that shows the greatest affinity for LSD is already involved; therefore, the resistance would be due to the fact that the substrate in question is already "busy" and, consequently, unable to react further to stimuli that are supposed to bear upon it by virtue of the circulating LSD. This explanation might be the same as that which would account for the common observation that psychotics rarely, if ever, change a psychosis, and that the development of one form of psychosis renders them "immune" to the development of another one. In this connection, an observation of Hoff and Arnold (45) may be pertinent. These authors have given LSD to patients with alcoholic psychosis. They have found that a great measure of resistance to LSD exists in subjects suffering from delirium tremens. In Korsakoff's syndrome, the reaction to LSD was the same as in normals so long as the midbrain and medulla were intact. In alcoholic psychoses, with more widespread damage (cortex, thalamus, hypothalamus, mammillary body, midbrain, and medulla), the LSD effect was nil. These data suggest that some structures in the diencephalon possess an LSD-sparing effect. Fabing (44) reported the LSD-antagonistic effect of the drug pipradrol, which, clinically, produces euphoria in depressed persons, and, therefore, one can assume that the point of its action is in the hypothalamus. Once again, therefore, it appears that if part of the critical substrate responsible for LSD psychosis is busy and under stimulation by another chemical, then LSD will not be able to dislodge or modify this effect and, therefore, some of the most important symptoms of LSD psychosis will not find expression.

Sketchy as the data so far available may be, they rather impressively point to a complex working mechanism. Interference with several enzyme systems would be one element of the LSD effect, and its selective embarrassment of that part of the central nervous system which subserves psychic function would be the other.

SUMMARY

d-Lysergic acid diethylamide (LSD-25) given to 25 normal adults produced widespread temporary alteration in psychic functioning which resembles most the undeteriorated schizophrenic reaction type.

Insight and detachment are sufficiently preserved to allow recognition of the split between thinking and feeling as reality control becomes disturbed.

Rorschach tests completed in 13 cases allowed a fairly good prediction of a psychotic-like change from the control to the drug test, though the type of model psychosis could not be reliably anticipated.

Paranoid-like reaction (14 cases) showed a better correlation with the occurrence of complex synesthesiae, especially when the cross influence involved the examiner's voice and thoughts, on the one hand, and the subject's thoughts and bodily sensations, on the other.

Theories aiming at elucidating the working mechanism of this drug point toward enzyme inhibition, on the biochemical side, and predominant vulnerability of the temporal lobe-diencephalic circuits, on the neurophysiological side.

References

1. Beringer, K. *Der Mezcalinrausch: Seine Geschichte und Erscheinungsweise*, Berlin, Springer-Verlag, 1927.

2. Stoll, A., and Hoffmann, A. Partialsynthese von Alkaloïden vom Typus des Ergobasins. *Helvet. chim. acta*, 26: 944, 1943.

3. Stoll, W. A. Lysergsäure-Diäthylamid, ein Phantastikum aus der Mutterkorngruppe. *Schweiz. Arch. Neurol. u. Psychiat.*, 60: 279, 1947.

4. Becker, A. M. Zur Psychopathologie der Lysergsäurediäthylamidwirkung. *Wien. Ztschr. Nervenh.*, 2: 402, 1949.

5. Fischer, R., Georgi, F., and Weber, R. Psychophysische Korrelationen: VIII. Modellversuche zum Schizophrenieproblem; Lysergsäurediäthylamid und Mezcalin. *Schweiz. med. Wchnschr.*, 81: 817, 837, 1951.

6. Rinkel, M., DeShon, H. J., Hyde, R. W., and Solomon, H. C. Experimental Schizophrenia-like Symptoms. *Am. J. Psychiat.*, 108: 572, 1952.

7. DeShon, H. J., Rinkel, M., and Solomon, H. C. Mental Changes Experimentally Produced by L. S. D. (d-Lysergic Acid Diethylamide Tartrate). *Psychiat. Quart.*, 26: 33, 1952.

8. Mayer-Gross, W., McAdam, W., and Walker, J. W. Psychological and Biological Effects of Lysergic Acid Diethylamide. *Nature*, London, 168: 827, 1951.

9. Hoch, P. H., Cattell, J. P., and Pennes, H. H. Effects of Mescaline and Lysergic Acid (d-LSD-25). *Am. J. Psychiat.*, 108: 579, 1952.

10. Savage, C. Lysergic Acid Diethylamide (LSD-25): A Clinical-Psychological Study. *Am. J. Psychiat.*, 108: 896, 1952.

11. Arnold, O. H., and Hoff, H. Untersuchungen über die Wirkungsweise von Lysergsäurediäthylamid. *Wien Ztschr. Nervenh.*, 6: 129, 1953.

12. Gastaut, H., Ferrer, S., and Castells, C. Action de la diéthylamide de l'acide d-lysergique (LSD 25) sur les fonctions psychiques et l'eletroencéphalogramme. *Confinia neurol.*, 13: 102, 1953.

13. Condrau, G. Klinische Erfahrungen an Geisteskranken mit Lysergsäure-Diäthylamid. *Acta psychiat. et neurol. scandinav.*, 24: 9, 1949.

14. Busch, A. K., and Johnson, W. C. LSD 25 as an Aid in Psychotherapy: Preliminary Report of a New Drug. *Dis. Nerv. System*, 11: 241, 1950.

15. Hoch, P. H., Cattell, J. P., and Pennes, H. H. Effect of Drugs: Theoretical Considerations from Psychological Viewpoint. *Am. J. Psychiat.*, 108: 585, 1952.

16. Belsanti, R. Modificazioni neuro-psico-biochimiche indotte dalla dietilamide dell'acido lisergico in schizofrenici e frenastenici. *Acta neurol.*, (Napoli) 7: 340, 1952.

17. Forrer, G. R., and Goldner, R. D. Experimental Physiological Studies with Lysergic Acid Diethylamide (LSD-25). *A. M. A. Arch. Neurol. & Psychiat.*, 65: 581, 1951.

18. Sloane, B., and Lovett Doust, J. W. Psychophysiological Investigations in Experimental Psychoses: Results of the Exhibition of d-Lysergic Acid Diethylamide to Psychiatric Patients. *J. Ment. Sc.*, 100: 129, 1954.

19. Sandison, R. A., Spencer, A. M., and Whitelaw, J. D. A. The Therapeutic Value of Lysergic Acid Diethylamide in Mental Illness. *J. Ment. Sc.*, 100: 491, 1954.

20. Anderson, E. W., and Rawnsley, K. Clinical Studies of Lysergic Acid Diethylamide. *Monatsschr. Psychiat. u. Neurol.*, 128: 38, 1954.

21. Frederking, W. Über die Verwendung von Rauschdrogen (Meskalin und Lysergsäurediaethylamid) in der Psychotherapie. *Psyche*, 7: 342, 1953.

22. Sandison, R. A. Psychological Aspects of the LSD Treatment of the Neuroses. *J. Ment. Sc.*, 100: 508, 1954.

23. Abramson, H. A., Jarvik, M. E., Kaufman, M. R., Levine, A., and Wagner, M. LSD-25: I. Physiological and Perceptual Responses. *J. Psychol.*, 39: 3, 1955.

24. Abramson, H. A., and Evans, L. T. LSD-25: II. Psychobiological Effects on the Siamese Fighting Fish. *Science*, 120: 990, 1954.

25. Abramson, H. A. LSD-25: III. As an Adjunct to Psychotherapy with Elimination of Fear of Homosexuality. *J. Psychol.*, 39: 127, 1955.

26. Witt, P. N. d-Lysergsäure-Diäthylamid (LSD-25) im Spinnentest. *Experimentia*, 7: 310, 1951.

27. Delay, J., Lhermitte, F., Verdeaux, G., and Verdeaux, J. Modifications de l'électrocorticogramme du lapin par la diéthylamide de l'acide d-lysergique (LSD-25). *Rev. neurol.*, 86: 81, 1952.

28. Rothlin, E., and Cerletti, A. Über einige pharmakologische Untersuchungen an Mausen mit congenitaler Drehsucht. *Helvet. physiol. et pharmacol. acta*, 10: 319, 1952.

29. Gaddum, J. H. Antagonism Between Lysergic Acid Diethylamide and 5-Hydroxytryptamine. *J. Physiol.*, 121: 15 P, 1953.

30. Clark, L. C., Fox, R. P., Bennington, F., and Morin, R. Effect of Mescaline, Lysergic Acid Diethylamide, and Related Compounds on Respiratory Enzyme Activity of Brain Homogenates. *Fed. Proc.*, 13: 27, 1954.

31. Woolley, D. W., and Shaw, E. Some Neurophysiological Aspects of Serotonin. *Brit. M. J.*, 2: 122, 1954.

32. Marrazzi, A. S., and Hart, E. R. Relationship of Hallucinogens to Adrenergic Cerebral Neurohumors. *Science*, 121: 365, 1955.

33. Block, W. Modellversuche um Schizophrenie problem, XIX International Physiological Congress, Montreal, 1953; Abstract of Communications 217.

34. Bercel, N. A. Automatic Analysis of Human Cortical Response to Sensory Stimulation. *Electroencephalog. & Clin. Neurophysiol.*, 4: 368, 1952.

35. Stoll, W. A. Rorschach-Versuche unter Lysergsäure-Diäthylamid-Wirkung. *Rorschachiana*, 1: 249, 1952.

36. Zeichner, A. M. Psychosexual Identification in Paranoid Schizophrenia. *J. Project. Techniques*, 19: 67, 1955.

37. Blickenstorfer, E. Zum ätiologischen Problem der Psychosen vom akuten exogenen Reaktionstypus: Lysergsäure-diäthylamid, ein psychisch wirksamer toxischer Spurenstoff. *Arch. Psychiat.*, 188: 226, 1952.

38. Brickner, R. M. A Neutral Fractionating and Combining System. *A. M. A. Arch. Neurol. & Psychiat.*, 72: 1, 1954.

39. Fischer, R. Factors Involved in Drug-Produced Model Psychoses. *Experientia*, 10: 435, 1954.

40. Mayer-Gross, W., McAdam, W., and Walker, J. Lysergsäure-Diäthylamid und Kohlehydratstoffwechsel. *Nervenarzt*, 23: 30, 1952.

41. Mayer-Gross, W., McAdam, W., and Walker, J. W. Further Observations on the Effects of Lysergic Acid Diethylamide. *J. Ment. Sc.*, 99: 804, 1953.

42. Liddell, D. W., and Weil-Malherbe, H. The Effects of Methedrine and of Lysergic Acid Diethylamide on Mental Processes and on the Blood Adrenaline Level. *J. Neurol. Neurosurg. & Psychiat.*, 16: 7, 1953.

43. Rinkel, M., Hyde, R. W., and Solomon, H. C. Experimental Psychiatry: III. A Chemical Concept of Psychosis. *Dis. Nerv. System*, 15: 259, 1954.

44. Fabing, A. D. New Blocking Agent Against the Development of LSD-25 Psychosis. *Science*, 121: 208, 1953.

45. Hoff, H., and Arnold, O. H. Die Therapie der Schizophrenie. *Wien. klin. Wchnschr.*, 66: 345, 1954.

46. Agnew, N., and Hoffer, A. Nicotinic Acid Modified LSD Psychosis. *J. Ment. Sc.*, 101: 12, 1955.

37

SCHIZOPHRENIA: A NEW APPROACH. II. RESULT OF A YEAR'S RESEARCH

ABRAM HOFFER, Ph.D., M.D., HUMPHREY OSMOND, M.R.C.S., D.P.M., AND JOHN SMYTHIES, M.B., D.P.M.

Saskatchewan Hospital, Weyburn, Saskatchewan

About one year ago, with the encouragement of the Editor-in-Chief, a short paper appeared in the *Journal of Mental Science* entitled "Schizophrenia; A New Approach" (18). In this paper it was noted that mescaline and adrenaline have a similar biochemical structure. It was suggested that one of the aetiological agents in schizophrenia might be a substance or substances lying between these two; with the psychological properties of mescaline but effective in concentrations nearer those of adrenaline. Dr. Harley Mason elaborated this suggestion from the biochemical standpoint. For convenience these hypothetical substances were called, collectively, M substance. If M substance occurred in the body, it would account for the group of illnesses usually referred to as schizophrenia better than any hypothesis so far advanced. It has been the good fortune of the co-authors of that first paper (J. R. S. and H. O.) to be able to join forces with the third author of this paper (A. H.) to test the hypothesis. It is with the ef-forts of the last year that this paper is concerned.

A proposition such as this sounds simple enough to test when sketched on paper, but once it is tackled in the laboratory and the ward, many difficulties soon appear. Money must be obtained, technical help sought, workers from other disciplines must be persuaded to give their support. When all this has been achieved, and it is no small achievement, one has not even started. First of all one must decide where to start. In the range of substances which lie between mescaline and adrenaline there are many hundreds perhaps thousands of compounds. Some of these have been made and are well known to pharmacologists, but many have found no place in medicine and are hidden away in obscure corners of the literature, or having no effect on a particular experimental animal have never been recorded in print. To make or obtain such a large number of compounds would be costly and laborious, but this work and expense would be but a tithe of the effort required

From the *Journal of Mental Science*, 100: 29, 1954.

to test them. For, since animals are unable to talk and so inform us of their experiences, testing must always be done on human volunteers.

So, a year ago, although we had received the keenest support from the Director of Psychiatric Services of the Provincial Department of Public Health, Regina, and although the Federal Department of Health and Welfare in Ottawa had secured a most generous grant for us from Dominion funds, putting us in a position to start work, there remained an unanswered question, "Where do we start?"

In order to answer this question an extensive survey of the literature was made in greater detail than had been possible for the first paper. We paid special attention to the chemistry and pharmacology of substances known to produce disturbances in perception, feeling, thought and behaviour without marked changes of consciousness. This survey showed that both Lindeman (13) and de Jong (11) had been aware that a chemical relationship existed between mescaline and adrenaline, but neither of them had linked this with Cannon's conception of stress, nor did they suggest that it might have special importance.

De Jong had, in order it appears to be "objective," made his jumping off place the occurrence of catatonia in small mammals and discovered that if large doses are given an almost unlimited number of substances can cause catatonia. He paid little attention to whether the catatonia was produced by large or small doses, or whether the substances themselves were likely to occur in the animal body. His findings were, therefore, unlikely to be of much assistance to those engaged upon a research into schizophrenia which is remarkable for being accompanied by few clearly demonstrable biochemical, anatomical or electrophysiological changes even when the psychological disturbances are most disastrous.

We, therefore, limited our enquiry to substances which could produce psychological disturbances similar to those found in schizophrenia without causing clouding of consciousness, confusion, or gross physiological disturbances.

Hallucinogens

As a working hypothesis we supposed that M substance was chemically closely related to adrenaline. This enabled us to narrow the search from hundreds of potential M substances to those lying on a continuum between mescaline and adrenaline. However, it was possible that the similarity in chemical structure between mescaline and adrenaline was purely due to chance. In order to test this inference we searched the literature to determine whether other compounds were able to produce psychological disturbances similar to mescaline and had a similar chemical structure.

When the literature is examined to catalogue these hallucinatory substances, which for convenience we have called the hallucinogens,[1] one is struck by their small number. Those that will produce their effects without being accompanied by other disturbing symptoms can easily be counted on the fingers of two hands and those whose chemical structure is known on the fingers of one hand.

We have so far obtained some information on five compounds which may be called the hallucinogens: mescaline, lysergic acid diethylamide, harmine, ibogaine and hashish. The active hallucinogenic principal in hashish has not yet been definitely established. The structure of the other compounds are shown below, with exception of ibogaine which is known to have an indole nucleus and is placed among the indole alkaloids, Mankse and Holmes (14).

These then are a group of compounds that have an indole nucleus in common, assuming that in mescaline the side chain can readily be fused by its amino group to form an indole compound. It might, therefore, be that the indole ring is associated with hallucinogenc properties, provided the compound is able to cross the blood brain barrier. This in itself did not bring us any closer to M substance since these compounds are all plant alkaloids and are unlikely to be present in the body.

Pink Adrenaline

Shortly after we completed our first paper an observation was made by one of us (J. S.) in curious circumstances. In the hopes of interesting a young and brilliant historian in our work so that he could be persuaded to take mescaline, he was invited to listen to a recording of a recent mescaline experience of H. O.'s. As the recording continued it became evident that the interest and curiosity which it had at first evoked was soon replaced by anxiety and alarm. At last the historian remarked, "I have also had such things happen to me." He then explained that for many years he had suffered from asthma, and that when he had a severe attack he would become "an adrenaline addict." He had experienced eidetic and hypnagogic imagery since childhood and had found that these large doses of adrenaline increased this imagery to an alarming extent and when his eyes were open "things looked different."

[1] One must always offer some excuse for coining a long new word, but there is really no other satisfactory one. It is not a good word but seems to us less obscure than eideticum or phantasticum and begs the question less than "schizogen" or "schizophrenogen." As Klüver has observed when we take these remarkable compounds we enter a world beyond language, so it is hardly surprising that they may be difficult to name.

This valuable piece of information combined with a careful scrutiny of adrenaline and its near neighbours suggested that if adrenaline could be deprived of its pressor qualities it might itself be a hallucinogen. A search was then started among people taking adrenaline medicinally

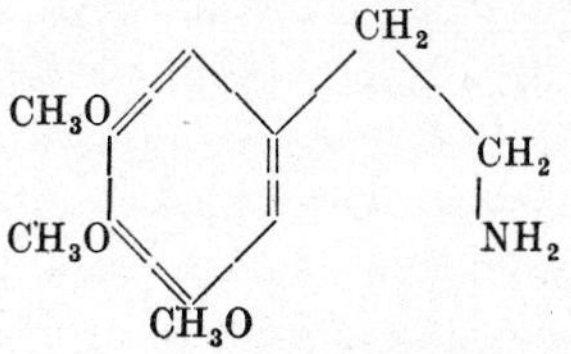

Mescaline.

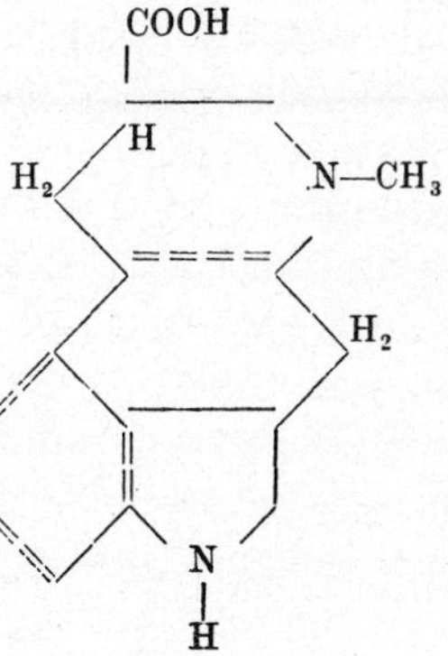

Lysergic acid.

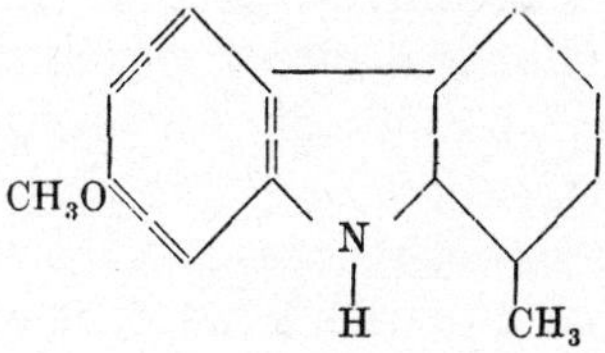

Harmine.

Fig. 1.

to see if they had similar experiences. We have discovered several. A young woman, asthmatic since she was seven, was controlled only by large doses of adrenaline. At the height of her adrenaline consumption she would have visual hallucinations of faces floating across the ceiling. These she related to the adrenaline injections and so did not endow them with any affect. Another woman with urticaria became frankly schizophrenic shortly after receiving an injection of adrenaline to control her allergic condition. The experience was of short duration. Another volunteer, who had the previous day taken lysergic acid diethylamide, was discussing his subjective impressions. He then volunteered that as a boy he had controlled his asthma by means of adrenaline sprays. Often after these sprays he had been aware of subjective changes very similar to this lysergic acid experience. Finally a young medical student reported that after receiving adrenaline to control his asthma he lost much of his ability to empathize; for instance, when driving, he is normally sensitive to the presence of children on the road who might be harmed. After adrenaline injection there was a tendency to allow the children to shift for themselves. Lindemann (13) showed that adrenaline injections markedly aggravated the symptoms of half the schizophrenic patients he studied.

At this point we were lucky enough to obtain another clue from Dr. Asquith, anaesthetist at the Regina Central Hopsital, who told one of us that when he was in England during the late war he had been forced, owing to shortage of supplies, to use adrenaline solution which was somewhat deteriorated. Anaesthetists discovered that, if much larger doses were injected than usual, pressor effects similar to those of the fresh solution could usually be obtained. This was thought to be satisfactory until it was noticed that there were more unfavourable "reactions" than with the fresh solution. It appears that some of these reactions were psychological disturbances, sometimes of an alarming sort. No special study of these psychological upsets were made because they were transient and it was considered necessary to avoid them rather than to investigate them. However, Asquith's observation drew our attention to "pink adrenaline."

At our first meeting in Saskatoon with our colleagues in the research, Professors Hutcheon, MacArthur and Woodford, we raised the question of "pink adrenaline" and put forward a suggestion about its composition. Hutcheon pointed out that "pink adrenaline" certainly contained among other things adrenochrome. In the exciting ten minute discussion which followed after Hutcheon drew the spatial formula of adrenochrome, it was shown that this substance was related chemically to every hallucinogen whose chemical composition has been determined.

The structure of adrenochrome is:

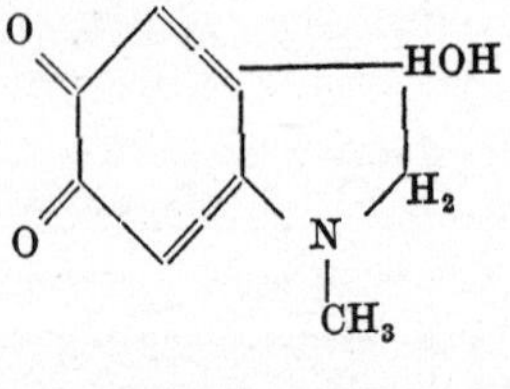

Fig. 2.

It is evident that we had stumbled upon a compound which has an indole nucleus in common with the hallucinogens, which is readily derived from adrenaline in the body, and which can be fitted into a logical scheme relating to stress. Under stress the quantity of adrenalin in the body will increase and this might be turned into adrenochrome in the schizophrenic individual.

Hutcheon agreed to synthesize and determine the toxicity of adrenochrome without delay. All our studies have been made with this synthetic adrenochrome.

It should be noted that adrenochrome, which is very unstable, is not the only substance which would be present in a decomposing solution of adrenaline. Such a solution could contain numerous degradation products of noradrenaline and adrenaline. This is the uncertain mixture that was given to patients who had been anaesthetized and possibly injected with morphine and atropine derivatives. Unfortunately, no study was made of these reactions so we can only speculate about the numerous possibilities.

Adrenochrome

This substance was discovered in 1937 by Green and Richter (10) who found that it played a role as an hydrogen carrier in concentrations that fall within the physiological range. It was found in skeletal muscle in a concentration of about 1×10^{-7} moles. There is still some doubt whether adrenochrome is present in the body. Beyer (4) completely ignores andrenochrome. However, Bacq (2) states "adrenochrome and its derivatives are certainly the most interesting oxidized derivatives of adrenaline. It is an error to consider adrenochrome as an inactive substance because it has completely lost its classical sympathomimetic action." Martin (15) states that adrenochrome is pharmacologically inactive but it is biochemically active.

There are three important bits of evidence for the presence of adrenochrome in the body: (1) Adrenochrome and its oxime (adrenoxyl) form excellent haemostatic substances and have been used therapeutically as vitamin P factors. They increase capillary resistance as well. When adrenaline is injected into a rabbit hemostatic activity appears after four minutes, is maximal after seven minutes and lasts for hours. Adrenochrome injection produces maximum hemostatic activity after three minutes. This is then evidence that the oxidized product of adrenaline may be the hemostatic agent, not adrenaline itself. (2) Adrenochrome being a quinone possesses many properties of the quinones. It oxidizes sulfhydril groups of glutathione, proteins and enzymes and thus is able to inhibit the activity of many enzymes of the glycolytic cycle, Meyerhoff and Randall (17) and the enzymes of the tricarboxylic acid cycle, Woodford (20). It has thus been found that adrenochrome inhibits the mitotic rate of growing cells probably because it interferes with the glycolytic cycle, Lettre (12). Bullough (6) found that, when mice were stressed by overcrowding, the adrenal medulla increased in size by 80 per cent, while the cortex increased 30 per cent. The epidermal mitotic rate fell 60 per cent. They also reported that *in vitro* adrenaline was not an antimitotic agent but that *in vivo* it was, whereas adrenochrome was antimitotic both *in vitro* and *in vivo*. They concluded that the antimitotic factor in the stressed mice was adrenochrome. (3) Martin, Ichniowski, Wisnasky and Ansbacher (16) found that paramino-benzoic acid inhibited the action of tyrosinase on adrenaline and this vitamin should, therefore, increase the sympatheic effect of adrenaline by blocking its conversion to adrenochrome. When administered to dogs it did increase their blood pressure and caused mild hyperglycaemia. This provides evidence that phenolases are active in the *in vivo* destruction of adrenaline.

There are at least five important ways, Bacq (2), in which the body detoxifies the rather large quantities of adrenaline that are produced by the adrenal medulla and the other sympathetic ganglia. These are:

(1) by excretion unchanged in the urine;
(2) by storage of active adrenaline within the cells;
(3) by deamination of the side chain to form oxidizable aldehydes;
(4) by esterification of the phenolic hydroxyls;
(5) by quinone formation to adrenochrome and its derivatives.

The deamination is catalyzed by the enzyme amine oxidase; the esterification is catalyzed by the enzyme sulfoesterase; and the quinone formation is catalyzed by the enzyme phenolase. Of the three main detoxification mechanisms amine oxidase forms compounds with no autonomic properties and which are easily metabolized. Sulfoesterase forms inactive adrenaline esters and these are so excreted in the urine. Phenolase forms adrenochrome which has no pressor properties but does have other important effects. If therefore one blocks either amine oxidase or sulfoesterase the adrenaline may be diverted into adrenochrome.

Substances that block amine oxidase should, therefore, divert adrenaline into adrenochrome formation. Amine oxidase is present chiefly in the liver, intestine, and central nervous system and converts adrenaline into 3, 4-di-hydroxyphenylhydroxyacetaldehyde. Burn (7) believes that amine oxidase plays a role in the sympathetic nervous system comparable to acetylcholine esterase in the parasympathetic system. The enzyme has been found around the sympathetic nerve endings in blood-vessels, the nictiating membrane and the iris of the cat. It destroys noradrenalin more quickly than adrenaline. Blaschko (5) made the interesting observation that compounds having the structure R — C — CH$_2$ — NH — CH$_3$ were inhibitors of amine oxidase. These findings have been supported by Beyer (3) who reported that phenylpropylamines having the amino groups on the terminal carbon were oxidized by amine oxidase, but that, if the hydroxyl groups were present on the ring, the compound was oxidized by phenolase. If the benzene ring contained no hydroxyl and, if the amino group were on the carbon adjacent to the terminal carbon, neither enzyme could oxidize it. The following compounds contain the grouping found to inhibit amino oxidase; cocaine, ephedrine, indole, indoleacetic acid, phenylisopropylamine, desoxyephedrine, pervitin, benzedrine, oxidized derivatives of adrenaline (adrenochrome), caffeine, nicotine, methedrine, and lysergic acid.

Electroencephalographic and other Studies of Adrenochrome

Woodford's (20) studies have shown that when adrenochrome gets into the cerebral cells it inhibits markedly intermediary metabolism of carbohydrates. Eade and Hutcheon's (8) studies on the lowering of body temperature by adrenochrome at the same time as body metabolism is increased, indicates that adrenochrome lowers body temperature by some central effect. This is suggestive evidence that adrenochrome can cross the blood brain barrier in contrast to adrenaline which is not able to do so. To test this possibility further intravenous adrenochrome was given to a series of volunteers (normals and patients) and E.E.G. records were taken on some. In epileptics with definite cerebral dysrhythmias the adrenochrome markedly increased the generalized arrhythmia within half an hour. The focal activity became more prominent. In people with a normal E.E.G. and a clinical history of epilepsy the adrenochrome clearly brought out the epileptic activity within half an hour better than metrazol does. In one schizophrenic subject the E.E.G. showed much dysrhythmia after adrenochrome whereas it was essentially normal before. A typical record before and after adrenochrome is shown below, Szatmari (19). This is further evidence that adrenochrome can rapidly cross the blood brain barrier and interfere with the oxidative processes of the cerebral cells. Further experiments are being made in animals with radioactive adrenochrome in order more definitely to localize the site of action of the adrenochrome.

We are now using adrenochrome as a routine in establishing the diagnosis of epilepsy since it so clearly brings out the epileptic activity.

We believe that this is the first time a substance thought to be present in the body has been shown to effect the E.E.G. so markedly. The implications regarding epilepsy are being explored by our research unit.

Effect of Adrenochrome on Cerebral Respiration

It has been shown that adrenochrome inhibits hexokinase (17) under anaerobic conditions. Naturally this would inhibit the entire oxidative system starting with glucose. Woodford (20) in confirmation reported that adrenochrome inhibited oxidation by brain tissue immediately upon addition to the system under aerobic conditions. Woodford (20) found that adrenochrome, in contrast to mescaline which requires a two to three hour preliminary incubation period with the brain tissue before consistent inhibitory results are obtained, shows inhibition immediately. Since the aerobic oxidation of both glucose and pyruvate is inhibited by adrenochrome, he interprets this as meaning that, in addition to hexokinase inhibition, an enzyme occurring below the pyruvate level is also blocked.

Some Pharmacological Experiments with Adrenochrome

Eade and Hutcheon (8) found that the LD_{50} of adrenochrome to be 137 mgm. per kg. Signs of intoxication included progressive paralysis of the hind limbs, dyspnoea, apathy and exophthalmia. They further found that adrenochrome has a hypothermic action in normal and adrenalectomized rats.

Some Psychological Effects of Adrenochrome

Once the toxicity of adrenochrome had been established in animals it was possible to begin trials in humans. It was uncertain how such an unstable substance should be given or what sort of dose would prove to have any psychological properties. On 9.x.52 two of us (A. H. and H. O.) therefore decided to start on ourselves using very small doses to begin with. Unfortunately, we later discovered that there was some doubt about the quantity of adrenochrome used in these first experiments because it was weighed out in a new and unfamiliar balance.

The first subject (A. H.) received what we supposed was .1 mgm. in 1 c.c. of water subcutaneously. This makes a fine port-wine coloured liquid. The injection was accompanied by a sharp and persistent pain at the site of injection. There were no recognizable psychological changes. Blood pressure and pulse readings taken every five minutes for half an hour showed no change.

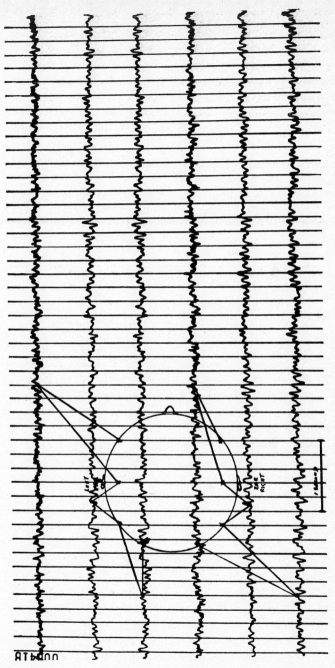

Fig. 3. (a) Epileptic subject interseizure pattern.

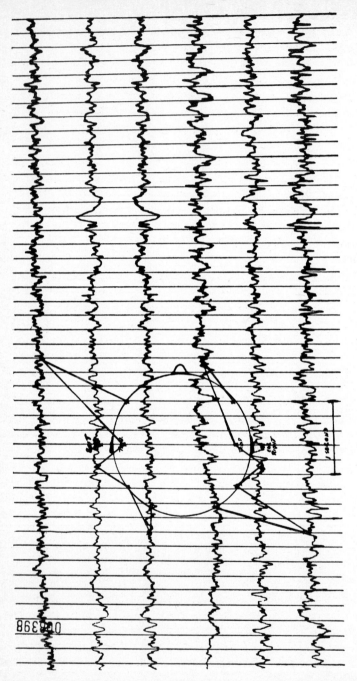

Fig. 3. (b) Same E.E.G. run 45 minutes after 10 mg. of adrenochrome (intravenous).

The second subject (H. O.) was given what we believed was .5 mgm. Again there were no pressor effects but there were marked psychological changes (see below).

Further experiments on our two wives and one of us (A. H.) using 1 mgm. subcutaneously produced some minor results, but by this time it seemed that our adrenochrome, which is very unstable, was beginning to deteriorate. On 16.x.52 5 mgm. of this deteriorating solution was given to H. O. and produced a response which was unpleasantly prolonged.

Since the subcutaneous injections were so painful, the first intravenous injection was given to a volunteer, Mr. C. R. Jillings, M.A., clinical psychologist. It was believed that adrenochrome given by this route would be much less painful. 1.0 mgm. of adrenochrome was, therefore, diluted with two 3 c.c. of sterile physiological saline and injected into the left antecubital vein. Almost immediately after the injection Jillings experienced a very severe pain which travelled up his left arm to the praecordium. This lasted about 10 minutes and was accompanied by pallor and sweating. There were no obvious psychological effects apart from alarm and dismay in the experimenters. It was later discovered that, if the adrenochrome solution is mixed with blood from the patient's vein, pain can usually be completely avoided.

Later A. H. and his wife both took 10 mgm. doses intravenously and had marked changes particularly in affect and behaviour. A. H. became overactive, showed poor judgment and lack of insight. R. H., his wife, became deeply depressed for four days and endured a condition which was indistinguishable from an endogenous depression. This unpleasant experience was aggravated by lack of insight, for she was unable to relate her depression to the injection of adrenochrome, although her change of mood came on immediately after it. An acute piece of observation by Dr. Roland Fischer, Ph.D. (9), suggests that this prolonged effect of adrenochrome was probably due to an attack of infectious hepatitis some years ago. It would, therefore, be prudent to enquire about previous liver disease before injecting adrenochrome or other toxic substances into an experimental subject.

To those who are familiar with mescal and lysergic acid we would emphasize that judging from the little experience which we have, it does seem that adrenochrome is more insidious than these two hallucinogens, its effects last longer and possibly in consequence of this its administration is accompanied by a loss of insight. Since this may have serious results experimenters should guard their subjects very carefully.

*Summary of an Account of an Adrenochrome Trial 9.x.52, 20–30
   hours approx.*
(Condensed from notes made at the time by the subject (H. O.).)

After the purple red liquid was injected into my right forearm I
had a good deal of pain. I did not expect that we would get any results from a preliminary trial and so was not, as far as I can judge,
in a state of heightened expectancy. The fact that my blood pressure
did not rise suggests that I was not unduly tense. After about 10
minutes, while I was lying on a couch looking up at the ceiling, I
found that it had changed colour. It seemed that the lighting had
become brighter. I asked Abe and Neil if they had noticed anything,
but they had not. I looked across the room and it seemed to have
changed in some not easily definable way. I wondered if I could
have suggested these things to myself. I closed my eyes and a brightly
coloured pattern of dots appeared. The colours were not as brilliant
as those which I have seen under mescal, but were of the same type.
The patterns of dots gradually resolved themselves into fish-like
shapes. I felt that I was at the bottom of the sea or in an aquarium
among a shoal of brilliant fishes. At one moment I concluded that I
was a sea anemone in this pool. Abe and Neil kept pestering me to tell
them what was happening, which annoyed me. They brought me a Van
Gogh self portrait to look at. I have never seen a picture so plastic
and alive. Van Gogh gazed at me from the paper, crop headed, with
hurt, mad eyes and seemed to be three dimensional. I felt that I
could stroke the cloth of his coat and that he might turn around in
his frame. Neil showed me the Rorschach cards. Their texture,
their bas relief appearance, and the strange and amusing shapes
which I had never before seen in the cards were extraordinary.

My experiences in the laboratory were, on the whole, pleasant but
when I left I found the corridors outside sinister and unfriendly. I
wondered what the cracks in the floor meant and why there were so
many of them. Once we got out of doors the hospital buildings, which
I know well, seemed sharp and unfamiliar. As we drove through
the streets the houses appeared to have some special meaning, but
I couldn't tell what it was. In one window I saw a lamp burning and
I was astonished by its grace and brilliance. I drew my friends' attention to it but they were unimpressed.

We reached Abe's home where I felt cut off from people but not
unhappy. I knew that I should be discussing the experience with
Abe and his wife but could not be bothered to do so. I felt no special
interest in our experiment and had no satisfaction at our success,
although I told myself that it was very important. Before I got to

sleep I noticed that the coloured visions returned when I shut my eyes. (Normally I have hypnagogic visions after several minutes in a darkened room when I am tired.) I slept well.

Next morning, although I had only slept a few hours, life seemed good. Colours were bright and my appetite keen. I was completely aware of the possibilities arising from the experiment. Colour had extra meaning for me. Voices, typewriting, any sound was very clear. With those whom I felt did not appreciate the importance of the new discovery I could have easily become irritable, but I was able to control myself.

H. O.'s Second Andrenochrome Experience 16.x.53 (p. m.)

I had 5 mgm. of adrenochrome this time because we thought that it was probably deteriorating.

I saw only a few visual patterns with my eyes closed. I had the feeling that there was something wonderful waiting to be seen but somehow I couldn't see it. However, in the outside world everything seemed sharper and the Van Gogh was three dimensional. I began to feel that I was losing touch with everything. My sister telephoned and, although I am usually glad to hear her voice, I couldn't feel any warmth or happiness. I watched a group of patients dancing and, although I enjoy watching dancing with the envious interest of one who is clumsy on his feet, I didn't have a flicker of feeling.

As we drove back to Abe's house a pedestrian walked across the road in front of us. I thought we might run him down, and watched with detached curiosity. I had no concern for the victim. We did not knock him down.

I began to wonder whether I was a person any more and to think that I might be a plant or a stone. As my feeling for these inanimate objects increased my feeling for and my interest in humans diminished. I felt indifferent towards humans and had to curb myself from making unpleasant personal remarks about them. I had no inclination to say more or less than I observed. If I was asked if I liked a picture I said what I felt and disregarded the owner's feeling.

I did not wish to talk and found it most comfortable to gaze at the floor or a lamp. Time seemed to be of no importance. I slept well that night and awoke feeling lively, but although I had to attend a meeting that morning, I did not hurry myself. Eventually I had to be more or less dragged out of the house by Abe. I had to get my car from a garage where it was being repaired. There was some trouble about finding it in the garage when at last I was seated in the driver's seat I realized that I couldn't drive it through traffic, although quite able to do so usually. I did not, however, feel anxious or distressed by this but persuaded the garage proprietor to drive me to my destination. I would, I believe, have normally found this a humiliating situation. I did not feel humiliated.

I attended the scientific meeting, and during it I wrote this note: "Dear Abe, this damn stuff is still working. The odd thing is that stress brings it on, after about 15 minutes. I have this 'glass wall other side of the barrier' feeling. It is fluctuant, almost intangible, but I know it is there. It wasn't there three quarters of an hour ago; the stress was the minor one of getting the car. I have a feeling that I don't know anyone here; absurd but unpleasant. Also some slight ideas of reference arising from my sensation of oddness. I have just begun to wonder if my hands are writing this, crazy of course."

I fluctuated for the rest of the day. While being driven home by my psychologist colleague, Mr. B. Stefaniuk, I discovered that I could not relate distance and time. I would see a vehicle far away on the long, straight prairie roads, but would be uncertain whether we might not be about to collide with it. We had coffee at a wayside halt and here I became disturbed by the covert glances of a sinister looking man. I could not be sure whether he was "really" doing this or not. I went out to look at two wrecked cars which had been brought in to a nearby garage. I became deeply preoccupied with them and the fate of their occupants. I could only tear myself away from them with an effort. I seemed in some way to be involved in them.

Later in the day when I reached home the telephone rang. I took no notice of it and allowed it to ring itself out. Normally, no matter how tired I am, I respond to it.

By the morning of 19.x.52 I felt that I was my usual self again.

Subject's Comment

I shall make no attempt to elaborate or discuss these two experiences. I am satisfied that they represent a model psychosis, but each reader must decide for himself on the evidence of what I have written and what my colleagues report.

Observations by A. H. and N. A. on Subject H. O.'s Reaction to Adrenochrome

Within 15 to 25 minutes of receiving the adrenochrome injection H. O. was preoccupied with the distasteful colour of the laboratory. He had never before made any comment concerning this. After he had described some of his experiences to us we showed him a reproduction of a Van Gogh painting which he observed very carefully for a long time. It was difficult to divert his attention toward some Rorschach cards we wished him to see. He stated they were not nearly as interesting. But when he did consent to examine these cards he refused to change cards until ordered to do so. Continual persuasion was needed to get a response. For this reason no complete evaluation of the protocol was obtained. However, in response to upper centre D section of card No. 10 he gave the response "these are shrimps, no they are statesmen — they are shrimp statesmen." This tendency toward contamination or the process of loosely combining two associations is not typical of H. O. who normally tends toward high F plus per cent. On the other hand, in word association tests under normal conditions, H. O. does give above average distant responses but is able to report the path of the associative process with no difficulty.

The change in H. O., marked by strong preoccupation with inanimate objects, by a marked refusal to communicate with us, and by strong resistance to our requests, was in striking contrast with H. O.'s normal social behaviour.

On the occasion of H. O's second trial the most noticeable objective change was his withdrawal from people. After the laboratory session we drove to the home of A. H. H. O. entered, found a chair where he sat for approximately one hour intently examining the rug. He did not greet the group of people who were at the house nor enter into the discussion.

H. O. was anxious and fearful on retiring and once was found wandering about. In the morning he was easily distracted. He required two hours to dress.

Briefly, the changes noted were preoccupation with inanimate objects, negativism, loosening of the associative process, anxiety and distractibility.

DISCUSSION

Adrenochrome is the first substance thought to occur in the body which has been shown to be a hallucinogen. Until it was discovered these peculiar properties had only been found in compounds derived from plants, whether from the peyotl (mescalin), or from an African bean (ibogaine), or from a jungle vine (harmine), or from rye rust (lysergic acid), or from the historic Indian hemp (hashish), or from that mysterious fungus *amanita pantherina*,[2] which has tempted so few

[2] Since this paper was written Mr. Aldous Huxley has given us an account of the preparation of *amanita pantherina* which may explain why it has not commended itself to western experimenters. The active principle is excreted in the urine of those who have ingested it. The hospitable Siberian chews the fungus himself and then offers his most

investigators, and whose active principle is completely unknown. The exotic nature of the hallucinogens catalogued here has made it possible for the sceptic to deny that anything like them could occur in the body, a rash assumption when we know that the body is capable of prodigious feats of chemical synthesis. It is now more difficult to assert that adrenochrome, or something like it, could not accumulate under certain circumstances, and produce devastating psychological disturbances long before any consistent physiological changes could be observed.

It is still a far cry from this to proving that overproduction of adrenochrome, or something like it, occurs in schizophrenia. However, we have shown that it could be adrenochrome, an immediate derivative of adrenaline.

At this point somebody usually says, "How can you explain such a complicated illness manifesting itself in so many ways, by such a simple mechanism?"

Those who put this question are often surprised to find that we have also thought about this. If one agrees that M substance could exist then there is no reason why it should not produce a wide variety of clinical pictures.

We have listed ten of the variables involved and there are probably more:

(1) The cultural setting.
(2) The personality of the patient.
(3) The age of onset.
(4) The rate of production of M substance.
(5) The quantity of M substance produced.
(6) The exact compound or compounds produced (small changes in chemical structure causes great differences in their physiological and psychological effects; e.g., adrenaline, noradrenaline, adrenochrome, amphetamine, mescaline).
(7) Specific localization of cerebral enzymes inhibited by M substance.
(8) The capacity of the body for storing M substance. (It is believed that some adrenochrome is stored in the red cells of the blood and other tissue cells (2).)
(9) The capacity of the body for detoxicating or destroying M substance.

---

favoured guest a brimming bumper of his urine. The hallucinogenic substance remains potent after four to five passages through the human body so that when one has enjoyed it one passes it on to someone else. Amongst the Siberians, less honoured guests receive the hallucinogen after it has been used by several others. It only remains now to carry out this experiment with schizophrenic urine.

(10) The success which the sick person has in dealing with the psychological disturbances produced by M substance. (This very important variable is partly determined by culture. A person who has a frame of reference which allows him to deal with astonishing experiences is less likely to disintegrate under the stress of a psychotic disturbance than one who has not.)

It would be possible to elaborate this but at this time it is not relevant.

Only when M substance has been isolated and identified can we begin to understand the mechanisms which produce schizophrenia. Once we understand these mechanisms it may be possible to design a rational treatment based upon exact knowledge, and not, as at present, upon guesswork.

Although we have answered our original question, in doing so we have posed many new questions.

There is the immediate question whether adrenochrome itself plays any part in schizophrenia. This in itself will be hard to answer because we have to search for a fairly unstable compound in a concentration of about one part in five million.

Then where exactly does adrenochrome inhibit cerebral metabolism? What is the meaning of the E.E.G. change which we have observed? What can we learn from the strange psychological changes in mood, perception, thinking and behaviour? And each of these questions, in itself, is the forerunner of a whole series of other questions. At present we cannot answer any of them, but perhaps as Archibald MacLeish pointed out:

> "We know all the answers, the answers,
> It is the questions we do not know."

The importance of a hypothesis may lie more in the questions which it allows us to ask than in the answers which we receive.

SUMMARY

Using a hypothesis first published in this journal last year the authors and their colleagues of the Saskatchewan Schizophrenia Research Group have shown that adrenochrome, a derivative of adrenaline, has psychological properties similar to those of mescaline and lysergic acid. This is the first time that a substance which probably occurs in the human body has been found to be active in this way. Adrenochrome has also been shown to produce E.E.G. changes in normal and epileptic people and to inhibit the aerobic and anaerobic respiration of brain tissue in the Warburg apparatus. Future work in this field is discussed. Those who wish to work with adrenochrome are warned of certain dangers.

Acknowledgements

The authors gratefully acknowledge the advice and support received from the members of the research unit and especially A. Szatmari, M.D., for permitting us to record E.E.G. tracings of work which will be published and N. Agnew, M.A. for participating in the psychological trials of adrenochrome and in reporting them here.

Appendix

For those who Intend to Work with Adrenochrome

If we are to learn more about schizophrenia, experiments with volunteers are essential, but these must be done with proper care. The toxicity of any sample of adrenochrome must, of course, be determined on animals, using the usual methods. Since it is a very unstable substance only freshly prepared solutions should be used. The solution should be mixed with the subject's own blood before intravenous injection; failure to do this results in great pain. We do not at present know why this should be.

It seems to us that adrenochrome's most dangerous properties are psychological ones. Subjects who have been given mescaline or lysergic acid cling to the essential experimental nature of their experiences, and derive considerable help by reassuring themselves that they will soon be over it. Those who have had adrenochrome appear to be liable to lose insight quickly and become unable to relate their experiences to the injection which they have received. It may be that the insidious nature of adrenochrome's action erodes insight, or perhaps it has some specific property which the others do not possess. Whatever the cause this loss of insight requires special care. Until we know more of this new model psychosis (to use Fischer's excellent term) produced by adrenochrome, it would be prudent to assume that it will be effective for at least 24 hours and to supervise the subject for that period of time. It is possible, though not certain, that large doses of niacin (1 gr. by mouth or 100 mgm. intravenously) may counteract the effect of adrenochrome.

In selecting volunteers we suggest that, until more is known about adrenochrome, those with a bad family background, who have history of liver disease or psychotic episodes, or whose Rorschach responses are suspicious should for the moment be excluded. Close supervision for 24 hours should include an absolute refusal to allow the subject to drive a car. We have some evidence that the capacity to relate time and distance may be subtly disturbed by adrenochrome. This could be disastrous.

We do not wish to appear alarmist, but believe that we should make other workers in this field aware of some of the troubles that we have encountered. It seems to us that we have a special responsibility to those who are prepared to trust us with the temporary custody of their minds and bodies to further man's knowledge of himself.

REFERENCES

1. Asquith, E. 1952. Private communication.
2. Bacq, Z. M. *J. of Pharm. Exp. Ther.*, 1949, 95: 1.
3. Beyer, K. H. *Ibid.*, 1941, 71: 151.
4. —— *Physiol. Rev.*, 1946, 26: 169.
5. Blaschko, H. *Nature*, 1940, 145: 26.
6. Bullough, W. S. *J. of Endocrinology*, 1952, 8: 265.
7. Burn, J. H. *Brit. Med. J.*, 1952, i: 784.
8. Eade, N., Hutcheon, D. E. 1952. Personal communication — to be published.
9. Fischer, R., Georgi, F., Weber, R., Piaget, R. H. *Schweiz. Med. Wchnschr.*, 1950, 80: 129.
10. Green, D. E., Richter, D. *Biochem. J.*, 1937, 31: 596.
11. De Jong, H. H. *Experimental Catatonia*, 1945. Baltimore: The Williams & Wilkins Co.
12. Lettre, H. *J. Clin. and Exp. Psychopath.*, 1951, 12: 241.
13. Lindemann, E. *Am. J. Psychiat.*, 1935, 91: 983.
14. Manske, R. H. F., Holmes, H. L. *The Alkaloids*, Vol. II, 1952. New York: Academic Press Inc.
15. Martin, G. J. *Biological Antagonism*, 1951. Toronto: The Blakeston Co., Inc.
16. Martin, G. J., Ichniowski, C. T., Wisansky, W. A., Ansbacher, S. *Am. J. Physiol.*, 1942, 136: 66.
17. Meyerhoff, O., Randall, L. O. *Archiv. Biochem.*, 1948, 17: 171.
18. Osmond, H., Smythies, J. *J. Ment. Sci.*, 1952, 98: 309.
19. Szatmari, A., 1952. Personal communication — to be published.
20. Woodford, V., 1952. Private communication — to be published.

38

THE IDENTIFICATION OF SMALL QUANTITIES OF HALLUCINATORY SUBSTANCES IN BODY FLUIDS WITH THE SPIDER TEST

PETER N. WITT

State University of New York College of Medicine at Syracuse

The term "hallucinogens" was introduced by Hoffer et al. (9) to characterize substances which produce hallucinations in man. The authors enumerate six substances as belonging to this group, namely mescaline, lysergic acid diethylamide (LSD), harmine, ibogaine, hashish, and adrenochrome.

No clear criteria exist which would be useful in the classification of the hallucinogens. Though many drugs like the barbiturates and alcohol may cause hallucinations if given to the right person at the right time in the right dose, they are not classified as hallucinogens. However, a substance like mescaline, if given in a dose of 400 mg., or 40 micrograms of LSD given subcutaneously invariably cause hallucinations (3, 20). Other substances are less reliable in this respect.

All of these drugs have effects in addition to their hallucinatory properties, particularly on the autonomic nervous system. These "side effects" might appear before, during, or after the phase of hallucinations and their relationship to the psychological symptoms is not known.

The psychological changes brought about by the hallucinogens are so subtle, the variations of symptoms from person to person so great, that it has never been possible to establish whether a substance invariably causes the same characteristic response pattern in all persons. It might well be that a preformed individual reaction pattern is released in each person. To put it differently: when a test is made and an unknown hallucinogen is given, it has not been possible to say which drug has been applied.

In recent years an hypothesis, to be elaborated below, has stimulated interest in the hallucinogens. The drugs have been used to produce so-called model psychoses in man. It has been observed repeatedly that the changes which appear after the application of these drugs have a striking similarity to acute deliria. These so-called symptomatic psychoses can become manifest during hunger, cachexia, fever, and after cerebral lesions. They appear also as hallucinatory episodes in chronic schizophrenia (4). In the pharmacological experiment a distinct relationship between the application of the drug to the person and the appearance of psychological changes can be seen, while in the case of acute deliria the symptoms might appear in the course of a chronic disease without apparent reason. The similarity of symptoms has led a number of observers to suspect that in acute deliria a substance similar to one of the hallucinogens might be present in the patient's body (10). A pathological metabolic pathway in the body of the diseased person might lead to the production of an abnormal substance in quantities sufficient to cause hallucinations. Such an hypothesis can only be substantiated if an hallucinogenic compound is found to be present in the patient.

Peters and Witt (14) have described a biological test which allows identification of most of the hallucinatory and some other psychotropic drugs. This method is at the same time sensitive enough to allow identification of small quantities of substances. A brief description and enumeration of results to date are in order.

The method uses differences in web-building behavior of the spider *Zilla-x-notata Cl.* before and after drug application.

The particular spider was chosen because it is commonly found in Switzerland and Germany where the method was developed. McCook (11) mentions its habitat in the United States as New England, New York, and California. It is easy to catch and lives outside its web in a self-made tube of thread. This tube is connected with the center of the web by means of a signal thread which transmits vibrations and tension changes from the web to the forelegs of the spider (Fig. 1). Whenever *Zilla's* web is destroyed it will build a similar web in the same place close to its old nest. In contrast, the common garden spider (*Aranea diademata*), which lives in the center of its web, falls down when the web is destroyed, and builds a new web at a new location.

The following method is used to catch the spider and make it settle down in the laboratory: as soon as the characteristic web of *Zilla* has been discovered (outdoors near a wall or window) the spider is enticed to come into its web. This can be done by throwing a fly into the mesh or by means of touching the threads with a vibrating tuning fork. While the animal looks around for the prey the signal thread is disengaged from the nest and attached to a little paper bag. When the disappointed spider now leaves the web, it proceeds along the signal thread directly into the paper bag. A new nest found in that way will be accepted by the spider without difficulty. The web is now cut and the spider brought back into the laboratory in the paper bag, which is fastened in an upper corner of a wooden frame measuring 15 x 15

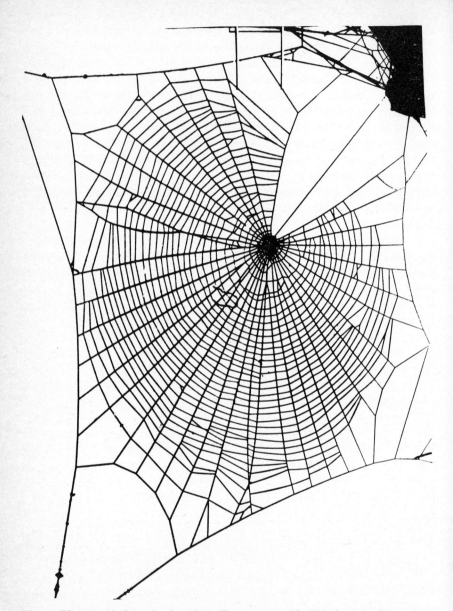

Fig. 1. Characteristic web of spider zilla-x-notata Cl. Thirty-six radii connect frame with hub; catching spiral leaves one sector free; signal thread divides free sector into two and connects spider in house at right upper corner via hub with all parts of web.

inches. If conditions are favorable and if the existing web is destroyed, a new web will be spun in this frame each night.

The method of catching described above indicates that the spider is an animal in which the sense of touch and vibration is predominant. The whole web may be regarded as an extended organ of touch, because the slightest change in its tension or a light vibration in the area of the net is transmitted via radii and signal thread to the spider. Predominance of the sense of touch and a poor sense of vision make spiders unable to discern between vibrations caused by a tuning fork and those caused by an insect. This was discovered by Boys in 1880 (6) and has since been used as a simple means of enticing spiders to come out of their house into the web. The animals recognize their error only when — expecting a fly — they bite into the metal of the tuning fork (12).

To prove the high specialization of the sense of touch Baltzer (2) performed another experiment: he showed that even an extremely hungry spider would not touch a fly that passed directly under its mouth if the fly's movements were not transmitted through a web. A spider sitting on a table or other solid surface would never attack its prey. Finally, Peters (13) eliminated the function of the eyes of some spiders by covering them with black lacquer. After this treatment the animals showed no change in behavior; they even built normal webs.

Thus it was shown that web-building as well as feeding is probably determined by the sense of touch alone. The spider measures distances by walking straight along a thread (21), it probes the tension of a thread by pulling it, and it orients the shape of the web according to gravity. The latter was shown by Peters (13), who turned the frame with the spider during the web-building. The web normally has its longer axis in the vertical direction. After it had been turned ninety degrees the spider added on in its new position until it was again longer in the vertical axis.

One of the purposes of the web is doubtless to bring the animal in touch with as much space as possible with as few threads as possible. But a web which could not catch and hold the insects which touch it would be useless. It actually provides the spider with all its food. This means that hunger is probably one of the stimuli that starts a spider on the web-building process. It has often been mentioned that satiated spiders will temporarily reduce the scale and frequency of their web-building, but no systematic investigation of this has been made. However, light and temperature also have a bearing on frequency of web-building. Spronk (19) put his spiders into a dark thermostat and found that web-building started during falls of temperature or at the nightly temperature minimum. Witt (25) showed that constant temperature and constant light reduced web-building activity; a group of spiders kept at temperatures and light which changed with day and night rhythm built significantly more webs than any of the controls. Under optimal light and temperature conditions, constant feeding with 1–3 drosophila flies a day (the quantity adjusted to the size of spider) produced regular new webs every day from each individual.

The animals have to go undisturbed through all phases of catching the insect before they will accept the booty and suck its contents. With an ingenious method, Wolff (27) has imitated the movements, surface and taste of the prey so that the spider will drink various solutions without even suspecting that anything is amiss. Sugar was found to disguise nearly every strange drug, its taste proving highly attractive to spiders. Drugs were therefore dissolved in sugar water, injected into the empty abdomen of house flies, thrown into the web, and made to vibrate by means of a tuning fork. The spider would then come out of its house, find the lure, wrap it up, bite it and drink part of the contents. After the spider has finished drinking, the rest of the fly abdomen can be taken out and weighed, the difference in weight before and after drinking indicating the amount that has been ingested by the spider. By knowing the concentration of the substance in the fluid, the amount of drug that was actually taken up by the spider can easily be calculated.

Inhalation of volatile drugs has also been tried successfully (7, 18). However, it is difficult to give drugs by injection, because the chitinous outer membrane of the spider is irremediably damaged by the needle. By using a microsyringe and very fine needles, Wolff and Hempel (27) were able to reduce the mortality of spiders after injection to about 50 per cent.

It has already been mentioned that there is a certain time at which webs are built. This time is constant for all spiders working on the same day under the same conditions, and it changes with the seasonal changes of sunrise. If we know how long it takes for a certain drug to reach its peak effect in spiders, we can apply it just long enough before web-building time so as to allow maximum effects to be seen in the web. On the other hand, by applying a certain drug at different times on different days, the onset, course and end of the effect of a certain drug can be determined.

Only if the sequence of events in the spinning of a web is known can its changes be interpreted. Much work has been done to establish this sequence and to analyze the influences which determine special patterns and proportions in a web. Descriptions can be found in Wiehle

(23), Peters (13), Tilquin (21), Savory (17), Witt (25); for the present purpose it is sufficient to remember that at first a Y-structure is made. This Y is suspended in a frame which consists of particularly strong threads. In the subsequent building period the spider connects the center or hub with the frame by means of a great number of radii (Fig. 2). Finally, it fills in the thin thread of the sticky spiral, begin-

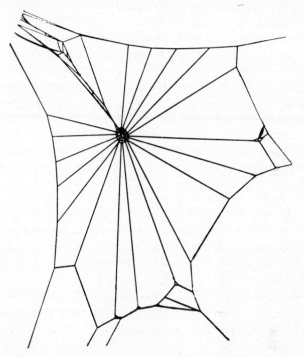

Fig. 2. Unfinished web of spider zilla-x-notata Cl. Frame, hub, and 18 radii have been built. Note house of spider in upper left corner.

ning at the outside and climbing from radius to radius until it gets near the hub. This spiral in its regularity and proportions is the most sensitive reagent to drugs (24).

The complete web is a fine record of the spider's movements during a certain period of time — normally about 20 to 30 minutes. By measuring and analyzing the web we actually measure the spider's movements. The movements again depend on the animal's ability to coordinate and translate incoming stimuli into outgoing signals. We measure possible lesions of all these functions in the web. The great number and complexity of functions involved in web-building is probably one of the reasons why relatively small doses of many drugs affect the web pattern.

A fresh web can hardly be seen and can easily be torn. It must therefore be made visible and preserved. In order to achieve the first purpose, little vessels with ammonia and hydrochloric acid are placed under the web. The rising fumes combine in the air and turn into ammonium chloride, forming a fine white film on the threads. We have now achieved good visibility without distortion. The pattern of each web is preserved on photographic film. The white threads stand out beautifully against a black background if light is directed onto the web from both sides. Care must be taken that the camera stands parallel to the web so that proportions are not distorted. With the help of enlarged or projected films, comparison of different webs built on different days by the same individual with or without drug influence can be made.

Statistical methods are used for evaluation of drug effects on web-building behavior. On any one day, some of the spiders receive the drug at a certain time; the others get nothing or only sugar water. The following two mornings the webs of all animals are again photographed,

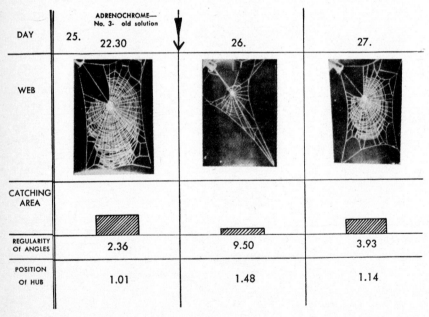

Fig. 3. Three different webs built by the same spider on three subsequent days; the drug was applied before the spider built the second web. Catching area, angles and position of hub were measured on the photographs and noted under each web (see text for further explanation). Note the similarity between web one and three and the abnormality of web two as a result of drug influence.

thus giving three photographs of three different webs per individual, one built before, one directly after, and one more than 24 hours after the drug administration (Fig. 3). Comparisons can be made among the three webs. Short-acting drugs, for instance, should cause a disturbance in the second web, while the first and third would be similar. By taking the mean figures of measurements made in the group of webs built under drug influence, we obtained reproducible effects of the drug independent of the individual. Comparing these with webs of spiders who built on the same days but did not receive any drug makes it possible to control for such influences as atmospheric changes.

A certain number of proportions, distances, and angles are known to recur fairly consistently in all webs, and standard deviations of these

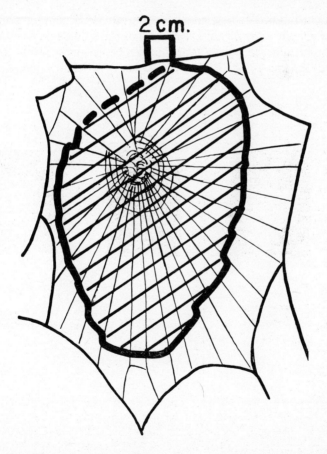

Fig. 4. The thick black line indicates the peripheral spiral thread which circumscribes the catching area. The "2 cm" mark on top was photographed together with the web so that original size can be calculated from the film.

figures have been calculated (25). Consistent deviations of one or more means have been found under the influence of certain drugs. The pattern of changed proportions is highly specific for each drug.

Measurements most frequently made in web photographs are:

1. The size of the catching area, measured with a planimeter along the peripheral turn of the spiral (Fig. 4). This area increases in size in the course of the spider's life, but is relatively stable from day to day.

2. The relationship between the horizontal and vertical diameter of the web. After drug application (Strychnine), changes have been observed in the value of the quotient of these two measures (27), as well as in the size of the standard deviations.

3. It has been observed that when the spider puts in radii it goes on doing this until it reaches the point where all angles are smaller in size than the sum of their two neighboring angles. After drug administration many oversized angles may be observed (Fig. 5). Their

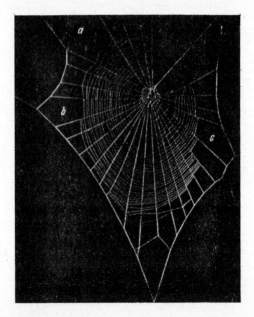

Fig. 5. In this web angles between radii at a, b, and c are called "oversized" because they are larger than the sum of their two neighboring angles.

number can be compared to the number of oversized angles in normal webs.

4. The size of neighboring angles between radii can be compared by calculating their quotient. If the angles are similar in size, the

quotient is one or near one. The means of all such quotients measured around the whole web should be near one in a regular web, higher or lower in drug webs.

5. The hub of the web may shift its position under the influence of drugs. This can be established by comparing the distance from nest to hub (a) to the distance from the hub to the opposite side of the web (b) in photographs taken before and after drug application (Fig. 6).

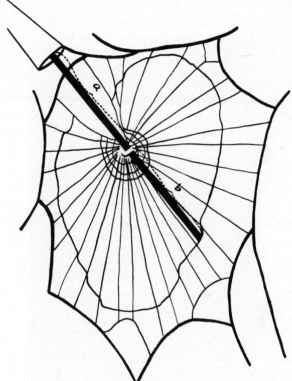

Fig. 6. Position of hub in web is calculated by dividing the length of (a) through that of (b).

6. The spiral is the finest indicator of the influence of any drug on the spider. Normally the distance between its turns decreases logarithmically from the periphery to the center (13) (Figs. 7 and 8). Slight disturbances can become manifest in the greater variation of distance from turn to turn (Pervitin, 15), while heavy disturbances lead to strangely deformed spirals with several centers or heavy digressions from the right direction (scopolamine, 27).

7. Finally, the frequency of web-building can be evaluated for each

spider. It has, for instance, been noted that a tranquilizer (chlorpromazine) interrupts the web-building totally for one or several days, the
length of the resting period depending on the dose (8). There are physiological interruptions in web-building, like the periods of molting,
which can be kept under control.

As soon as the method was published, investigations were started
in a number of laboratories, applying the technique to problems in
the chemistry of schizophrenia. Particular attention was given to the
questions of whether the spider test could detect small amounts of hal-

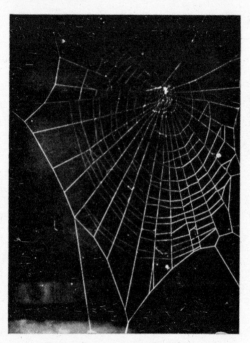

Fig. 7. Web built under the influence of mescaline; note increasing distance
between turns as spiral approaches hub. Compare with Fig. 1.

lucinatory substances in the body fluids of mental patients, and what
effects these substances have on behavior. That the spider test could
detect the presence of behavior disturbing substances in the urine and
that these substances could be recovered was suggested by two preliminary observations.

In one instance mescaline was added to a urine specimen. In the
usual extraction process from 50 to 70 per cent of the mescaline was
recovered.

At another time the urine of a patient had clearly shown the presence
of a substance which disturbed the spider's web-building. A thorough

check showed that the patient had received 0.75 mgm. scopolamine on the previous evening. This finding was regarded as an indication that a substance like scopolamine, if present in the patient, could be recovered in the urine and identified by the spider test.

The following summarizes the procedure and results of two groups

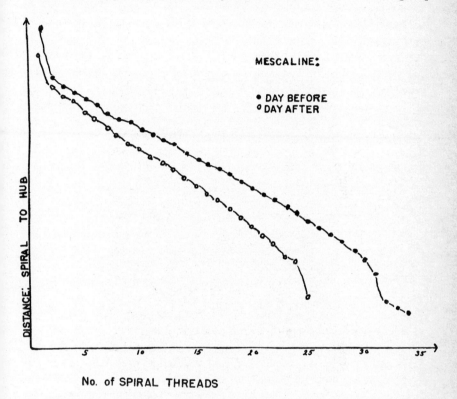

MESCALINE:

• DAY BEFORE
○ DAY AFTER

DISTANCE: SPIRAL TO HUB

No. of SPIRAL THREADS

Fig. 8. Graphic comparison of distances between turns of spiral of normal and mescaline web built by the same spider. The graph shows the greater steepness of the spiral near the hub after mescaline. Compare with Fig. 7.

of experiments. The first was done by the author in cooperation with Dr. Manfred Bleuler, head of the department of psychiatry at the University of Zurich, and Dr. Rolf Weber, biochemist at the Theodor Kocher Institute of Medical Research at Bern (26). Dr. Bleuler chose from among his patients three subjects and two controls who had the same diet. Patient Number One was a chronic alcoholic with hallucinations; Number Two showed a symptomatic psychosis after an accident which had occurred two years earlier — he was semicomatose with hallucinations; Number Three had shown a sudden marked deterioration and had received a diagnosis of chronic schizophrenia with hallucinations.

Having established that the patients had not had any drug for 24 hours or more, we waited for their acute hallucinations and then took about 500 ml. of urine. The fresh urine was immediately frozen in order to avoid deterioration of labile substances. By means of ion exchange resins and other extraction methods, the urine was concentrated to 400 mgm. of solids consisting mainly of basic amines. It is interesting to note at this point that the urine of the three patients yielded between 200 and 400 mgm. of dry substances, while the urine of the control persons yielded about 30 mgm. substances each. Directly before the substance was given to the spiders it was dissolved in sugar water and a quantity corresponding to 1/150 of the total fed to each spider 6 or 11 hours before the time of web-building.

In the second group of experiments (16), the urine of a great number of patients was collected over many days, cooled and chemically separated into several fractions. This was done in the Basel Psychiatric Hospital by Dr. Georgi and co-workers under the assumptions that the illnesses of the patients were basically similar and that they had similar chronic metabolic disturbances. This increased sample enabled us to feed far more than 1/150 of the content of the urine to each spider; one assumed consequence of the increased dose was an increase in the amount of the hypothetical substances contained in the dose which each spider received. One difficulty with this procedure is the assumption that the same substance was present in all patients all the time with or without manifest hallucinations.

The spider test revealed no difference between the urine of the controls and the patients' urines in either experiment (26, 16). These results do not support the recent set of optimistic statements appearing in the press and popular magazines. The most recent of these appeared in *Time* magazine of May 6, 1957 and in a United Press release, in connection with the work of Nicholas A. Bercel. I quote: "Spiders fed with serum taken from patients suffering from the catatonic form of schizophrenia . . . seem to become catatonic too . . . the webs they spin are like the last vestiges of ragged lace. The spider's reaction, like that of human volunteers injected with schizophrenic serum (*Time*, May 14) shows that this disease is associated with a disorder in blood chemistry."

Certainly we may state that the urine of the three patients after their hallucinations contained smaller or no amounts of the known hallucinatory substances or substances of similar activity, than those known to disturb the spider's web-building. It is an advantage of the method that we can extend our statement to substances of similar activity. It is a disadvantage that inactivated breakdown products of the active substances would not have been detected. A comparison of the minimal effective doses of certain substances in man to the dose that would have been detectable with the spider test is made in Table 1.

TABLE 1

Drug	Minimal effective dose * in gamma individual		The amount in gamma that would have been detected in the urine with the spider test **
	In spider	In man	
D-Lysergic Acid Diethylamide	0.03	10	9
Chlorpromazine	1.0	37 500	300
Adrenochrome (9)	4	500	1 200
Scopolamine	5	500	1 500
Pervitin	10	5 500	3 000
Strychnine	30	2 000	9 000
Xylopropamine (22)	40	2 500	12 000
Nembutal	40	50 000	12 000
Mescaline	100	400 000	30 000
Caffeine	100	100 000	30 000

* This dose is a rough approximation because the minimal effective dose varies considerably from one individual to the next, it depends on the criterion used for evaluaton, and it has never been clearly established for some of the drugs. The table gives the lowest dose which has shown an effect.
** The figures in this column are the figures in column 1 times 300. If we assume (according to the model experiment with mescaline) that 50 per cent of any amine that was in the original urine is still in the extract, and if we take into consideration the drinking of 1/150 of the total extract by each spider, a change in web-building behavior through the extract would have been caused by 1/300 of the quantity that was in the total urine. Each figure in column three that is smaller than the corresponding figure in column two shows that the minimal effective dose in man was not in the patients' urine.

Assuming that the patients in their severe toxic state contained more of the hypothetical substance than the minimal effective dose, considerable amounts might have been excreted and would have been identified by the spider test. This was clearly not the case.

The major aims of this paper were to present a new biological test and to apply that test to pertinent issues in the chemistry of schizophrenia. The evidence so far leads to confidence in the general technique. With regard to the essentially negative finding from the urine of patients and its relationship to the hypothesis of toxicity, the following questions come to mind.

1. Is it necessary to postulate a toxic substance or could we not just as well assume lack of a normal substance or substances? This is reminiscent of the serotonin hypothesis (28).

2. Is this hypothetical substance evenly distributed over all extracellular water of the body and is it excreted in the urine?

  a. Could it be produced and destroyed locally like acetylcholine?

  b. Could it be excreted in the urine in inert form?

  c. Could it be excreted in the urine but not extracted by our method of preparation?

d. Could it be active only as long as it is bound to proteins? (Mescaline, 5)

e. Could it be a substance that is active in man but not in spiders? These are only a few points that must be taken into consideration when interpreting our results. However, at the moment, there seems to be only one way to test the hypothesis, namely, to go on looking for the substance in urine, blood and maybe cerebrospinal fluid of many patients at many different times.

REFERENCES

1. Bacq, Z. M. *Pharmacol. Rev.*, 1: 1, 1949.
2. Baltzer, F. *Mitt. Naturforsch. Ges. Bern*, 24, 1923.
3. Beringer, K. *Der Meskalinrausch*, Springer, Berlin, 1927.
4. Blickenstorfer, E. *Arch. Psychiat. u. Z. Neurol. u. Psychiat.*, 188: 226, 1952.
5. Block, W., Block, K., and Patzig, E. *Hoppe-Seyler's Z. physiol. Chem.*, 290: 160, 1952; 290: 230, 1952; 291: 119, 1952.
6. Boys, C. V. *Nature* (London), 23: 149, 1880.
7. Epelbaum, F. *Arch. intern. Pharmacodynamie*, 104: 241, 1956.
8. Heimann, H., and Witt, P. N. *Monatsschr. Psychiat. Neurol.*, 129: 104, 1955.
9. Hoffer, A., Osmond, H., and Smythies, J. *J. Mental Sci.*, 100: 29, 1954.
10. Keup, W. *Monatsschr. Psychiat. Neurol.*, 128: 56, 1954.
11. McCook, H. C. *American spiders and their spinningwork*, Philadelphia, 1889.
12. Peters, H. M. *Z. vergleich. Physiol.*, 19: 47, 1933.
13. ——— *Z. Morphol. Oekol. Tiere*, 36: 179, 1939.
14. Peters, H. M., and Witt, P. N. *Experientia*, 5: 161, 1949.
15. Peters, H. M., Witt, P. N., and Wolff, D. *Z. vergleich. Physiol.*, 32: 29, 1950.
16. Rieder, H. P. and Witt, P. N. *Monatsschr. Psychiat. Neurol.*, in press.
17. Savory, T. H. *The spider's web*, F. Warne & Co., London, 1952.
18. Schwarz, R. *Arch. intern. Pharmacodynamie*, 104: 339, 1956.
19. Spronk, F. *Z. wiss. Biol. Abt. C*, 22: 604, 1935.
20. Stoll. W. A. *Schweiz. Arch. Neurol. Psychiat.*, 60: 1, 1947.
21. Tilquin, A. *La toile géométrique des araignées*, Presses Universitaires de France, Paris, 1942.
22. Weber, H. J., and Pellmont, B. *Schweiz. med. Wochschr.*, 85: 1166, 1955.
23. Wiehle, H. *Z. Morphol. Oekol. Tiere*, 8: 468, 1927.
24. Witt, P. N. *Behaviour*, 4: 172, 1952.
25. ——— *Die Wirkung von Substanzen auf den Netzbau der Spinne als biologischer Test*, Springer, Berlin, 1956.
26. Witt, P. N., and Weber, R. *Monatsschr. Psychiat. Neurol.*, 132: 193, 1956.
27. Wolff, D., and Hempel, U. *Z. vergleich. Physiol.*, 33: 497, 1951.
28. Woolley, D. W., and Shaw, E. *Science*, 119: 587, 1954.

Part V

PSYCHOPATHOLOGY AND THE SOCIAL CONTEXT

39

SOCIAL CLASS DIFFERENCES IN ATTITUDES TOWARD PSYCHIATRY

F. C. REDLICH, M.D., A. B. HOLLINGSHEAD, Ph.D., and
ELIZABETH BELLIS, B.A.

Yale University, New Haven, Connecticut

In a series of recent studies exploring social structure and psychiatric disorders, a significant relationship between social class and prevalence of treated psychiatric disorders was established. We were particularly impressed with the more frequent prevalence of treated psychoneuroses in the higher social classes and of chronic schizophrenia in lower classes (5, 12, 13). An important finding was the fact that patients of higher classes (classes I and II) more frequently receive psychotherapy, particularly so-called insight therapy, than lower classes (classes IV and V), who are more likely to receive supportive psychotherapy, organic treatment, or no therapy (12). A study in a psychiatric dispensary, where ability of the patient to pay was a controlled factor, demonstrated that social status is closely related to 1) acceptance for therapy, 2) length of therapy, 3) duration of therapy sessions, and 4) choice of therapist (8, 15).

With these facts in mind, we asked ourselves whether or not social class influenced the attitudes of neurotic patients to psychiatric therapy and whether or not it influenced the therapists' attitudes and the course of therapy. The importance of such an exploration was previously stressed by Redlich (11). The following report deals with the investigation of attitudes in relation to social class.

Only a few studies have been made of the relationship between social class and level of information about psychiatry and of the relationship between social class and attitudes toward mental illness and psychiatric treatment. An analysis by Redlich reports the responses of small lay groups to a sentence-completion test and to a multiple-choice type of questionnaire about mental health. He noted a possible class difference in information level. This paper also contains a bibliography of earlier publications (10). A study by Hollingshead surveyed a representative sample of newly married couples in New Haven, using an interview approach. A decided class difference in willingness to utilize psychiatric

From the *American Journal of Orthopsychiatry*, 25: 60, 1955.

help for marriage difficulties and a class difference in respondents' familiarity with psychiatry were apparent (4). Class differences in attitudes have also been emphasized by Dollard and Miller, who assert the existence of different attitudes to homosexuality and other psychopathological phenomena in the different classes (2).

The various polling surveys have noted a relationship between educational level and attitudes toward psychiatry. The better-educated respondents are "more humanitarian" and "more scientific" in their ideas about mental illness and treatment than are those with less education (3, 16). These surveys, however, deal chiefly with responses people say they would make in hypothetical situations. Questions which tap present attitudes are more likely to yield responses indicating a certain amount of prejudice and lack of understanding about mental illness even among those who are supposedly well informed and who are in the higher social levels, for instance, among specialized panels of lawyers, clergymen and teachers. Over a third of the medical men showed similar prejudices (14). In an analysis of cartoons about psychiatrists, Redlich concluded that persons in the higher social levels show fear and hostility toward the psychiatrist at both the conscious and unconscious level (9).

In sum, large segments of the public are uninformed about various aspects of mental illness and treatment. Although the better-educated and those in higher social levels seem better informed than the general public, they also reveal areas of prejudice and misunderstanding about some aspects of psychiatry.

METHOD

Following Hovland, Janis and Kelly (6), we use the term "attitude" to designate an intervening variable inferred primarily from action responses to situational stimuli. The action responses are participation in psychiatric treatment; they are responses to various stimuli, such as behavior, situations, thoughts, affects and fantasies around psychiatric illness and treatment. We infer attitudes wherever we can from a real situation and not from a hypothetical question. We wish to stress, too, that in this report we are almost exclusively concerned with overt verbal and nonverbal behavior and make only cautious and occasional reference to unconscious attitudes, simply because our material does not permit such inference.

We attempted to explore: 1) Attitudes of neurotic patients inferred from the nature of the chief presenting complaint. 2) Attitudes of neurotic patients inferred from source and method of referral of patients to psychiatrists. 3) Attitudes of neurotic patients inferred from knowledge prior to contact with psychiatrists and changes of such knowledge during contact with psychiatrists. 4) Attitudes inferred from sentiments expressed by neurotic patients at first contact with psychiatrists. 5) Attitudes inferred from the nature of communication between neurotic patients and their therapists during treatment. 6) Attitudes of therapists to neurotic patients.

Our data were collected from 50 psychiatric patients, who were selected according to the requirements of a stratified sample on the basis of the following criteria: 1) sex, 2) age, 3) diagnosis, and 4) social class position. We selected 25 males and 25 females between 22 and 44 years of age who had been diagnosed as psychoneurotic or schizophrenic and who were from classes III and V. Patients were chosen from nonadjacent classes because we were interested in attempting to assess the influence of class position on various aspects of mental illness. We focused upon classes III and V for three reasons: they represent 40 per cent of the population of the New Haven community; they have different rates for "treated prevalence"; these classes have not been studied carefully in previous psychiatric research.

Social class was determined by Hollingshead's *Index of Social Position*. This index utilizes three factors: occupation, education, and ecological area of residence, from which, after appropriate statistical analyses, each individual can be assigned to one of five social classes. Class I stands at the top of the socioeconomic scale, class V at the bottom. Occupationally, class III is composed, in large part, of proprietors of small businesses, white-collar workers, and skilled manual workers. Educationally, it consists predominantly of high-school graduates. Residentially, these people live in flats and single family dwellings in widely scattered areas. The composition of class V is almost exclusively unskilled and semiskilled workers who have an elementary education or less and who live in the most crowded areas of the New Haven community.

Patients with known psychosomatic complications were excluded from the sample. Additional qualifications for inclusion in the survey were: 1) the patient had to be willing to enter the study; 2) members of his family had to be willing to cooperate; and 3) his therapist had to consent to have the patient studied. The sample was drawn largely — by reason of class status — from clinics, state and VA hospitals. The 50 cases were gathered over a year and a half so that patients were at various stages of treatment during the interviewing. Each patient was interviewed at least three times by two different psychiatrists. The sociologists interviewed the families, including a spouse, sibling, and at least one parent. The therapist in charge of each case was interviewed also by a psychiatrist on the project. Following completion of this field work, two separate teams composed of a sociologist and a psychiatrist evaluated each case. After we completed the field work on all the cases, we found, by statistical analysis, that our sample was representative of neurotic and schizophrenic patients in our census study who were between the ages of 22 and 44 and who were in classes III and V.

The tables and the examples in this paper are derived chiefly from direct statements by the patient and therapist. Many of the ratings were made by more than one judge; the agreement varied but was always high. We have not attempted to deal with preconscious or unconscious attitudes. In this particular paper, we make use primarily of material obtained from the 25 neurotic patients, although we do refer to our previously reported census study.

FINDINGS

Attitudes inferred from chief complaint of neurotic patients. Our neurotic patients presented a great variety of complaints at their first psychiatric interview. We divided these into somatic complaints and emotional and interpersonal complaints. Emotional and interpersonal complaints could not be clearly differentiated. In most of our patients the two types of complaints coexisted. Thus, we had to make judgments as to definite predominance of one of the types of responses. Findings are presented in Table 1.

It would seem that class III patients present their complaints in terms of emotional and interpersonal difficulties more frequently than class V patients, who usually present themselves with "somatic" symptoms. Scrutinizing our records, we were impressed with the fact that prior to any contact with psychiatry, many patients in both classes considered their difficulties as an expression of organic illness. Patients expressed their organic bias during therapy by asking their therapists for "pills" and "shots" and expressing their lack of confidence in a "talking" treatment. Class III patients, as will be demonstrated later, seem more inclined than class V patients to accept the notion of psychogenic etiology in the course of treatment.

Attitudes of patients inferred from source and method of referral. From our psychiatric census study, we noted that neurotic patients in both classes showed a high frequency of referral by physicians. Class III patients were usually referred by general practitioners in the community whereas class V patients were referred by the staff of a medical dispensary or of an emergency room. Social agencies played a larger role in the referral of class V patients, and a considerable number of class V neurotics were committed. Self-referrals in class V were absent, but 20 per cent of our class III patients came to treatment on their own initiative.

Attitudes of patients inferred from knowledge prior to contact with psychiatrists and changes of knowledge. In general, knowledge about

TABLE 1. PREDOMINANT TYPE OF PRESENTING COMPLAINT BY CLASS

Type of Complaint	Class III	Class V
Somatic	2	9
Emotional and interpersonal	11	3
Total	13	12

$\chi^2 = 6.74$; $p < .01$

TABLE 2. LEVEL OF PSYCHIATRIC KNOWLEDGE OF NEUROTIC PATIENTS BEFORE TREATMENT

Class	Fair	Poor	None
III	5	2	6
V	—	—	12
Total	5	2	18

$\chi^2 = 6.5021$; $p < .02$

psychiatry on the part of all our patients was quite inadequate. Our ratings were based on molar judgments, using three categories: fair, poor, and none. In making such ratings we relied on direct statements by neurotic patients to our investigators, as well as on evaluation of the patients' communications during treatment. See Table 2.

Actually, we found that few patients before entering treatment understood any of the principles of dynamic psychiatry, and even those patients whose knowledge we rated as fair usually knew little more than that psychiatry deals with mental illness, that psychiatrists heal their patients not only by medicine or surgery but also by "mental" methods. During psychotherapy, some of our patients learned something about the "human mind," about unconscious conflict, about mental mechanisms expressing themselves in psychological and somatic symptoms, and how obtaining and applying insight to their problems can help. Again, we found a definite, though not a statistically significant, class difference among those who gained in knowledge and those who did not. See Table 3.

Attitudes inferred from sentiments by neurotic patients upon entering therapy. Most of our patients were averse to the idea of psychiatric intervention. We were not able to measure or rate differences in hostility and anxiety expressed by class III and class V patients. In many instances, hostility was rooted in fear and shame, as illustrated by such typical comments as, "People think you are crazy when you

TABLE 3. INCREASE IN INFORMATION OF NEUROTIC PATIENTS
DURING TREATMENT

Class	Moderate	Slight	No Increase
III	3	4	6
V	—	2	10
Total	3	6	16

$\chi^2 = 2.3040; \ p < .20$

come to see a psychiatrist" or "Psychiatry is fine for crazy people but it can't help me." It was difficult for all our patients to accept the idea of exploring their own emotions. Even among those who seemed most willing to talk about their problems, a number were apparently complying in the hope that after the "talking" would come the "treatment." In some of these patients this hurdle was never overcome and therapy came to a standstill.

Most of the neurotic patients started treatment rather passively. Even after they were in treatment, with the exception of the few who "got the idea," patients remained hesitant and unable to utilize psychiatric help. They tended to retain their rigid attitude and considered the psychiatrist as a magical doctor who could miraculously cure their physical ills; they expected "pills and needles," sympathy and warmth, and they were disappointed at not having such demands gratified. Even when therapists decided to change from insight therapy to supportive treatment, their patients tended to be disappointed in not getting sufficient practical advice about how to solve their problems and how to run their lives. Table 4 indicates that such inability to change was more apparent in class V patients than in class III patients.

Communication between therapists and neurotic patients by class. We attempted to make a molar rating of communication between therapists and patients (Table 5). Such a rating, using categories of "good," "intermediate," and "poor" after psychotherapy was under way, was based on whether or not therapists and patients were relating meaningfully to each other on the verbal level and whether or not the patient understood the principal intent of the therapist. Many of our patients, particularly those in class V, neither understood nor accepted the notion that psychological conflict may reveal itself in physical symptoms. In one of our class V cases, the therapist thought that after six months of "insight therapy," the patient accepted the idea that his troubles were not caused by his "bad teeth" but by his unresolved anxieties and frustrations. When our investigators interviewed the patient some time later, he still clung to the "theory" that his teeth had poisoned his system and made him weak. If the

TABLE 4. CHANGE OF ATTITUDE BY NEUROTIC PATIENTS
DURING TREATMENT BY CLASS

Class	No Change	Change
III	2	11
V	8	4
Total	10	15

$\chi^2 = 4.86$; $p < .05$

TABLE 5. LEVEL OF COMMUNICATION BETWEEN THERAPIST AND
NEUROTIC PATIENT BY CLASS

Level of Communication	Class III	Class V
Good	4	—
Intermediate	3	—
Poor	6	12
Total	13	12

$\chi^2 = 6.50$; $p < .02$

therapeutic intent was treatment through insight, it was not grasped by any of our lower class V patients, nor by approximately half of the class III patients. For instance one patient said about "insight therapy," "The doctor teaches me to forget things in my past." "Talking therapy" struck some patients as "silly and ridiculous" or, as one said, "Talking about my troubles makes me feel worse."

Attitudes of therapists to neurotic patients by class. In considering whether attitudes toward mental illness and psychiatric treatment affect the process of diagnosis and therapy, the attitudes of the therapist toward his patients must be taken into account. We interviewed 17 therapists: 3 private practitioners, 9 residents, 2 medical students, and 3 psychologists, who were rather evenly distributed by social class of their patients. By direct interview and by scrutinizing the records, we tried to assess judgments of therapists about their patients — whether they held views and values similar to those of their patients, whether they noticed social differences between themselves and their patients, whether they could cultivate them as friends, whether generally they liked or disliked the patients. Our rating of such "surface" attitudes is expressed in Table 6. The numerical differences by class in such a gross rating are striking. Much of the "dislike" of these patients, particularly of the lower class patients, is due to the frustration of the therapist who had to work with a "bad case" in which desperate environmental difficulties made therapeutic gains unlikely. In many cases, the value systems pertaining to therapeutic interaction were far

TABLE 6. THERAPISTS' ATTITUDES TOWARD NEUROTIC
PATIENTS BY CLASS

Therapist's Attitude	Class of Patient			
	III		V	
	#	%	#	%
"Liked" patient	9	(61.5%)	2	(16.6%)
"Disliked" patient	3	(23.1)	9	(50.0)
Intermediate or unclear	1	(15.4)	1	(33.3)
Total	13	(100 %)	12	(99.9%)

$\chi^2 = 4.66$; $p < .05$

apart. In a number of class V patients the therapists disapproved of their sexual and aggressive behavior, their lack of discipline and responsibility. While our therapists often enough rejected class III values they at least understood them; in contrast to this, they were at a loss to understand values of class V patients.

Most of the therapists were strongly motivated to carry out and learn insight therapy and felt disappointed when their plans failed. Moreover, a lack of personal feeling and understanding for the lower class patient was apparent. Therapists were irritated by overwhelming demands or the patient's inability to comprehend therapy. The following are illustrations of such attitudes: "Seeing him every morning was a chore; I had to put him on my back and carry him for an hour"; or, "He had to get affection in large doses; this was hard to do"; or, "The patient was not interesting or attractive; I had to repeat, repeat, repeat"; or, "She was a poor, unhappy, miserable woman — we are worlds apart." Most of the male therapists were somewhat more tolerant of female patients than of male patients in the same class.

DISCUSSION

Like other investigators, we were impressed with the widespread fear of mental illness, hostility toward psychiatrists, and ignorance of the subject matter of psychiatry. Certainly, fear and reluctance, whether openly expressed or inferred from preconscious or unconscious fantasies, such as demonstrated in the paper on the psychiatrist in caricature (9), are not limited by class.

In our controlled case study, the differences in attitudes of class III and class V patients were definite but relatively small. However, the social status differences in our patients were small, too, as some of our class III patients actually came from class IV families. We know that social mobility is an important factor influencing attitudes toward psychiatry, particularly if attitudes are inferred from empathy and communication between psychiatrist and patient. This aspect of the problem will be treated in detail in another paper.

From experiences with class I and class II patients, not cited in our findings, we know that conscious attitudes toward psychiatry are more favorable in these classes and that knowledge of modern psychiatric principles is more susbstantial among such patients. The essential values underlying insight therapy are more likely to be shared by psychiatrists and upper class patients. Good therapy takes a good therapist, and at this stage of our knowledge also a good patient capable of some empathy with his psychiatrist. Such patients, it seems, are more frequently found in the upper classes. As we gain knowledge in psychotherapeutic techniques the patients' empathy will become less and less necessary.

Although the existence of unconscious processes and psychodynamic considerations was difficult for most of our patients to conceive, such notions had the least reality for the class V patient before and during treatment. This is not surprising as class V persons have less formal education and are less rewarded for verbalization and for thinking, particularly for thinking about symbolic and interpersonal processes which are crucial in grasping concepts and methods of dynamic psychiatry. Books and lectures on psychiatry have reached — at least superficially — the upper and middle social classes, but they have not had any impact on class V individuals. The occasional use of movies and modern mass media of communication have had as yet little effect on this population. From our material, it would seem that the Armed Forces are the greatest educators of the lower classes in understanding psychiatry and mental hygiene.

At this time insight therapy is less likely, in our opinion, to be grasped by the lower classes than physical therapy or a therapy employing "magical methods." This should not be construed as a recommendation of "supportive" or "suggestive" techniques but as a challenge to find appropriate methods for all kinds of patients. We are just interested in paving the way for a rational method of emotional re-education for lower class patients. Maxwell Jones (7) has been pioneering in developing such techniques in a hospital setting. What has been said about therapy may be applied to prevention, too. Ideas of prevention, based on the propositions of dynamic psychiatry, and carried out by the Mental Hygiene Movement, have not penetrated to the lower classes. Much education and a search for new and better techniques need to be undertaken before the largest segments of the population can be reached. Kingsley Davis came to similar conclusions (1).

As we stated before, the lack of rapport and communication found between our therapists and patients, particularly class V patients, is partly due to the fact that most of the therapists in our controlled case study were beginners. But, for the most part, these *are* the therapists who will be dealing with class V patients and with many of the class III patients, also. We wish to stress our belief that psychotherapy of class V patients is by no means impossible; but such techniques need to be developed. Psychotherapists who are able to devise therapeutic techniques for children and schizophrenics should be able to do the same for lower class patients. To achieve this, they will have to learn more about the way of life of these patients, their ethnic and social values and attitudes; and they will have to overcome some of their own social prejudices. Such understanding will be important in arriving at more efficient and rational methods of psychotherapy for lower class patients, who are more in need of help than any other group.

Summary

Patients in class III and class V shared similar outlooks toward mental illness and psychiatric treatment, but some qualitative and quantitative differences in these areas are apparent and seem to be related to social class status.

1. Although patients of both class III and class V had a tendency to conceive of their difficulties as somatic, class V patients were more likely to do so than class III; and class V patients were less likely to correct their somatic biases during treatment.

2. Class V patients were less likely than class III patients to come to treatment on their own initiative and more likely not to change their attitudes toward psychiatry once in treatment.

3. Class V patients knew less about psychiatry than class III patients, as expected, and were less likely to pick up information during the course of treatment.

4. Therapists were superficially aware of social differences between them and both class III and class V patients. With their class V patients, however, they more frequently "disliked" the patients, did not understand their values, and often had difficulty in understanding them as persons. Therapists disliked the class V patients' lack of responsibility and discipline, their dependency and ineptness at facing and correcting their emotional problems. Many of the therapists became discouraged in treating class V patients, especially when extremely difficult reality situations were added to other difficulties.

5. Communication between therapists and many patients of both class III and class V was poor, though this was decidedly more marked

with class V patients. These patients were less likely to understand what their therapists were driving at and more likely to accept the therapist's authority than class III patients. They wanted relief from misery but did not comprehend how understanding themselves could have any bearing on their life situations.

6. Practical implications from our findings in terms of more adequate methods of psychotherapy for lower class patients are mentioned.

REFERENCES

1. Davis, Kingsley. Mental Hygiene and Class Structure. *Psychiatry*, 1: 55–64, 1938.

2. Dollard, J., and N. E. Miller. *Personality and Psychotherapy: An Analysis in Terms of Learning, Thinking, and Culture*. McGraw-Hill, New York, 1950.

3. Felix, R. H., and J. S. Clausen. The Role of Surveys in Advancing Knowledge in the Field of Mental Health. *Publ. Opin. Quart.*, 17: 61–70, 1953.

4. Hollingshead, A. B. The New Haven Marriage and Family Study. (Unpublished.)

5. Hollingshead, A. B., and F. C. Redlich. Social Stratification and Psychiatric Disorders. *Am. Sociol. Rev.*, 18: 163–169, 1953.

6. Hovland, C. I., I. L. Janis, and H. H. Kelly. *Communication and Persuasion*. Yale Univ. Press, New Haven, 1953.

7. Jones, Maxwell. *Social Psychiatry: A Study of Therapeutic Communities*. Tavistock, London, 1952.

8. Myers, J. K., and L. Schaffer. Social Stratification and Psychiatric Practice: A Study of an Out-Patient Clinic. *Am. Sociol. Rev.*, 19: 307–310, 1954.

9. Redlich, F. C. The Psychiatrist in Caricature: An Analysis of Unconscious Attitudes Toward Psychiatry. *Am. J. Orthopsychiatry*, 20: 560–571, 1950.

10. ——— What the Citizen Knows about Psychiatry. *Ment. Hyg.*, 34: 64–79, 1950.

11. ——— The Concept of Normality. *Am. J. Psychotherapy*, 6: 551–576, 1952.

12. Redlich, F. C., A. B. Hollingshead, et al. Social Structure and Psychiatric Disorders. *Am. J. Psychiatry*, 109: 729–734, 1953.

13. Robinson, H. A., F. C. Redlich, and J. K. Myers. Social Structure and Psychiatric Treatment. *Am. J. Orthopsychiatry*, 24: 307–316, 1954.

14. Roper, Elmo. People's Attitudes Concerning Mental Health. A Study made in the city of Louisville, September 1950 (unpublished).

15. Schaffer, L., and J. K. Myers. Psychotherapy and Social Stratification: An Empirical Study of Practice in a Psychiatric Out-Patient Clinic. *Psychiatry*, 17: 83–93, 1954.

16. Woodward, J. L. Changing Ideas on Mental Illness and Its Treatment. *Am. Sociol. Rev.*, 16: 443–454, 1951.

40

A COMPARISON OF THE INCIDENCE OF HOSPITALIZED AND NON-HOSPITALIZED CASES OF PSYCHOSIS IN TWO COMMUNITIES

BERT KAPLAN, ROBERT B. REED, AND WYMAN RICHARDSON

University of Kansas, Harvard University, University of North Carolina

In recent years a number of studies[1] have presented data suggesting that there is an inverse relationship between socio-economic status and mental illness. To workers interested in the epidemiology of mental disorders these findings are of great importance since they imply that certain social patterns play a significant etiological role in the mental illnesses.

Socio-cultural factors, related as they are to psychological development, are precisely the kind of environmental conditions which could explain especially high rates of psychiatric disorders. The suggested relationship between socio-economic level and the occurrence of mental illness is therefore one of the first results of the applications of the epidemiologic method to understanding of the mental disorders. The next step, that of explaining the basis for the relationships, should be a very productive one for both psychiatry and social sciences.

Before advancing to the phase of theoretical explanations, however, it seems necessary to consider alternate explanations of these findings. One such explanation is that the findings are based on rates of admission to mental hospitals; yet several surveys have indicated that a substantial percentage of those who become psychotic do not enter mental hospitals.[2] It would seem therefore that evidence supporting

From the *American Sociological Review*, August 1956.

[1] Robert E. Clark, "The Relationship of Schizophrenia to Occupational Income and Occupational Prestige," *American Sociological Review*, 13 (June, 1948), pp. 325–330; Robert E. L. Faris and H. Warren Dunham, *Mental Disorder in Urban Areas*, Chicago: University of Chicago Press, 1939; August B. Hollingshead and Frederich C. Redlich, "Social Stratification and Psychiatric Disorders," *American Sociological Review*, 18 (April, 1953), pp. 163–169; Robert W. Hyde and Lowell V. Kingley, "Studies in Medical Sociology I: The Relation of Mental Disorders to Community Socio-Economic Level," *The New England Journal of Medicine*, 231 (October, 1944), pp. 543–548; Clarence W. Schroeder, "Mental Disorders in Cities," *American Journal of Sociology*, 48 (July, 1942), pp. 40–48.

[2] Paul Lemkau, Christopher Tietze, and Marcia Cooper, "Mental Hygiene Problems in an Urban District," *Mental Hygiene*, 25 (1941), pp. 624–646; Lemkau, *et al.*, "Mental Hygiene Problems in an Urban District, II," *Mental Hygiene*, 26 (1942), pp. 100–119;

the hypothesized relationship is based on only a part of the total number of cases of psychosis. Since it cannot be assumed that non-hospitalized cases are distributed in the same way as hospitalized cases, it seems very possible that if the additional cases of non-hospitalized psychotics were also considered, the alleged relationship might be altered.

The specific questions asked in this study were: When only hospitalized cases are considered, does a comparison of incidence at two different socio-economic levels support findings of studies in other regions that there is a lower incidence of hospitalization for psychosis at the higher socio-economic levels? What is the incidence of non-hospitalized cases of psychosis in the two study areas described below? Does this incidence rate vary with socio-economic status in the same way as does the incidence of hospitalized cases? If the hospitalized and non-hospitalized cases are combined, is there still a difference in the incidence rates between the two areas? And finally, is the case finding method used here epidemiologically useful?

PROCEDURES

The comparative values of incidence and prevalence studies have been the subject of much controversy. Since our concern in this study was to investigate the relationship between the factors influencing the occurrence of mental disorder rather than the factors influencing its duration, the incidence figure is clearly more relevant.

Several different periods were used for targets. In Wellesley, a predominantly upper and upper-middle class suburb of Boston, the fifteen year period 1936–1950 was chosen for hospitalized cases. The study did not include the more recent years because records for the last two or three years were incomplete. For the non-hospitalized cases only the last five years (1946–1950) of this period were used because information about earlier years is considerably less reliable and complete. In the Whittier Street area of Roxbury, a lower and lower-middle class neighborhood in Boston, the study of the hospitalized cases covered a one year period, 1949, because this area had a population of about 68,000 and an adequate number of cases could be gathered for comparison in this one year. The search for non-hospitalized cases, however, covered a five year period, 1948–1952, since a large turnover of informants, the main sources of information, made it advisable to study the most recent five year period. To compare rates during these different target periods it was necessary to estimate

William F. Roth, Jr. and Frank H. Luton, "The Mental Health Problem in Tennessee," *The American Journal of Psychiatry*, 99 (March, 1943), pp. 662–675.

the number of person-years in each age group by sex. In Wellesley the total population for each year was estimated by counting the yearly List of Residents for every third year, and estimating for the intervening years by straight line interpolation. The percentage distribution by age and sex was estimated for each year by linear interpolation of 1940 and 1950 census figures. On the basis of these two facts, person-years over the fifteen year period were obtained. A similar technique was used to estimate the person-years for the non-hospitalized case study. In the Whittier Street area census findings were utilized. The incidence of hospitalized psychosis was determined by searching admission records of all private and state mental hospitals in Massachusetts.

The community case finding survey was carried on by the senior author, a psychologist. The method consisted of interviewing individuals in the community who were in positions or roles which made it possible for them to know of mentally ill persons. The informants were asked to review their contacts during the target period and describe new cases of mental illness they might have encountered. The clergy, medical practitioners, social workers, public health nurses, welfare department workers, nursing home workers, school nurses, local health officers, and psychiatrists provided potential informants. We reasoned that if a person became mentally ill, most families would seek some kind of outside help. The few who did not seek aid might be known to individuals such as our informants who had a good knowledge of the community and what was happening in it. This method is relatively economical, although it leaves the researcher with some uncertainty whether he has found all the cases. Even if his survey has been fairly complete and accurate, he has no way of knowing or demonstrating it.

In Wellesley work was facilitated greatly by our connection with the Human Relations Service. This agency, under the sponsorship of the Harvard School of Public Health, had been attempting over a five year period to develop a program of preventive psychiatry in Wellesley. Its excellent relations, especially with local physicians and clergy, greatly facilitated the present study. During the interview the informant was asked to describe the symptoms and behavior of persons who had become psychotic for the first time during the years under study. It was explained that our definition of psychosis meant serious mental illness of the kind that might ordinarily lead to hospitalization. It was also made clear that we were not interested in neurosis, in the feebleminded, in alcoholism or in people who just "had problems."

The problem of diagnosis has been mentioned as one of the great difficulties in doing epidemiological research. It has been thought that since criteria for the diagnosis of psychosis vary so much, it would be difficult to say what any particular incidence figure meant. It is our feeling that this problem did not prove to be a crucial one in the present study. There were, to be sure, a number of cases which seemed borderline. However, they were a relatively small group of cases and our diagnostic procedures with respect to them were standard in the two areas. In the majority of the cases, psychosis was easily recognized by symptoms such as delusions or paranoid trends, which were present in most cases of diagnosed psychotics. There were two diagnostic problems of greater difficulty. One concerned senile psychosis, the other the depressions. Although patients are admitted to mental hospitals with all degrees of senility, it seemed to us good psychiatric practice to differentiate between senility and senile psychosis. The former we defined as intellectual changes of not too great severity accompanying old age. In order to establish the latter diagnosis we looked for severe intellectual deterioration with disorientation, lack of recognition of family, excitements, living in the past, severe emotional upset, or delusions accompanying intellectual changes. The other difficult diagnostic problems involved the depressions. Here we attempted to distinguish between the neurotic and the psychotic depression.

The final decision whether a person was psychotic or not was made by a psychiatrist not connected with the study.[3] He examined the notes of the field worker and on the basis of the evidence contained in them, separated the cases into four categories: the "certain" cases, the "probables," the "improbables," and the "certainly not" cases. He was then asked to examine the "probables" a second time and to divide them into two groups, those he thought had a high degree of probability and those he thought had a lower degree. The former group was then combined with the "certains." We believe this was justifiable because these were not borderline cases, but cases in which it was difficult to get information. The information available strongly suggested the diagnoses which were made.

The Communities

The town of Wellesley (population, about 20,000) is a fast growing suburb of Boston. It is known as one of the three or four wealthiest towns in the area and attracts persons of well above moderate means. The town is, however, by no means homogeneous in this respect and does contain groups of quite different socio-economic levels.

[3] Gerald Caplan, Lecturer on Mental Health, Harvard School of Public Health.

The Whittier Street area is not a political entity but a section of Boston proper. Varying socio-economic and ethnic characteristics of the residents divide the eleven census tracts into three fairly distinct sub-districts: In the "R" area less than 25 per cent of employed persons are "white collar" workers; the majority of people in the area are non-white and are largely native born. About one-fourth of the residents are less than 15 years of age. The median rental in this area is $25, and 37 per cent of the housing is dilapidated. The "S" area is, in its economic characteristics, mid-way between the "R" and "K" sub-districts. Of the resident workers, 30–53 per cent are "white collar" workers; 33–45 per cent of the adults are high school graduates. The population is predominantly Irish in ethnic origin. Median rentals in this area vary from $25 to $41, and there is a marked variation in type of housing from well-maintained, older, single family structures to dilapidated, multi-family structures. The "K" sub-district is the site of many institutions. Compared to the other sub-districts, there are fewer children (families in this economic stratum are known to move to suburban homes when children are born); the residents are predominantly native-born white, and the majority are high-school graduates pursuing white-collar occupations. Median rentals range from $42 to $61; there are many apartment houses in the district and only about 4 per cent of dwellings are dilapidated or without running water. The population for individuals over 15 years of age is 56,303 in the combined eleven census tracts.

RESULTS

Hospitalized Cases of Psychotics (First Admission). There were 203 new admissions for psychosis to mental hospitals from the Wellesley area in the 15-year target period, 1936–50, and 90 cases from the Whittier Street area in the one-year target period, 1949.

Analysis of admissions by age and sex (Table 1) shows that in Wellesley there was no significant variation in the age-incidence rate in either sex under 65 years of age, but in both sexes there was a significant increase after the age of 65 years, and this increase was higher in males than in females. In Roxbury, a similar increase in incidence was noted over 65, but the sex incidence in older persons was reversed, in that a higher rate was found among females over 65 years of age. The sex reversal in persons over 65 years of age is not statistically significant. Because of the comparative similarity between sexes and between age groups under 65 these cases are grouped in subsequent analysis.

The Whittier Street area shows a higher incidence of hospitalized psychosis than does the Wellesley area. Within each of the two areas, there are also marked differences in incidence rates, apparently associated with socio-economic characteristics. The number of cases in each sub-district in Wellesley is too small to justify statistical comparison, but incidence rates are lower in the sub-districts rated highest socio-economically and highest in those at the lower level of the scale.

The differences in hospitalized psychosis incidence are even more dramatic if the higher socio-economic areas in Wellesley are compared to the lower socio-economic areas in Roxbury, as is shown in Table 2. The same marked difference is found between these populations in all age groups.

TABLE 1. FIRST ADMISSIONS FOR PSYCHOSIS BY AGE AND SEX

Age	Wellesley, 1936–1950				Whittier Street Study Area, 1949			
	Male		Female		Male		Female	
	Cases †	Rate *	Cases	Rate *	Cases	Rate *	Cases	Rate *
15–24	13.6	8.4	16	8.6	3.	5.2	6.	9.1
25–44	21.8	7.0	32	7.5	17.	17.4	14.	12.3
45–64	18.4	7.1	32	9.2	9.	13.6	10.	11.2
65 and over	30.0	43.4	36	27.8	9.	31.9	22.	49.9

* Cases per 10,000 person years of exposure.
† Cases appear in fractional numbers because the ages of a small number of cases were unknown. They were distributed among the four age groups in the same proportions as was the population at large.

TABLE 2. FIRST ADMISSIONS FOR PSYCHOSIS FOR WELLESLEY AND WHITTIER STREET

	15 and over		15–64		65 and over	
	Cases	Rate *	Cases	Rate *	Cases	Rate *
Wellesley Total † (Wellesley exclusive of the lowest socio-economic areas — IIB-IIC)	199.8	10.5	133.8	7.9	66.0	32.4
	139.6	9.3	92.9	6.9	46.7	30.6
Whittier Street Total ‡	90.0	16.0	59.0	12.0	31.0	42.9
Whittier Street (minus highest socio-economic areas)	64.	22.8	40.	16.2	24.	70.3

* Cases per 10,000 person years of exposure.
† During 15 year period, 1936–1950.
‡ During one year period, 1949.

Incidence of Non-Hospitalized Psychosis. A comparison of the incidence of non-hospitalized psychosis in Wellesley and the Whittier Street area (Table 3) indicates a reversal of the results shown for hospitalized cases. A lower incidence rate of non-hospitalized psychotics was found in the Whittier Street area than in Wellesley (2.0

cases per 10,000 person years exposure in Whittier Street and 6.7 cases per 10,000 person years of exposure in Wellesley).[4]

If incidence rates for hospitalized and non-hospitalized cases are added (Table 4), total incidence of psychosis in the Whittier Street area is higher than in Wellesley in all adult age groups. (24.8 cases per 10,000 person years of exposure in Whittier Street; 17.2 cases per 10,000 person years of exposure in Wellesley.)

DISCUSSION

In summary, we found that when only hospitalized cases of psychosis are considered, incidence rates were considerably higher in a lower and lower-middle class area than they were in an upper-middle and upper class area. Comparisons of sub-areas in Wellesley and Roxbury indicate that for hospitalized cases the same relationship between

TABLE 3. TOTAL INCIDENCE OF NEW CASES OF NON-HOSPITALIZED PSYCHOSIS, BY AGE FOR WELLESLEY AND WHITTIER STREET

	15 and over		15–64		65 and over	
	Cases	Rate *	Cases	Rate *	Cases	Rate *
Wellesley						
New cases of non-hospitalized psychosis ‡	47 †	6.7	26	4.3	21	21.8
Whittier Street (highest socio-economic areas omitted)						
New cases of non-hospitalized psychosis §	29 †	2.0	12	1.0	17	9.9

* Cases per 10,000 person years of exposure.
† One-half of cases in which we were not certain of year of onset were included. Six were added in Wellesley and five in the Whittier Street Area.
‡ During 5 year period, 1946–1950.
§ During 5 year period, 1948–1952.

incidence rate and socio-economic level holds. The incidence of new non-hospitalized cases is much lower in the lower and lower-middle class area than in the upper-middle and upper class area. When both types of cases are combined, the difference between the two areas is reduced. However, a considerable difference remains with the lower socio-economic area revealing a higher psychosis incidence rate.

Before venturing an interpretation of these results, it is necessary

[4] It will be noted that in Table 3, rates for Wellesley are given excluding sub-areas IIB and IIC, the lowest socio-economic areas, and for the Whittier Street area excluding the census tracts which were at relatively high socio-economic levels. The purpose was to make the groups being compared more homogeneous with respect to socio-economic status. In Tables 3 and 4 the Wellesley rate is given for the whole community since non-hospitalized cases could not be located by sub-areas and therefore a separate rate could not be computed for Wellesley minus the lowest socio-economic areas.

to consider whether the fact that a greater incidence of non-hospitalized cases was found in Wellesley than in the Roxbxury area is an
artifact reflecting a greater difficulty of finding cases in the latter
area. Does the paucity of cases in the Roxbury census tracts result
from a lack of co-operativeness on the part of our informants? This
does not seem to be the case. Although only 29 cases were finally
counted, over 175 cases were discussed. Sixty-five of these were judged
to be psychotic and not hospitalized, but two-thirds of the cases either
began before the five-year period in which we were interested or lived
just outside of the area. Our informants in Roxbury were as co-operative
as those in Wellesley, but two-thirds of the cases they knew about could
not be counted in our study.

There is some reason to suspect, however, that the search in Wellesley was more complete than that in Roxbury. Perhaps the best indication of this is the fact that in Wellesley many cases were known
to two, three, four or five informants, while in Roxbury only rarely
was a case known to as many as two informants. This suggests that
Roxbury informants were each scrutinizing some small part of the
whole area, while the Wellesley informants tended to be looking at
the same population, because the number of people was smaller and
the area was a political entity. It may be seen that there is a much
greater chance for gaps in our research to develop in the former situation than the latter. It is entirely possible that even in Wellesley
certain groups evaded the scrutiny of any of our informants. In Roxbury we had a strong feeling that this was the case. In the light of
these facts it is necessary for us to admit that the search in Roxbury
in all probability underestimated the actual incidence rates.

It is difficult to know to what degree our Roxbury count is inac-
curate. We would have to have found three times as many cases as
we did if the real rates in Roxbury were to approximate those in Wellesley. It is inconceivable to us that this number could be found. Furthermore, we have undoubtedly underestimated the Wellesley rate
as well so that to equal it an even greater number should be found
in Roxbury.

How can the result that the Roxbury area has twice as high a hospitalization rate as does Wellesley, but a rate of non-hospitalized psychosis which is only about one-third as large, be explained? We believe
the answer lies in different attitudes toward hospitalization for mental
illness. In Wellesley the field worker frequently encountered the attitude that the mentally ill person should be kept out of the state hospital
at any cost. This is partly due to the general perception of the state
mental hospital as a "snake pit" and commitment of a relative there,
equivalent to abandoning him to the worst possible kind of treatment.

Table 4. Total Incidence of Psychosis and First Admissions for Psychosis by Age for Wellesley and Whittier Street

	15 and over		15–64		65 and over	
	Cases	Rate *	Cases	Rate *	Cases	Rate *
Wellesley						
Total Incidence of Psychosis †	....	17.2	....	12.2	....	34.7
First Admissions for Psychosis †	199.8	10.5	133.8	7.9	66.0	32.4
Whittier Street (highest socio-economic areas omitted)						
Total Incidence of Psychosis ‡	....	24.8	....	17.2	....	80.1
First Admissions for Psychosis §	64	22.8	40	16.2	24	70.3

* Cases per 10,000 person years of exposure.
† During 15 year period, 1936–1950.
‡ Number of cases could not be added since the two categories were based on different time periods, and no totals are given.
§ During 1 year period, 1949.

In part, also, it is related to a reluctance on the part of upper-middle class families to use public hospital facilities since these are regarded as institutions established to serve the poor rather than those families in the $7–15,000 a year category. Even these levels of income, however, are insufficient to maintain a relative for prolonged periods of time in a high-cost private mental hospital.

In Roxbury, on the other hand, there is a pattern of extensive utilization of public hospital facilities, frequently for illness which private physicians ordinarily handle in homes. Nearby are two large state hospitals which are known to most people in the area, and while it would be an exaggeration to say that there are no barriers between hospitals and the community, there are probably less than in Wellesley where there is no mental hospital. We believe there is a much more casual acceptance of hospitalization in the Whittier Street area than in Wellesley.

Complementing those attitudes toward hospitalization as an explanation of our findings, is the equally important fact that Wellesleyites are better able to care for psychotic individuals in the home. Their households are less crowded and they are better able to afford the extra nursing care needed. It may be easier in Wellesley houses to isolate the mentally ill person on a separate floor or at least in a separate room. In Roxbury there is overcrowding and usually no way for the patient to be isolated. Perhaps most important, in Wellesley it is possible, indeed it is a frequent pattern, to have old people who have become senile cared for in a private nursing home. Roxbury residents could rarely afford such care.

Our explanation, then, of the disparity of incidence rates of non-hospitalized psychosis is that <u>Wellesley residents try, to the limit of their abilities, to keep family members from being committed to mental hospitals, and they have real abilities in this respect</u>. In Roxbury, on the other hand, while somewhat similar attitudes exist, it is our impression that they are not held so strongly, <u>that families are more prone to hospitalize their members when it is indicated</u>. Even where there is a strong desire to keep a family member out of the hospital, <u>it is ordinarily very difficult or impossible to provide the necessary facilities and nursing care</u>.

If we accept this explanation of our results as reasonable and adequate, there is the very strong implication that many cases who in Wellesley might have been found in the non-hospitalized group, were in Roxbury found to be hospitalized. <u>Even when the hospitalized and non-hospitalized cases were combined, the Wellesley community had a lower incidence rate than did the Roxbury area</u>. The discovery of <u>more Roxbury cases would increase this difference. We may say, therefore, that the inverse relationship between the socio-economic status and the incidence of mental disorder is verified, although the inclusion of non-hospitalized psychotics reduces the height of the correlation</u>.

Let us for a moment assume the language of the statistician and say that any study of the incidence of mental illness is bound to discover a certain amount of variance among groups at different socioeconomic levels. If the study has been based on records of hospitalization alone, we can say on the basis of this investigation that a certain amount of the variance can be explained by the fact that a large number of people who become psychotic do not enter mental hospitals and that proportionately more of these cases are found at the upper socio-economic levels than at the lower levels. We believe that another factor explains much of the remainder: the direct consequences of the system of social stratification on the psyche of the individual. Our theory is that the whole network of prerogatives, attitudes, and expectations surrounding any class position has important consequences for the individual ego structure which in turn is an important factor in determining resistance to mental illness. By ego structure is meant the complex of factors concerning the ego — the self picture, self esteem, feelings of adequacy, and most important of all, the ego strength which prescribes on the one hand the amount of impulse control and on the other hand the degrees of successful management of the environment.

A number of considerations lead us to this belief. George Mead and many others have shown the extent to which the individual accepts the public definition of his self. If society says he is superior, he feels that he is superior; if it views him as inferior, then he feels himself to be inferior. While we do not mean to imply that the self picture is given in its entirety by these public definitions, we do maintain they are accepted to a considerable extent by the individual and incorporated into the ego system. If they are of a beneficial bolstering kind, we can expect that the stability and resistance of the individual will be increased. The plain fact of social stratification does not operate alone however; the social superiority feelings of the upper-middle and upper classes are ordinarily accompanied by child rearing and education patterns which have the effect of reinforcing them. It is true that individuals with low self esteem and ego strength are found in great numbers at all class levels and it would be incorrect therefore to hold that these characteristics are determined by class position. Our argument is only that they may sometimes, in some cases, be influenced by it and that if all other factors were constant, or varied randomly, the influence of class position on the ego system and on the resistance to mental illness could be discerned.

Summary and Conclusions

Incidence rates of hospitalized psychosis were compared in two communities in the Metropolitan Boston area and were found to be significantly higher in the lower-middle socio-economic area than in the upper level socio-economic community. This finding confirms other studies which suggest an inverse relation between social environment and mental disorder.

An etiological relation between lower socio-economic conditions and mental illness cannot be accepted, however, until we explore the possibility that cases of psychosis may be hospitalized at differing rates in the upper and lower levels of society, so that studies of hospitalized psychosis alone do not give a true picture of incidence.

The lower socio-economic community revealed a significantly lower incidence of non-hospitalized psychosis than did the higher level community. We believe this fact can be explained by differing attitudes toward hospitalization of mental illness in the two communities. Residents in the higher social community resisted hospitalization for their mentally ill family members. Because they had more money and more spacious housing, they were better able to keep ill members of the family at home.

Comparison of sub-areas in the two communities indicates that the same inverse relation between hospitalized psychosis incidence rates and socio-economic levels persists within the individual communities.

A description and discussion of our case-finding procedure for non-hospitalized psychosis is given. The method does not reveal accurately the number of non-hospitalized cases of psychosis in an area but it indicates within the limits of the method, that incidence rates of non-hospitalized psychosis vary differently with socio-economic status than do rates of hospitalized psychosis.

The difference in the incidence of hospitalized psychosis in high socio-economic and low socio-economic communities, found by previous investigators and confirmed by this study, is reduced by including non-hospitalized psychosis in the two areas. But there remains a significant inverse relation between socio-economic circumstances and mental illness. This finding may be the direct consequence of a system of social stratification on the psyche of individuals. In addition the possibility exists that more intensive case-finding methods for non-hospitalized psychosis would reveal even more non-hospitalized cases in the upper level community, thus reducing the differences in total psychosis rates to the point that incidence is the same for the two communities.

41

THE CONCEPT OF A THERAPEUTIC COMMUNITY

MAXWELL JONES, M.D.

Belmont Hospital, Surrey, England

Applied to a psychiatric hospital the term "therapeutic community" implies that the responsibility for treatment is not confined to the trained medical staff but is a concern also of the other community members, i.e., the patients. How far can patients usefully participate in the treatment of other patients and how will this participation affect them? How far can they in turn be helped by other patients?

The importance of staff tensions as they affect treatment have long been recognized and the work of the Chestnut Lodge group has had a profound effect on the thinking and practice of psychiatric nursing and we hope of psychiatrists themselves. This subject has been ably discussed in the recent publication by Stanton and Schwartz (1). Relatively less attention has been paid to the social life of patients when staff are not present and the therapeutic possibilities this social interaction may have. Attention has been drawn to this subject by the interesting experiences of Caudill, a social anthropologist, who was admitted to a mental institution for 2 months as a patient in order to study the social situation from the patients' point of view. He states (2):

While the staff exercised control over the patients, they did not give recognition to the patient world as a social group, but rather,. they interpreted the behavior of the patients almost solely in individual dynamic-historical terms. The patient group, thus lacking an adequate channel of communication to the staff, protected itself by turning inward, and by developing a social structure which was insulated as much as possible from friction with the hospital routine. Nevertheless, such friction did occur, and the subsequent frustration led to behavior on the part of the patients which, although it overtly resembled neurotic behavior arising from personal emotional conflicts, was, in fact, to a considerable extent due to factors in the immediate situation.

If a therapeutic community with active patient participation is to be established in any psychiatric treatment unit a drastic revision in existing staff and patient roles and role relationships will be called for. It is clear that the changes that might be attempted will depend

From *The American Journal of Psychiatry*, February 1956.

on many factors, including the type of patient, the treatment goals, the previous training of the staff, the degree of self-determination and freedom of action granted to the center, the culture of the adjacent hospital, if any, the culture of the wider community, economic factors, etc. In this presentation, however, we are assuming positive sanctions from higher authorities, complete freedom shared by staff and patients alike to organize the community, and a single therapeutic goal, namely the adjustment of the individual to social and work conditions outside, without any ambitious psychotherapeutic program.

Detailed description of all the role changes and social reorganization which, in our experience, are necessary cannot here be undertaken (7); however, certain main points can be discussed. The psychiatrist has, like all doctors, been given and accepts many of the qualities of the witch doctor. His greater knowledge is assumed in all treatment situations whether individual or group. The patient understandably enough wants to feel that the doctor knows what he is doing and by his attitude contributes to what is often an illusion. The doctor maintains many of the symbols of his office even when they have no immediate usefulness, e.g., the traditional white coat, prominent stethoscope, and, in the U.S.A., the peculiarly ugly framed official qualification found in most doctors' offices. Moreover, in America the status of psychiatry is higher than its proved usefulness merits. How far do factors such as these create barriers to free communication between doctors and patients? How honest are we in admitting our limitations to our patients, nursing staffs, etc., and how readily do we turn to them for help? To give a simple illustration, how often is the wrong patient sent from an open to a closed ward in an attempt to resolve a tense ward situation? The fact is that we do not know and unless we attempt to analyze the disturbance we cannot find out. Such an analysis will usually involve the whole ward community and may be difficult or impossible to carry out without free communication between patients and staff and between the individual members in both groups. If, however, it is possible to institute a ward meeting and to achieve some degree of communication it may be possible to learn a great deal about the patients' feelings, their attitudes toward the staff, and so on. It has been our conscious aim to develop the freest possible communication between patients and staff and this has necessitated a reorganization of the doctors' time-table. Increasingly less time has been spent in individual interviewing and proportionately more in group and community meetings so that at present ⅓ of the day is spent in the former and ⅔ in the latter. A group meeting usually comprises about 10 patients, a psychiatrist, and several members of the nursing staff. These meetings are run on analytic lines but techniques vary with the personality and training of the psychiatrist. Every patient attends his group meeting (one hour) daily. By a community meeting we mean a discussion group involving the entire population of the unit (100 patients of both sexes, 4 psychiatrists, 1 psychiatric social worker, 1 psychologist, 1 social anthropologist, 4 workshop instructors, and a nursing staff of 15).

A community meeting epitomizes the function of a therapeutic community. The aim is to achieve the freest possible expression of feeling by both patients and staff. This is a departure from the usual role of staff members in the familiar therapeutic group of 8 to 12 persons. In the latter it is the patients only who verbalize their feelings and the staff use such communications as seem therapeutic but do not reveal (at least not intentionally) anything of their own feelings. In a community meeting the staff are free to verbalize their own anxieties where they relate to the community, e.g., the growing hostility of the hospital authorities and local residents to the drunken behavior of certain patients. This threat may have been unknown to the patients but is now fed back to the total community by the staff. The community is thus faced by a social problem which has meaning for everyone. It has taken us 8 years to arrive at the point where the patients no longer attempt to sidestep their responsibility in tackling both the therapeutic and administrative aspects of such a problem in collaboration with the staff. The meaning of the individuals' need to turn to alcohol is the major problem and can be discussed as a current event with the other patients who participated in the outing. This can be implemented by further communications from the patients' own doctors, the P.S.W., members of their groups, and so on. Moreover, the timing of a particular alcoholic "binge" can often be seen in response to some current tension, say a general feeling of antagonism to the supposedly authoritarian behavior of certain staff members or to a state of unresolved tension in the staff members themselves. This in turn may uncover some of the deeper feelings of antagonism toward parental figures and highlight some of the transference or counter-transference difficulties. Thus the emphasis may be on uncovering therapy, on group dynamics, on education, or it may become clear to some staff members or patients that at least one factor in the situation is a response, often unconscious, by patients to unresolved staff tensions. In the latter eventuality the current practice is to postpone discussion of this tension to a later staff meeting, but we feel that a time may soon arrive when such discussion will constantly occur in the presence of the patients themselves. Already we are aware of the extraordinary sensitivity of some patients to such tensions and the probable advantages in accepting their participation, as we do in dealing with patient problems. We have already gone some way in this direction by admitting freely that the staff frequently display neurotic defenses and have casualties luckily only of a minor kind. These neurotic manifestations are usually commented on by the patients and when my own emotional difficulties begin to get out of control the patients show a most touching solicitude and desire to treat me, or an obvious pleasure in my discomfiture, depending on the particular patient! Someone will be probably be heard to say that it is time I talked about my difficulties or more specifically that I have a work problem! In addition, the patients are fully aware that we have frequent staff meetings to deal with our own group and interpersonal tensions. Thus we are patently at one with them in constantly needing treatment. The only reason for separating the two treatment areas (patients and staff) is to give the patients the feeling that our difficulties refer to immediate problems particularly in the field of learning, e.g., the training of new staff members and are not of such magnitude as to warrant the term "illness." Clearly patients want to feel that the staff can cope with their own problems, if they are going to be able to treat them competently, so it is probably better to hold staff groups separately until such time as community techniques have reached the point of perfection when patients can safely be told the whole truth.

The community meeting is a sort of general feed-back and clearing house for current problems from both patients and staff. A problem relating specifically to a particular subgroup, say a workshop or a ward, may be left for later discussion by the particular subgroup. More often, however, it will touch off a more general problem and lead to an immediate discussion. Sometimes the community's current anxiety centers around a particular patient and the whole hour is spent in discussing this patient. It may be that the patient is acting out in so disturbing a way that a decision must be made about his possible transfer to a mental hospital where there are adequate facilities for the supervision of individual patients.

Take the case of an adolescent behavior problem in a girl who has been resorting to excessive amounts of Benzedrine by eating the contents of inhalers that she can buy in any chemist's shop in England. In addition to this, she set fire to a roller towel in the kitchen of her ward. The cause of the fire was at first unknown and it was only as a result of various group meetings that the factors became known and could be fed back into the community meeting. In working through many aspects of this girl's problem — her early rejection, her illegitimacy, orphanage upbringing, the development of her criminal activities, etc. — the whole community became involved and informed about her problem in some depth. She was able to say why she wanted to burn down the hospital and needed to take Benzedrine; that she hated her doctor and could

not communicate with him in individual interviews because he reminded her
of the magistrate who had sent her to a corrective institution. Moreover, it
soon became clear that no matter how kind the community might be the only
real friends she had ever known belonged to the criminal fringe and she felt
almost as strong a desire to return to them as to get well.

This type of problem involving adaptation to a new set of values and
the whole concept of health is probably best handled in the community where many other patients are preoccupied with similar problems
bearing on social values.

The constant verbalization of problems and working them through
in daily group and community meetings lead to the development of
a rather sophisticated and articulate community. Visitors are constantly surprised by the patients' understanding and insight in handling their problems in collaboration with the staff. Social attitudes
come in for frequent discussion, e.g., such problems as informing, discipline, etc., which have such sinister association for patients — many
of whom have been in prison — and have obvious importance in relation to the establishment of free communications, as do the various
attitudes patients adopt toward the general topic of "treatment."
How many patients in psychiatric hospitals have clear ideas on this
subject? One is tempted to ask the same question in relation to hospital staffs. To staff members who are prepared to recognize this
problem we can recommend the advantages of discussing the topic in
community with the patients. A surprising amount of mutual education can result. The trained staff member is forced to review some
of his traditional attitudes and is unable to retreat to his safe position
of omnipotent silence. For instance, in most psychiatric hospitals sedatives are used in large amounts. Stimulated by the frequently occurring problem of drug addiction and the tensions produced by the
"acter-outers" in demanding sedatives from the night staff, we have
found it necessary to discuss this problem on many occasions. The community has slowly changed its attitude until it is now accepted by everyone that our previous practice of giving sedatives was in the main a defense against difficulties (both patient and staff) which were much
better dealt with by verbalization or other forms of acting out in the
group or community meetings. Little distinction is made by the patients between the use of sedatives and of alcohol. The latter is seen
in the main as a regressive symptom of the patient whereas sedation
is seen as a symptom in this case not only confined to the patient but
frequently involving the staff as well. The staff's need to give sedatives has been freely discussed and was seen to reflect the anxieties
of doctors and nurses at least as much as it was used as a specific
therapeutic procedure. I know of only one other hospital where the

use of sedatives has been discontinued and this again was the result of a careful analysis of the staff motivations in prescribing drugs.

We have developed another community technique which gives us some insight into the patients' attitude toward treatment and the unit generally. Every Friday morning we have a 2-hour seminar with any professional visitors who care to attend. The majority of the staff is present and the patients are represented by 8 different volunteers each week. The average number of visitors is 20 and we avoid any temptation to structure the meeting. The usual pattern is that the patients start talking about their current tensions or seek information about the visitors, their particular professions, reasons for studying the unit, and so on. As the visitors are drawn from the social science and medical fields they may well touch off some controversy, *e.g.*, between probation officers and patients with an antisocial background. The patients are frequently openly hostile to the unit or staff members; this draws the staff into the discussion and the situation becomes very similar to the daily community meetings. Usually, however, at some point the visitors' need for specific information leads the patients to express their own views about treatment, the social organization of the unit, and similar subjects. In this way we learn a great deal from the interdisciplinary seminar and not only can test the patients' concept of the unit culture but can learn something of the reaction of trained outsiders.

There is nothing particularly new in the concept of a therapeutic community. John Wesley had something like this in mind when he formed his "bands" some 200 years ago. The field of juvenile delinquency has produced experiments like those of Aichorn (3), Bettelheim (4), and Redl (5), and it is not pure chance that our own recent experience has been largely in the field of "adult delinquents" or the "acting-out disorders." I feel strongly that we psychiatrists have largely failed to meet the treatment challenge of the antisocial patient, whatever his classification. These patients need specially trained staff and a therapeutic community if their antisocial attitudes are to be modified. To the best of my knowledge the social rehabilitation unit at Belmont Hospital is the only one of this kind with the possible exception of some prison communities. I have deliberately left any mention of the antisocial patient to the end and avoided writing specifically about this problem, as there seems to be an equally good case for the application of the general principles of a therapeutic community in most, if not all, psychiatric hospitals.

Thanks to the courtesy of Professor Bob Matthews, I was able to spend the month of February 1954, visiting the department of psychiatry at Louisiana State University, and also several of the state mental hospitals. This experience has been reported elsewhere (6) but briefly it helped to confirm my impression that many of the principles of a therapeutic community are equally relevant to a psychiatric hospital and social rehabilitation unit such as ours.

REFERENCES

1. Stanton, A. H., and Schwartz, M. S. *The Mental Hospital*, New York: Basic Books, 1954.
2. Caudill, W., et al. *Am. J. Orthopsychiat.*, 22: 314, 1952.
3. Aichorn, A. *Wayward Youth*, New York: Viking Press, 1935.
4. Bettelheim, B. *Love is Not Enough*, Glencoe, Ill.: Free Press, 1952.
5. Redl, F., and Wineman, D. *Controls from Within*, Glencoe, Ill.: Free Press, 1952.
6. Jones, M., and Matthews, R. A. *Brit. J. Med. Psychol.* In Press.
7. Jones, M. *The Therapeutic Community*, New York: Basic Books, 1953.

42

A THERAPEUTIC MILIEU

BRUNO BETTELHEIM, Ph.D., and EMMY SYLVESTER, M.D.
The Orthogenic School, University of Chicago

This paper describes the treatment of emotionally disturbed children in an institutional setting. The clinical material on which this discussion is based concerns a syndrome developed in non-therapeutic institutions which may be called "psychological institutionalism." For the purpose of showing how these children are rehabilitated at the Orthogenic School, two cases will be presented in full.

Psychological institutionalism may be regarded as a deficiency disease in the emotional sense. Absence of meaningful continuous interpersonal relationships leads to impoverishment of the personality. The results of this process are observed in children who have lived in institutional settings for prolonged periods of time, but it is not limited to them. It also occurs in children who are exposed to a succession of foster homes or to disorganized family settings.

Non-institutional living *per se* will therefore not cure or avoid institutionalism. Neither can psychotherapeutic measures be effective which neglect the core of the disturbance. Only measures arising from benign interpersonal relationships among adults and children can combat the impoverishment of the personalities of children who suffer from emotional institutionalism. Since behavior disorders in the common sense do not necessarily form part of the clinical picture, the factors which cause impoverishment of personality are only rarely subjected to psychiatric study. Understanding these factors furnishes leads to the construction of a therapeutic milieu.

A frame of reference that consists of depersonalized rules and regulations may lead the child to become an automaton in his passive adjustment to the institution. There is no need for independent decisions because the child's physical existence is well protected and his activities arranged for him. Compliance with stereotyped rules rather than assertive action constitutes adequate adjustment, but does not allow for spontaneity. Reality testing is not extended to variegated life conditions. Complete determination by external rules prevents the development of inner controls. Emotional conflicts cannot be utilized toward

From the *American Journal of Orthopsychiatry*, 18: 191, 1948.

personality growth because they are not intrapsychic conflicts, but only occasional clashes between instinctual tendencies and impersonal external rules. The cause of these serious deviations in personality development — the absence of interpersonal relationships — is also responsible for their remaining unrecognized. The child lives in emotional isolation and physical distance from the adult. Even in instances where the child lives in proximity of touch and experience with adults, such closeness does not serve the purpose of personality growth if the significant characteristics of the normal child-adult relationship are not maintained. Frequent change in the personalities and absence of proper and consistent dosage of the adult's distance from and closeness to the child, turn into shadowy acquaintance what should be intimate relationships. This "not knowing" the adult deprives the child of images of integration.

In a therapeutic milieu, on the contrary, the child's development toward increasing mastery must be facilitated. Training in skills and achievements, specialized programs and activities, are of peripheral importance only. They are therapeutically justified solely if they originate from the central issue of the therapeutic milieu. A therapeutic milieu is characterized by its inner cohesiveness which alone permits the child to develop a consistent frame of reference. This cohesiveness is experienced by the child as he becomes part of a well defined hierarchy of meaningful interpersonal relationships. Emphasis on spontaneity and flexibility — not to be misconstrued as license or chaos — makes questions of schedule or routine subservient to the relevance of highly individualized and spontaneous interpersonal relationships. Such conditions permit the emergence and development of the psychological instances, the internalization of controls, and the eventual integration of the child's personality. It may be assumed that these milieu factors which determine the children's rehabilitation in the therapeutic milieu, have validity for the institutional care of children in general.

The personality defects which result from the absence of these factors in an institutional setting are clearly demonstrated by a control group of six to eight year old children who were not considered disturbed by their environment. The reason for the psychiatric study was a "purely administrative one" — they had reached the age limit of the residential institution in which they had spent the greater part of their lives. They arrived at the clinic in groups and presented themselves as physically well developed, neat and well-groomed youngsters. Their behavior in the waiting room was rather striking: they seemed to have an unusual amount of group spirit and had completely accepted their respective positions in the group as leaders, followers, protectors, or proteges.

This apparent social maturity was in marked contrast to their behavior in the individual contact with the psychiatrist, in whose office many were excessively shy whereas others became aggressively demanding. These forms of behavior were fixed. Lack of the flexible adaptability which even disturbed children show during the course of a psychiatric interview, characterized these children. The shy ones remained shy throughout the interview. Others were unable to modify their demands which appeared in two different and mutually exclusive varieties. They took the form of "toy hunger" in the children who had interest in toy material only, and of "touch hunger" in those whose need was exclusively for physical contact. The children who were not overwhelmed by rigid shyness entered conversation readily, and it was possible to get a picture of their subjective world.

In spite of psychometrically good intelligence, all conception of coherence of time, space, and person was lacking. Their lives were oriented to washing, dressing, eating, and resting, experienced as pleasurable and unpleasurable purely in terms of their own bodies, and only loosely connected with the adults responsible for their care. Hardly any of the children referred to the staff by name. Some were able to distinguish individual staff members according to the functions of physical routine they supervised. For many children, there existed one exception in this nameless world: the nurse in charge of the sickroom. This seems significant, since she was the only person who, temporarily at least, was in full charge of all the needs of the child.

The automaton-like rigidity of these children, their egocentric preoccupation with functions of their own body, their inability to master a one-to-one contact with an adult, are indications of a serious lag in personality integration.

The deviation in personality development shown by these children allows important conclusions. It demonstrates the dangers of rearing in a setting where a number of adults take care of isolated functions of the child rather than of the whole child, and stresses the necessity of giving each child the opportunity for a continuous central relationship to one adult in the institution.

Upon admission to the School, the children, whose personality development in the therapeutic milieu will be presented, showed striking similarities to this control group. While the severe psychopathology of the patients will become obvious in the description of their gradual rehabilitation, it should be kept in mind that none of the children in the control group were considered in any way abnormal by those who managed the institutional environment in which they lived.

The following case material demonstrates the slow and gradual emergence of personality structure in two children who showed all the characteristics of emotional institutionalism when they were admitted to the School. Here, the simple activities such as eating, bathing, and going to bed, which had also been provided in the non-therapeutic institution, are carried out within meaningful interpersonal relationships. Thus they become essential therapeutic tools for personality rehabilitation.

Case 1:[1] A ten year old boy of superior intelligence had lived in various institutions since his birth. His adjustment demanded psychiatric attention only when self-destructive tendencies of long standing culminated in a suicidal attempt. His life had been characterized by scarcity and tenuousness of personal ties. During the process of rehabilitation, it became obvious that his self-destructive act was more a desperate than a pathological effort to break through his isolation. This he revealed in a situation which was characteristic for him in the beginning of treatment at the School. An explosion of rage had followed his awkward and ineffectual attempt to get close to other children by provoking their aggression. It was then that he said, "I went up on the Empire State Building and jumped off. After that everybody was my friend."

Although he had always lived in proximity to others, he had never experienced the structured hierarchy which differentiates children from adults and thus permits their interaction. He neither knew how to react to adults nor how to get along with children. For him, adults were those who were bigger than he, individuals who by virtue of greater strength and size enforced rules, inflicted punishment and prevented children from "bothering them."

One counselor devoted herself particularly to him. Though he was for a long time unable to reciprocate the offered relationship, he immediately utilized the additional comfort which the contacts with the counselor offered. Toward the end of the first month, he expressed his first appreciation of her devotion when he snuggled against her and said, "I am a laughing hyena." He could express happiness only by coloring his incorporative tendencies with primitive feeling tones of joy. It took another month before he was able to ask any personal questions of her, the person whom he knew best. Once, when he had assured himself of his hold on his special counselor who had let him cling to her arm, he asked her were she lived. Although it was clear to all other children that the counselor's room was three doors from their dormitory, his deep isolation had to lift before he could envisage her as a living, personal entity.

[1] Credit for most of the direct work in the rehabilitation of this boy is due to Miss Gayle Shulenberger and Mrs. Marianne Wasson.

This breaking through of his isolation was apparently meaningful to him and he feared its return because his ability to maintain contact was still very tenuous. The arrival of a new boy in the dormitory became an immediate threat to him. However, he found means of reassuring himself; he asked his counselor to come over to his bed and asked to kiss her good night for the first time. He then told her a story which he called a "joke": Two people had started to go somewhere but soon found themselves back in the same place from which they had started. His insecurity and fear that the newcomer would set him back with his counselor to where he had started showed that he still lacked faith in the reliability of human ties which he had just learned to appreciate.

He became more aloof for several days, but then realized that his fears of abandonment were not justified. This gave him the courage to display regressive behavior for the first time. Though prompted by the threat of a newcomer, this regression was actually progress, since he experimented actively with his ability to cope with vicissitudes in human contacts. Only with his counselor did he begin to act like a small child. In baby talk he called her his mother, saying, "My mamma washes my hands for me. She gets me clean socks." He asked her to help him dress and to spoon-feed him. He was permitted to experience this primitive child-adult relationship. Two months later, baby talk and desire for spoon-feeding were given up spontaneously and new aspects appeared in his relationship with his favorite counselor. Formerly he could maintain contact with her only as his expectations of immediate and tangible gratification were fulfilled. Now the relationship to her became time-structured. His helplessness, the primitivity and urgency of his needs made him desire the permanency of her support. While walking close to her he said, "I am going to hang on to your arm for the rest of my life." It took a whole year for him to develop a feeling of closeness to two adults, his counselor and his teacher. With the rest of the staff, he got along without conflict since he recognized that they served useful functions.

The relative freedom in the therapeutic milieu remained unacceptable to this boy so long as he lacked inner control and the ability for self-regulation. For many months after entering, he complained that the School was not strict enough. Everyone, including himself, was being too spoiled. He praised the disciplinarian spirit of the orphanage from which he had come. In this way, he expressed the fear of his own as yet unintegrated impulses which at the School were no longer controlled completely by outside rules.

In his eating habits, he experimented with gratification and control of primitive impulses. In addition, through these eating habits he tested the attitudes of the significant figures of his new environment toward his needs.

The boy, who had been well fed and of normal weight upon admission to the Orthogenic School, began to overeat, to suck his thumb, and complain that the staff tried to starve him. Gratification of primitive needs alone gave him a sense of security and means of emotional expression. In eating he also found compensation for the barrenness of his existence, which had to remain limited so long as he could not avail himself of the opportunities for satisfaction offered in the therapeutic milieu. He either insisted that the adults force him to eat, or he ate incessantly. Awareness of his lack of inner control and judgment made it necessary for him to have his devouring tendencies constantly permitted and regulated by others.

He had to check up on the food supplies in kitchen and store rooms to make sure that he could expect continued gratification. This evidence had to be tangible. When he noticed once that the milk supply was lower than usual, his doubts could not be dispelled by verbal assurance; he had to wait around until the milk was delivered.

After he had overcome his starvation fear, he became secure enough to regress once more, and actually recapitulated to the feeding of an infant. He had the courage to discover a baby bottle with nipple which had been on the kitchen shelf since his arrival, and said, "What about that bottle?" When asked, "What about it?" he answered, "I thought I might put some milk in it." He was not prevented from doing it; he used the nipple, then discarded it, but persisted for several days in drinking out of the bottle. Then he began to suck milk out of bottles through straws and for a long time carried a milk bottle around in school and on the playground.

For nearly a year his incorporative needs had been met unconditionally in quantity and form of gratification, before he showed spontaneous attempts to control his gluttony. He began to show some discrimination with regard to food, then he refused second servings, often of dishes he liked best. With self-imposed limitations, his wish for adult control of his eating disappeared. He had begun to have mastery over his primitive desires.

Certainty of unconditional gratification by others and his trust in his ability to master his impulses had to be firmly established before he showed awareness of the needs of others, which is essential in establishing any true interpersonal relationship. Such awareness first centered around eating, the function of such great importance to him. He began to arrange tea parties in which he himself prepared and served all the food. He showed great concern that everybody should have enough to eat. These parties were at first limited to his favorite counselor, the person who for a long time had satisfied all his desires. Then he stopped grabbing food from the plates of the other children and gradually included them in his parties.

Since there had never been any pressure on his table manners, the spontaneous changes in this area are significant indications of his inner changes. His greed, his noisy smacking and sucking, gave way to the eating habits of a normal child. Thumb sucking was relinquished for the socially more acceptable chewing of gum. Personality changes paralleled this process of arriving at mastery of primitive needs through their unconditional gratification. While initially his time was spent mostly in daydreaming, he gradually began to participate in active sports, learned to swim and play baseball and showed pleasure in these achievements.

After two months at the School, his artistic ability spontaneously came to light. His first artistic productions had a bizarre quality and were mainly elaborations of death and cemeteries. While he had up to then continuously disturbed the classroom by hyperactivity, noisiness, and frequent temper tantrums, he now began to isolate himself in painting when the pressure became too great. This temporary and self-chosen isolation was permitted. It made his classroom experience more acceptable to him and to the others. The topic of his drawings changed; while he still needed occasional retreat from the classroom situation, he no longer drew cemeteries but maintained some contact with the class by elaborating on the topics of the moment by painting farmers in the field, Indians, and animals in an aquarium.

His painting lost none of its imaginative and creative qualities. He derived much personal prestige when the principal asked him for one of his paintings for his office; and on the next day he offered paintings to others, indicating that he had accepted the status they were ready to give him. He began to show interest in his clothes and accepted his counselor's suggestion to select them personally. In the store, he showed fear of this personal responsibility which had been delegated to him, but immediately utilized the experience of being respected as an individual. During this shopping expedition he talked about his fears for the first time and told his counselor that he often asked her to sit on his bed at night because he worried about death at that time.

Gratification of primitive needs had made possible the emergence of sublimation. He was permitted to use his artistic talent to master the classroom situation. He received prestige and praise for his painting. These freed his intellectual abilities, and in ten months he made academic progress equivalent to fourteen months.

The inability to connect present action, past experience, and future expectation led to many instances of confused and explosive behavior because regular repetition of routine at the orphanage had made the boy's life an "empty" continuum. In the absence of meaningful experiences, his existence had not been structured into past, present, and future.

Maturation as a historical process can proceed only if the child's life experience is structured in the dimension of time. Although in the therapeutic milieu children are not overwhelmed with too many activities, still the boy complained that there was too much to do. Holidays are made enjoyable in a casual way, to avoid over-excitement. Instead, small everyday activities are made carriers of interpersonal relationships. Although he did not yet know what made one day different from another and was still unable to react to the events that structure everyday life, he responded to the major event of Easter. He accepted the present and took part in the egg hunt. He was cautious and not too enthusiastic, but for the first time expressed concern about a future event: he wondered about Christmas and asked whether it would be possible for him to participate in its celebration and what it would be like. He could already envisage an event in the future but was able to tolerate it only on the assumption that it would be similar to the experience in the present which he could accept. He wanted to be sure it would not necessitate new adjustments.

Hallowe'en he enjoyed tremendously. He now took the sources of pleasure in his present existence for granted. On Thanksgiving Day he complained that while living in the orphanage, he had had no fun on holidays. He was now able to appraise his present life in terms of his past, and said, "This is my first real Thanksgiving." He went on to complain that at the orphanage the children "never did anything." They just had a meal like any other day. Then he reminisced about Hallowe'en. His story was rather jumbled but he had begun to see his life in the therapeutic milieu as a sequence of meaningful and variegated events which he had the courage to face. He looked forward to Christmas as a new "different" holiday. Structuralization of his existence into present, future, and past was taking shape.

In the service of mastery of the new situation, all mechanisms that had proven their adequacy were activated. New clothes had begun to give him security through prestige. Accordingly, on Christmas morning, he was the only boy who took great care to dress in his best outfit. His tolerance at seeing others receive gratification and the ability to postpone his own gratifications, were recent acquisitions. His behavior was in line with them. He went to the fireplace where the stockings were hanging, and instead of grabbing his presents, he insisted on telling the other children about what he found in his stocking and admiring what they found in theirs. Then he very slowly repacked all the presents in his stocking. It seemed to the adults that he had not noticed a sled and some other presents and they pointed these out to him. He replied harshly and ran out of the room, muttering to himself, "This is enough. I cannot stand more of this." Later, in the afternoon, he unpacked some of his toys and started to play with them.

In a previous step of his rehabilitation, unconditional gratification of his seemingly boundless needs had been therapeutically indicated. This permitted recapitulation and gratification of infantile expectations and established the basis for personality growth. Once he had learned that food is always made available and that presents do not disappear, he could make a further step. His new capacity to permit himself gratification was a new achievement. It represented ego growth even if guilt about receiving it may have prompted him to postpone gratification.

Therapeutic response from the adult had to be in line with the status of his ego development. Because he was not forced to deal with his gifts according to conventional adult expectations of gratitude, he was really able to enjoy the gifts — in his own time. Thus the adults' respect for the patient's self-set limitations again represented unconditional recognition of his autonomous tendencies. Through such attitudes of the adult, the boy derived a sense of personal integrity from incidents in his everyday life. This modified his conception of himself and established self-esteem. He became able to face the "bad" past and also developed trust in a benign and manageable future, while he took his present existence for granted.[2] Two successive dreams which he spontaneously related to his counselor illustrate this.

In the first dream, he was king of the universe, Superman. He had a million dollars and ruled everyone. In the second dream, he went to visit the orphanage. He was in the pool (where the older children had thrown him into the water and never given him a chance to learn to swim). He showed them how well he was able to swim and dive. All the children sat around the pool and admired him and liked him very much.

The first dream shows how he attempted to compensate for his lack of personal status in the orphanage by ideas of omnipotence. In the second dream, his recently acquired real achievements, swimming and diving, give him prestige among those with whom he used to have none. Thus the new strength permitted him a more assuring perspective on past and future. While the past had been bad, a similar situation would not again find him helpless.

[2] It should be mentioned that in children whose past experiences have been less malignant, the same process leads to the emergence in memory of the positive factors in their past lives.

He learned to see his past in a light which no longer overwhelmed him. Trust in his ability to master situations which once had over-powered him made his outlook of the future realistic and therefore more optimistic. A similar change occurred in his daydreams: instead of being a great dictator and Superman, he now daydreamed about becoming a street car conductor after having lived in a nice foster home for quite a while.

During the year of his stay at the School, the boy made significant steps in personality growth. Environmental attitudes which made such development possible were to him personified in the first counselor who had gratified his dependent needs, permitted him defensive activity, and mediated between him and the outside world whenever he needed such help. As he experienced the implications of interpersonal relation-ships in his contacts with her, his total human environment began to take on shape and structure.

When he came to the School, all he knew about people was that there are small children, and big children who tell the small ones what to do. Human interaction was a matter of domination through strength or material possessions. For a long time, contact with other children con-sisted in forceful attempts to take their toys. This behavior was dented when, on St. Valentine's Day, he unexpectedly received valentines from some of the other children. He was happy that he should have made friends. Gradually, he became able to share his toys occasionally, and there was a lessening of the inner struggle which first arose with such performance.

He was surprised that he had found a new *modus vivendi* with other children and searched for an explanation of their kindness. He came to the conclusion that "the children here act right because the grownups treat them right." This was his first recognition of a benign hierarchy of human inter-relations. Such awareness was possible only because he had experienced it explicitly in his contacts with the counselor.

Since he was no longer isolated, the slowness and blocking dis-appeared which had been equivalents for depressive reactions. The desire and ability to communicate gave new meaning to his artistic creations; he discovered spontaneously that personal ties were the source of his new strength. He told the psychiatrist that he had much more energy now and explained, "Before, I thought that I could get energy and strength from food only; now I know that I get energy from other children, counselors, baseball, swimming, and drawing, that is, if I make a picture for somebody."

In a later interview, about one year after admission to the School, he expressed his contentment in a fictitious telephone conversation. As the chairman of the board of directors, he called the School's principal to check up and offer help. He asked, "What do you need for your children? Candy, paper, paint, crayons, nothing? They know you have all they need? That is good. Good bye."

He became eager to understand the relationship of grownups to one another, since he now knew what adults have to offer children and what children may mean to each other. Their relationships were no longer empty or overwhelming and threatening, and he could therefore accept them. He stated with great pride that he now knew what grownups were — they "act like ladies and gentlemen. They go to college, they care for children, they like children. I will be a grownup too someday, but not for a long time." He had acquired a well defined reference frame and can be expected to proceed further in growth.

Case 2: [3] This case, like the first, is also characterized by a child's desperate effort to cope with an unbearable reality. The outward signs of this struggle for mastery were hyperactivity, destructiveness and stealing, severe inhibition of intellectual functioning, and extreme suspiciousness. These symptoms appeared first when Mary was six years old. She had been transferred to a foster home from the nursery where she had lived after her parents had deserted her at the age of three. While at the nursery, she had not presented any manifest problems, but in the foster homes her behavior became progressively more difficult and led to many changes in homes until she came to the Orthogenic School at the age of nine. Her disturbed actions were only the surface ripples of her megalomaniac fantasies, evidence of the unavoidable clashes between external demands which she could not fulfill, and her magic world to which she could no longer successfully retreat.

Psychiatric study before admission to the School showed that she was quite detached from the many adults and children with whom she had lived. She was utterly confused about their identity. Physiological activities like eating and sleeping were not gratifying experiences, but duties imposed by rules or the wishes of others. She hardly knew what playing meant. She said, "Where I live, there is a doll buggy, but I must not touch it." She explained, "Once I was a baby, but I was never wheeled in a buggy."

When asked where she lived, she answered, "In a place where you get clean clothes after playing. Then you take a nap and eat sometimes." She was unable to name any of the children or adults in the orphanage. When asked whether she had a friend, she said, "They tell me that John is my friend." When asked who took care of her, she replied, "A nurse, that is a lady, any lady."

A large segment of her life was spent in <u>autistic fantasy</u>. She said

[3] Credit for most of the direct work in rehabilitating this girl is due to Miss Marjorie Jewell and Miss Joan Little.

that she was a good girl because she did not bother anybody. Nothing bothered her either since she, and everything around her, was magic. She only had to open her window, say goodbye to the children, then she could fly to God who was nice always.

A few days after admission Mary said she liked the School. "It is like in the nursery before, but it is better, because it is all in one. The school is just here and not five blocks away." Through simplification in denial of any difference, distance, or discrepancy between the constituents of her outside world, she reduced her new environment to manageable proportion. In the foster homes she had had to protect herself from being overwhelmed by the multitude of external events, since the empty existence of her early years had not equipped her to deal with them adequately. But the autistic mechanisms which she applied did not help her to master the persistent demands of reality; when she attempted to withdraw more deeply, her inadequacy only increased and anxiety resulted. Her confusion which led to constant misinterpretations and contaminations seemed to reduce her intellectual functioning to a near feebleminded level.

In the School her need to avoid anxiety determined the nature of her initial adjustment. This need was met as her spontaneous methods of mastery remained unchallenged by external pressure. At that stage, the existence of actual sources of satisfaction and stimulation in the therapeutic milieu was of value for her only because she was not forced to combat external pressure. Still, the presence of such factors was essential from the beginning for her rehabilitation. They had to be available when she was ready to take advantage of them. Opportunity for stimulation and gratification distinguished the therapeutic milieu from the barrenness of nursery life which had led to impoverishment of her personality, while freedom from the pressure which had made her foster home experiences so deleterious, precluded necessity for further confusion and withdrawal.

Since she could not, *a priori*, expect conditions in the external world to be different from her past experiences, she had to apply her old mechanisms of mastery in the new environment. Her courage to explore reality had first been severely curtailed by lack of stimulation in the orphanage, and later by her experiences in foster homes. Protective withdrawal into a world of all-powerful magic was therefore maintained at the School until she developed sufficient confidence in herself and trust in others gradually to modify her defenses.

Mary had not learned to live without magic protection, and now met benign, relatively powerful figures. In proportion to the abject degree of her helplessness, she needed protective figures of such strength as could only be furnished by endowing them with magic powers. Under the aegis of these figures, she could venture forth to test reality with greater comfort and security. Thus, in a way, she tried to establish magic contact with what seemed to her the most important figures in her new environment, the principal and the psychiatrist. In order to be able to retain them as "magic" figures, all realistic contact with them had to be avoided, and they had to be both depersonalized and unified. To do so was also in line with her past efforts to organize her world by recognizing persons only as carriers of useful or dangerous functions. This tendency she demonstrated by depriving the two figures, the principal and the psychiatrist, of the only personal characteristics of which she was aware, their names. She contaminated them into "Dr. Bettelster." Whenever she used this contamination, it designated both of them in the magic and protective functions she assigned to them. She refused to recognize them as persons and avoided personal contact. Because she rebuffed their efforts, contact was discontinued.

She began to approach the principal about one of his functions with which she had become familiar — his role as mediator. She established a routine of complaining to him, remaining aloof at the same time. She did this in line with her magic expectations, and not in terms of a realistic interpretation of his function. She invariably expected him to take her side, protect her, and punish the others. The fact that she received protection only when she needed it, and that other children were not reprimanded just because she complained about them, did not change her conviction of his role as her special protector. When other children expressed fear about events which were beyond control, she reassured them with the statement, "It cannot happen here because of Dr. Bettelster." Gradually, after she had established personalized contacts with her favorite counselor, she separated the psychiatrist from the principal, still adhering to the conviction of their inherent identity: she then called the one Dr. Bester and the other Dr. Vester. Much later, after she had finally found true security in the relationship to her counselor, it became possible for her to divest them of some of their presumed magic characteristics, to accept them tentatively as real, and recognize them as two different persons with different names.

Under the magic protection of the most powerful figures that she had created for herself, she was able to explore segments of reality and to approach a relationship with her counselor. In the meantime, the other children had to remain anonymous and unreal because to acknowledge their presence would have interfered with her need to claim her counselor for herself.

Gratification of her most urgent needs became the basis for her human contacts. For many months she over-ate, staying in the dining room after the others had left and scavenging for food in spite of the large helpings she had already eaten. After every meal, she wrapped food in a napkin to take with her for fear she might be hungry before the next meal. Whenever a course was put on the table, she jumped up excitedly and looked at her counselor for reassurance that she would get more food. Frequently she ate directly from the plate without utensils in order to finish in time for a third and fourth helping. No limitations were put on her needs. After a month she required fewer helpings of food. Now her eating habits did not reflect greed but became distinctly babyish. She sucked her food and occasionally spat it out. Then she started to carry a small jar with her in which she kept a ration of candy. Her eating habits changed only after she had formed individualized relations to her counselor and to some of the children.

She did not tolerate any closeness and had to be permitted to "float around" in School for some time. Out of the confused anonymity of her existence, familiarity with carriers of useful functions emerged slowly.

Children remained anonymous to her much longer than adults. A friend was a child who was "bigger and can beat you up; you go to her bed." But she was hardly able to distinguish one child from another. To her, they were nameless and existed only if tangibly present. She spoke to them as "that girl," and the only way she called to them was "Hey, you."

On a walk with a counselor, two of the other children ran ahead and were out of sight for a few minutes. When the rest of the group caught up with them, she said without any sign of being perturbed, "Oh there they are. I thought they were dead."

When she began to individualize the children, it was in terms of their attitudes toward the counselor to whom she had become very attached. She consistently expressed her dislike for some children who called this counselor names. In her first attempts to make friends, she adopted toward other children those attitudes which she expected from her counselor in fantasy, and had to be restrained from giving away all of her possessions. Her tendency to concede to any demand made by other children was inappropriate and had to be modified.

Confusion had been the outcome of her attempts to orient herself toward people around her. Similar disorientation showed her helplessness in other areas. Since she had lived in many parts of the city without sufficient awareness of reality ever to find her way about, she was utterly lost in the neighborhood of the School. She showed pseudologic attitudes when she claimed to know every person and every building, in attempting to compensate for her overwhelming ignorance by such confabulation about persons and places. She claimed to recognize old acquaintances and insisted that she had lived on that or the other street. Isolated actual recollections appeared later and then in connection with functions and activities she had begun to master at the School.

Conventional concepts of time meant nothing to her and she manipulated time purely in terms of her own needs and tensions. On July 10th, she recalled that her birthday had been on "June two and three" (June 23rd). This meant to her that her next birthday would be "in two or three days." Whenever she acquired any valid and usable knowledge, she used it compulsively to orient herself. When she was already sufficiently settled at the School to wish to remain, reassurance that she could stay as long as she wanted was insufficient. She had to orient herself by applying the terms of the seasons she had just learned about in class, and asked repeatedly: "Will I be here in the summer? Will I be here in the winter?" repeating the seasons many times. In this way, she sifted her new knowledge in terms of its value for the reassurance she needed. Facts were accepted and retained only after she had tested their usefulness for her immediate needs.

When she first began to experience activities and events in the external world as more gratifying than complete immersion in fantasy, she could not stand the tension of any delay in the succession of external occurrences. If she wanted to buy something, she could not accept the fact that stores were closed in the evening. She could not stand any moment without activity and continuously asked: "What are we going to do now?" Before an answer could be given, she had already wandered to some other subject and she was unable to comprehend what was said to her.

The same pressure appeared in her manner of talking. While she had been quiet and uncommunicative when she first came to the School, with turning to reality, her speech became rapid and explosive. She deleted syllables and ran words together, so that her talk was difficult to understand. Of this, she was initially unaware. Then she became frustrated about her inability to express herself. Her sentences became even less comprehensible as she now interspersed them with recurring exclamations of disgust. She finally realized this when she stopped herself in the middle of a sentence, looked apologetically at the counselor and said, "I can't even speak the English language. I can never say what I want to."

A process of gradual organization started in and around her daily contacts with her special counselor. At first her counselor was a nameless one of many. Her appreciation was unspecific as to source and form of gratification. She said, "I like them, they are good to you." A few weeks later, she dimly recalled her counselor's name; but she still could describe her life at the School only in a stereotyped enumeration of activities which were related solely to herself, such as eating, bathing, going to bed. She mentioned other children only in terms of their interference or non-interference with these activities.

After about a month, contacts with the counselor centered around such simple activities as Mary initiated herself. She demanded to be carried, to be cuddled and fed. When she saw the counselor after a short absence, she shouted, "I love you," hugged her and playfully bit her. Her attitude then did not yet express the interpersonal relationship of a nine-year-old, but was the possessive clinging of an infant.

After about six months, her haunted, sober expression occasionally gave way to real smiling at her counselor. In these moments, she seemed to be in contact, her voice was natural, she finished her sentences and could be reached by the counselor's reply.

It was then, in her contacts with the counselor that she energetically and actively went about the task of getting order into her immediate world. Temporarily her activities assumed a compulsive character. She was first concerned with the order of things around her and started her new activity around eating situations. She cleaned her candy box repeatedly, stacked candy bars according to color and size, counted them and said spontaneously, "This is fun." Then she cleaned her shelves vigorously, arranged and rearranged her toys and wanted her clothes laid out exactly and neatly for the next morning. Her bed had to be perfect and she liked to sweep the floor around it and even underneath. It was as if orderliness in objects related to her had to precede inner order.

Her counselor made some comment about the amount of cleaning she did and she replied that she liked to clean, and added, "Then when I grow up," and stopped. When asked to go on, she said, "Well, it was silly and I know it is not true, but I thought that I would have all my cleaning-up done by the time I grow up." Thus she experimented with her ability to comprehend and master the objects around her in their relation to each other and to herself. In this experimentation with external order, she achieved mastery over one sector of the outside world. As she became able to internalize this achievement, she made her first steps in integration.

It should be kept in mind that her activity emerged spontaneously within the setting of her contacts with the counselor in which, within a reference frame of predictable and maintained interest, she had already experienced not only order, but also unconditional gratification.

Conclusions. The aim of any psychotherapeutic procedure is to help the patient toward adequate mastery over inner and outer forces.

The importance which milieu factors have for causing emotional disturbances in childhood is well established. It is also realized that manipulation of milieu factors can be used toward the rehabilitation of emotionally disturbed children.

In direct psychotherapy of children, recognition is given to the fact that shaping the individual's biological needs in the earliest years is of decisive importance for later personality structures as well as for prognostic considerations. When distorted growth processes can be recapitulated within the benign setting of the psychotherapeutic relationship, symptoms become unnecessary, personality structure changes, growth phenomena appear, and psychotherapy can be considered successful.

Similarly, emotionally disturbed children can be helped through living in a milieu which is aware of the factors that promote restoration of function growth, and new integration. The two children described improved in the particular therapeutic milieu because there insight was translated into uninterrupted action extending over twenty-four hours a day. The children showed improvement because they lived in an environment which, from the start, provided them with a stable frame of reference. While the adults maintained the interpersonal hierarchy in all their dealings with the children, their actions always remained spontaneous within the indications set by the psychological reality of the individual child. This was the spirit in which every child received such gratification as his instinctual and defensive needs dictated at any given moment.

The use of the continuously maintained one-to-one relationship within a therapeutic milieu as one of the many aspects of milieu-psychotherapy is stressed.

43

CLINICAL OBSERVATIONS ON THE EMOTIONAL LIFE OF CHILDREN IN THE COMMUNAL SETTLEMENTS IN ISRAEL

GERALD CAPLAN

School of Public Health, Harvard University

The communal settlements in Israel are socialistic aggregations of people. They have been in existence about twenty to twenty-five years, and are composed of individuals who, because of ideological reasons, have decided to live together and to eschew the capitalist principle of private property. They live together in groups of from 200 to 1,000 adults, mainly in agricultural areas which were originally barren. The settlement and all its property is owned communally, and nothing belongs to the private individual. The organization of the commune resembles that of an early Greek democracy: Government is by decision of the plenary session of all the members, which delegates authority to elected committees and there is no single leader. Each committee has an elected chairman, who serves a term of office and then moves on to some other job. The men and women are members on equal terms, and work on equal terms, although the heavier work in the fields is usually done by the men. Both men and women work in agriculture, and in housework.

This interesting social experiment has a complicated background, the discussion of which is not relevant to our topic of today. Very briefly, it arose out of the Zionist socialist movement, the goal of which was the return of the Jewish people to Palestine to form a national home, and to found what eventually became the State of Israel. Most of the settlers came from eastern European bourgeois families, and chief among their ideals was the "return to the soil."

However, the reason they founded these settlements was only partly based on socialist ideology. It was also partly a reaction to economic necessity, and it was a very practical arrangement for poor immigrants, who had to settle in barren areas often surrounded by hostile Arab forces. It was a program of uniting in order to accomplish a dif-

From *Problems of Infancy and Childhood*, ed. M. J. E. Senn, New York: Josiah Macy Jr. Foundation, 19.

ficult job of work. When they started, most of these settlements were extremely poor, but in the last 20 years many of them have gradually become rich. The movement, at the present time, is rapidly altering many details of the organizational framework, especially with regard to the changes in the country as a whole which followed the establishment of the State of Israel in 1948.

The original settlers were, on the whole, highly selected people. They were called "pioneers," and have well deserved this name since they have formed the real backbone of the Jewish return to Israel. Until recently, they represented the hero stereotype of the nation. This has begun to change, and I shall say a word or two about that later on.

What interests us here, and links with Dr. Bowlby's earlier discussion, is that in these settlements the children are taken care of communally from birth, and the family as the central unit of society is quite designedly set aside. The reasons for this were many, prominent among them being the fact that most of the first settlers were in their early twenties, and in coming to the new land they were revolting not only against the bourgeois life of their parents in eastern Europe, but also against their parents personally. They were very conscious of their own emotional shortcomings, and they ascribed these to the defective upbringing they had experienced from their parents. In other words, they had a pretty low opinion of parents as child rearers.

In planning their new way of life, they decided that when their own children came along they would give them the benefit of the latest advances of modern psychology. They would engage professional well-trained workers to take care of them, and not leave matters to chance by allowing them to be brought up by the biological parents who had so little knowledge of child rearing, and who also had so little time to devote to children, in this hard-working communal life.

In addition there was another reason, of a deeper sociological kind. In order to perpetuate their system of communal living, they felt they had to move the family out of the center of the stage in order to avoid the identification of children with their parents in regard to life interests and occupational choice. In other words, the children had to be brought up to accept more readily the ideals of the commune rather than the ideals of the individual parents.

I am not too sure how conscious of this factor the early settlers were in their planning, but certainly when we look at the communal settlements today it is obvious that, from a sociological point of view, one of their greatest strengths in perpetuating themselves lies in the fact that the grown-up children identify with group values rather than with the values of their families. Usually when there is a conflict between the interests of the group and those of the family, the children brought up in this way will support the group.

The majority are born in hospitals outside the communal settlement. There is no rooming-in in these hospitals, so right from birth they are separated from their mothers. When they return to the settlement, the infants are housed in the communal nursery, and from then on the child is housed separately. For the first year he lives in the communal nursery; he then moves to the communal toddler house where he stays until the age of three. After that he moves to the kindergarten house, and later to the schoolhouse.

Walser: There is no breast feeding, either?

Caplan: Breast-feeding is neither encouraged nor discouraged. I wish to emphasize, however, that there is considerable variation in regard to child-rearing practices in the different settlements, and what I am presenting here is an average pattern of the details.

Israel is a country of very rapid growth, and there is a tendency for pendulum swings in regard to slogans. I hesitate to compare it with this country, but in certain respects it is not dissimilar. That is to say, during one year breast-feeding might be fashionable, the next year feeding from a bottle might be the vogue, and the following year the fashion might swing to feeding from a cup. It depends on which expert has been on a lecture tour at that time!

The infants from birth to one year are taken care of in groups of five or six by one trained worker, and then, between one and three, two groups coalesce so that one worker has ten or twelve children under her care. From three onwards, there is usually one adult for about fifteen children.

The mothers have a vacation for the first six weeks after delivery before returning to work. They do not care for their children, but they come into the nursery to feed them, whether by breast, bottle, or cup and spoon. The feeding takes place in groups: that is to say, the five women come in and nurse their children together in the same room. During these times the fathers often come in, too. The usual rule is that the babies should not be visited at other than feeding times, but since the mothers are not working and have nothing else to do, they often manage to break this rule during the first six weeks.

At the end of this period the mother returns to work, and she is given time off to feed the baby, either by breast or formula, until the baby is four or five months old. After that the feeding is taken over by the professional workers in the nursery. From this time on, the parents visit their children for only about two hours at the end of their day's work, and for longer periods at weekends. When the parents visit, they often bring the child's siblings along with them, having picked them up from the kindergarten or schoolhouse. This is interfered with by quarantines for infectious diseases: especially polio, which is becoming a serious problem in Israel. Because of this the baby houses are often closed to siblings for months at a time.

As the child grows older, the parents begin to take him for little walks in the settlement during the two-hour visiting period, and they often take him to their own room for a visit. Gradually this habit of taking him back to the parents' room increases. Formal contact between parents and children is limited to this period, although in the smaller settlements, when the children are old enough to roam about, they are able to see their parents going about their work. All the practical care of the child, such as feeding, habit training, etc., is in the hands of the professional women workers, some of them with children of their own, who have expressed interest in this work. Many of them are volunteers, though not all.

All of the jobs in the communal settlements are deputed. A Work Committee delegates the jobs to the different members, and the latter accept the work because of their allegiance to the group. The baby nurses, who care for the infants up to one year, usually are given about a year's training, or even more in certain cases. The people who take care of the toddlers usually have much less training: perhaps a short course of a few months, with one or two weeks of refresher courses every year or so.

You can see that although the early settlers decided that their children would be brought up by highly-trained professional workers, the exigencies of the situation — the shortage of money and training facilities — have resulted in few highly-trained workers, apart from exceptional cases.

Trainham: You said that some of the child care workers volunteer; others are assigned. Is some screening method employed to assist in placing workers where they can function most effectively in meeting the children's needs, and also their own?

Caplan: No. It is done in a quite haphazard way.

Baumgartner: Once trained, do they stay in that work, or are they sometimes called out later to do agricultural work, or something else?

Caplan: There may be a tour of duty: some move out of it into other aspects of the commune's activity, and some carry on in this work for years.

Wolf: Is there any possibility that the mother would be such a professional worker; that is, is it possible that somebody is chosen as a professional worker who then would take care of her own child in a group of additional children?

Caplan: That happens, but very rarely. Usually if she is a child care worker, she takes care of other children. They do not like to have a mother taking care of her own child.

Escalona: Do the children think of themselves as so-and-so's child, or are they merely identified by their own names, with relatively little emphasis on who their parents are?

Caplan: They are all called by their first names, but in regard to their feelings about their family, I should like to take that up later when I discuss the emotional life of the children.

Fremont-Smith: Do they sleep in the nursery or child house? You said as they begin to walk they go more and more to the parents' rooms.

Caplan: Only during the visiting period.

Fremont-Smith: They always go back?

Caplan: Yes, they live separately from their parents all their lives.

Fremont-Smith: So there never is a family other than husband and wife, in our cultural sense?

Caplan: I have been describing the original situation, which was almost universal in these settlements until some ten years ago. We have a generation of children who were brought up in this manner. In the last few years, however, the social pattern has begun to change, and in some settlements it has been moving more and more from this pattern toward the encroachment of family interests and family values.

Baumgartner: How much continuity is there in the care of one baby with a professional worker? Does the same worker tend to stay with her group? If they are sent out on a tour of duty, when does that interruption take place?

Caplan: There is an interruption at one year, and at three years. At one year the child is moved away from the infant house worker to the toddler house staff, and at three years to the kindergarten house with its staff. There may or may not be interruptions in between these times, according to whether individual workers change their jobs. It is not considered desirable to change workers between times.

Benjamin: Did the professional organization, as originally set up twenty-five years ago, keep records on the behavior of mothers and children, and on all these variations which you implied when you said you were giving us an average?

Caplan: There are very good historical records, in most of these settlements, with regard to organizational matters. They were directed by committees, which kept minutes of their meetings. Little details of organization were often argued for days. However, it is rare to find any worth-while records of the behavior of the children.

I should say here that my knowledge of this subject is derived from four years' residence in Israel. During my first year, I was advisor in

Mental Health to the Government, and I travelled widely in the country, visiting many of the settlements, or Kibbutzim. The Hebrew word for communal settlement is "Kibbutz"; the plural, "Kibbutzim."

During the last three years, I was in charge of a mental hygiene organization which worked in the Kibbutzim, but not with the Kibbutz children. We were responsible for supervising the mental health of immigrant children, many of whom were cared for in the Kibbutzim. Our workers went into most of the settlements in the country, and as part of our work we felt we had to study the general cultural milieu of the Kibbutz, but this was not a specific research project. We did make one systematic, but rather small, survey of their child-rearing practices, of which you will find a very good account in *Human Relations* (1). The article is by Elizabeth Irvine, one of our casework supervisors, who wrote it primarily for Dr. Bowlby's World Health Organization survey.

Parks: What is the usual attitude of the mothers toward pregnancy and childbirth?

Caplan: Here again there has often been a conflict between the interests of the family and the natural instincts of the mother on the one hand, and the interests of the group on the other. When the settlement is new and poor, they cannot afford children because they insist on providing them with proper facilities. Even in young Kibbutzim the children's houses are built of brick or stone, and cost a lot of money. They contrast with the dwellings of the adults which are often tents or wooden shacks. Children therefore involve the investment of a good deal of capital for the settlement, so pressure is brought to bear on the individual families not to have children until the group can afford them. In the newer Kibbutzim there is a sort of rationing system in regard to the number of families who are allowed children, and most of them abide by the rules. There have been cases of settlers who have defied the group in this connection: for instance, a friend of mind had five children, and she is known throughout the settlement movement as a very naughty person!

Parks: What type of medical care do they receive? What about anesthesia and analgesia? Are the mothers completely narcotized at the time of delivery?

Caplan: It depends on the individual hospital. On the whole, in Israel, there is no anesthesia, and little analgesia, during delivery, but I doubt whether you would call it natural childbirth.

Walser: How far away from the settlements is the hospital?

Caplan: Usually not more than from two to four hours' journey.

Walser: Do they go there ahead of time and wait?

Caplan: No, they usually go when they are in labor.

Walser: Do they walk?

Caplan: No, they go in an ambulance, or by car. All of these settlements have means of transportation.

Butler: What importance does the commune attach to the job of rearing children? Do they say: This is a very important job; hence we assign very competent people, or do they consider it to be a minor job, which may be handled by less competent people?

Caplan: It is regarded as one of the most important jobs in the commune. The reason that the workers are sometimes poorly trained is not because of a lack of appreciation of the importance of the work; it is just that training facilities are not available. Whenever it is possible to provide better training, they do so.

Baumgartner: Do they regard children as a potential source of economic strength in the commune? In a country that needs agricultural workers, as I assume Israel does, one might expect that they would try to increase the population, and yet you say they are very strict about limiting the number of children.

Caplan: It is because they are so very poor. They certainly do not regard children as only a source of economic strength; they are more interested in perpetuating their idealistic way of life, and increasing their political strength.

McLendon: How do the mortality and morbidity rates compare with other countries?

Caplan: I have no definite figures on that, but offhand I would say that they compare favorably with those of Australia, which is pretty good. I think I should warn you not to be prejudiced by looking at this culture pattern with preconceived ideas although I know it is very difficult not to be prejudiced. Let us try to realize that we are prone to bias in regard to this subject. As I listen to myself talking today, I realize that I, too, am prejudiced.

Washburn: Isn't it true that in the Kibbutzim there was originally a high level of education and intelligence, which is a little different from some of the cruder rural experiments?

Caplan: The adult founders of the Kibbutzim on the whole belong to an extremely high intellectual class. It is not unusual to go into their fields and find professors, and even physicians, doing agricultural work. I say "even physicians," not because a physician has a higher status than a professor, but because physicians should be practicing medicine. Some physicians in the Kibbutzim are raising chickens and tilling the soil because they feel that the return of the Jews to the soil is a great ideal. They feel that Jews have for too long been professional people and middle men. They want to turn the clock back and make a fresh start. Especially in the smaller settlements there is quite an active intellectual cultural life, with talks and debates. Some of these little places out in the wilds have excellent record collections of classical music.

I should now like to talk a bit about our observations of the emotional life of the children brought up as I have described in these settlements, and I shall also say a little about the effect of this life on their parents. So far, there has been no valid scientific investigation carried out on the emotional life of the Kibbutz children, and what I am going to say is based on the clinical impressions of my colleagues and myself, while visiting the settlements. It is also based on our experience as mental health consultants to one of the big groups of Kibbutzim in relation to their emotionally disturbed children. They brought their problem children to us for investigation and advice over a period of three years, and we got a good deal of information that way. We have had a few Kibbutz children in psychotherapy, but not very many. I fancy that the psychoanalysts in Israel have analyzed a number of children who have grown up in the Kibbutzim, but I have not been able to obtain any consensus of opinion of their findings, and I do not think they have published any relevant material.

Of course the main thing that interests me, and probably all of us, is what the effect on the emotional life of the children has been, during the partial separation from parents which characterizes their upbringing. It is almost of the same order as in children brought up in institutions, where frequent visiting is permitted. Does it pervert their personality development?

These are our findings: Children below the age of from about five to seven, and particularly the toddlers, manifest symptoms which, in our Western culture, we would feel to be signs of emotional disturbance. There is a tremendous amount of thumb sucking, temper tantrums, and general lack of control over aggression — much more so than among children raised in families. Enuresis is endemic. We did a study of children in their fifth year, and we found that in Kibbutzim in different parts of the country, the average incidence of enuresis was from 30 to 50 per cent.

When you observe the young children, especially the toddlers, they look like deprived children in institutions. Because of the shortage of workers, the toddlers spend a lot of time during the day on their own. They are kept in enclosures with wire netting around them and with very few toys, because if they had toys they would harm each other with them. They are quite aggressive to each other. When a visitor comes to the edge of one of these enclosures, the children all throng to that side; lay visitors find this behavior entrancing, and go away talking about the beautiful friendly children of the Kibbutzim. However, to me this experience was only too much like the feeling one has when one walks into a long-stay children's institution. The children in Israel, up to the age of five or six, look puny and small despite the fact that they get a pretty good diet. When the adults in the settlement are practically starving, they still make sure that the children are well fed. Whenever I have seen them my impression has always been that they are suffering from some kind of low grade upper respiratory, or naso-pharyngeal infection, since there is so much evidence of running noses, coughing, and so on.

Trainham: Do they actually ingest a good diet? Is the apparent poor nutrition the result of faulty metabolism, or of food refusal?

Caplan: I do not know. I think there is considerable difficulty in feeding certain children, but I feel that on the whole they eat reasonably well.

From what I have said so far, you can see that up to the age of about six the Kibbutz children look as though they are suffering from maternal deprivation. But — and this is the very interesting thing — when they get above that age, the incidence of signs of disturbance falls, and it falls more and more rapidly as the children approach adolescence. By the time they reach the age of about ten or eleven, the signs of emotional disturbance among these children appear only about as frequently as they do among children brought up in our culture. If we drew a graph of incidence of disturbed children in the two cultures, the Kibbutz line would start higher and begin falling at about age six. At age ten it would cross the line of our culture, and from then on it would reveal progressively less disturbance among the Kibbutz children than in our own. They have a much smoother adolescence than our children, and as young adults they are remarkably non-neurotic. The young adult of the Kibbutz is a remarkable specimen: He is very sociable, and has excellent interpersonal relationships. He is a stable, phlegmatic individual — rather extroverted, and is prepared to sacrifice himself for his group to a notable degree. He does not make egotistical demands on the group, and he is everything the original settlers wanted their children to be. However, if you talk to one of the old-timers when he is off his guard, he will confess to you, "These young fellows do not look like Jews; we miss the idealistic thinking, the interest in spiritual matters — the philosophical bent."

During the Arab war I had some experience with the treatment of psychiatric casualties of the Israeli army. The Kibbutz graduates formed the shock troops of the Israeli striking force. They were the real heroes who fought against tremendous odds with inadequate weapons, and they were always in the thick of the fighting. Yet I never saw a Kibbutz war neurotic. Apparently these men did not break down under stress, or at least if they did, they got killed. Their behavior in battle was extraordinary. They would perform deeds of outstanding valor with a complete disregard for their own personal safety.

Another interesting thing is that in the groups of Kibbutz graduates there is very little bickering. There are no jealousies: at least as far as an outsider can see. They live together extremely harmoniously, and this observation applies also to relationships between the sexes.

This is the picture, and the question is how can one explain this quite extraordinary state of affairs? It is easy enough to explain the signs of deprivation in the younger children, but why the fall in the graph, and why do children who look as though they were going to become neurotics, develop into remarkably stable individuals?

Butler: Maybe they are going through their struggles then, instead of being spoiled and having to face them later.

Caplan: I think that is one possible explanation, except that in our culture, if our theories are correct, we would expect that children brought up in this way would not turn out so well afterwards.

Butler: That is our theory, but we have no evidence.

Caplan: The question is whether this particular social experiment throws our theories out of line or not. I think it is quite important to know.

Sylvester: They are perhaps the kind of individuals who are described in such novels as *Brave New World*, by Aldous Huxley, and seem to be distinguished by certain negative characteristics. The absence of neurotic manifestations might indicate some kind of flattening in the course of adaptation.

Caplan: It might, but our observations show that in fact that is not the case. It is true that they are not philosophers, and they are not as interested in the high spiritual values as their neurotic and introverted parents, but they do lead a very full life.

Sylvester: To what extent is there an elimination of individual differences between these children? Do all the children brought up in the same group resemble each other?

Caplan: My feeling is that they do, to a considerable extent, but this is an area about which I can give you only very vague impressions. In order to study this question, we would have to carry out an intensive psychological investigation of many individuals, which I was not able to do.

Sylvester: Has a second generation already been born there?

Caplan: Yes, but unfortunately I can give you no information about them because the number is still very small. The practical situation also makes such a study difficult, but it would certainly be a very interesting project to undertake.

Fremont-Smith: Do they have artistic expression in music, painting, and so forth, or is this lessened by a certain loss of individuality?

Caplan: As far as one can tell they seem quite average in this regard. Their education is along the lines of good progressive schools in this country, and they use the project method as a routine. Their individuality is fostered in this and other ways, and is not entirely lost by any means.

Baumgartner: What observations have been made on their behavior when they leave their own group? For example, what were they like in an army where there were other people not reared in that way?

Caplan: My impression is that wherever they go as individuals, they quickly join a group. If people from their own Kibbutz are not available, they join a group from other Kibbutzim.

They all have a high school education, and go to school until they are eighteen. This is in line with the socialistic ideal that all men are equal, so that all the children, whatever their intelligence, are given an equal chance of higher education. Many of them go to the university in Jerusalem. The Kibbutz sends them as individuals, and in Jerusalem they live in houses belonging to the Kibbutz movement. They live with young people from the other Kibbutzim, and move around together in groups.

Sylvester: Has anyone made any observations as to how these children react to newcomers, such as the immigrant children who are put into the Kibbutz for the purpose of being absorbed there?

Caplan: This was done in the early days of immigration of unaccompanied children. Some of these children were placed in groups of Kibbutz children with the idea of achieving their quicker integration into the new country. The experiments almost all failed; the immigrant children just could not make the grade. It was not so much because of the social pressure of the Kibbutz children forcing them out; it was because of the tremendous disparity in intellectual attainment.

Sylvester: Do you think their relative lack of individuality has something to do with their capacity to tolerate differences in others?

Caplan: They do tolerate differences in others. However, they realize that other people are not like them, and they regard themselves as the elite. If other people treat them kindly, they are charming, but they become quite aggressive if attacked.

Benjamin: In the case of those who go to the university, have you any data on their choice of courses compared with that of a family group?

Caplan: No, but from my general knowledge of the situation, I believe that they do not in fact choose what courses they will take; but are given the duty of learning certain things according to the needs of the Kibbutz.

Escalona: Is it possible that the present graduates from this way of life were different, as young children, from the ones being trained now under similar circumstances? We do not have direct evidence as to what these adults were like in the preschool ages. Is it conceivable that there have been subtle changes in the experience of the children over the years; and that this present generation may grow up different?

Caplan: That is certainly a valid objection. I did not see these adults when they were young children, but information gathered from a large number of different sources, of all political trends, indicates that the emotional pattern in the young children has been a consistent one.

Walser: Is there any real lack of competitiveness?

Caplan: I would rather say that they show a positive cooperativeness; that is to say, competition among members of a group practically does not exist.

Walser: For school grades also?

Caplan: Yes, that fits in with the ideals of the adults as well as the children.

Fremont-Smith: It is interesting how many of our questions, including my own, have been directed to finding the weak spot in this system. Almost a hundred per cent of the questions that have been asked have been culturally oriented by us against this intrusion into our hallowed ways.

Spock: The narcissism of every one of us is threatened.

Montgomery: I was interested in the frequency of enuresis in children from five to seven. Could you say something about the degree of coerciveness in their bowel and bladder education?

Caplan: That varies from place to place, and I am sure that the incidence of enuresis is related to the type of habit training. I am sorry we do not have the information and figures which might show a direct correlation. As I indicated previously, the bowel and bladder training is undertaken by the professional workers and not by the parents, and this is also of considerable significance.

The other thing to consider is that because of the shortage of professional workers, habit training has to be regimented. Years ago in many Kibbutzim, they started bowel training at five or six months of age, but lately most of them have adopted newer procedures in this regard. By and large they do not start, nowadays, until the child is about one year old, but since in the toddler years there are about ten children per adult worker, it is quite clear that there has to be considerable regimentation. In some places the children sit on the stools for quite a long time, and in one place we visited we found them tied on because they could not sit properly for the time felt to be necessary. Another factor is the change of environment which takes place at the age of one, and again at three, when the children move from nursery to toddler house, and from there to kindergarten.

The incidence of enuresis varies, but the average is about three times as great, among five-year olds, as we found in a survey of kindergarten children in Jerusalem, where the incidence of reported enuresis was 10 to 15 per cent.

Moloney: I think we have to be cautious in accepting these post-adolescent products of the Kibbutzim as being emotionally mature individuals. We know that the conformistic character is quite an infantile character, and the products of the Kibbutzim conform to an abstraction. The ideology of the Kibbutzim may be a consistently tyrannical and intolerant abstraction for the mother. The ethos could be as tyrannical, and just as intolerant, as a flesh-and-blood mother figure.

We know the consistent training by a tyrannical mother can produce a neurotic character structure. A character neurotic becomes one by virtue of the fusion in his personality of his superego with his ego. Anxiety is bound by the fusion, and therefore free-floating activity becomes insignificant. A characteristic feature of the mature person is an appropriate spontaneity manifested in all situations.

In the service, we saw individuals who became psychotic when they were lifted out of an environment that permitted them to gravitate to the type of living which would give them the greatest amount of security. These individuals, displaced to a military situation, often became psychotic overnight. A similarity in the Kibbutzim group indicates to me a possible lack of individuality and flexibility.

We know the history of their hostilities exhibited during the first four or five years of their lives. As they become aggressors, or warriors, they have a permissible target for the discharge of the pent-up resentments and hostilities. It is a question whether, after they leave the service, they will have to continue to have a target for the discharge of their cumulative resentments in order to maintain their balance. I am thinking of the Nazis, for instance, who had to have such a target, which in their case became the Jews themselves.

Caplan: I wish to emphasize that my report was based on clinical impressions, and I would not claim scientific validity. On the other hand, they are the impressions of experienced clinicians who spent a number of years on the spot, and who were on the lookout for all the kinds of things which have been mentioned here.

I should warn you against trying to alter the facts, as reported, in order to suit a theory. I think we must be prepared to accept them as being more or less true. I cannot say that I found the people in the Kibbutzim to be like machine men, or that they seemed to be emotionally flattened. To me, they looked like healthy people, and I know them well enough to feel confident that they are indeed reasonably healthy from a psychological point of view. Let us see whether we cannot try to understand what is going on, instead of attempting to alter the facts to suit some preconceived ideas.

In regard to the question of hostility, I found that under peacetime conditions these people do discharge their aggression, but not in hostility to other people. They find very fitting, and I think healthy and positive, avenues for the discharge of their aggression in the pioneering work they do in clearing swamps and turning rocky mountainsides into agriculturally productive fields, and so on. They live a very hard life, and when they grow up they go in small groups to found new Kibbutzim, usually on the borders of the country or in the southern desert. They do a remarkable job, not only as warriors in wartime, but also as constructive settlers. So they have adequate outlets for their aggressive energy.

Baumgartner: Have any of them who have gone out to industrialize an area worked in industry, or do they all do agricultural work?

Caplan: The early Kibbutzim were all entirely agricultural, but more and more of the settlements have added small industries to their economy.

Baumgartner: Are there any differences?

Caplan: Not really, except that on the whole the older and larger Kibbutzim are the ones which have developed most industrial undertakings.

I might here say a word about membership of the Kibbutzim. In order to become a member they have to go through a procedure not dissimilar to the admission formalities of a professional organization, or an artisan guild. There is a period when the candidate is under observation, and approval is necessary for promotion. It takes some years to be accepted as a full member.

Butler: In our discussion of the separation of infant from mother, I wondered how much of what we spoke of as the effect of separation was actually due to the misfortune in the family that had resulted in the separation. It seems to me that Dr. Caplan has had an opportunity to study the separation of infant from mother without separation by other factors.

Kris: I think that we underrate changes in the individual coming about after early childhood. All that happens to a child after infancy is being considered a frustrated follow-up of an already molded form, and there is no clinical evidence of that being so. There is a lot of clinical evidence for the relevance of earliest impressions, if not corrected by later impressions, but the question to which extent they can be corrected by later impressions has, to my mind, not even seriously been asked.

We have heard about hospitalism necessarily creating psychiatric conditions. We have a recent follow-up study by Beres and Obers (2), in which it is shown that this is not so. Numerous experiences from elsewhere suggest that there is a gap in our knowledge. This is due to the fact that our data come from a psychoanalytical perspective in which by necessity we focus on the influence of the past on the present. However, lately we have been able to understand that early distress may produce not only negative, but also positive effects in personality, and we have learned to study, not only conflict, but also the areas outside conflict.

A case report was published two years ago by Anna Freud and Sophia Dann (3). This concerns a group of children from concentration camps who had been brought to England. In this group, attachments to parental figures were substituted by intergroup attachments; certain types of behavior developed, and others remained undeveloped. The group was disorganized by the fact that predominant adult figures, namely, nurses, were introduced. Although the children did not look well, nevertheless before the introduction of the adults their performance was, in many ways, superior to that of any such age group in our experience, as far as mutual help and in-group sentiment were concerned.

I imagine what happened with the Israeli children was not only related to the fact that the parents were possibly in a somewhat special position — that is, they were there and not there — but that at a very early age, the "elite" feeling became a significant factor. It would be fascinating to make an analytical study of such individuals. I know we would probably analyze the misfit among the elite, but I do not think that would matter because even in the misfit one can see the healthy. In our psychiatric experience we have learned to see in the healthy, the neurotic. I think probably we are now, to some extent, going in the opposite direction, and may become able to see productive capacities in the sick. I think we do already, to some extent.

Frank: It has long been accepted that there are no new problems in adolescence, but merely a revival of the problems of early childhood, especially of relations with parents. Dr. Caplan's Kibbutzim children might be explained in this way: if the young child is not in contact with parents, who are so often responsible for early problems, then there is nothing to be revived later in adolescence.

Another point: what about the English nannie who more or less takes over the mother role in the family?

Bowlby: She is very rare in these days.

Frank: Today, yes, but for a good many years she played a considerable part in the rearing of English children.

Bowlby: Oh, yes.

Frank: What did that do to the character structure and personality, particularly of the boys who went off at seven or eight to a boarding school, and saw their families for only a short time during the year? That is one group upon which there should be a considerable number of observations and clinical material, since some of them must have been under psychotherapy.

We have also had experience in this country of the Indian children who have been taken away from their families quite early, and then have gone back from government schools to their homes. Before the recent war, there were reports that many Chinese intellectuals were putting their babies in orphan asylums so they could devote their whole time to saving their country. We might enlarge our sample by taking into account other cases where the usual mother-child relationship has been interfered with.

Moloney: As Dr. Kris said, psychoneurosis is not the only yardstick by which we can measure emotional maturity in any culture; there are others. For instance, character neuroses, or the amount of crime occurring in a culture, are also factors to take into consideration in measuring emotional maturity. To illustrate, I have been told that in Ireland they have much juvenile crime, but adult crime is at a minimum. Is it a consequence of the fact that the number of institutionalized adult insane is 600 per 100,000, which is 200 per 100,000 more than is recorded for the United States? Also, if we were to use the absence of a psychoneurosis as a measuring stick for emotional maturity, then the Japanese would be very emotionally mature, since they have only 50 per 100,000 committed or institutionalized insane. However, according to Rempei Sassa's study, they have a death rate from arterial hypertension of over 9 per cent in Tokyo (4, 5). He believed this figure to be the highest for any metropolis in the world.

Butler: What is your explanation of their hypertension?

Moloney: I think it is the result of the rigidities in their character. The Japanese people are unable to express themselves flexibly and spontaneously. They swallow their angers, hostilities, and individualistic aggressions (6); this fact has been fairly well established. But in Tokyo, where they have a population of 5,500,000, this high death rate from hypertension is all the more phenomenal when one takes into consideration that in 1949, according to Brigadier General Crawford Sams, of the American Military Government (7), ten per cent of the Japanese suffered from tuberculosis, which usually occurs in persons with low blood pressure.

Walser: I wonder which disease comes first in that case, since low blood pressure does not cause tuberculosis.

Caplan: To go back to the communal settlements: I feel it is not necessary either to deny the facts or our psychological theories. I think if we look more carefully at the phenomena underlying the graph of high incidence of disturbance up to six, and then at its subsequent fall, that it is possible to explain it without altering our theoretical basis at all.

In trying to think out an explanation I was very much impressed by Anna Freud's paper (3) already mentioned by Dr. Kris. We have to explain, not only the much higher incidence of disturbed young children, but also the progressive fall in incidence round the ages from five to seven. I am not sure whether we should use the term "latency period" in this case, or not. The fall does appear to coincide with the beginning of the latency period, but we need more evidence before we can say whether this is significant.

Foord: Dr. Caplan, in order to give us a better picture of these children would you describe the progress of their physical growth and development? You mentioned that up to six they are puny, and prone to have upper respiratory infections.

Caplan: As they pass beyond the critical age of about six, they begin to improve physically, as well as emotionally, and as adolescents and young adults they are very well developed in both respects. If you have heard stories about the excellent physique of the Kibbutz children, they are true, but they refer to the older children.

For the young Kibbutz child there are three important sets of love objects, as compared with the one important set of love objects for a child in our culture. The first is his parents, and although he only sees them for a couple of hours a day, there is no doubt that he is attached to them and shows signs of deprivation when he is separated from them. If the parents go away from the Kibbutz, the child grieves. If one of the parents dies, the child mourns. I saw a group of children from one of the Kibbutzim who had been evacuated from the front line to Haifa during the Arab war. Many of them were without their parents, and they were showing the same kind of reactions to the separation which I saw in English children during the wartime evacuation.

Fremont-Smith: Were they separated from the Kibbutz also?

Caplan: No, they had their group, including the child-care workers, with them, but the parents were left behind.

If one of the parents was killed, or went off permanently for some reason, there seemed to be a sort of cushioning in their mourning reaction. I felt that although their relationships with their parents seemed like child-parent relationships in our culture, it was actually of lower intensity. When they lost a parent, they fell back on the secondary love object, which was the professional worker. There is no doubt that these children have very strong emotional attachments to the professional workers.

Fremont-Smith: Is there one special one?

Caplan: Yes, there usually is.

Fremont-Smith: So there is a real mother substitute.

Caplan: Yes. Up to the age of one year there is one adult for five children, and between one and three there is one adult for every ten children.

Trainham: Does this mother substitute operate throughout the 24-hour period?

Caplan: She functions just as a mother usually does. She works with the children all day, and at night the children sleep by themselves. She may sleep in another room in the same house.

Trainham: But she is the mother person for her group 24 hours daily, and seven days a week?

Caplan: She acts as the mother person during the daytime. She has her off-duty when the children go to their parents during visiting hours. You can see that she works very hard, and for long hours, but so does everyone in a Kibbutz.

In addition to these two sets of objects, the parents and the professional workers, there is a third object and that is the peer group of the other children. Until recently, children were grouped with others of their own age. More recently some Kibbutzim have started the experiment of mixing the young children as far as ages are concerned. They have organized children of mixed ages into family type groups, under the influence of Anna Freud's work in the Hampstead Nursery.

The group of children becomes an important love object, if you can call it that, around about the age of two. Our observations indicate that even at that age children can make fairly strong and continuing emotional attachments to other individual children, and to the children's group as a whole. This was rather surprising because normally one would not expect that to happen until later. Anna Freud and Sophia Dann (3) refer to signs of very close attachments in their group of concentration camp children, which took place as early as 18 months of age. The group of children is, at the beginning, not a gratifying object, especially at the toddler age. The child has appetitive needs and wants gratification from the group, but at this stage gets very little fulfillment of these needs.

So if we compare Kibbutz children with children brought up in our culture, we can say that statistically the former, having three sets of love objects, stand about three times the chance of suffering from a lack of gratification. I do not know whether you are prepared to follow me in this argument, but in addition to the group which we know is not gratifying, the Kibbutz child has the chance of nongratification both by his parents and the professional workers.

Also, there is the emotional burden of the split allegiance between parents and workers. This is probably less of a problem than it would be if the child-care workers were more carefully chosen and had better training. I can imagine that a child seeing his parents only two hours a day, and being in contact the rest of the time with well selected, highly-trained professional workers, might have difficulty deciding where his primary emotional attachment was directed. In practice, this seems to be a rare dilemma for most children, and there seems but little doubt that their primary love is directed towards their parents, although they see them for so short a time during the day. You hear them bragging about "my daddy" and what he did when the Arabs attacked. They idolize their fathers and love their mothers. On the other hand, they also talk about "my Sarah" or "my Rebecca" when referring to the professional worker who is a love object of the second order.

These factors taken together explain the high disturbance rate in the younger age group, but if we turn our attention to the relationship between the individual child and his peer group, we find an interesting change with increasing age. As the children grow older the peer group becomes more and more effective as a gratifier of the needs of the individual members. One reason for this is that the children perceive the cooperative communal life of the adults by whom they are surrounded, and they identify with the values and methods of group organization. They do not, at this age, perceive the individualistic difficulties of the adults, such as the jealousies and intrigues which obstruct their cooperation, and they mould their own groups on the ideals of the adults, rather than on the actual conditions of their lives.

Kris: Are you assuming that gratification is identical with libidinal gratification? There is also the satisfaction of aggressive tendencies, and these children can fight with each other much more intimately than with anybody else.

Caplan: I think that is certainly a valid point which is open to debate, but I was not referring to that. In talking of libidinal gratification, I was referring to their need for love, which is partly fulfilled by the group as an entity.

I should like to say a few more words about the peer group as a gratifier of the individual's love needs. As they pass the 6-year-old level, these groups become progressively more gratifying. The group as a whole is very jealous for the rights of every individual member, and it does not impose on the individual members. Like the group described by Anna Freud and Sophia Dann (3), it comes to the assistance of those of its members who are backward, or who fall behind in their activities. It does not develop or impose group ideals and values which are inimical to the individual rights of its members, which makes it a very special kind of group formation.

Another factor of significance to our inquiry makes itself felt between the ages of about six and eight. The adults in the Kibbutz begin to reduce their individual demands on the children, and they give more and more autonomy to the children's group. At this age too, there is a lessening of the turbulence of the child's feelings towards its parents, and both they and the professional workers begin to adopt a permissive attitude towards the peer group, along the lines of "you will decide for yourselves." An example of the attitude of adults to mid-latency children in a Kibbutz, is that a teacher will not enter the children's room without asking permission from the group. If the children were to say, "you must not come in here," the adult would not go in. By the time these children reach adolescence, the adults of the commune give the children the right, as a group, to make all kinds of decisions about their own welfare, which in our culture we would certainly not give to children. Some of us, who know how savage groups of children in our culture can at times be to individuals, might be frightened of the consequences of leaving the power of control and punishment in the hands of the children. But we find that these Kibbutz groups are rarely cruel to their members because they appear to be very sensitive to the susceptibilities of the individual.

An interesting topic for inquiry would be the nature of the superego structure in these children, and I am sorry that I have no valid evidence to bring before you on this point. I do suggest, however, that the Kibbutz child introjects the values developed by his peer group, and if this is the case he grows up in a peculiarly secure emotional environment. He is surrounded continually by members of his group who exert external control on his behavior, which is in line with his internalized controlling superego forces. This culture therefore produces a situation which is similar to certain types of group psychotherapy which we prescribe for disturbed children.

Baty: How long do they stay in these groups, and when do they begin to divide by sexes?

Caplan: The usual thing is for them to stay in their groups all their lives. If a group of young adults branches off to form a new settlement, it is usually composed of clusters of the original units of five, ten or fifteen who were brought up in the same children's houses.

Their behavior in regard to sex and marriage is very interesting. There is complete coeducation in the Kibbutzim — more than in any other situation which I have observed. Boys and girls are treated with complete equality: they sleep in the same room, bathe in the same shower, and move naked quite freely in front of each other. The adults have imposed this framework on their children with almost a religious fervor, because they feel that the smuttiness of sex in bourgeois society is largely due to separate education of boys and girls, and because of false modesty in regard to sex matters. The adult Kibbutz members point with great pride to the absence of perversion and sex play among their children. In fact very little sex play does take place, and the children seem to develop sexual morality without the adults ever having overly inculcated morals into them. Masturbation is regarded as a normal and natural, but childish, habit. When adolescence is reached, the children are urged not to masturbate, in the same way as smoking and ballroom dancing are vetoed as unbecoming to members of an elite leader class.

The question is: what does this kind of upbringing do to their sex life, and why is there no sex play in so permissive an atmosphere? A finding, which throws some light on this subject, is that marriages rarely occur between members of the same group. It appears as though the group of fifteen or so behave toward each other like siblings, and an intense incest taboo seems to develop. When they marry, they find their mate in another group, or in other Kibbutzim.

Fremont-Smith: Is there not just one group in another Kibbutz?

Caplan: In a big Kibbutz, it may be another group in the same settlement; but in smaller Kibbutzim they marry someone from another Kibbutz.

An important question is what kind of passionate love relationships they make in marriage, and unfortunately I do not have the information to answer it. All I can say is that they appear to have a satisfying sex life, but what it means to them in the way of passion and romantic love, as we find it in our culture, I just do not know. It is an area which would be difficult to explore, but would certainly be a profitable field of inquiry.

Bowlby: I am extremely interested in Dr. Caplan's data, and I am sufficiently well acquainted with him to know that he does not overlook any of the obvious things which any ordinary psychoanalyst would think important.

I think he has already answered Dr. Butler's question as to whether some of the separation responses which I described earlier were not really due to what I called the associated variables — in other words that separation itself was not the important thing. We have given considerable thought to this, and we do not think the associated variables are responsible for these phenomena, but we can not be absolutely sure.

Of course, the Kibbutz children are brought up in completely different circumstances from the children I described. They are certainly not children without any substitute mothering: they have a complex of love objects, which may answer Dr. Frank's point about English nannies, and possibly also black mammies. This business of multiple love objects is a complex area which we do not know much about, but it is clearly very different from the situation in which a child has no love object whatever.

As to the point which Dr. Kris raised: the follow-up study of Beres and Obers (2) in which they observed the results in children of separation experiences in early life, showed that various personality structures developed later. We ourselves have done an analogous follow-up study and have found the same thing. One or two of the school children who had been in a sanatorium for a long time before their fourth birthday are well-adjusted personalities so far as one can tell. This differential outcome presents a tremendous problem.

Also, because I attach great importance to early experience, I do not underestimate the importance of later experience, and I would not be a psychoanalyst if I did because, after all, psychoanalytic treatment is a later experience. At the same time, I think there are reasons to suppose that certain sorts of early experience may have a nearly irreversible effect. The experimental work on behavior under stress shows that in conditions of intense stress, peculiar sorts of responses develop and become stabilized. It is certain that many young children in a separation environment are under intense stress, and it may be that the experimental work on stress responses is relevant to our understanding of why some children seem to perseverate in making very pathological responses.

Fries: The split in the libidinal attachment recalls the situation in the "extended family" of the Navahos (8). In such a family, certain functions that we would consider to belong to the parents are split off and assigned to other relatives, e.g., much of the discipline is taken over by the mother's brothers and the grandparents. The mother's sisters are called "mother," and in many ways can substitute for her. The result of this system is that the libidinal attachments are greater in number, and less intense in quality; dependence is less on one or two relatives, and the ambivalence tends to be divided among different individuals, authority being identified with the relatives, rather than the father and mother.

Another point about the Navahos is that the children know exactly how to behave towards an uncle, a maternal cousin, and so forth. This behavior, being culturally determined, makes life simpler in this respect compared with our system of each one working out his own relationships with each member of the family. I think there are similarities between the Navahos and the Israelis.

I might mention also, that among the Navahos around Ramah, before they were acculturated, the young children up to the age of five all had a mild respiratory infection, and one saw them with a continuously discharging nose.

Caplan: It is interesting that the parents in the Kibbutz do not have to frustrate the children very much; they seem to have the role of gratifying parents. There appears to be a split in the child's ambivalence, which in our culture develops towards the parent. In the Kibbutz the ambivalence develops in regard to the child-care workers, and going to the parents is a holiday. This leads to considerable tension between the professional workers and the parents, because the former feel that they do all the dirty work, and literally they do, and that the parents just gratify the children.

Bartemeier: Like grandparents.

Caplan: Yes, the attitude of the parents is really like grandparents in our culture.

Kris: Some months ago there was a private discussion by a group of us, including Miss Freud. One of the questions we raised was this: the large family unit of rural communities offers, as in the case of the institution, various substitute objects such as older siblings, and grandparents, with a distribution of feelings of importance, and also restricted functioning. In the usual urban, two-child family, there is a scarcity of opportunity for displacement, and there is a high concentration of conflict on key objects. I have looked over the literature to see whether there were any data on large families in relation to the incidence of neuroses. I have not found any, although I may not have looked carefully enough.

Bowlby: I do not think there is very much.

Kris: Dr. Caplan, you spoke about the coeducational life in these groups, and you contrasted family groups and groups of peers. Is it a group of peers you speak of, or a group in which all children are of the same age? An age group is not necessarily a group of peers. Also, three-year-olds are not all three-year-olds: even if they are born on the same day, they may not all be of the same maturity. Are there any other criteria except chronological age?

Caplan: To my knowledge no, except in a large settlement where there would be a large number of children to divide into groups of five. It is conceivable that they might mix the bright ones together, or mix the dull ones together, except that since they do the mixing at birth, they would not really know.

Kris: I do not necessarily mean bright. Maturity has many aspects.

Caplan: But the selection is at birth, and once they are in that group they stay there.

Kris: I am speaking of the capacity of the group to gratify the individual. For instance the group is a place where aggression may be discharged without deep conflict.

Escalona: If I understand correctly, Dr. Caplan, you said that because there is more than one set of love objects in the experience of these young children, the probable frequency of frustrating moments is greater. I am not sure that is so. One can be frustrated only a certain number of times a day in the course of ordinary experience, and I think the fact that there is a wider range of possibilities for frustration only means that the distribution is greater — not that it is a more frequent occurrence.

Caplan: I did not mean the frequency per day, but the frequency per hundred children of being frustrated by parents or child-care workers.

Escalona: That does not seem to me to hold either. I do not think that the fact there is more than one set of love objects automatically increases the total number of occasions when frustration is likely to occur. It seems to me that it is the significance of frustration that is important to the child, in so far as it involves a threat to the important relationships in his life.

Caplan: Without wanting to labor the point, I would say that if you are correct, these children should from an early age appear more stable than the children in our culture, whereas they appear less stable. They show the signs which we usually associate with lack of gratification.

Escalona: I would not go as far as you do in that, and I am not sure that it is a matter which can be discussed in terms of quantity. The frequency of frustration does not seem to me to be the same thing as the depth or sufficiency of gratification. I could easily imagine that under the circumstances you describe, important kinds of gratifications would be less frequent or altogether lacking, which would not mean that there would be more frustration.

Caplan: I'm sorry, the difficulty is in my use of the term "frustration." I was using the term loosely as a synonym for lack of gratification in regard to their need for love from objects.

Baty: Are you not talking about two different things? Dr. Caplan is talking about attachment to an individual, like the mother-child attachment, and Dr. Escalona is talking about other frustrations. Isn't that the difference?

Caplan: Yes, I believe it is.

Benjamin: Dr. Caplan, you have a certain assumed *a priori* probability in each of your three frustrations, but you also have an assumed probability of gratification, and thinking of it in the simple algebraic fashion that you did, you have exactly the same increase in the possibility of gratification that you have in the lack of gratification. If you make the assumption that there is a half probability for each of your three — which would be highly artificial — you would come out exactly the same in the end. In other words, I do not think this can be handled on an algebraic basis at all, but on the differential and field equations in relation to gratification and frustration. I should recommend that the number "three" be left out, because in order to give it plausibility you would have to select a most artificial *a priori* probability in each of your three groups of frustration. If you can find it, you could select the numbers so as to arrive at three.

Another point: it seems to me we are having an interesting theoretical discussion on the valuable data you have given us, and you have clearly described to us the limitations of these data. I think in order to deepen the significance of discussion, it would be helpful if you could tell us more. Are there further significant details which you could give us about the adult finally produced by the Kibbutzim? You told us that they were less philosophical and spiritual; you also gave us some positive statements about their group cohesiveness.

Caplan: All I can say is that this is a fascinating field for inquiry, and given the money and personnel, I think research could certainly be done. The information I gave you was gathered on the side, as it were, and not as a central part of my assignment in the country. That explains why my report contained more problems than solutions.

Benjamin: So far you have given us the feeling that there are a great many positives, but we have very little idea of what the sacrifices would be. You have given us the impression that there is less variation from individual to individual than we would see in our culture, although you say you do not have much data on the subject.

Butler: There are variables here other than the communal living: the conditions under which they live are very primitive as compared with ours, and there is no wealth, leisure, or luxury. Those are the factors that would affect artistic development, philosophical interest, etc., as well as the mere fact that they are living in a communal society.

Benjamin: Right. I was merely asking for more data descriptively.

Baumgartner: Would you say that the people who founded these groups were highly intellectual — more so than average educated people?

Caplan: I am sorry, but I just do not have the data. In my presentation I tried to be as cautious as possible and to indicate how impressionistic my information was, but in regard to this point I would not even venture a generalization. It would be, as you realize, a rather difficult generalization to make. For instance, I would find it very difficult, after spending some time in this country, to say how Americans differ from Englishmen. In order to obtain sufficient data for theoretical conclusions, a lot of intensive psychological research would be needed.

Benjamin: Right, Dr. Caplan, I have the impression that one would encounter unusual difficulties, if an attempt were made to conduct an intensive psychological investigation in this case, because of the fear, on the part of the Israelis, that it might involve criticism of their experiment. Do you think that would be the case?

Caplan: Yes, entry into the field for a serious investigation might be resisted at first, but I think this obstacle could be overcome. However, I think this field as a research laboratory will soon be obscured by changes in the development of the social system. There is evidence that the Kibbutzim, in their original form as I have described them, are rapidly changing their pattern, and the reasons are many. There are economic, sociological, and political reasons, and some of them are connected with the establishment and development of the state.

One of the main tasks of this project has been the incorporation of very large numbers of new immigrants: the Jewish population of the country has more than doubled in the last five years. In this work of central importance to the nation, the Kibbutzim have played a very minor part. This is just what might be expected, because the Kibbutzim are closed groups, and although they welcomed new immigrants as guests, they did not wish unselected strangers to become members. The new immigrants, on their part, had no interest in joining communal settlements, since they had had more than enough of group living in concentration camps or ghettos. A high proportion of them immigrated from oriental countries, and they did not take kindly to this product of European ideology.

So the national prestige of the Kibbutzim has fallen, because they made little contribution to the task of absorbing the exiles, and their numerical ratio to the population as a whole has decreased. There is one exception to this, however, and that is that they have taken immigrant children with the idea of educating them to their way of thinking, so that later on, as adults, they will choose the Kibbutz way of life. In this they are succeeding to a considerable extent.

Another factor is one I referred to earlier; namely, the conflict between the family and the group. This has become more evident with the passage of time, and I would compare it with the little I know of the history of the Hutterites, with which some of you may be familiar. This was a Christian sect, originating in Germany centuries ago. They have at present, in this country, about 8,000 members, who live in communal settlements very similar to the Kibbutzim. In the past they also reared their children communally, but as they developed there was a growing tension between the family and the group in regard to the care of their children, and nowadays the children are brought up in the care of the family. This sect is held together by a very strong religious feeling, and this brings me back to a question raised by Dr. Fremont-Smith about the religious attitudes in the Kibbutzim. Some of these settlements are religious, and some nonreligious. What interests me is that in the nonreligious, or antireligious, Kibbutzim they have invented forms of social custom and ceremonial which very much resemble those of orthodox religion, such as festivals similar to those in the Jewish religion, which in certain cases are like pagan festivals. It looks as though the settlements which have denied orthodox religious practices have been forced to invent a substitute.

Let me come back for just a minute to the tension between the family and the group: There have been a number of adult members who have left the Kibbutzim over the years. This has usually been due to the pressure of the wife, and her dissatisfaction has usually been an expression of the revolt against the edict of the Kibbutz that she cannot care for her children herself. There has also been a growing tendency in recent years for parents to take their children back to their room at visiting times, and there to set apart a children's corner, with special toys and furniture, where the child is given a meal on the occasion of his visits. This development has now reached the stage where in some Kibbutzim — mainly the older and richer ones — the parents are given an adjoining room for their children, and after the age of six or seven the children live with their parents.

Benjamin: Are these wives all Kibbutzim products themselves?

Caplan: No. I am talking about the original Kibbutz members, mainly people from Europe. In some Kibbutzim, the new ruling is that a baby will spend the first few weeks of life in the parents' room, until the mother returns to work. In such cases, of course, this leads to trouble, because the mother often becomes strongly attached to her child, and when he finally has to go into the communal nursery there will be a succession of quarrels between her and the child-care workers.

Kris: You mean to say evolution can only be prevented by purge?

Caplan: It can be prevented by something else; that is, the Kibbutz graduates apparently do not have these conflicts. The parents who were themselves reared in the Kibbutz, do not seem to suffer from these tensions with the group. They do not cause trouble, and they often look down on the "complexes" of other parents. However, they sometimes break away from the settlement and found a new Kibbutz of their own.

Benjamin: You know of no cases of Kibbutz graduates who, as mothers, have rebelled against the commune?

Caplan: It is practically unknown for anyone born and brought up in a Kibbutz to give up that way of life.

Butler: If someone in the group wishes to start a new Kibbutz, how does he acquire the necessary financial backing?

Caplan: This has unfortunately been a topic of considerable interest in Israel during the past couple of years. One of the large organizations of Kibbutzim was composed of members belonging to two separate political parties: extreme left-wing socialists, and more liberal socialists of approximately the same political color as the British Labour Party. The members of the two parties lived together in each of the Kibbutzim in reasonable amity until the establishment of the state. Then questions of power politics came to the fore, and the erstwhile friends began to quarrel. About a year ago they decided that the partnership must break up because each side wished to impose its own political ideology on the school system. They pay very great attention to the political education of their children, and the members of the extreme left did not wish their children to be taught by teachers of the middle left. The membership of many Kibbutzim has consequently split. What often happens is that the smaller group exchanges with a group of the opposite party seceding from another Kibbutz. If this is not possible they have to divide the property, and this is usually a rather difficult procedure.

Spock: Dr. Bowlby wondered why some children do very badly in severe separation situations, and others not so badly. At the time of my pediatric residency, in 1932, when practically no one in pediatrics realized that children had emotional needs, most of the residents and nurses were somewhat scornful of any staff member who showed open affection for children on the wards. Yet every once in a while there was a child so appealing that he could extract a warm smile from the most hard-boiled resident of them all.

We have been talking as though altruistic love on the part of a young child for others were a strange and abnormal substitute for being sufficiently loved by parents. I am not sure that early altruism is not normal, although it may be exaggerated when a child is deprived of parents. In American pediatric and psychiatric practice, we are accustomed to parents who are so concerned with their children, and are so dominating in family relationships, that it may be too little initiative is left to the children in establishing affectionate relationships with other children, which may be off the norm in the opposite direction. When Dr. Caplan was speaking of the children of the Kibbutz who, as they grew up, seemed to find a security from each other that they may have missed in the nursery, I was thinking of the hundreds of irresponsible, impulsive psychopaths whose histories I wrote up in the Navy. Every once in a while there would be one who, like the others, had been deprived of love in early childhood, had been in trouble all through the school years, had a poor work record, and a poor police record. But then, unlike the others, he married a woman with some stability and devotion, had children, and abruptly settled down into a relatively hard-working and responsible existence. I thought of such a patient as having belatedly achieved a sense of belonging, so that he grew up in a family he had created, instead of the one into which he was born.

Foord: We have noted that these Kibbutz children, and English and American children reared by nannies, mammies, and governesses, have at least one thing in common; namely, two love objects. It seems to me that to the child, who has parents but is cared for by someone else, the important thing is the kind of parent-child relationship which actually exists. To what extent is he deprived: is he accepted by his parents, and does he know and feel this?

You said that some of the mothers did revolt. You also said that these children were rationed, a factor which should make for a higher percentage of "wanted" children. But can you give us more data on the relationships established between parents and children? Does the system in general block the establishment of any close relationship? I realize that these children see relatively little of their parents, but I should like to know more about what happens when they do see them.

Caplan: So far as I could make out, all the possibilities for disturbed parent-child relationships are present, even though they are together only for a brief period, and in the young children one observes most of the effects of such disturbances, just as they are seen in family children. It is also true that many children do not accept the situation of separation from their parents very kindly. For instance in regard to habit training, it is not uncommon for a child to want to have a stool in the parents' room, as well as in the communal nursery, and to want to perform for his parents, which they very often resent. The children also make all kinds of extra demands in regard to eating when they visit, which the parents cannot completely gratify. The expression of the natural impulses of the children, and those of the parents, often leads to situations such as we see in families on holiday in our culture.

It is true the parents have plenty of time and nothing to do, and they should be relaxed and happy; but it is not unusual to find scenes of turmoil between parent and children on such occasions, and this you find in the Kibbutz, also.

Bowlby: Drs. Fries and Benjamin have both raised the question of whether there is any sacrifice in personality development and if so, what? I, myself, am chiefly concerned as to whether these Kibbutz graduates grow up to become intolerant and totalitarian characters. Is the Arab war an opportunity for masking this at the present time?

Caplan: The direction of the present Arab war is not in the hands of these people. By and large, there are few persons of national leadership caliber in Israel. There are relatively few adult Kibbutz graduates, and they play little part in the leadership of the country.

With regard to the question of totalitarianism in their personalities, I have formed the impression, which may be biased but I think not, that it does not exist to any obvious degree. To tell the truth, I have never moved in Nazi or similar circles, so it is hard to compare them, but I did not find more intolerance among people reared in the Kibbutzim than among other children in Israel.

The Jews who are born in Israel and have been brought up there, whether in a Kibbutz or in a town, have a certain intolerance of people from the outside, because this is a young and very rapidly growing country, and they feel they are reacting against the troubles the Jews have suffered for centuries. Also, it is a small country cut off from its neighbors, and people tend to be a bit intolerant of strangers in any small place. But I do not think the Kibbutz graduates are any different from the others in this respect.

Butler: Perhaps we should ask the question a little differently: is the Kibbutz organization maintaining a democratic character, or is it being taken over by a few dominant people, and thus tending to become totalitarian?

Caplan: No, absolutely not. It is a very democratic organization, and sometimes appears to be a bit too much so; the arguments at committee meetings, plenary sessions and movement conferences seem to go on for days and weeks!

REFERENCES

1. Irvine, E. Observations on the aims and methods of child rearing in communal settlements in Israel. *Human Relations*, 5, 247 (1952).

2. Beres, D., and Obers, S. J. The effects of extreme deprivation in infancy on psychic structure in adolescence: a study in ego development. *Psychoanalytic Study of the Child*, Vol. V, New York, Internat. Univ. Press, 1950 (p. 212).

3. Freud, A., and Dann, S. An experiment in group upbringing. *The Psycho-*

analytic Study of the Child, Vol. VI, New York, Internat. Univ. Press, 1951 (p. 127).

4. Moloney, J. C. *Battle for Mental Health*, New York, Philosophical Library, 1952.

5. Sassa, R. Klinisch-statistische Studie über Apoplexie. *Psychiat. neurol. jap.*, 42, 41 (1938).

6. Benedict, R. *The Chrysanthemum and the Sword; Patterns of Japanese Culture*, Boston, Houghton Mifflin, 1946.

7. Moloney, J. C. A study in neurotic conformity: the Japanese. *Complex*, (Spring, 1951), p. 26.

8. Leighton, D., and Kluckhohn, C. *Children of the People; the Navaho Individual and his Development*, London, Oxford, and Cambridge, Harvard Univ. Press, 1947.

44

ASIAN PSYCHOLOGY AND MODERN PSYCHIATRY

ALAN W. WATTS

American Academy of Asian Studies, San Francisco

At the basis of Asian culture there are certain traditions and ways of life which have the outward appearance of religions. However, when one investigates such phenomena as the Vedanta, Yoga, Buddhism, and Taoism more deeply, and becomes familiar not so much with their popular application as with the thought and practice of their most advanced exponents, one discovers disciplines which are neither religion nor philosophy in the Western sense. For, unlike Christianity or Judaism, they only rarely involve "beliefs" — that is to say, adherence to positive, formulated opinions about the nature and destiny of man and the universe based on revelation or intuition. And, unlike Western philosophy, their *modus operandi* is only quite secondarily the construction of a verbal and logical description or explanation of man's experience.

Oriental "philosophy" is, at root, not concerned with conceptions, ideas, opinions, and forms of words at all. It is concerned with a transformation of experience itself, and it would seem that one of the things most akin to it in Western culture — akin by form rather than content — is psychotherapy. For this is the one major area in which the West has developed disciplines which aim at transforming the actual processes of the mind, and, through them, of the ways in which we experience the world, usually without commitment to any metaphysical or philosophical theory. Thus the curing of a psychotic or neurotic person, the transformation of the way in which he thinks and feels, is to a large extent the best Western analogy of the special concerns of Oriental philosophy. In many respects, then, it is more accurate to speak of such a phenomenon as Buddhism as psychology, rather than philosophy or religion. But this requires at least two reservations: that in *popular* practice it has many of the characteristics of a religion, and that its ultimate concerns are, as yet, hardly within the scope of Western psychology.

From the outset, there is one notable difference between the "psychotherapy," the transformation of the mind, envisaged by an Oriental

From the *American Journal of Psychoanalysis*, 18: 25, 1953.

psychology, on the one hand, and Western psychiatry, on the other. In the West we are chiefly pre-occupied with the transformation of mental states which are peculiar to relatively few individuals, and which arise out of certain special conditioning circumstances of the individual's history. But Asian psychology interests itself in the transformation of states which are common to mankind as a whole, and is thus, as it were, a psychotherapy of the "normal" man. It proposes to change patterns of thought and feeling which are characteristic of the society as well as of the individual, though this does not amount in practice to an attempt to change the society as a whole. For it is recognized that in any given society relatively few individuals seem to have the capacity and the interest to liberate themselves from patterns of conditioning common to all.

It follows that for an Oriental psychology, "normalcy" could never be a standard of mental health — where "normalcy" means the ways of thinking and feeling, the conventions and life-goals, acceptable to the majority of persons in a particular culture. Likewise, the diseases of the mind are not recognized in terms of deviation from the normal. From this (Oriental) standpoint, there is a clear absurdity in trying to achieve the "happy adjustment" of an individual to the conventions of a society which is largely composed of unhappy people. Thus an Oriental psychology such as Buddhism is concerned, not with the peculiar frustrations of the neurotic individual, but with the general frustration, the common unhappiness (*duhkha* in Sanskrit), which afflicts almost every member of the society.

Buddhist and Hindu psychology agree in ascribing this general unhappiness to *avidya* — a Sanskrit term for a special type of ignorance or unconsciousness, which is the failure to perceive that certain desires and activities are self-contradictory and "viciously circular." The victims of *avidya* are thus described as being in the state of *samsara* — the "round" or "whirl" — a life-pattern which, having set itself a self-contradictory goal, revolves or oscillates interminably to the increasing discomfiture of those involved. Thus, self-contradiction rather than deviation from the cultural norm becomes the criterion of mental disease, for which reason this basic difference between Oriental and Western psychology requires some explanation.

Self-contradiction is technically described in Buddhist and Hindu psychology as the human mind in a state of *dvaita*, which is duality or dividedness, a concept rather more inclusive than the approximate Western equivalent of "internal conflict." One of the simplest examples of *dvaita* and its attendant self-contradiction is the making of one's life-goal the acquisition of pleasure and the avoidance of pain. It is pointed out that pleasure and pain are relative experiences, such that a life consisting wholly or even principally of pleasure is as far beyond any possibility of experience as a world in which "everything is up" and nothing down. To the degree that one avoids pain one also eliminates pleasure, and so achieves a way of life that is merely indifferent and boring. Consequently a life devoted to the pursuit of pleasure or happiness is devoted to a self-contradictory goal, because, in so far as one succeeds in gaining pleasure, there is necessarily a proportionate increase in some form of pain — often the simple, but most unpleasant, anxiety of losing what one has gained.

Buddhist psychology, in particular, emphasizes as perhaps *the* major form of self-contradiction a division of experience into subject and object, thinker and thought, feeler and feeling. According to Buddhist psychology, the notion that "I" am in some way different from the feelings which I now feel or the thought which I now think, the notion that man's psycho-organism contains an ego as the enduring subject of a changing panorama of sensations, is an illusion based on memory (*smrti*). The notion of the ego arises because of the apparent phenomenon of self-consciousness, of knowing that one knows, or feeling that one feels. But it is pointed out that, in fact, we are never actually self-conscious. While thought A exists, we are not aware *that* we are aware of thought A. "I am aware that I am aware of thought A" is no longer thought A, but thought B. Every attempt to be aware of being aware is an infinite regress, a vicious circle, like trying to bite one's own teeth. Thought B is not thought A; it is the memory of *having had* thought A, so that one is never aware of an ego which actually "has" (present tense) an experience. There are simply memory-traces of past experiences, and these suggest a continuous ego as a whirled light suggests a continuous circle of fire.

Thus the self or ego of which we claim to be conscious is in fact an abstraction from memory. The real substratum or content of the ego-experience is the memory of what has been, and not the knowledge of what *is*. In fact, then, I am not different from my present complex of thought-feeling-sensation. The difference between "I" and "my experience" is a misinterpretation of the difference between two kinds of experience — memory and immediate awareness. In fact, there is no "I" *apart* from the present, immediate experience. But contradiction arises when we try to make the abstract, conventional, and actually non-existent "I" *do* something. For example, let us suppose that the present feeling is one of acute anxiety. If I "feel" that, apart from this anxiety, there is some separate, subjective ego which "has" this state of mind, efforts of will are made to fight the anxiety or to escape from it; the "I" is opposed to the anxiety. The result, however, is the familiar vicious circle of worry, because the effort to get rid of the anxiety is not

the work of some independent, controlling "I": it is the anxiety itself
— in a state of self-contradiction which only aggravates it.

THE "EGO" AS AN ABSTRACTION

But when it is realized that in fact there is no "I" to be rescued from
anxiety, there follows a psychic relaxation in which the anxiety itself
subsides. This realization is not, of course, a matter of mere theoretical
perception, for it arises, not so much through intellectual self-analysis,
as through a total awareness (*samyaksmrti*) of what and how one
actually feels *now*. Buddhist "psychotherapy" values nothing more than
simple attention to the actual, immediate content of sensation and feeling — as distinct from the verbalized abstractions which thought constructs *about* it. Thus it is understood that "ego" is an abstraction,
and not a content of the immediately perceived world. It is a convenient
abstraction if treated, like the equator, as imaginary. But if treated as
real, as an effective agent, it is only a source of confusion and psychic
self-contradiction.

From the foregoing it might seem that there is one respect in which
Buddhist psychology contradicts itself. It states that the pursuit of
pleasure and the flight from pain is an illusory and impossible life-goal,
and yet it proposes a deliverance from the "general unhappiness" called
duhkha. This reveals an important aspect of the technique of Buddhist
psychology. Stated verbally and formally its "goal" is release from
duhkha, but in actual practice it dispenses with psychological goals
entirely. "Goal" implies futurity, and the object of Buddhist psychology is not future. The object is complete attention to what one feels
now, complete *presence* of mind. This involves the falling away of any
notion of a psychological goal, because it dissipates the sense of the
"I" distinct from the present feeling, and hence of the possibility of
changing or escaping from it. Finding itself "trapped," totally unable to
choose to be other than the "now-state" of the mind, the "I" gives up
or expires (*nirvana*). But this is a case of *stirb und werde* (die and
come to life), of the familiar paradox of the law of reversed effort, of
the creative freedom which comes through "self-surrender."

In our seminar, participants trained in some forms of Western psychotherapy often objected that this "surrender" of the ego would imply
the mere abandonment of the psyche to the lawless direction of the unconscious, and that it was an attempted reversion to the undifferentiated
state of "primitive mentality" in which the conscious and the unconscious are still confused. But such an objection rests on a confusion
between "ego" and "consciousness." For in practice this dissipation of
the ego comes about, not through unconsciousness, but through very

intense consciousness, through the clearest awareness of the present realities of psychic life. Furthermore, the various types of Oriental psychology are not at all afraid of the "lawless direction" of an "unconscious" which has become capable of so great a clarity of consciousness. This may sound paradoxical if it is not understood that in Oriental psychologies such as the Hindu, Buddhist, and Taoist the unconscious is recognized as the source of consciousness, as *that* which is conscious. There should be no difficulty in understanding this when put into its simple physical parallel: we are conscious *with* the brain but not *of* the brain. We simply do not know how we are conscious, how we remember, how we reason, abstract, and perceive *gestalten*. We only know that the autonomic nervous system, for example, effects miracles of organization so complex that the conscious intellect is baffled in attempting to understand them. Oriental psychology feels, then, that the direction of life is basically from those unconscious processes which have thus far organized the marvelous complexity of the human form, and which constellate not only the autonomic nervous system but consciousness, memory, and reason itself. One might ask, then, *what* directions we are to trust if we cannot trust these!

The following quotations from the Chinese Taoist philosopher Chuang-tzu (c. 400 B.C.) aptly express the Oriental attitude to this unconscious process (*Tao*):

Your body is not your own: it is the delegated image of Tao. Your life is not your own: it is the delegated harmony of Tao. Your individuality is not your own: it is the delegated adaptability of Tao. You move, you know not how; you are at rest, you know not why. These are the operations of the laws of Tao.

Things are produced around us, but no one knows the whence. They issue forth, but no one sees the portal. Men one and all value that part of knowledge which is known. They do not know how to avail themselves of the unknown in order to reach knowledge. Is not this misguided?

Tao is not "God" in the personified or conceptualized sense of the West — not a definite *thing*, but a negative concept analogous to the *un*conscious. Chuang-tzu's mentor, Lao-tzu, said: "The Tao which can be defined (lit., tao-*ed*, made its own object) is not the regular Tao." Tao is thus the total process of life which cannot be defined nor made conscious because no standpoint of observation exists outside it.

The foregoing considerations, which were but a few of the topics reviewed in our seminar, suggested two points of application for Western psychotherapy. The first was the therapeutic value of the subjective abandonment of any psychological goals, in the future, coupled with the gentle but persistent focusing of attention on the immediately present totality of feeling-sensation — without any attempt to explain, diagnose, judge, or change it. Oriental psychologies do not particularly value rationalized explanations of *how* a person has come to feel the way he feels, in terms of his past history and conditioning. They do not stress the idea that the perception or understanding of a causal chain, running from the past to the present, effects release from it. For the task of unravelling the conditioning of the present by the past is infinite, since it leads not only to conditioning of the child by the parents, but also to the conditioning of the parents — and the child — by their entire social context. By such means, a thorough psychoanalysis would have to go back to Adam and Eve!

WESTERN "WRONG-AWARENESS"

Their feeling is rather that we are conditioned unconsciously by the past because of an incomplete and incorrect awareness of the present. Such "wrong-awareness" (*avidya*) underlies, in their opinion, one of the basic assumptions of Western thought and science: namely, the whole notion that the past contains the entire explanation of the present, that the understanding of what-is-now is complete in its mere history. For Oriental thought, the past exists only conventionally. It has no real existence, being a logical inference from present memory — an abstraction, and not a real, concrete experience. Therapy consists in releasing the mind from treating the abstract as the concrete, without, however, losing the power of abstraction.

The second point of application goes hand-in-hand with the first. Clear awareness, clear feeling, of one's real and present experience involves, as we saw, the realization that the ego — the continuing "I" as the substratum of changing experiences — is an abstraction and thus not an effective agent.[1] It can no more perform an action or effect a psychological change than, say, an inch or the number three. Yet Western science, and especially applied science (technology), is based on the assumption that its immediate objective is always the understanding and *control* of the environment by the ego. Western culture as a whole rests on the feeling that man, as ego, is the independent observer and potential controller of a world which he experiences as profoundly *other* than himself. Yet it is for this reason that Western technology leads us repeatedly into vicious circles. For if this split between the ego and the environment is unreal, the whole effort of technology

---

[1] It must be understood that we are not here using the terms "I" or "ego" to designate the total human organism. In ordinary speech, as well as in psychological jargon, they are seldom so used, but refer rather to a supposed center of consciousness for which other parts of the organism, such as the glands or the limbs, are objects which the "I" *has* or *uses.*

is like the attempt of a hand to grasp itself. Its ultimate issue is the (almost) totally controlled or planned society — the totalitarian state — which is precisely the breakdown of society because it is based on mutual mistrust. It is the maximum effort of everyone to control everyone and everything else. "Am I my brother's policeman?"

Generally speaking, psychiatry shares most of the unexamined assumptions of Western science. Thus it tends to represent the unconscious as a mass of irrational and chaotic "drives" which have to be organized and controlled by the ego, the conscious. However, the method of control is not that of Protestant Puritanism or Catholic moral theology — the method of whip and spur. It is the much improved method of the humane horse-trainer, who "loves his animals" and gently coaxes them into obedience with lumps of sugar rather than whippings. But from the standpoint of Oriental psychology this is still a quazi-schizoid state of mind. It gives inadequate practical recognition to the fact that consciousness is a function of the unconscious, however much this may be admitted in theory. Man is not dual, the horse and its rider. The relationship of conscious and unconscious is perhaps better represented by the centaur. For it is surely absurd to conceive the unconscious as an un-intelligence, a generator of nothing but colossal blind urges with which "we" must somehow come to terms, for we do not actually know *how* we reason or "will," or attain creative insight — which is only to say that these are, at root, unconscious functions.

"Inspired Spontaneity"

The second point of application is, then, a recognition of the fact that therapy is not the increase of conscious control over the unconscious by the ego. It is rather an integration of conscious and unconscious, preparatory to a type of living, thinking, and acting which in Zen Buddhism is called *mushin* (*mu* "no", *shin* "mind"). *Mushin* is a kind of "inspired spontaneity." It is the art of making the appropriate responses to life without the interruption of that wobbling and indecisive state which we call "choosing." In other words, *mushin* is when acts and decisions are "handed over" to the same unconscious processes which organize the ingenious structure of the body. Ordinarily, our breathing, circulation, hearing, and seeing all happen *mushin* — without the necessity of conscious direction and control. But there are also times when we make a witty remark or get an extremely important idea by the same mysterious process. We did not "try"; it just "came."

Buddhist psychology proposes to facilitate this process to the point where inspired spontaneity is not the exception but the usual mode of thought and action. But as in many other arts, this comes about through a process of growth and a subtle kind of "effortless discipline." It is by no means to be confused with acting wildly — saying or doing the first thing that comes into one's head. Yet thinking or acting "wild" or at random is indeed the starting-point, though, like free-association in the analyst's office, it occurs in a context (i.e., some sort of *ashram* or school) where the resultant vagaries are accepted. In due course, one learns to use *mushin* as a way of action just as one learns the use of any other instrument or faculty which, at first try, seems erratic and unreliable.[2]

In Western psychology, free-association — the nearest thing to *mushin* — has a different objective. The Freudian or Jungian analyst is primarily interested in *what* associations, symbols, and other diagnostic materials are produced in free-association. It is a way of exploring the unconscious in order to control it. In Buddhist psychology the point of interest is rather *that* spontaneous images and symbols are produced. The preliminary vagaries of *mushin* are not analyzed, for *mushin* is being brought into play as a way of life rather than a diagnostic technique. Herein, I believe, is reflected the wide difference between Eastern and Western psychology, the one trusting the unconscious and attempting to liberate the full depth of its wisdom, and the other trying to arrange a treaty wherein the unconscious accepts the control of the ego in return for a certain recognition of its blind demands. But there are signs that this difference is decreasing. Of late many of us have noted the growth of a remarkable humility and readiness to admit ignorance in Western psychiatric circles. For in the course of scientific research there is a long preliminary stage of rapid progress and easy over-confidence, until a point is reached where every addition to our knowledge reveals, at the same time, a new universe of ignorance. Through such knowledge we come to the place of which Chuang-tzu said, "He who knows that he is a fool is not a great fool."

[2] For further information about the techniques of *mushin* see Suzuki, D. T., *The Zen Doctrine of No-Mind* (London, 1949) and *Zen Buddhism and its Influence on Japanese Culture* (Kyoto, 1938), esp. ch. 4. Interesting discussions of the same phenomenon from the standpoint of Western psychology will be found in three articles by E. D. Hutchinson in *Psychiatry*, vols. 2, 3, and 4 (1939, 1940 and 1941) respectively entitled *Varieties of Insight*, *The Period of Frustration in Creative Endeavor* and *The Nature of Insight*.

45

INDIVIDUAL AND SOCIAL CHANGE IN A COMMUNITY UNDER PRESSURE: THE OATH CONTROVERSY

R. NEVITT SANFORD

Vassar College

My concern in this paper is with the role of individual character in producing social change, and with the effects upon the individual of changes in the groups and communities of which he is a part. At the same time, I join those who have urged that the large organization or the small community — a university for example, offers special advantages as a unit for study. This unit is not so large but that the necessary observations can be made, but large enough, and sufficiently complicated in its structure, so that some generalizations derived from its study might hold for the whole society. It is to be urged, however, that this can be true only if the relations of the organization to the larger society are understood and specified.

The University of California, during the period of the so-called Loyalty Oath Controversy, seems to me to lend itself well to such a study. Social and political forces present in the nation at large — in the world at large — forces which could not be described or understood without references to past and current history, were brought directly to bear upon the university, resulting in changes in the social structure as sweeping as they were profound. Yet, if one put his mind to it, it was still possible to keep track of individuals. Some, it appears, had important roles in furthering the major totalitarian trend, others in resistance to it; all were required to adjust, and this for many involved drastic internal reorganization. These adjustments in individuals led directly to changes in social structure — changes which in their turn required new individual adjustments.

The Oath Controversy: A Factual Review

The briefest review of the major events of the crisis will suffice for the present purpose. In March, 1949, the President of the University recommended to the Board of Regents that, in view of apparently

From *The Journal of Social Issues*, 9: No. 3, 1953.

impending attacks upon the university by groups within the state legislature, all employees of the university be required to sign, in addition to the constitutional oath of loyalty, an oath having special reference to the Regents' anti-Communist policy. This recommendation was unanimously adopted by the Board. In June, the Academic Senate (Northern Section) met to consider what action to take. Although there appeared to be much unity of feeling in opposition to the special oath, there were many differences of opinion about grounds for opposition and about what was to be done. Finally, a resolution was passed requesting the president to ask the Regents that the special oath "be deleted or revised in a manner mutually acceptable to the Regents and members of the Academic Senate." The Senate's Advisory Committee (advisory to the president) was instructed to consult with the president "with a view to working out a solution." No solution was immediately forthcoming; and there followed a period — about a year — of negotiation, dispute and compromise. During the first five or six months the faculty marshalled its strength and showed increasing firmness, but the Regents remained unyielding; and then, under great economic pressure and in the absence of widespread public support, the faculty began a slow retreat from its earlier idealistic position and was finally routed altogether when the Regents dismissed 45 of its members.

The dispute was then taken into the courts, where it remained until November of 1952. The final result might be termed a limited victory for academic freedom. But, as so often happens in such cases, so much history had intervened that the final decision had an aspect of anticlimax, if not irrelevance. (The special oath was ruled out, and the dismissed professors were reinstated on the condition that they sign a new oath required of all state employees.)

It needs only to be added that immediately after the defeat of the faculty's political efforts, when they were in a position, so to speak, of having "nothing to lose but their chains," they showed that they were quite unbowed; by their ringing denunciation of the Regents' action, by their rejection of the principle of cooperation against conscience, by their practical steps to support their colleagues who had been dismissed, they recaptured the moral position on which they had first taken their stand.

Virtually all of the facts that are needed for the present purpose have been set forth in *The Year of the Oath* by George Stewart and others.[1] The present paper may be regarded as an effort to add a few footnotes to that work. Naturally it is impossible to do more than touch upon a few aspects of the whole changing picture. As story

[1] George Stewart, *The Year of the Oath*, New York: Doubleday, 1950.

material, I am sure the whole thing is old hat. In another sense, however, it is very much alive; for I believe we have here excellent examples of social processes of wide generality and considerable significance. I should like to make one effort to exploit some of this material for social science before it fades altogether from my mind.

The social changes to which my title refers include such practical matters as decline in the output of research and in the quality of teaching, such formal organizational matters as changes in routes of communication and in the occupancy of committee chairmanships, such social matters as the splitting of the community first into two groups, then into several, and finally into numerous splinter groups, or the increased cohesion in some departments and the disruption in others, and finally, such changes in the organization of social roles as the decline and disappearance of some leaders and the emergence of others, the breaking up of some friendship groups and the formation of others, changed attitudes toward the president, changed attitudes of students toward professors, and so on. Various social science disciplines have at their disposal the means for describing with some precision states of affairs in all these areas; I am reasonably sure that a systematic study of the California incident in its temporal aspect would yield many hypotheses concerning the conditions of change; and that in a recurrence of a similar incident it would actually be possible to *predict* changes in formal organization, in role structure, and so on.

As for what happened to individuals, *The Year of the Oath* reports, on the basis of systematic interviewing: worry, depression, fatigue, fear, insomnia, drinking, headache, and indigestion; failure to function well, worsening of relations with colleagues, suspicion, distrust, loss of self-respect. One might say that we were offered a remarkable opportunity to study the dependence of mental health, and ill health, upon factors in the contemporary situation. For myself, accustomed to focus mainly on historical (life history) determinants of ill-health, the experience was an eye-opener.

Unfortunately, it is not possible to go very far into these matters in the space at our disposal or from the limited perspective of a psychologist. I have chosen to confine myself to three general topics, first, personality factors as determinants of the individual's role in the production of social change; second, personality factors as determinants of the ways in which other individuals and groups are perceived in a crisis, and of the role requirements made upon them; and, third, some changes in the inner household of the individual attendant upon conflict and disruption in the social groups of which he is a member.

PERSONALITY FACTORS AS DETERMINANTS OF ROLE SELECTION

The chapter entitled "Life in the Ivory Tower" in *The Year of the Oath* begins with a rather charming analogy. The academic community at Berkeley is likened to the Indian tribe who used to inhabit that same area, and the onslaught of the University's regents is seen as analogous to the encroachment upon the Indians of the all-powerful Spaniards. The councils in the sweathouse might well have resembled some of those which took place in our Faculty Club. "Doubtless some of them, uncompromising, counseled resistance, and others pointed out that resistance against such power was mere suicide. Doubtless some advised flight; others, abject submission. . . . If the period of strain was long extended . . . we can only believe that many tribesmen became acutely depressed, that old friends quarreled, that certain renegades went over to the enemy, and that a kind of general disintegration set in . . ."

This analogy, though subject to revision as we shall see, has the very great merit of regarding the California dispute as but an instance of something that is very general; it invites us to seek the general laws of group conflict and of group change under pressure. More than that, it invites us to consider the role of individual character in determining the course of events; for surely the tribesmen who were advising this or that kind of action were governed largely by their individual personality structures.

Our book on *The Authoritarian Personality* [2] was published in the midst of the loyalty oath controversy. A colleague, from the Department of Speech, who knew this work — and who was evidently mistaking an outward calm for scientific disinterestedness — said to me, "This must be a perfect laboratory set-up for you." Many of us psychologists, in casual conversation, have spoken of the California incident as if the community had suffered an infestation of authoritarian personalities, or as if those authoritarian personalities normally to be found in such a setting, among Regents and academicians alike, had somehow got the upper hand. At the same time, however, some reviewers of our book have stated that this research represented a "personality approach," in contradistinction to some other kind of approach — presumably an historical or a social or economic one. The question, of course, is how far do factors of personality enter into matters such as this Loyalty Oath Controversy? And granting that they do enter in, how do they take their place within the framework of history and socio-economic process?

[2] T. W. Adorno, Else Frenkel-Brunswik, D. J. Levinson, and R. N. Sanford, *The Authoritarian Personality*. New York: Harper, 1949.

Let us consider, first, some hypotheses concerning the behavior of the Regents. It may be that in requiring the special oath they behaved wisely, with a full grasp of the realities of the situation. This hypothesis need not detain us, however, for the fact remains that they acted in such a way as to get large sections of the faculty up in arms; and finding themselves opposed, they resorted to policies and tactics that were unmistakably totalitarian.

It must be pointed out first —and this is the main trouble with the analogy of the Indian tribe — that the Regents were actually a part of the university community. They certainly belonged with the tribe rather than with the Spaniards; strictly speaking, or constitutionally speaking, they were the tribal chiefs. To use another analogy, they were very important members of our "university family." (If you suspect that this analogy will be overworked before we are through, I am afraid you are right.) The attack on the University from outside was apparently building up among the Spaniards in the state legislature. The Regents and the University Administration, acting in their role of tribal chiefs, sought to ward off the attack by appeasement, or even by collaborationist activities. Hence, we never did see in the California dispute that drawing together of the whole community such as we expect to see when the enemy is outside and clearly perceived. Instead we saw a deep division within the ranks, such as occurs in modern states whose wars are not only tribal or nationalistic but ideological; everybody, Regents and Faculty alike, had to be concerned with internal as well as external enemies. More than this, those members of the Faculty who wished to fight the external enemy found themselves opposed by established authority, and had thus to engage in activity of a revolutionary sort. George Stewart remarks at another place that if the Regents had chosen to *lead* a fight against the outside enemies of the University, they would have found the Faculty behind them to a man. The struggle in fact was essentially a civil one, and hence more complicated and disturbing; the emotional implications of such strife go very deep, divisions within the social group or body politic leading inevitably to divisions within the individual personality. This is a matter to which we shall revert later on.

The attribution of authoritarianism to the Regents seems at first glance justified on two grounds: they adopted an attitude of authoritarian submission toward an imagined public opinion — the outside enemy; and they adopted an attitude of authoritarian aggression toward those under their governance. Yet I believe we should be exceedingly cautious about the assignment of personality determinants of these actions, and we should reject altogether the easy supposition that these authoritarian actions were merely the work of authoritarian personalities.

To dramatize the issue somewhat I should like to suggest that it is very instructive to consider the California dispute from a Marxist point of view. George Stewart's valuable research on the individual members of the Board of Regents makes it very easy to apply to them the "ruling class" concept. And the whole course of events, from the beginning up to the time of a lower court's decision in favor of the Faculty, seemed to be toward a polarity, with the Regents as representatives of established economic power at one pole, an economically dependent, spiritless, "proletarianized" group of academic employees at the other. This movement certainly had an appearance of inevitability, and it must be said that some people on our side seemed ready to adapt themselves to, if not to help along, this historical arrangement of forces.

The major fault with this version is the consideration that a group of small business men, small farmers, labor leaders, professional men, and former academicians or university presidents — to approximate George Stewart's ideal board — would probably have behaved very much as our Regents did. They would now have been men in public life, and in the prevailing circumstances, they could not have afforded to permit their anti-Communist valor to become suspect. Moreover, there was no evidence to suggest that any of the Regents consciously attempted to manipulate things in such a way as to serve immediate economic ends; there were political motives, to be sure, but here what was to be observed was sensitivity to that public opinion in which they themselves participated even as they helped to create it.

As the struggle proceeded the Regents, of course, became more and more totalitarian in their actions. This, I think, is best understood in field-theoretical terms. They were in a position corresponding somewhat to that of a teacher before a rebellious and misunderstood class. The more things threatened to get out of hand the more rigid they became, and the more rigid they became the greater was the actual danger of a break-out somewhere, and so on.

This view of the Regents' behaviour tends to de-emphasize group membership determinants and to accent the general psychology of response to social role, to the momentary face-to-face group situation and to trends of opinion in the country at large. Farther back in the history of the dispute, when threats to the university were building up in the state legislature, the matter would be otherwise, for there, it seemed clear, some classical authoritarian types could be seen at work. As far as the Regents' behaviour is concerned, the most that can be said for authoritarianism in personality is that it probably gave rise to certain susceptibilities and readinesses, e.g., the stronger the authoritarian disposition the earlier did a Regent adopt a rigid attitude toward the rebellious faculty. If, however, a program for selecting regents or trustees on the basis of psychological tests were to be adopted, then some sort of equivalent of our scale for measuring authoritarian trends ought probably to be included in the battery.

When it comes to the faculty and other members of the university staff, the matter is much the same. Probably few who knew the university would disagree with George Stewart's statement that "the faculty was representative of the general population, exhibiting the same range of political opinion and social outlook." This means that had a scale for measuring authoritarianism been administered to our faculty a wide range of scores would have been obtained. And, I suppose, one might have expected a relationship between amount of authoritarianism and the stage at which the oath was signed. But such a relationship could not have been very close, for a great variety of potent factors, including especially factors other than personal inclination, operated to determine when a given individual would sign the oath. One might say that had the mean F-scale been high, and dispersion slight, there would have been no controversy in the first place; so large a proportion would have signed at the start that organized opposition would have been impossible. But it is doubtful that a corresponding low mean score would have made a crucial difference.

The point to emphasize is that we are concerned here with a more or less normal distribution of authoritarianism, with a mean probably lower than would be found in the population at large. The question is, how do authoritarian trends in personality exert their influence in such circumstances as we are considering? A general formulation might be as follows. In the whole complex of events, situations arise which act as stimuli for the authoritarianism latent in us all; in such circumstances the more authoritarian personalities are the first to respond, and they carry other slightly less authoritarian personalities along with them; then, they proceed to help transform the situation in such a way that the stimulus for authoritarian response is greater than it was before. Meanwhile, those who have responded, under strong stimulation, in an authoritarian way find it very difficult to get back to where they were in the first place; a certain commitment has been made, and they find themselves involved in an authoritarian structure. Those who cannot adapt themselves tend to leave the field, and the structure becomes self-perpetuating.

Let us return to the first meeting of the Academic Senate, in June 1949, when the strong resolution that the special oath be deleted suffered amendment and the Advisory Committee was instructed to consult with the President with a view to working out a solution. Concerning this meeting George Stewart and his collaborators have this to say. ". . . The faculty makes an important parliamentary mistake, which is to vex them later and perhaps fatally to injure their cause; viz., certain members believe the Advisory Committee has been entrusted with power to act, while other members believe that the Committee has been given power only to *consult* and refer the matter back to the Senate" and, in another place, "If the faculty had firmly asked in June what it asked in September, or in September what it asked in November, the controversy might have ended at that point."

How did it happen that despite great unity of feeling in support of a clear and firm resolution, the faculty actually emerged from the meeting formally on record as indecisive, willing to consider compromise on principle, and deeply divided? There were, to be sure, technical and accidental factors, such as the unfamiliarity of liberal members — who, as might be expected, had attended too few faculty meetings — with Senate rules and parliamentary procedure, but there is strong evidence that the main trouble was psychological. Amid the rousing speeches in defense of democratic rights, there was occasionally heard a voice urging caution; e.g., "The Regents would not have proposed this if they had not had good reason," or "We must not declare war on the Regents," and when it came to the question of just how to proceed, these voices grew more confident; "We must go through regular, established channels." These voices, for the most part as it seemed, came from men who were in some sense close to the administration, or who held important administrative posts, or who had done notable work as members of important committees. They were the voices of soundness, of conservatism. We must not be hasty with the diagnosis of authoritarian personality trends. There are role determinants to be considered. It seems very likely that some men, in urging caution, were doing no more than fulfilling the requirements of their roles within the university structure. And that in the acceptance of these roles authoritarianism within the personality was of no particular importance. Yet, the occasion was heavily charged with emotion; men were most certainly responding in accordance with reaction systems that went pretty deep. In so far as there were authoritarian personalities among us, I do not think we need doubt which way they were inclined. But *most* of us listened to the words of caution; we didn't want to do anything foolish; perhaps we didn't want to be identified with those among us who seemed a little too eager to engage in an all-out war against the Regents. We wanted to be "reasonable." I suppose it is no longer news that totalitarian movements gain their staunchest supporters, in time, from the ranks of the law-abiding citizens, and probably it is in just such situations as this, situations in which various accidental factors could seem to have dictated the choice, that irrevocable steps are taken.

What I am really suggesting, then, is that in situations of this kind we should focus not so much on particular personalities as on *kinds of behaviour*. It may be granted that mistaken actions will orginate more readily in some personalities than in others, but it is *actions* — their determinants and their consequences — that should command our first attention, for there is the danger that they will be evoked in any of us.

Unconscious Factors as Determinants of How Others Are Perceived

One of the major factors making for strain throughout the California controversy was our inability to predict what was going to happen. We rarely had the satisfaction, the ego-supporting experience, of seeing things go according to expectations. We were forever being surprised, taken aback; unable to anticipate happenings, we had to be prepared for anything — which amounted to being fully prepared for nothing. These, of course, are the circumstances of panic. Fear, such as would have been appropriate to real danger, tended to be replaced by anxiety, and accordingly, the reaction systems of early childhood were aroused and tended more and more to influence our imagery of those about us — the Regents, the president, colleagues, students, the general public. The more such imagery came to dominate our perceptions, the less well were we able to predict. A vicious circle was complete.

The Regents of course were central in all this. Our whole strategy depended essentially on how we sized them up. Now there was — and is — a standing order of the Regents that no member of the faculty may communicate directly with a Regent; and since for a very long time the Regents had caused no special trouble, they were in the minds of most of us very shadowy figures. And so, as feeling mounted in the June meeting, the stage was well set for projection. It was apparent from the speeches that were made that imagery of the Regents varied widely. At one extreme was the imagery of them as wise and benevolent "elder statesmen" who would do nothing but what they, after sober thought, had decided was best for the University. At the other extreme was imagery of them as erstwhile "robber barons," who had now cynically taken on a garb of respectability and public service, while remaining hand-in-glove with the powerful economic interests of the state. The prevailing view, and the one that was too crucially determining, was that they were at least reasonable men, and that a "mature" approach was not to go off half-cocked, but calmly to talk things over with them. If we behaved ourselves we would be treated with justice; with some sternness perhaps, but certainly with justice.

This imagery of the Regents persisted for a long time; it withstood several striking demonstrations that as a group they deviated very considerably from what was imagined. There were, no doubt, a number of men in important faculty positions who had already come to terms with power and were for peace with the Regents at any price, but in my opinion their influence would not have been very important but for the very widespread and deeply rooted feeling that good behaviour would be rewarded — that the Regents in the end would enact the role of judicious authority. We cannot doubt but that men have to be sorely tried before they will undertake to throw off the restraints of constituted authority. The cry "we must put our trust in the good faith of the Regents" lasted beyond the time when objective evidence argued to the contrary.

As the Regents, by their actions, moved into the unmistakable position of "the enemy" there appeared a tendency to dwell in fantasy upon their overwhelming power and ruthlessness. During some months of the controversy an important question for strategy was how many non-signers of the oath would the Regents fire rather than retreat from their position. *Five hundred* was a more or less official estimate at one time — the estimate of a committee selected to lead the faculty's fight. I think it is fair to say that men — I mean here *men* and not women (who were less prone to this kind of persecution imagery) who had earlier over-estimated the "good father" aspects of the Regents were the very ones who tended now to over-estimate the ruthless power aspect. The two kinds of imagery are not unrelated. At one meeting a professor, in urging his colleagues to sign the oath and thus accept a compromise proposed by his committee, asserted that the Regents would fire 500 before they would give in *and* that all should put their trust in the good faith of the Regents.

At the start and for a long time the Regents were conceived as a unit; after a number of Regents' meetings had been reported in the press, it became apparent that they themselves were sharply divided. Here we seemed to borrow a page from Melanie Klein. We conceived of "bad" Regents who would give no quarter at all, and "good" Regents who supported the position of the majority of the faculty. It now became possible to hate the "bad" Regents and love the "good" ones. This was an aid to our internal equilibrium. But the greatest care had to be taken lest in opposing the "bad" Regents someone would go too far and alienate the "good" Regents.

The analogy — one might almost say the fact — of the "University family" once again seems more fitting than the analogy of the Indians and the Spaniards. The family analogy was employed in a rather striking way by the leader of the "bad Regents." At one stage of the dispute — a fairly late stage — a compromise appeared to have been reached. The arrangement was that the non-signing professors were to have hearings by the Faculty Committee on Privilege and Tenure, whose recommendations for firing or retention were to be followed by the Regents. Protesting this arrangement Mr. X angrily exclaimed, "They will tell their brothers, but they won't tell us." This traditionalist has a right to bemoan the fact that in so far as we in America are moving in the direction of totalitarianism, the instrument for enforcing conformity becomes more and more the peer culture rather than traditional authority; but Mr. X ought to realize that the major fault lies with him and his kind; instead of exercising the father role to lead us toward worthy objectives which we all can share, they too often exploit our natural trust, in the interests of power and security for themselves alone.

It would, of course, be wrong to attempt to describe the controversy mainly as a family drama. There were no doubt other determinants, in our culture and in the climate of opinion, of how the Regents were perceived, and there was, after all, reality. The present thesis is simply that such emotional undercurrents as I have indicated were always there — to favor misperceptions and to render clear thinking difficult. As pressure mounted and frustration increased, as any way out seemed increasingly remote, as one's identity as a professor was threatened, then perceptions of the scene tended increasingly to be influenced by unconscious fantasies.

We find a very similar state of affairs when we come to consider imagery of the President. Abraham Flexner quotes a man whom he describes as a "wise philanthropist, head of a great business, and trustee of a University" as saying, "A man may be president of a trans-continental railroad, an international banking corporation, a far-flung business, but the presidency of a great university is an impossible post." Sociology has provided us with a nice under-statement of the case: the post involves by its very nature a conflict of roles. One might suggest, again borrowing from sociology, that we have to do here with a "cultural lag." The post seems to have been nicely designed in the beginning for an educator with a philosophy of his own who could lay down conditions for accepting the post, win the support of his faculty and push through a program. But the day of the "strong president" seems to be about over. (How many of us could name more than 4 or 5 university presidents? The smile is familiar, but I can't remember the name! The situation seems to be somewhat better with the colleges.) Either of the president's roles — appointee and voting member of the Regents or chairman of the Academic Senate would seem to be enough to all but dominate a strong personality. The university president today seems usually to be enmeshed in a vast machinery; decisions of necessity tend to be purely administrative or political.

And yet the emotional need for a strong president persists. Just as on the national scene the President remains as the vehicle for the hopes and aspirations of the people, despite his steadily decreasing freedom of movement, so with faculties in times of crisis: the need is for a sanctioned leader behind whom all can rally. So I think it was with us anyway. We kept hoping the President would do something; we cherished the illusion that he *was* doing something, long after our better judgment should have told us that we were asking for the impossible. Our hopes went up or down as reports filtered out of the Regents' meetings that he had been weak or strong, had stood up well or poorly. There were efforts to exempt him from the skullduggery that was frequently ascribed to "the administration." In short, I think there was a widespread tendency to project onto the President imagery of the "good father." Or, perhaps, somewhat more realistically, on the part of some, that of the "elder brother." The Regents, of course, had more or less pre-empted the role of "bad father," but at times when it appeared that the President was their ally, he too shared in this projection. I would not exclude the possibility that the President stood, in some of our minds, as a "mother figure." This hypothesis might, as a matter of fact, help explain the persistent hope and belief that the President could somehow intercede with the Regents, or take some sort of lead in the struggle for democratic rights. Perhaps our training in American culture was such that it was difficult to believe that mother could get nowhere with father or would not sooner or later speak up for idealism. The precise nature of the imagery would, of course, make little difference; the point is that in our somewhat regressed state, deeper emotional trends influenced the role requirements made upon others and distorted our perceptions of them, thus interfering palpably with the effective pursuit of our purpose.

What "public opinion" is — what "the people" think or will do — is, I suppose, always an excellent screen for projection. In the present instance it was generally assumed that the public would feel little sympathy for our cause, and in a sense this was correct, for within two years the voters of the state were to support a loyalty oath rather overwhelmingly. But this does not mean that we had any special insight into the workings of the public mind, or that we — many of us — were not right for the wrong reasons. In general, I think we committed the unpardonable political error of over-estimating popular information and under-estimating popular intelligence. For tactical reasons, no effort was made to carry the issue to the public until very late in the day; and then rather gingerly, cautiously, defensively. "Don't make any public statements" became an almost daily warning to non-signers; there was the implied danger that if they sounded off about democratic rights the people would think they *were* Communists. Yet, so complete was our pre-occupation with the dispute, we tended unconsciously to assume that others knew about it too. In my own experience I never encountered anyone outside the academic community who had more than the vaguest notion of what the dispute was about, but who could not be brought to see, after five minutes' explanation, the justice of our cause. (This is not to say, of course, that he would have voted on our side.)

As members of the academic profession we permit ourselves, from time to time, a certain measure of contempt for other people, not so much for the "mass" of people, as for the semi-educated, perhaps especially for the alumni — the products of our work! — who do most to determine policy in our country. We thus have reason to suppose that the feeling is mutual. And we are well aware, from both subjective and objective evidence, of a traditional hostility toward "teacher." These things, combined with such knowledge as we had about the general climate of opinion, were enough to make us suspect general disapproval. Once a man had fully identified himself with the opposition to the oath he felt himself to be in the role of a non-conformist, so far as the general public was concerned. The tendency toward contempt was now reinforced, for it served as a mechanism of defense.

As evidence that unwarranted assumptions about public disapproval actually injured our cause I may cite the following. Lawyers on our faculty spoke frequently in our meetings, and almost always, it seemed to me, to the effect that we would not stand a chance in court — and especially not if we stood on constitutional grounds. Now since our state constitution says clearly that the university shall be kept free of political influence and that there shall be no oath of office other than the long-standing constitutional one, the clear implication was that the court would somehow be guided by a prevalent public opinion. When the appellate court decided for the faculty, and with a clear stand on constitutional ground, the lawyers had no recourse but to say it was a poor decision from a legal point of view. But the damage had been done. The persistent thought that we had no chance in court had a depressing effect upon morale.

I am not saying that an all-out campaign of publicity could have won the day (though I keep thinking of how the Alien and Sedition Laws were repealed); but it does seem that we worried ourselves more than was necessary with our imagery of the general public, and that we expressed less faith in democracy than is healthy.

It is remarkable how little, in the various discussions of the California dispute, has been said about the students. One might suppose that in a study of a University community, students would have a very important role. Actually, in the California incident student opinion counted not at all. If the student was a teaching or research assistant and so had to sign the oath, he was lost in the shuffle; his, so to speak, was a second class conscience. Perhaps, this is a reflection of the tendency in our culture to prolong adolescence, and to regard college students as in no important sense grown up. Our students, like most, were either somewhat radical or generally passive, that is to say, conservative. The best ones, that is, those in whom we could see something of ourselves, were, of course, more on the radical side. They, therefore, represented those parts of our personality that urged us to do something bold and foolish — and noble. They made us anxious. They had, of course, to be held in check, lest they arouse anger in the "bad regents" or timidity in the "good ones." Naturally, they made many of us wonder whether we were being true to ourselves.

Changes in the Individual

We may now turn to consider briefly some effects of changes in the community upon the internal structure of the individual. The outstanding fact about a special oath is that it necessarily creates a conflict of conscience both in those who take it and in those who do not. This was pointed out to us at our first meeting by a European colleague who had witnessed the destruction of the German and Italian universities — very largely with the use of oaths — under Hitler and Mussolini. In our case a number of people signed the oath more or less right away. There were various reasons. Some regarded it as "Just a piece of paper," some sympathized with the Regents' action, some — perhaps most — thought with good reason that economic sanctions would be immediate, some, in the general confusion of that first summer, thought that the Academic Senate had officially approved the oath. When it became clear that the faculty, as an organized body, was going to make an issue of it, these men were immediately divided within themselves. On the one hand, there were the demands of loyalty to one's colleagues, and on the other, the need to justify one's action or to uphold the principles that had led to signing the oath. Some warded off guilt feelings by working long and hard to effect the repeal of the oath and supporting their non-signing colleagues to the end; others, though working for repeal of the oath, were perhaps overeager for a settlement, and thus too ready to compromise the principles which others were upholding; still others — relatively few, I think — repressed the guilt feelings and grew increasingly impatient with uncompromising colleagues; at least one went over completely to the Regents, writing a letter to show his solidarity with them and his rejection of the faculty position.

Non-signers of the oath had, I think, during the first months of the controversy a relatively easier time of it. They had the satisfaction of having taken a conscientious position in defense of traditional principles of freedom, and they had the support not only of their most highly respected colleagues but of the voting majority in the Academic Senate. But as time went on their position became increasingly difficult. As the Academic Senate began voting in favor of compromises with the Regents, non-signers began to find themselves not only without the full support of their official body, but actually divided among themselves. After the Academic Senate had voted, when the dispute was about nine months old, to uphold the Regents' policy excluding Communists from positions in the University, thus giving up the principles of "no political test" and "no guilt by association" (in the belief that this would end the controversy), those individuals who still felt bound to stand on these principles found themselves in dissent not only from the Regents but from the great majority of their own colleagues. And even those who preferred to remain uncompromising with respect to the principle that only teachers may judge the competence of teachers, or who had other good reasons for not signing the oath, found themselves becoming increasingly isolated from the larger academic community. At times when some particular strategy or some particular compromise was being urged by the leadership of the Senate, the appeal to the non-signers was on the basis of faculty unity or "love of the university," i.e., signing the oath at a particular time, it was urged, would spare the university the worst damage. Here then, there was conflict between the demands of individual conscience or, as some would have it, pride, and the need for conformity with the immediate and highly valued group. In other words the non-signer was forced to wonder whether in insisting on the luxury of a clear individual conscience he was not letting his colleagues down.

We might say, then, that both signers and non-signers suffered from moral unsupport. (It might be inserted here that the distinction between signers and non-signers should not be over-drawn. Whether or not a person signed the oath, and when, was a function of many factors; not least, economic ones. Hence, when it comes to assigning virtue, as you and I would conceive it today, the signer-non-signer dimension would be far from a complete guide. What mattered most psychologically, as it seemed, was whether or not —and the degree to which — a person was allied in spirit with the non-signers.) Almost everybody involved, let us say, suffered moral unsupport; and I think we may say that in almost everybody changes — conflict or splitting — in internal object or agency followed immediately upon, and were determined by, conflict and splitting in the surrounding community.

We are, of course, accustomed to the idea that the establishment of a strong conscience requires a long series of reinforcements by external agencies; which reinforcements presumably decrease in importance as the individual matures. Many of us, however, have not been accustomed to paying much attention to the continuous reliance of the more or less mature and enlightened conscience upon external reinforcing agencies. Perhaps in times of relative social stability the phenomenon is not easy to observe; and it is rare that we have the opportunity to observe what happens under social disorganization. In recent years we have been much enlightened, I think, by the observations made within the concentration camps, by Bettelheim and others. The author of *Dungeon Democracy*,[3] for example, remarks that men whose nations were still fighting in the war stood up better, in the concentration camp, than men whose nations had gone down through occupation or internal collapse. In the present instance, I think the same processes were at work, though in a situation far less extreme.

But we seem hardly to have accounted in full for the serious internal disturbances that occurred. The split within the faculty community was the more serious for the individual the more exclusively he had come to rely on that community. And such reliance was made necessary for most, it seemed, not only because they were opposing the authority of the Regents but because of the disapproval, real or imagined, of the public at large. It was probably this latter, as much as anything, that threatened one's identity as a professor; and if one's professional colleagues were going to be divided and therefore weak where could strength be found? I am afraid that today the first question the typical professor asks himself in a moral crisis is: what are the others going to do?

Can we in this day and age conceive of an individual conscience that is both enlightened and so firmly internalized that it can endure without external support? Can we without resorting to the concepts of psychopathology? I should doubt it. The present episode did not provide a crucial test of this question, and let us hope that we never see the experiment undertaken. There were, as we have seen, men and women who held out against the oath despite the power of the Regents, the disapproval — real or imagined — of the general public, the impatience of the faculty leadership, and even the solicitous urgings of respected

[3] Burney, C. *Dungeon Democracy*. New York: Sloan and Pearce, 1946.

colleagues. But they were not, I think, without external support. They had each other, they had staunch friends outside the university, they had the support — and knowledge of the hopes and expectations — of colleagues at other universities and colleges; they, in many cases, had their wives or husbands, and they had the remembered promptings of admired figures in more remote times and places. Last ditch non-signers sometimes joked among themselves about the interesting psychological study they as a group would make. But I am not aware that this needed research was ever undertaken. One hypothesis may be suggested: that they were all in some sense *inner directed*, to use David Riesman's term. And another thing: I think most still had roots in some other community or culture than mid-century Berkeley; some had not been at Berkeley long enough to become fully integrated into the university community, others perhaps were just not altogether capable of being integrated. There was also the factor of having other identities besides that of university professor. And finally there was the factor of knowledge, at least a sense of familiarity with what was going on, than which there is no greater supporter of the ego; this, it seems safe to say, was greater on the average in this group than in the faculty at large. Perhaps it was not so much knowledge as an irresistible impulse to take an analytic view of things. One professor, who has published a statement about the controversy and his position in it, lists among his reasons for not signing the oath his curiosity about what would happen to him.

On the whole, it seems to me, the events I have described lend support to those theorists who have sought to conceptualize the internal community, the personality, in terms that could also be applied to the external community. You will have noticed some attempts at this kind of thinking in this paper.

Since in taking an oath, if one does so seriously and willingly, one gives over part of his individual conscience to those who require the oath, it follows that one is not the same afterward; one has introjected a new object; and it is reasonable to say that that agency, group or institution *is* conscience, and it is not so important any longer to say whether it is inside or outside the individual. The Regents, who those who opposed them, were clearly an external persecutor, but since response to them depended on how they were perceived, and how they were perceived depended on what was projected onto them, one might say that the external persecutor was also inside the personality. I needn't remind you of the projected father, mother, and sibling imagery, or of the spirited students who had to be responded to as if they were some of our own impulses. And as we have just seen, the "good conscience" which could make us joyful or depressed, depending on whether we felt it was for us or against us, tended more and more as the pressure increased to find residence in external representatives.

Just one more example. *The Year of the Oath* reports many instances of suspicion — founded and unfounded — among the opponents of the oath. This suspicion centered mainly on colleagues or members of the administration who might have "gone over to the enemy" or who seemed not to be doing their part in the struggle although they appeared to be friends. Now, in so far as a man had tendencies to defection which he could not accept in himself he would be disposed to see such tendencies in others. Thus, one might say, if there had been no traitors it might well have been necessary to invent them. But there *were* traitors. As one colleague pointed out, "You can't call it paranoia when one's suspicions are in accordance with the fact." But you can say that the presence of real external traitors made the internal one the more difficult to manage, and that the amount of hostility directed to the external traitor depended in part on the strength of this internal "bad object."

I still say it is difficult to apply these concepts in the analysis of ordinary human relations, or to human relations in ordinary times. Surely they would never have been thought of had their creators studied only smoothly functioning adult communities. It is in children that the boundaries between the inner and the outer worlds are vague and highly permeable; in children, and in men who have been so reduced by real pressure that modes of reaction appropriate to childhood begin to make their appearance on the scene.

The *Year of the Oath* is replete with slightly apologetic references to our lapses in judgment, our inability to think clearly. In my opinion, it is not too much to say that at times we went so far as to take over the methods of "the enemy" — the Regents. This was particularly apparent in faculty demands for unity — no matter what the basis — and in the arrangement by which our Committee on Privilege and Tenure was to get men to "tell their brothers what they would not tell their father." Psychoanalytic theory, like the Greeks, has a name for this: identification with the aggressor. It seems pretty clear that this process was at work. But it must also be borne in mind that as the professor behaved more like the administration and the administration more like the Regents and the Regents more like the politburo the similarities in behavior may have been due to similarities in the stimulus situation. Still, I think Thomas Mann was right! The worst evil of totalitarianism is that it forces its victims to adopt its methods.

CONCLUSION

I shall close with a comment about the role of social science and of psychology in matters such as the loyalty oath controversy. At one point in the struggle, when the faculty was rather desperately engaged, a colleague proposed a novel strategy. Everybody would sign the oath except two or three "honorary non-signers," men of great distinction and unquestioned ideological purity. This would rob the Regents of numerous attractive victims and offer them, if they held their ground, only the most unpalatable fare.

This strategy was not only very clever; it had a fascinating conspiratorial quality. But it was hooted down by the assembled non-signers. "Why," they asked, "if we cannot, because of principle, sign the oath for the Regents, should we sign it for the sake of this dubious strategy?" Later, of course, many of these same non-signers were to be forced to accept the principle implicit in this strategy — the principle that it is all right to sacrifice a few individual consciences for the good of the group. As I have said, however, this principle was rejected by the faculty in the end.

Now, what I wonder is whether it was more than an accident that the man who proposed this strategy was a social scientist. I wonder, indeed, if we do not see here a weak spot in the social science outlook, the spot where regression begins when pressure is applied. Social science easily acquires the habit of considering individuals as members of groups; it frequently seems to argue that individuals should lose themselves in groups; how often will it end by casually sacrificing a few individuals for the sake of the group?

Social science is never completely detached from value. It is perfectly proper to ask how social science might be instrumental in the realization of democratic values. But I would suggest that we pay at least as much attention to the values as to the instruments. It is all right for the social scientist to ask how a university might rid itself of a loyalty oath. (It is not all right for social science to lend itself to those who wish to impose one. This would be to say not only that science has nothing to do with value but that science has no interest in humanity.) But suppose we have accepted the task of countering by scientific means the attacks upon the universities. We should strive, it seems to me, to include within our considerations the broadest possible context of values; human affairs being, to say the least, very complex, we as social scientists have to be very careful lest in our efforts to achieve by the means of science a particular end we do not endanger, or impair, other values which have some necessary, if obscure, relation to our means. Events such as the loyalty oath controversy offer great opportunities for observations *in medias res*. But they do not favor the detachment that is necessary. The next time a situation such as that which prevailed in Berkeley in June 1949 seems about to develop, a team of social scientists, not attached to the university in question and with ample foundation support, should appear on the scene immediately. They would not, of course, be unconcerned about the outcome; but they would view matters in the largest perspective, entertaining a great variety of hypotheses, including outrageous ones. In our situation such scientists might have asked, for example, whether individual liberty might not have been better preserved had there been no organized opposition to the oath at all. Their answer would probably have been in the negative — but there is no certainty.

As for the role of psychology — it would be out of keeping with the whole spirit and direction of this paper if I did not conclude by saying that psychology can make its major contribution, not by planning an over-all strategy, but by recognizing, and pointing out, those instances in which reaction systems brought over from infancy intrude themselves, to interfere with the best laid plans of normally reasonable men.

46

AN OPERATIONAL CONCEPTION OF CRIMINAL RESPONSIBILITY

RICHARD G. BOARD, M.D.

Washington, D. C.

In the Isaac Ray Award book, *The Psychology of the Criminal Act and Punishment*, Gregory Zilboorg summarizes a long-standing situation regarding criminal responsibility:

. . . yet no solution of the problem has yet been found. We all, or almost all, agree that the method under discussion is deficient, but no sufficiently workable change has as yet been suggested. Here is an example of our earnest but inefficient groping in the matter.

This passage describes a kind of puzzlement we feel when attempting to solve a problem without adequate conceptual tools — the kind of puzzlement we might feel, for example, in trying to solve problems regarding motion without knowing the concept of acceleration. The example of inefficient groping referred to was a fairly recent suggestion by a leading physician in England.

The time is surely come to determine afresh in what circumstances mental illness should mitigate criminal responsibility.

Like most of our endeavors in this area, this suggestion directs our attention toward establishing new criteria for determining criminal responsibility rather than toward investigating the logical content of the concept of criminal responsibility itself. This venerable concept has remained essentially unanalyzed since our ancestors first formulated it. We cannot hope to dispel the appalling prejudice that envelops this subject until we have attained a logical analysis of criminal responsibility which places us on firm theoretical ground. This article attempts such an analysis.

The Monte Durham Decision, recently rendered by the District Court of Appeals of the District of Columbia, holds that a person whose criminal act was the result of mental illness or defect cannot be regarded as criminally responsible. The court was explicit in its statement that establishing criminal responsibility has always been concerned with rendering a moral judgment of the criminal:

From *The American Journal of Psychiatry*, October 1956.

. . . we permit it [the jury] to perform its traditional function which . . . is to apply our inherited ideas of moral responsibility to individuals prosecuted for crime. Juries will continue to make moral judgments still operating under the fundamental precept that "our collective conscience does not allow punishment where it cannot impose blame."

The sequence to judgment is this: If an individual is criminally responsible, he is morally responsible, and if he is morally responsible he can be judged morally guilty. Consequently a judgment of guilty currently means 2 things: (1) The accused committed the crime; (2) the accused was morally guilty in committing the crime. All of the law's endeavors to establish criteria for determining criminal responsibility, from the M'Naghten rule to the Durham decision, have as their purpose the selection of those who can be appropriately subjected to a moral judgment. In its historical context, criminal responsibility is equatable to moral responsibility, an idea having a metaphysical content dealing with free choice between the values of good and evil or a theologic content dealing with the struggle between heaven and hell.

Whatever the necessity of values and value judgments in guiding human endeavor, the mundane task of administering the law constitutes an operation exclusively confined to the natural world of cause and effect. In such a situation, trying to use a metaphysical or theological concept like moral responsibility will inevitably prove embarrassing. The bankruptcy of our present position in this regard is exemplified by the following two quotations from prominent legal minds. The first advocates an ostrich position in the sands of action:

From any objective point of view the escape of the law from reality constitutes not its weakness but its greatest strength. If judicial institutions become too sincere, too self-analytical, they suffer the fate of ineffectiveness which is the lot of all self-analytical people.

The second quotation portrays the cynicism resulting from such strength:

. . . a lay jury as well as lay witnesses are far more competent to determine "responsibility" than the experts. The experts are incapable of reaching a moral judgment which is responsive to the question the jury must answer; for they are strangers to the "folklore" of human behavior. If one does not believe in the existence of witches, he can hardly be of much utility as a witch-hunter.

Despite its viewpoint, the above calls a spade a spade. It becomes obvious that the modern inquisition, the discernment of moral responsibility in the accused, relies on the psychiatrist rather than the medieval torturer to extract information necessary to brand the accused as "normal" enough to be morally responsible. Only now it is the mentally ill who are exempt from being witches, a strange turn in history. Were a psychiatrist to write a book entitled "Determining Normality in Criminals," we would have in hand a modern *Malleus Maleficarum.* This is an ironic and pathetic situation for psychiatry to be in. We have had the alternative of abandoning the courtroom or of trying to work along as best we can, liberalizing the criteria regarding criminal responsibility by our cooperation. The latter seems the course of wisdom if we are not deluded into the view that science can ever establish criteria which have any rational connection with this metaphysical inquisition concerning moral responsibility. Liberalized criteria for establishing criminal responsibility, as represented by the Durham decision, for example, are but siren songs, luring the psychiatrist from his deterministic science to pose as an expert on theological matters. Where in the range of psychodynamics does moral responsibility suddenly or gradually appear? No scientist can answer that because moral responsibility is an idea belonging to a realm of discourse foreign to science. Asking the psychiatrist to ascertain the presence of moral responsibility in criminals is like asking the surgeon to dissect out the soul or the astronomer to locate heaven.

If the procedure of establishing criminal responsibility is to be other than a euphemistic disguise for the inquisition of moral responsibility, we must delineate what actual consequences result from determining criminal responsibility and understand why and if these consequences are necessary or desirable. By studying the procedure of establishing criminal responsibility like any other phenomenon in society we discover the operational meaning or "cash value" of the concept. For the sake of brevity I shall present this operational analysis of the concept of criminal responsibility in deductive fashion.

Criminal law is administered in accordance with several value judgments:

(1) Society is entitled to protection from further malfeasance by the criminal. A subsidiary value judgment is that a degree of punishment or isolation can be imposed on the criminal as a method of securing this protection.

(2) Society is entitled to protection from potential criminals, from first offenders as well as repeaters. A subsidiary value judgment is that apprehended criminals can be punished by society to create deterrent examples before the law as a warning to potential criminals.

(3) Society is best served by humane administration of the law consistent with the humane purpose of the law.

These value judgments can be condensed into 3 aims in administering criminal law: (1) preventing further malfeasance by the criminal; (2)

deterring others from committing criminal acts; (3) humaneness toward criminals.

Other aims such as vengeance toward the criminal are rejected as unworthy of society, although they persist as contaminants in the judicial process. Administering criminal law involves striking a balance between the 3 general aims just mentioned, a very difficult procedure sometimes. Methods of achieving these aims are now briefly reviewed.

The aim of preventing further malfeasance by the criminal can be accomplished by isolating him from society through imprisonment, hospitalization, or execution. Another way of preventing a criminal from committing more crimes is to rehabilitate him into a good citizen, either through psychiatric treatment, in or out of hospitals, or by punishment, in or out of prison. Punishment as a method of rehabilitation is given in the same educative spirit as in punishing a child.

The second aim in administering criminal law, deterring others from criminal acts, is accomplished by creating deterrent examples before the law by punishing criminals in hand as a warning to potential criminals.

The third aim, humaneness, is accomplished by inflicting no unnecessary punishment upon the criminal. "Necessary" punishment is that punishment sufficient either to rehabilitate the criminal by teaching him a lesson or sufficient to adequately deter most others from violating the law, or sufficient to accomplish both at once. The advantage of imprisonment is that it can provide punishment sufficient for both rehabilitation and determent while also isolating the criminal from society.

Whether or not criminals can be efficiently rehabilitated by punishment is a question of fact. The present assumption in law is that the fairly "normal" criminal is amenable to being taught a lesson by punishment. On the other hand, the law also recognizes that many psychotics and neurotics are so compulsively driven by psychopathology that no reasonable punishment will succeed in altering their behavior. Two factors are involved: the type of punishment and the psychodynamics of the punished.

Whether or not punished criminals make efficient deterrent examples before the law is also a question of fact. The answer hinges on the psychology of those to be deterred. The law currently operates on a rather simple rule of thumb which describes the psychology involved: Those most like ourselves usually make the best deterrent examples for us. The most impressive way to learn the lesson that we will be punished if we commit a crime is to learn by the sad experience of being punished for a transgression — learning by experience. A more efficient but less impressive way is to learn by example. Examples most like ourselves come closest to learning by experience and are therefore the best examples. Whatever we may think of this theory of determent psychology, it is the implicit theory with which criminal law is now operating.

With the above in mind, the problem arises as to which criminals will be the best deterrent examples for warning those to be deterred. Another problem concerns the determination of which criminals can be efficiently rehabilitated by punishment. The shotgun technique of punishing all criminals strikes us as inhumane since exercising some selectivity permits us to avoid inflicting unnecessary punishment on inefficient deterrent examples and inefficiently punishable criminals. In other words, we want to balance the aim of humaneness to criminals with the aims of preventing further malfeasance by the criminal and by potential criminals.

Most psychotic and many neurotic criminals fail to appear enough like the average to make good deterrent examples before the law. Nor are they good deterrent examples for those most like themselves, other psychotics, since such persons are too lost within themselves to be amenable to any deterrent examples. Consequently we wish to exempt these inefficient deterrent examples from punishment for purposes of determent. Usually these same persons are also inefficiently punishable — *i.e.*, punishment will not rehabilitate them.

In regard to determent, it is interesting to note that it is merely the appearance of the criminal, how his overt behavior impresses the population to be deterred, which is of crucial importance. This complex problem is currently handled by relying on a rather random sampling of the general population, 12 jurors tried and true, to reflect the psychological response of the general population by deciding whether or not the criminal strikes them as "normal" — *i.e.*, (implicitly) enough like themselves to make a good deterrent example. It is only in connection with considering the probability that punishment may rehabilitate the criminal that all of the details of his psychodynamics become important.

It now becomes clear that when we try to distinguish between mentally ill and "normal" criminals or between those who know right from wrong, or by using other criteria for criminal responsibility, ostensibly to determine whether or not they are morally responsible, we are really trying to decide whether or not the criminal is sufficiently normal to be enough like the rest of us to serve as an efficient deterrent example before the law and whether or not he is normal enough to mend his ways if taught a lesson by punishment. The entire content of the concept of criminal responsibility, as far as the natural world is concerned, is contained in the following definition: criminal responsibility is deterrent efficiency and/or efficient punishability. Deterrent efficiency is the degree of effectiveness of the criminal serving as a deterrent example before the law in deterring most others from crime. Efficient punishability is the susceptibility of the criminal to being adequately rehabilitated, as regards asocial acts, by the method of reasonable punishment.

In many cases of "temporary insanity" and in crimes resulting from "adequate provocation," it is the circumstances leading up to the crime rather than the personality of the criminal that are too unusual to require making the person an example before the law. Also, the circumstances may be regarded as so provocative that the average person in this situation would be as impervious to determent as the psychotic. So determent seems unnecessary and impracticable. Regarding rehabilitation of the criminal, the circumstances of the crime may be so unusual that it is highly improbable that the criminal will ever be exposed to them again. Consequently it is pointless as well as ineffective to try to rehabilitate him to an extent that he would behave differently if he ever encounters this unusual situation again. The assumption is that he will not be a criminal in usual circumstances. So again, punishment for purposes of rehabilitation is too unnecessary and ineffective to be humanely administered to these "normal" personalities who have committed crimes because of very unusual circumstances.

The concepts of deterrent efficiency and efficient punishability are quantitative although not currently measurable. They deal only with matters of complex but ascertainable fact in the natural world. They are consistent with the determinism of causal or stochastic (probability-type) principle and have no reference to the metaphysical concept of moral responsibility. They are the key to the effective administration of criminal law and represent what we have implicitly been doing right for the wrong reasons during our long preoccupation with the illusory relation between mental illness and moral responsibility. They furnish a firm guide as to the kind of questions a psychiatrist can answer in the courtroom without departing from science into metaphysics. These questions are:

1. Is the accused capable of adequately participating in his defense?

2. Was the accused psychologically capable of or motivated toward committing the crime?

3. What are the probabilities of the criminal repeating crimes under the following conditions: (a) after punishment (*i.e.*, is he efficiently punishable); (b) after psychiatric treatment in a hospital; (c) after no punishment, treatment, or rehabilitation; (d) while living in society during attempts at rehabilitation?

4. What are the probabilities that the punished criminal will make an efficient deterrent example before the law? — *i.e.* what is his deterrent efficiency?

5. What are the probabilities of the criminal again getting into cir-

cumstances similar to those precipitating his criminal act? Were these circumstances essentially happenstance or did he seek them?

6. What latitude of circumstance is sufficient to precipitate criminal behavior by this criminal?

7. What are the probabilities that the average person might find himself in circumstances similar to those of the crime?

8. What is the probability that the average person would respond to these circumstances with a criminal act?

It must be apparent that some of these questions require the consultation of the sociologist or criminologist as well as the psychiatrist. Questions 3 and 4 deal with criminal responsibility and 5 through 8 deal with "temporary insanity" and "adequate provocation."

DISCUSSION

Criminal responsibility historically has been identified with moral responsibility. Moral responsibility is a metaphysical or theological term about which no science, including psychiatry, can say anything scientific. Establishing psychiatric criteria for determining the presence of moral responsibility in criminals is a logical impossibility. In this article criminal responsibility is divorced from moral responsibility and is redefined as deterrent efficiency and/or efficient punishability, quantitative concepts dealing with the effectiveness of a punished criminal as a warning to others and the susceptibility of a criminal to rehabilitation through punishment. Regarding criminal responsibility, the psychiatrist can appropriately answer only questions bearing on these 2 complex problems of fact. These are the questions he is really answering when he gropes around in the scientifically meaningless search for moral responsibility in criminals. This article attempts to furnish the psychiatrist with adequate conceptual tools for a positive alternative to the law's antique preoccupation with the metaphysical concept of moral responsibility. This alternative is: Criminal responsibility is a concept concerning discriminations of fact in the natural world. These discriminations of fact are necessitated by our attempts to balance three aims in administering criminal law, prevention of further malfeasance by the criminal, deterrence of potential criminals from crime, and humaneness toward criminals. These 3 aims derive from value judgments regarding society's entitlement to humane protection. While these value judgments may have metaphysical origins, carrying them out requires scientific rather than metaphysical conceptions. Moral responsibility and judgment are misplaced metaphysical conceptions quite inappropriate to the administration of law in the natural world, an area that requires scientific rather than metaphysical conceptions.

Moral values embodied in the laws must be applied in the natural world through concepts appropriate to that world. The revised conception of criminal responsibility meets this necessity.

Besides providing the ground for understanding the reasons behind previous criteria of criminal responsibility, the operational concept of criminal responsibility entails several changes in the judicial process. By disqualifying the state as a moral judge of individuals, the separation of church and state is confirmed. Abandoning the moral judgment of individuals removes another obstruction to the government of acts by law rather than of individuals by men. The redundancy inherent in compounding the moral judgment of acts embodied in the law with the moral judgment of individuals who violate the law is avoided. Finally, it permits us to recognize that determining criminal responsibility involves the problem of what to do with an individual who has violated the law rather than the establishment of his guilt. Determining criminal responsibility is currently a prelude to pronouncing a judgment regarding guilt only because of the confusion about moral responsibility. It is operationally a part of the sentencing procedure. This is why the psychiatrist should be an adviser to the court regarding sentencing rather than a controversial participant in establishing moral guilt.

SUMMARY

If the operations stemming from a concept comprise its meaning, the meaning of criminal responsibility is defined as deterrent efficiency and/or efficient punishability, quantitative, operational concepts without the metaphysical connotations of moral responsibility. As a consequence, the role of the psychiatrist in the courtroom is specifically revised.

REFERENCES

1. Zilboorg, G. *The Psychology of the Criminal Act and Punishment*, New York: Harcourt Brace, 1954.
2. Brain, W. R. Letter to the Editor, London Times, Sept. 1, 1952.
3. Hill, W. P. *Univ. of Chicago L. Rev.*, 22: 380, Winter 1955.

INDEX

ACTH. *See* Adrenocorticotrophic hormone
Abbott, J. A., 311
Abraham, K., 348
Abramson, H. A., 606, 626
Abstract attitude, 561–62, 570–71
Acetylocholine, 623
Acklesberg, S. B., 561
Adaptation, loss of, 174. *See also* Habituation
Adaptation energy, 174
Adorno, T. W., 766n
Adrenal glands, 175, 178f, 185, 223, 239; cortex, 171–76, 179, 330; medulla, 223, 225, 231
Adrenalectomy, 172–85 *passim*; 240
Adrenalin, 223, 225, 226, 230, 240, 298, 329, 474, 641–47; and mescaline, 640. *See also* Epinephrine
Adrenergic agents, 298
Adrenocorticotrophic hormone (ACTH), 175–87 *passim*; 329–30
Adrenoxin, 628
Affect, 102–4, 123; loss of, 364. *See also* Emotional reactions
Affectionless character, 10
After-image persistence: in brain injured, 530; and LSD–25, 618, 629
Aggressive behavior: amydalectomy, 510–18; in hospitalized children, 60–68; as response to frustration, 83, 96
Agnew, N., 630
Aichorn, A., 705
Aita, J. A., 573
Alarm reaction, 171, 174, 178
Alexander, F., 123, 198
Allen, R. M., 569
Altschule, M. D., 330, 339
Amanita, 497–98, 499, 655
Amaral, M. A., 587
Ambivalence, 351
Amino acids, 625–26
Amobarbital sodium (Amytal), 289–90, 620, 629
Amygdalectomy, 509–18
Anal stage, 349
Anderson, A. L., 568, 572, 574
Anesthesia: in obstetrics, 154, 163; operations on children, 42
Anger, physiology of, 223–33
Angyal, A., 329
Animism, 558
Ansbacher, S., 646
Anxiety: conditioning, 275–87; and cortical excitability, 298; in hospitalized children and parents, 58–72; and lysergic acid, 615, 621; and mescaline, 631; objective, 74–75; in psychotherapy, 416; in schizophrenia, 330, 408–11, 420, 452; separation, 361; situational, 285; unconscious, 275
Anxiety neurosis, 86, 231, 292
Anxiety scale, 284
Anxiety state, 292, 296
Aphasia, 563
Apnea: and neurological disorder, 154, 162
Arnold, O. H., 630, 636
Arousal reaction, 476, 478
Artemidorus, 258
Arteriosclerosis, cerebral, 560, 562
Arthritis, rheumatoid, 185
Asch, S. E., 521
Ashby, W. R., 587
Asphyxia: at birth in human infants, 154; experimentally produced in guinea pigs, 154–56; effect in later life, 158–63
Asquith, E., 644
Association: in dreaming, 260–61; serial, 275–77
Asthma: allergens, 209, 220; experimental psychogenic attacks, 209–22
Atropine, 240
Attention: in brain-injury, 520–21, 566–67; following psychosurgery, 583
Attitudes: in treatment, 485; social class and psychiatry, 678, 680; influencing psychiatric hospitalization, 695–96
Atwell, C. R., 570, 583
Austen, Jane, 263
Australian Aboriginal, The, 234
Authoritarian Personality, The, 766
Autism, early infantile, 3–24; and brain damage, 8, 22, 559; case histories, 9, 18–20; and childhood schizophrenia, 3, 4, 5, 21; EEG, 7; etiology and development, 5, 7, 11; follow-up studies, 6, 15–24; genetic factors, 5, 8, 11, 21; interpersonal relationships, 4, 6, 7, 23; language and communication, 7, 15, 17; and mental deficiency, 4, 7; organic factors, 15; parents, 4, 8, 10, 11, 16; pathognomonic features, 3, 4, 5, 15; treatment, 7, 17, 21; ritual and repetition, 4, 559
Autoerotism, 363
Autonomic lability score, 279
Autonomic nervous system, 102, 223–24
Autonomic responses, conditioning, 275–87

INDEX OF CONTRIBUTORS